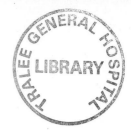
HEMATOLOGY IN CLINICAL PRACTICE

third edition

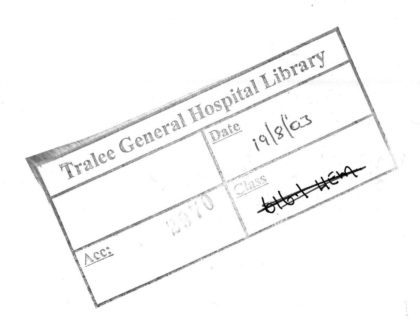

A Lange Medical Book

HEM
CLIN ... ICE

A Guide to D

third edition

ROBERT S. HILLM
Past Chairman, Depa
Maine Medical Center
Professor of Medicine
University of Vermont

KENNETH A. AUL
Scientific Director
Maine Medical Center
Associate Professor o
University of Vermon

McGraw-Hill
Medical Publishing Division

New York   Chicago   San Francisco   Lisbon   London
Milan   New Delhi   San Juan   Seoul   Singapore   Sy

McGraw-Hill

A Division of The McGraw·Hill Companies

HEMATOLOGY IN CLINICAL PRACTICE, Third Edition

Copyright © 2002, by The **McGraw-Hill** Companies, Inc. All rights reserved. Printed in The United States of America. Except as permitted under the United States Copyright Act of 1976, no part of this publication may be reproduced or distributed in any form or by any means, or stored in a data base or retrieval system, without prior written permission of the publisher. Previous editions copyright © 1999, 1996, 1993, 1989 by Appleton & Lange.

345678910   DOC/DOC   098765432

ISBN: 0-07-137502-3

This book was set in Adobe Garamond by Rainbow Graphics.
The editors were Martin Wonsiewicz and Scott Kurtz.
The production supervisor was Richard Ruzycka.
The cover designer was Mary McKeon.
The index was prepared by Stephen Shimer.
The printer and binder was R. R. Donnelley and Sons, Inc.
This book is printed on acid-free paper.

Library of Congress Cataloging-in-Publication Data

Hillman, Robert S., 1934–
    Hematology in clinical practice / Robert S. Hillman, Kenneth A. Ault.—3rd ed.
        p. ; cm.
    Includes bibliographical references and index.
    ISBN 0-07-137502-3
        1. Blood—Diseases. I. Ault, Kenneth A. II. Title.
        [DNLM: 1. Hematologic Diseases. WH 120 H654h 2002]
    RC636 .H46 2002
    616.1′5—dc21   2001044038

Contents

Color Plates appear between pages 214 and 215

Preface

Hematology in Clinical Practice, Third Edition, is written specifically for clinicians—students, residents in training, primary care internists or family practitioners, and clinical hematologists/oncologists. It is a practical guide to the diagnosis and treatment of the most common disorders of red blood cells, white blood cells, and hemostasis. Each disease state is discussed in terms of the underlying pathophysiology, clinical features that suggest the diagnosis, the use of state-of-the-art laboratory tests in the diagnosis and differential diagnosis of the condition, and current management strategies. For the student, specific chapters discuss a systematic approach to the workup of a patient with hematologic disease, providing a foundation for clinical training.

We would like to thank James McArthur and John Bolles of the University of Washington's Health Sciences Center for Educational Resources for the color photographs selected from the American Society of Hematology National Slide Bank; Catherine Hartung for the artwork; and Jacqueline Hedlund for her editorial assistance.

HEMATOLOGY IN CLINICAL PRACTICE

third edition

PART I
Red Blood Cell Disorders

Normal Erythropoiesis

The oxygen required by tissues for aerobic metabolism is supplied by the circulating mass of mature **erythrocytes** (red blood cells). The circulating red blood cell population is continually renewed by the erythroid precursor cells in the marrow, under the control of both humoral and cellular growth factors. This cycle of normal erythropoiesis is a carefully regulated process. Oxygen sensors within the kidney detect minute changes in the amount of oxygen available to tissue and by releasing erythropoietin are able to adjust erythropoiesis to match tissue requirements. Thus, **normal erythropoiesis** is best described according to its major components, including red blood cell structure, function, and turnover; the capacity of the erythroid marrow to produce new red blood cells; and growth factor regulation.

STRUCTURE OF THE RED BLOOD CELL

The mature red blood cell is easily recognized because of its unique morphology. At rest, the red blood cell takes the shape of a biconcave disc with a mean diameter of 8 μm, a thickness of 2 μm, and a volume of 90 fL. It lacks a nucleus or mitochondria, and 33% of its contents is made up of a single protein, hemoglobin. Intracellular energy requirements are largely supplied by glucose metabolism, which is targeted at maintaining hemoglobin in a soluble, reduced state, providing appropriate amounts of 2,3-diphosphoglycerate (2,3-DPG), and generating adenosine triphosphate (ATP) to support membrane function. Without a nucleus or protein metabolic pathway, the cell has a limited lifespan of 100–120 days. However, the unique structure of the adult red blood cell is perfect for its function, providing maximum flexibility as the cell travels through the microvasculature (Figure 1–1).

Membrane

A. INNER AND OUTER LAYERS:

The shape, pliability, and resiliency of the red blood cell is largely determined by its membrane. The structure of this membrane is illustrated in Figure 1–2. It is a lipid sheath, just two molecules thick, that consists of closely packed phospholipid molecules. The external surface of the membrane is rich in phosphatidylcholine, sphingomyelin, and glycolipid, whereas the inner layer is largely phosphatidylserine, phosphatidylethanolamine, and phosphatidylinositol. This asymmetry is maintained by two transporters—**flipase,** an ATP-dependent aminophospholipid translocase that rapidly transports phosphatidylserine and ethanolamine from the outer to the inner membrane, and **flopase,** which moves phospholipids more slowly in the opposite direction. The normal asymmetric distribution of membrane phospholipids can also be rapidly disrupted by a calcium-activated "**scramblase**" present in the membrane. Interference with these transporters results in a relocation of phosphatidylserine to the cell surface with a resulting increase in the thrombogenic potential of the cell surface. Moreover, accumulation of excess phosphatidylserine on the red cell surface plays a role in macrophage destruction.

Approximately 50% of the red blood cell membrane is made up of **cholesterol** that is in equilibrium with the unesterified cholesterol in the plasma. Because of this, the cholesterol content of the membrane is influenced by plasma cholesterol levels, as well as by the activity of the enzyme lecithin cholesterol acyltransferase (LCAT) and bile acids. Patients with liver disease who have impaired LCAT activity accumulate excess cholesterol on the red blood cell membrane, which results in abnormal red blood cell morphology (**targeting**) and at times a shortened survival.

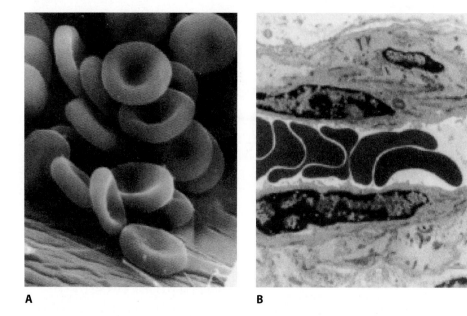

A   B

Figure 1–1. **Red blood cell morphology. A:** Adult red blood cells are characterized by their lack of a nucleus, and biconcave disc shape. Each red blood cell has a diameter of approximately 8 μm and a width of 2 μm. Red blood cells are extremely pliable as they pass through small vessels and sinusoids. **B:** The section of a small blood vessel demonstrates the ability of red blood cells to undergo major shape distortions. (Scanning EM photographs used with the permission of Dennis Knuckel, Ph.D., copyright © 1993, American Society of Hematology National Slide Bank.)

B. RETICULAR PROTEIN NETWORK:

The outer lipid membrane layer is affixed to a reticular protein network consisting of **spectrin** and **actin.** As shown in Figure 1–2, the integral proteins glycophorin C and Band 3, which function as anion exchangers, extend vertically from the spectrin lattice work through the lipid layer to make contact with the cell surface. Spectrin heterodimers interact horizontally with protein 4.1 and complementary spectrin heterodimers to form a hexagonal lattice framework under the lipid bilayer. Defects in the vertical structure of the membrane (deficiency of spectrin, ankyrin, or band 3, or loss of lipid) result in spherocyte formation. Damage to the horizontal spectrin framework results in severe red cell fragmentation or mild elliptocytosis.

The integral proteins and surface glycosphingolipids are also responsible for the cell's **antigenic structure.** More than 300 red blood cell antigens have now been classified with the ABO and Rh blood group antigens, being of primary importance in typing blood for transfusion (see Chapter 37). Autoantibodies against minor blood group antigens can result in increased red blood cell destruction by the reticuloendothelial cells.

Hemoglobin

The red blood cell is, basically, a container for **hemoglobin**—a 64,500 dalton protein made up of 4 polypeptide chains, each containing an active heme group. Each heme group is capable of binding to an oxygen molecule. The **respiratory motion of hemoglobin,** that is, the uptake and release of oxygen to tissues, involves a specific change in molecular structure (Figure 1–3). As hemoglobin shuttles from its deoxyhemoglobin to its oxyhemoglobin form, carbon dioxide (CO_2) and 2,3-DPG are expelled from their position between the β-globin chains, opening the molecule to receive oxygen. Furthermore, oxygen binding by one of the heme groups increases the affinity of the other groups to oxygen loading. This interaction is responsible for the sigmoid shape of the oxygen dissociation curve.

Inherited defects in hemoglobin structure can interfere with this respiratory motion. Most defects are substitutions of a single amino acid in either the α- or β-globin chains. Some interfere with molecular movement, restricting the molecule to either a low- or high-affinity state, whereas others either change the valency

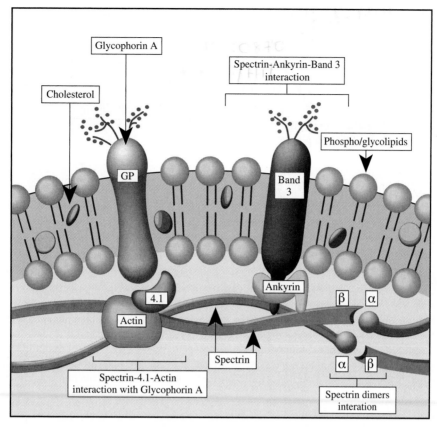

Figure 1–2. **Red blood cell membrane structure.** The red blood cell membrane consists of a two-molecule–thick lipid sheath fixed to an intracellular protein network. The outer lipid layer is rich in phosphatidylcholine, sphingomyelin, and glycolipid; the inner layer is made up of the phosphatides of serine, ethanolamine, and inositol. Almost half of the lipid layer is cholesterol. The membrane proteins, glycophorin C and band 3, penetrate the lipid sheath and make vertical contact with the reticuloproteins, spectrin, protein 4.1, actin, and in the case of band 3, ankyrin. Spectrin heterodimers provide a horizontal framework by bridging protein 4.1 to complementary spectrin dimers.

of heme iron from ferrous to ferric or reduce the solubility of the hemoglobin molecule. Hemoglobin S (sickle cell disease) is an example of a single amino acid substitution that results in a profound effect on solubility.

The normal red blood cell contains approximately 32 pg of hemoglobin [mean cell hemoglobin (MCH) = 32 ± 2 pg]. **Normal hemoglobin synthesis** requires an adequate supply of iron and normal production of both protoporphyrin and globin (Figure 1–4). Protoporphyrin synthesis is initiated in the mitochondria with the formation of delta aminolevulinic acid from glycine and succinyl-CoA. Synthesis then moves to the cell cytoplasm for the formation of porphobilinogen, uroporphyrin, and coproporphyrin. The final assembly of the protoporphyrin ring is carried out by the mitochon-

dria, after which iron is incorporated under the control of the cytoplasmic enzyme, ferrochelatase, to form heme.

Globin chains are assembled by the cytoplasmic ribosomes under the control of two clusters of closely linked genes on chromosomes 11 and 16. The final globin molecule is a tetramer of two α-globin and two non–α-globin chains. In the adult, 96–97% of the hemoglobin is made up of two α-globin and two β-globin chains (**hemoglobin A**) with minor components of hemoglobin F and A$_2$. The final assembly of the hemoglobin molecule occurs in the cell cytoplasm. Small amounts of iron, protoporphyrin, and free globin chains remain after hemoglobin synthesis is complete. The iron is stored as ferritin, whereas the excess porphyrin is complexed to zinc.

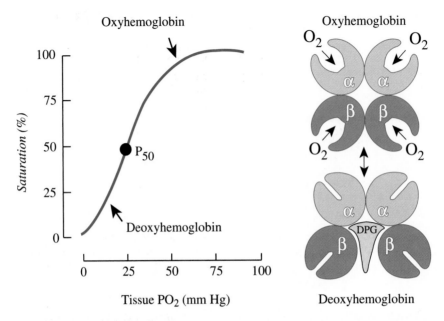

Figure 1–3. Hemoglobin-oxygen dissociation curve. Hemoglobin is capable of a respiratory motion where oxygen loaded at the lung is unloaded at the tissue level. To accept oxygen, 2,3-DPG and carbon dioxide are expelled, salt bridges are ruptured, and each of the four heme groups opens to receive a molecule of oxygen. Oxygen release to tissues reverses the process; salt bridges are reestablished and both 2,3-DPG and carbon dioxide are accepted. The complex interaction of the four heme groups is responsible for the sigmoid shape of the hemoglobin-oxygen dissociation curve.

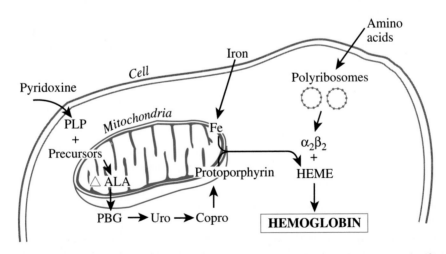

Figure 1–4. Hemoglobin synthesis. Normal hemoglobin synthesis requires an adequate supply of iron, amino acids, and pyridoxine (vitamin B_6). Porphyrin production is the responsibility of the mitochondria, whereas globin production is controlled by ribosomal RNA. The formation of the complete hemoglobin molecule involves the assembly of heme from protoporphyrin and iron and the union of a heme molecule with the two α and two β-globin chains that comprise the globin component.

This complex series of reactions is triggered by erythropoietin stimulation of red cell progenitors. With precursor differentiation, there is a coordinated transcriptional induction of heme biosynthesis, globin synthesis and transferrin receptor expression, which is required for iron transport (see Chapter 5). **The rate of hemoglobin synthesis** is determined by the availability of transferrin iron and level of intracellular heme. Hemoglobin synthesis is maximal in more mature marrow erythroblasts but persists to a lesser degree in the marrow reticulocytes. The cessation of heme synthesis is heralded by a decrease in membrane transferrin receptor expression, followed by a downregulation of heme and globin synthesis.

Cellular Metabolism

The stability of the red blood cell membrane and the solubility of intracellular hemoglobin depend on four glucose-supported metabolic pathways (Figure 1–5).

A. EMBDEN-MEYERHOFF PATHWAY:

The **Embden-Meyerhoff pathway** (**nonoxidative or anaerobic pathway**) is responsible for the generation of the ATP necessary for membrane function and the maintenance of cell shape and pliability. Defects in anaerobic glycolysis are associated with increased cell rigidity and decreased survival, which produces a hemolytic anemia.

The Embden-Meyerhoff pathway also plays a role in supporting the methemoglobin reductase, phosphogluconate, and Luebering-Rapaport pathways.

B. METHEMOGLOBIN REDUCTASE PATHWAY:

The **methemoglobin reductase pathway** uses the pyridine nucleotide-NADH generated from anaerobic glycolysis to maintain heme iron in its ferrous state. An inherited mutation of the **methemoglobin reductase enzyme** (also referred to as **NADH-diaphorase** or **cy-**

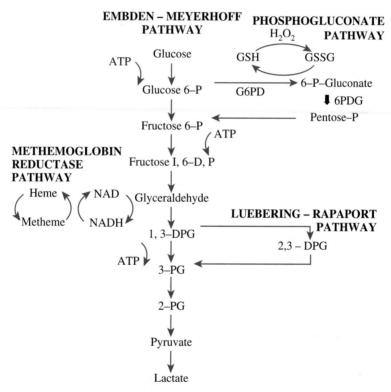

Figure 1–5. Red blood cell metabolic pathways. The red blood cell depends on four metabolic pathways to keep hemoglobin in solution and maintain membrane integrity. The Embden-Meyerhoff pathway is responsible for the generation of high energy phosphate (ATP) for membrane maintenance, whereas the other pathways support hemoglobin function. The methemoglobin reductase (NADH-diaphorase) pathway is required to maintain hemoglobin in a reduced state. The phosphogluconate pathway helps counteract environmental oxidants and the Luebering-Rapaport pathway generates intracellular 2,3-DPG.

tochrome b$_5$ reductase) results in an inability to counteract oxidation of hemoglobin to methemoglobin, the ferric form of hemoglobin that will not transport oxygen. Patients with Type I NADH-diaphorase deficiency accumulate small amounts of methemoglobin in circulating red cells, whereas Type II patients have severe cyanosis and mental retardation.

C. PHOSPHOGLUCONATE PATHWAY:

In a similar fashion, the **phosphogluconate pathway** couples oxidative metabolism with NADP and glutathione reduction. It counteracts environmental oxidants and prevents globin denaturation. When patients lack either of the two key enzymes, **glucose 6 phosphate dehydrogenase (G6PD)** or **glutathione reductase (GSH)**, denatured hemoglobin precipitates on the inner surface of the red blood cell membrane, resulting in membrane damage and hemolysis.

D. LUEBERING-RAPAPORT PATHWAY:

Finally, the **Luebering-Rapaport pathway** is responsible for the production of 2,3-DPG. It is tied to the rate of anaerobic glycolysis and the action of the pH-sensitive enzyme **phosphofructokinase**. The 2,3-DPG response is also influenced by the supply of phosphate to the cell. Severe phosphate depletion in patients with diabetic ketoacidosis or nutritional deficiency can result in a reduced 2,3-DPG production response.

REGULATION OF OXYGEN TRANSPORT

Red blood cells play a central role in oxygen transport. At the cellular level, oxygen supply is a function of red blood cells perfusing the tissue and their hemoglobin oxygen-carrying capacity. The unique physiology of the hemoglobin-oxygen dissociation curve allows an onsite adjustment of oxygen delivery to match tissue metabolism. At the same time, components such as pulmonary function, cardiac output, blood volume, blood viscosity, and adjustments of regional blood flow are also important contributors to oxygen transport.

Hemoglobin-Oxygen Dissociation Curve

Under normal conditions, arterial blood enters tissues with an oxygen tension of 95 mm Hg and a hemoglobin saturation of better than 97%. Pooled venous blood returning from tissues has an oxygen tension of 40 mm Hg and a saturation of 75–80%. Thus, only the top portion of the hemoglobin-oxygen dissociation curve is used in the basal state (Figure 1–6). This provides a considerable excess capacity for increased oxygen delivery to support increased oxygen requirements. The sigmoid shape of the hemoglobin-oxygen dissociation curve also helps in this regard by releasing oxygen more easily as the tissue PO$_2$ falls below 40 mm Hg.

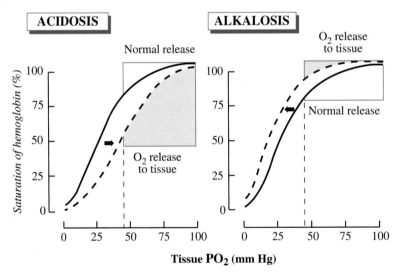

Figure 1–6. pH and hemoglobin-oxygen affinity. Oxygen delivery responds to tissue metabolism and blood pH—the Bohr effect. When acid products are released at the tissue level, the hemoglobin-oxygen dissociation curve of red blood cells in the vicinity immediately responds with a shift of the curve to the right. This shift has the effect of releasing more oxygen to tissues and opening hemoglobin to receive additional amounts of CO$_2$. Alkalosis has the opposite effect. It shifts the hemoglobin-oxygen dissociation curve to the left and effectively reduces the amount of oxygen released to tissue.

The affinity of hemoglobin for oxygen is also influenced by temperature, pH, CO_2 concentration, and by the level of red cell 2,3-DPG. As shown in Figure 1–6, the position of the hemoglobin-oxygen dissociation curve is affected by the rate of tissue metabolism, CO_2 production, and blood pH (**the Bohr effect**). When a tissue generates increasing amounts of CO_2 and acid metabolites, the resulting acidosis shifts the dissociation curve to the right. This shift permits the release of more oxygen for the level of tissue PO_2. The reverse is also true. With an increase in pH such as with an acute respiratory alkalosis, the hemoglobin-oxygen dissociation curve shifts to the left, reducing the amount of oxygen available at any tissue PO_2.

The Bohr effect is instantaneous and can be highly localized to a specific site. For example, the blood perfusing an exercising muscle will be able to deliver 75% or more of its oxygen because of the low tissue PO_2 and the acidosis-induced Bohr effect. Oxygen unloading simultaneously lowers the CO_2 tension in the red cells (**Haldane effect**), thereby facilitating its diffusion from metabolizing tissues. This reciprocal interaction promotes optimal exchange of oxygen and carbon dioxide during exercise.

When the amount of oxygen removed by tissues continues at a high level (**widened arterial-venous difference**), the resulting increase in deoxyhemoglobin in the cell stimulates an increased production of 2,3-DPG. This situation will be true regardless of whether the cause of the hemoglobin desaturation is hypoxia, cardiac failure, or anemia. The rise in intracellular 2,3-DPG sustains the shift of the dissociation curve to the right and provides significant compensation for a chronic anemia or hypoxia.

2,3-DPG metabolism also responds to **systemic acidosis** or **alkalosis**. The initial shift of the curve to the right in a patient with acidosis will be corrected over the next 12–36 h by a compensatory reduction in the 2,3-DPG level. The Bohr effect is reversed by the lower 2,3-DPG and the curve shifts back to normal. Although this readjusts the level of oxygen delivery to match tissue requirements, it can create a problem if the acidosis is suddenly corrected. Because it takes a number of hours to replace the intracellular 2,3-DPG, a sudden return to a normal pH will shift the oxygen dissociation curve to the left owing to the lower than normal 2,3-DPG level.

Hemodynamic Factors

The **self-regulating capacity of the oxygen dissociation curve** takes care of most of the variation in tissue oxygen requirements in the basal state. With maximal exercise, the untrained subject will reach a limit determined not by oxygen loading but by a low maximal cardiac output resulting in poor oxygen delivery to tissues. In contrast, highly trained athletes have a greatly increased cardiac output, so that pulmonary loading and peripheral transport determine their limits. To maximize performance, they must tolerate both arterial hypoxemia and marked metabolic acidosis.

A. ANEMIA:

The oxygen dissociation curve will also compensate for an anemia of moderate severity. However, once the hemoglobin falls below 9–10 grams per deciliter, components such as changes in blood volume, cardiac output, and regional blood flow come into play. Both the pulse rate and stroke volume increase in patients with severe anemia and there is a redirection of blood flow to vital organs. These hemodynamic changes are often appreciated by patients. As their anemia worsens, they are increasingly aware of the force of ventricular contraction and often complain of pounding headaches, especially with physical exertion.

B. OXYGEN SUPPLY:

Impairments in lung function also affect oxygen supply. Although the sigmoid shape of the hemoglobin-oxygen dissociation curve does counterbalance reductions in alveolar PO_2, there is a limit to this compensation. Moreover, desaturation of hemoglobin results whenever unsaturated venous blood is shunted through areas of damaged lung tissue. The physiologic response to a decreased oxygen tension in ambient air, as for example the oxygen tension at moderately high altitudes (3000–4000 m), is an increase in 2,3-diphosphoglycerate to raise the P_{50}, that is, shift the oxygen dissociation curve to the right. Moderate exercise will still further elevate the P_{50} via the Bohr effect to maintain oxygen delivery to tissues. Under conditions of more marked hypoxia (altitudes greater than 4000 m), reflex hyperventilation results in a reduced PCO_2 and respiratory alkalosis. The latter shifts the oxygen dissociation curve to the left with a reduction in oxygen delivery to tissues. Still, high hemoglobin affinity for oxygen provides a physiological advantage for acclimatization to high altitudes. Subjects born with a high-affinity hemoglobin such as hemoglobin Andrew-Minneapolis (P_{50} 17 mm Hg) demonstrate normal arterial oxygen saturations at altitudes up to 4000 m, smaller increases in heart rate, and little or no increases in erythropoietin when compared with normal individuals. Animals that normally live at high altitudes also have high-affinity hemoglobins.

C. BLOOD VISCOSITY:

Sustained hypoxia usually results in a compensatory rise in the red blood cell mass and hematocrit. Although this increases the oxygen-carrying capacity of blood, it also increases blood viscosity. The interaction of the hematocrit level and blood viscosity is discussed extensively in Chapter 12. Tissue oxygen delivery is maximum at a hematocrit of 33–36% (hemoglobin of 11–12 grams per deciliter), assuming no changes in cardiac output or regional blood flow. Above this level, an increase in viscosity will tend to slow blood flow and decrease oxygen delivery. This effect is relatively minor until the hematocrit exceeds 50%, at which time blood flow to key organs such as the brain can be significantly reduced.

REGULATION OF ERYTHROPOIESIS

RBC Production

The **rate of new red blood cell production** varies according to the rate of red blood cell destruction and tissue oxygen requirements. Changes in the oxygen delivery to tissue are sensed by peritubular interstitial, fibroblast-like cells in the kidney. A decrease in the oxygen content of hemoglobin (pulmonary dysfunction), the hemoglobin level (anemia), or the hemoglobin affinity for oxygen (shift in the oxygen dissociation curve) will stimulate an increased production of erythropoietin by renal interstitial cells. This is accomplished by recruitment of new cells to initiate transcription of erythropoietin messenger ribonucleic acid (mRNA) by a single gene on chromosome 7. The **mechanism of regulation** involves the sensing of oxygen tension by a flavoheme protein that controls the level of **hypoxia inducible factor (HIF-1)**. The latter interacts with response elements in nuclear DNA to activate erythropoietin gene expression.

The erythropoietin then travels to the marrow, where it binds to a specific receptor (**EPOR**) on the surface of committed erythroid precursors. This receptor is a 508–amino acid glycoprotein coded by a gene on chromosome 19. Within hours, there is a detectable increase in deoxyribonucleic acid (DNA) synthesis. This is followed by a proliferation and maturation of committed stem cells to produce an increased number of new red blood cells. Erythroid progenitor apoptosis is also inhibited. The **full marrow response** takes several days. Given a sustained increase in erythropoietin stimulation, a rise in the reticulocyte index will not occur for 4–5 days and a detectable increase in hematocrit will take a week or more.

A. MEASURING THE ERYTHROPOIETIN RESPONSE:

The erythropoietin response to anemia can be directly measured by assaying the serum erythropoietin level (Figure 1–7). Once the hemoglobin level falls below 12 grams per deciliter, there is a logarithmic increase in the serum erythropoietin level. At the same time, it is important to note that with mild anemia (a hemoglobin level greater than 12 grams per deciliter), the erythropoietin level is not increased. This probably reflects the compensation of the 2,3-DPG–induced shift in the hemoglobin-oxygen dissociation curve combined with the sensitivity level of the renal sensor. Physiologically, it may reflect that a hemoglobin level of 12 grams per deciliter is best for maximum tissue oxygen delivery.

B. OTHER FACTORS INFLUENCING ERYTHROPOIETIN LEVEL:

Although the erythropoietin response is primarily a function of the severity of anemia or hypoxia, other factors, such as the erythroid marrow mass and levels of inflammatory cytokines, will influence the serum erythropoietin level. Erythropoietin binds avidly to ery-

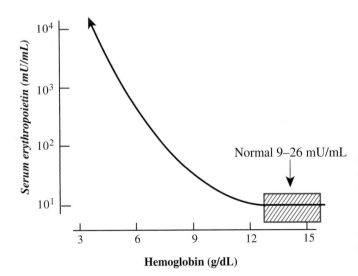

Figure 1–7. **Erythropoietin production and anemia.** Once the hemoglobin level falls below 12 grams per deciliter, the plasma erythropoietin level increases logarithmically. Patients with renal disease or the anemia associated with chronic inflammation show a lower than predicted response for their degree of anemia.

throid progenitors and is removed from circulation. Therefore, with **aplastic anemia,** extremely high levels of serum erythropoietin reflect both an increased production and a decreased clearance. In contrast, with **chronic hemolytic anemias,** the expansion of marrow erythroid precursors results in a more rapid clearance of erythropoietin from circulation and, therefore, a lower serum level.

Inflammatory cytokines, including interleukin-1, tissue necrosis factor (TNF-α), and transforming growth factor β, also play a role in regulating erythropoietin production and erythroid progenitor proliferation. They are responsible for the lower than normal erythropoietin response in patients with inflammatory disease states (see Chapter 4). Finally, direct suppression of the erythropoietin response is seen in patients receiving certain drugs (chemotherapeutic agents, cyclosporin A, and theophylline) or who are infected with human immunodeficiency virus (HIV).

Two other factors, **angiotensin II** and **insulin-like growth factor-1 (IGF-1),** may also play an erythropoietin-like role in certain settings. The erythropoietin-independent growth of erythroid progenitors in polycythemia vera may involve a hypersensitivity to IGF-1, whereas hypoxia has been shown to induce IGF-1 binding protein. Evidence for a role for angiotensin II is indirect. Post renal transplant erythrocytosis can be reversed by the administration of angiotensin converting enzyme inhibitors, without changing the serum erythropoietin level.

ERYTHROID MARROW PRODUCTION

Erythroid marrow production can be defined for the basal state and in terms of its capacity to increase in response to anemia. Patients who experience acute blood loss or sudden hemolysis of circulating red blood cells can show increases in new red blood cell production of 2 to 3 times normal, that is, the release of 40–60 mL of new red blood cells per day. With a chronic hemolytic anemia, even higher production levels can be attained. This capacity to compensate for anemia is as much a normal characteristic of the erythroid marrow as its steady-state characteristics.

Measurement

The level of production can be assessed from several measurements of red blood cell production and destruction (Table 1–1). Clinically, the marrow E/G ratio and reticulocyte index are of the greatest value. The **marrow E/G ratio** (the ratio of erythroid to granulocytic precursors) is determined by inspecting a stained smear of aspirated marrow particles. As long as the granulocyte production of the marrow is normal, it is

possible to estimate the proliferation of erythroid precursors. In the basal state, there will be approximately one erythroid precursor for every 3–4 granulocytic (myelocytic) precursors. With anemia and high levels of erythropoietin stimulation, the number of erythroid precursors increases dramatically to give ratios of 1:1 or greater. The morphology of the precursors is also important. Normal proliferation shows a balanced increase in erythroid precursors at all stages of maturation. If the number is skewed toward a younger population, especially a population with abnormal morphology, this suggests a defect in DNA synthesis or cytoplasmic maturation. These defects can result in a failure of cells to mature and early death in the marrow, so-called **ineffective erythropoiesis.**

Effective red blood cell production is measured clinically by counting the number of **reticulocytes** (new red blood cells containing increased amounts of RNA) entering the circulation. Although both the E/G ratio and reticulocyte count are at best semiquantitative, they do provide sufficient information for clinical diagnosis. A measurement of radioiron incorporation into red blood cells (**erythron iron turnover**) can provide a more accurate measurement of red blood cell production. This technique was used originally to define and classify red blood cell disorders as defects in either marrow proliferation (hypoproliferative anemias), precursor maturation (ineffective erythropoiesis), or red blood cell destruction (hemorrhagic and hemolytic anemias).

The performance of the erythroid marrow can also be extrapolated from studies of red blood cell destruction. **Clinical indicators of red blood cell destruction** include the serum lactic dehydrogenase level, the indirect bilirubin, and observation of the rate of rise or fall of the hematocrit over time. **Research measurements** that are more accurate in defining levels of red blood cell destruction include carbon monoxide (CO) excretion, stool urobilinogen, and a direct measurement of radiolabeled red blood cell survival (^{51}Cr red blood cell survival). The latter has been used clinically to define both the rate and

***Table 1–1.* Measurements of red blood cell production and destruction.**

Production	Destruction
Marrow E/G ratio	Change in hematocrit
Reticulocyte index	Indirect bilirubin
Erythron iron turnover	Lactic dehydrogenase (LDH)
	^{51}Cr—red blood cell survival
	CO excretion/stool urobilinogen

the site of destruction, whether in spleen or liver. The other measurements are not as practical.

Basal and Stimulated Erythropoiesis

The ability of the erythroid marrow to increase red blood cell production in response to anemia or hypoxia is a basic characteristic of the normal erythron. Thus, normal erythropoiesis is defined not only for the basal state but also for acute and chronic anemia (Table 1–2).

A **normal 70-kg adult** has a circulating red blood cell mass of approximately 2000 mL (300×10^9 red blood cells per kg). Since red blood cells have a lifespan of 100–120 days, 1% of the red blood cell mass, approximately 20 mL of red blood cells, is destroyed daily and replaced by new red blood cell production. This steady state is clinically appreciated from the **E/G ratio** of 1:3 and the **reticulocyte index** (the reticulocyte count corrected for hematocrit and reticulocyte shift; see Chapter 2). With an **acute anemia** secondary to hemorrhage or hemolysis, the marrow will respond with a threefold increase in cell production within 7–10 days. This can be detected from the increase in the E/G ratio to 1:1 or higher and a rise in the reticulocyte index to three times normal. With a **chronic hemolytic anemia**, red blood cell production can increase further, reaching levels of five to eight times normal. These patients show E/G ratios greater than 1:1 and reticulocyte indices greater than five times normal. The highest levels of red blood cell production in patients with hemolytic anemias require an expansion of the erythroid marrow mass to new areas of the marrow cavity. This process takes time and is most prominent in patients who have congenital, lifelong hemolytic anemias.

Several factors play important roles in defining the **marrow's response to anemia or hypoxia.** Obviously, the severity of the anemia or hypoxia and the adequacy of the erythropoietin response are extremely important in setting a level of "expectation." A chronic hypoproliferative anemia develops when, for example, a patient cannot produce increased amounts of erythropoietin because of renal damage.

Factors that determine the marrow's responsiveness include its anatomical structure, the presence of a normal pool of stem cells, and the supply of essential nutrients. The anatomical structure of the marrow is organized to provide a nurturing environment for cell development. Erythroid precursor cells are maintained in a network of reticular cells and fibers in close proximity to vascular sinusoids. The marrow syncytium is designed to sustain the developing cells in a nutrient-rich environment while they proliferate and mature. Cells lining the sinusoids have the ability to regulate the exit of cells from the marrow into circulation, allowing only those cells that have completed maturation to leave.

The **importance of these marrow characteristics** cannot be overemphasized. An abnormality in marrow structure, as seen with radiation damage or myelofibrosis, significantly impairs new red blood cell production. Overgrowth of other cellular components, as with myeloid leukemias or infiltrating tumors or lymphomas, will decrease red blood cell production by occupying the space required for red blood cell precursor growth.

The **supply of nutrients** to the marrow is also important. The most important nutrient is the iron required for hemoglobin formation. The level of the normal marrow's response to a hemorrhagic or hemolytic anemia is essentially a reflection of iron supply (Figure 1–8). In response to a hemorrhagic anemia, a normal individual with normal iron stores will be able to maintain a serum iron level sufficient to support a production increase of up to 3 times normal. As shown in the figure, this level of production is attained as the hematocrit falls to levels between 20% and 30%. More severe anemia with a greater erythropoietin response does not result in a greater marrow production response. The cause of this plateau is the limitation of iron delivery from normal stores.

Figure 1–8 also shows the effect of variations in iron supply. With **iron deficiency,** the erythroid marrow will be unable to respond, despite a high level of erythropoietin stimulation. The patient with iron deficiency appears to have a hypoproliferative anemia even though the erythropoietin level is increased and the marrow morphology appears to be normal. In contrast, patients

Table 1–2. **Normal response to anemia.**

	Basal (Hgb > 13 g/dL)	Anemia (Hb < 8 g/dL)	
		Acute	Chronic
Marrow—E/G ratio	1:3	1:1	1:1
Reticulocyte index	1.0	2–3	3–8

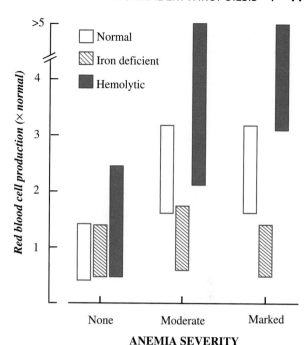

Figure 1–8. **Red blood cell production and iron supply.** The ability of the erythroid marrow to increase production is a direct reflection of iron supply. With worsening anemia, a normal individual with 500–1000 mg of reticuloendothelial iron stores can increase red blood cell production twofold to threefold. An individual with iron deficiency will be unable to increase production above basal levels. In contrast, patients with chronic hemolytic anemias show production levels in excess of 3–5 times normal, with moderate to marked anemia.

who have **hemolytic anemias,** where the destruction of adult red cells provides a major source of iron for recycling to the marrow, can have marrow production that increases to levels well above three times normal. Chronically, these patients can achieve production levels in excess of 5 times normal.

BIBLIOGRAPHY

Beutler E, et al: *Hematology,* 6th ed. McGraw-Hill, 2001.

Goodnough LT, Skikne B, Brugnara C: Erythropoietin, iron, and erythropoiesis. Blood 2000;96:823.

Hillman RS, Finch CA: *Red Cell Manual,* 7th ed. FA Davis, 1997.

Hsia CCW: Respiratory function of hemoglobin. N Engl J Med 1998;338:239.

Ponka P: Tissue-specific regulation of iron metabolism and heme synthesis: Distinct control mechanisms in erythroid cells. Blood 1997;89:1.

Zwaal RFA, Schroit AJ: Pathophysiologic implications of membrane phospholipid asymmetry in blood cells. Blood 1997;89:1121.

Clinical Approach to Anemia

The presence and nature of an anemia may be apparent from the clinical presentation. Acute blood loss, when severe, can be expected to produce a hemorrhagic anemia; chronic blood loss will generally result in an iron deficiency anemia. More often, however, the laboratory provides the first clue to an anemia. Routine measurement of the complete blood count (CBC) provides a sensitive method for both detection and diagnosis. Thus, the clinical approach to an anemia involves both a bedside evaluation and the skilled use of the laboratory.

CLINICAL PRESENTATION

The signs and symptoms of an anemia are a function of its severity, its rapidity of onset, and the age of the patient. Mild anemias produce little in the way of symptoms other than a loss in stamina and an increase in heart rate and dyspnea with exercise. This reflects the ability of the hemoglobin-oxygen dissociation curve to compensate for modest reductions in the hemoglobin level in the basal state. It also shows the loss of the capacity of the hemoglobin-oxygen dissociation curve to respond to situations of increased demand once it is used to compensate for the anemia.

With more pronounced anemia, the patient's exercise capacity can be markedly reduced. Any exertion is accompanied by palpitations, dyspnea, a pounding headache, and rapid exhaustion. In younger individuals, these symptoms and signs do not appear until the hemoglobin has fallen below 7–8 grams per deciliter (hematocrit of less than 20–25%). However, older individuals, especially those with atherosclerotic cardiovascular disease, can become symptomatic with more modest anemia (a hemoglobin of 10–12 grams per deciliter). This can include worsening of ischemic manifestations, including angina and claudication. Moreover, anemia can precipitate heart failure in the older patient with underlying heart disease.

The rapidity of onset of the anemia is also important. Although the hemoglobin-oxygen dissociation curve can rapidly compensate for modest falls in the hemoglobin level, cardiovascular compensation for more severe anemia takes time. This situation is worsened if the anemia is the result of **acute blood loss** (a deficit in both red blood cells and plasma volume). The

reduction in total blood volume jeopardizes the cardiovascular response. Patients with acute hemorrhagic anemias are at risk for signs and symptoms of both tissue hypoxia and acute vascular collapse. In contrast, patients with long-standing anemias are able to expand their total blood volume and compensate with an increase in cardiac stroke volume and changes in regional blood flow.

CLINICAL EVALUATION

The cause of anemia may be suggested from the history and physical examination. Ongoing blood loss is an obvious and dramatic clue to the cause of the patient's anemia. The history can be equally revealing in diagnosing other types of anemia. A documented history of anemia that reaches back to childhood is highly suggestive of a hereditary disorder, especially a congenital hemolytic anemia. The sudden onset of a pancytopenia in an otherwise healthy individual may be explained from the patient's history of occupational or environmental exposure to toxic chemicals. Race can also be an important clue, because many of the hemoglobinopathies and enzyme deficiency states follow racial lines.

History

The patient should be questioned extensively regarding the timing of the onset of symptoms, transfusion history, past blood count measurements, nutritional habits, alcohol intake, and any associated symptoms of acute or chronic illness such as weight loss, fever, or night sweats. A few complaints are unique to specific types of anemia. For example, the adult iron-deficient patient may report craving ice, whereas children may be observed eating dirt (**picophagia**). Complaints of a sore mouth and difficulty swallowing are expressed by patients with vitamin B_{12} and iron deficiency. The sickle cell anemia patient will have a lifelong history of episodic bone and joint pains.

Physical Examination

The physical signs of an anemia depend very much on the acuity of onset. The patient with acute blood loss will show signs of hypovolemia and hypoxia. A loss of more than 30% of the blood volume in less than 12 hours cannot be compensated by the normal mechanisms of venospasm and redirection of regional blood flow. Such patients will show signs of hypovolemia, including postural hypotension and tachycardia with exertion. Once the acute volume loss exceeds 40% of the total blood volume, the patient will exhibit all the symptoms and signs of hypovolemic shock, including anxiety, confusion, air hunger, diaphoresis, rest tachycardia, and hypotension even while supine. The appearance of symptoms and signs of a hypoxia in such patients is as much a result of inadequate perfusion of vital organs as a reflection of their anemia.

When an anemia develops gradually so that the plasma volume has time to increase, compensation is accomplished by a combination of the shift in the hemoglobin-oxygen dissociation curve, an increase in cardiac output, and a redistribution of blood flow (Figure 2–1). By physical examination, it is possible for one to detect the changes in cardiac output and blood flow. The patient demonstrates a more forceful apical impulse, a wide pulse pressure, and tachycardia with exertion. Flow murmurs secondary to increased blood turbulence are frequently heard as mid- or holosystolic murmurs at the apex or along the sternal border with radiation to the neck.

An anemia may also be suggested from the patient's general appearance. In fair-skinned patients, skin and mucous membrane pallor are relatively good indicators of anemia. However, skin color is a less reliable measure of the hemoglobin level in heavily pigmented patients, or in those with marked vasoconstriction or dilatation. Marked edema as seen in patients with nephrotic syndrome or myxedema can also interfere with anemia detection. To avoid these confounding variables, it is best for one to look at the conjunctiva, mucous membranes, nail beds, and palmar creases of the hand when assessing the hemoglobin level.

Laboratory Evaluation

Although the history and physical examination may point the way to the presence of anemia and suggest its cause, a thorough laboratory evaluation is essential to the definitive diagnosis and treatment of any anemia. The routine hematology laboratory offers several tests relevant to anemia diagnosis: the more routine tests such as the CBC and reticulocyte count as well as studies of iron supply that serve both as screening tests and a jumping-off point to diagnosis (Table 2–1). A larger number of more specific tests come into play when one is confirming the diagnosis of specific conditions.

A. COMPLETE BLOOD COUNT (CBC):

The CBC includes determinations of the hemoglobin, hematocrit, red blood cell count, red blood cell volume and hemoglobin content, platelet count, and white blood cell count. These measurements are provided by

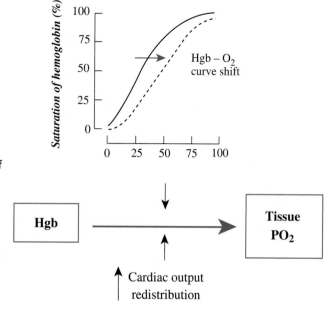

Figure 2–1. Tissue oxygen supply. Delivery of oxygen to tissues is a function of the hemoglobin level, the hemoglobin-oxygen dissociation curve, and the characteristics of tissue blood flow. With anemia, the hemoglobin-oxygen dissociation curve shifts to the right so as to deliver additional oxygen for a level of tissue PO_2. As the anemia worsens, cardiac output increases and there is a redistribution of blood flow to critical organs.

Table 2–1. **Routine laboratory tests in anemia diagnosis.**

Complete blood count
  Red blood cell number—Red blood cell count, hemoglobin, hematocrit
  Red blood cell indices—Mean cell volume (MCV), mean cell hemoglobin (MCH), mean cell hemoglobin concentration (MCHC), red blood cell distribution width (RDW)
  White blood cell count, white blood cell differential
  Platelet count
  Blood film morphology—cell size, hemoglobinization, anisocytosis, poikilocytosis, polychromasia
  Reticulocyte count—reticulocyte production index
Marrow examination
  Marrow aspirate—E/G ratio, cell morphology, iron stain
  Marrow biopsy—cellularity, morphology
Iron studies
  Iron transport—Serum iron, total iron binding capacity
  Iron stores—Serum ferritin, marrow iron stain, serum transferrin receptor

any of the common automated counters, including the Model S Coulter Counter, and instruments manufactured by TOA and Technicon. Newer instruments not only measure the white blood cell count but also perform a 3- or 5-part automated white blood cell differential. Instruments do vary in their technology, using a highly focused light source, an electric field, or a radiofrequency wave to discriminate between cells.

Automated instruments are not only fast but extremely accurate. The coefficient of variation (measurement error) of an automated counter is usually less than 2%, and each of the major measurements, including the hemoglobin level, hematocrit, red blood cell count, and mean cell volume, can be standardized independently with commercial red blood cell and hemoglobin standards. A printout of a Coulter counter blood count is shown in Figure 2–2. A range of normal values with 95% confidence limits is provided as a part of the report.

B. Hemoglobin/Hematocrit:

The hematocrit and hemoglobin level are used interchangeably in identifying the presence of an anemia. The Coulter counter directly measures the hemoglobin and calculates the hematocrit from measurements of the red blood cell count and mean cell volume (MCV). Other counters measure the hematocrit from the red blood cell size-distribution curve. This can make the hemoglobin measurement somewhat more accurate, since artifacts introduced by cell agglutination can increase the MCV and falsely elevate the hematocrit.

To diagnose an anemia, any patient value must be compared with a "normal" reference value. Table 2–2 summarizes the mean normal values for hemoglobin and hematocrit according to age and sex. At birth, the hemoglobin averages 17 grams per deciliter with a hematocrit of 52%. These values then decrease during childhood only to recover during adolescence until a mean hemoglobin level of 16 grams per deciliter (hematocrit of 47%) is reached in adult men and 13 grams per deciliter (hematocrit of 40%) in menstruating women.

These are mean values, however, and any normal population of men or women will vary around the mean in a Gaussian distribution (Figure 2–3). Therefore, it is common practice to state 95% confidence limits (2 standard deviations [SD]) for the mean normal value. For the adult male hemoglobin level, this is 16 ± 2 grams per deciliter; for the hematocrit, it is $47 \pm 6\%$. For the adult female hemoglobin level, it is 13 ± 2 grams per deciliter and for the hematocrit, it is $40 \pm 6\%$. When a patient's hemoglobin or hematocrit falls within these limits, it is most likely normal. As shown in Figure 2–3, however, the actual probability that the patient's hemoglobin/hematocrit is normal or abnormal will depend on the incidence of disease in the population. When the prevalence of anemia is high, the overlap of abnormal and normal populations will increase, thereby reducing both the sensitivity and specificity of the hemoglobin and hematocrit measurements. Of course, the lower the patient's hemoglobin value, the more likely it represents a true anemia.

Normal values for the hemoglobin and hematocrit are influenced by several environmental and physiologic factors. Populations living at higher altitudes have predictable increases in their hemoglobin levels of approximately 1 gram per deciliter of hemoglobin for each 3–4% decrease in arterial oxygen saturation. The same effect is produced by smoking since carbon monoxide decreases the hemoglobin-oxygen saturation. A patient who smokes more than one pack of cigarettes per day will show an increased hemoglobin level of between 0.5 and 1 gram per deciliter. Slightly lower hemoglobin levels are seen in black populations, 0.5 gram per deciliter below those of whites. During normal pregnancy, there is a steady decline in the hemoglobin level to 11–12 grams per deciliter during the second and third trimesters. This decline is caused by an expansion of plasma volume and does not represent a true anemia. Actually, the pregnant woman's red blood cell mass is increased late in pregnancy.

C. Mean Cell Volume (MCV):

Automated counters produce a size-distribution curve for the red blood cell population (Figure 2–4), which is then used to calculate an MCV. The normal MCV is

Sample results for
a patient with
a normocytic/normochromic anemia

WBC count	**9.8**	WBC x10³	7.8 ± 3
RBC count	**3.09**	RBC x10⁶	M 5.4 ± 0.7 F 4.8 ± 0.6
Hemoglobin	**9.5**	HGB g	M 16.0 + 2 F 14.0 ± 2
Hematocrit	**29**	HCT %	M 47 ± 5 F 42 ± 5
Mean red blood cell indices	**91**	MCV μ³ (fL)	90 ± 9
	30	MCH pg	32 ± 2
	33	MCHC %	33 ± 3
RDW - CV	**13.5**	RDW	M – F 13 ± 1%
RDW - SD	**48**	RDW	42 ± 5 fL
Platelet count and platelet volume	**150**	PLT x10³	M – F 140 - 440
	7.5	MpV μ³ (fL)	M – F 8.9 ± 1.5

Normal values

Figure 2–2. **CBC results.** Direct measurements on the Coulter counter include the white blood cell count, red blood cell count, hemoglobin, MCV, platelet count, and the mean platelet volume. Calculated values include the hematocrit, MCH, MCHC, and RDW.

Table 2–2. **Normal hemoglobin/hematocrit values.**

Age/Sex	Hemoglobin (g/dL)	Hematocrit (%)
At birth	17	52
Childhood	12	36
Adolescence	13	40
Adult man	16 (±2)	47 (±6)
Adult woman (menstruating)	13 (±2)	40 (±6)
Adult woman (postmenopausal)	14 (±2)	42 (±6)
During pregnancy	12 (±2)	37 (±6)

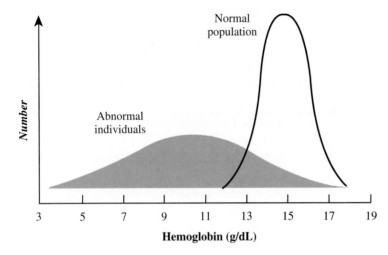

Figure 2–3. **Distributions of normal and abnormal hemoglobin values.** The shaded area shows the expected distribution for a normal population of adult males. Patients with red blood cell disorders may or may not fall outside this normal distribution. Very anemic patients will have hemoglobin values well below the normal distribution, whereas those with less severe disease may fall within the normal range.

90 ± 9 fL and generally coincides with the peak of the Gaussian distribution of red blood cell size. The MCV accurately detects any general increase (**macrocytosis**) or decrease (**microcytosis**) in red blood cell volume. It is less sensitive to the presence of small populations of microcytes or macrocytes, because they have little impact on the mean. To detect small numbers of abnormal cells, the clinician should look at the size distribution curve provided by the counter, inspect the stained blood smear, or both.

Although the MCV is both accurate and highly reproducible, errors may be introduced by red blood cell agglutination, distortions in cell shape, the presence of very high numbers of white blood cells, and sudden osmotic swelling. The latter is seen in patients with very high blood glucose levels or, rarely, with hypernatremia, when the red blood cell sample is diluted for counting. Since the diluent is isotonic, cells containing excess glucose or sodium will act as tiny osmometers and swell.

D. Mean Cell Hemoglobin (MCH):

The automated counter provides a calculated mean cell hemoglobin (ie, the hemoglobin level divided by the red blood cell count). The normal MCH is 32 ± 2 pg. This is an excellent measure of the amount of hemoglobin in each individual red blood cell. Patients with iron

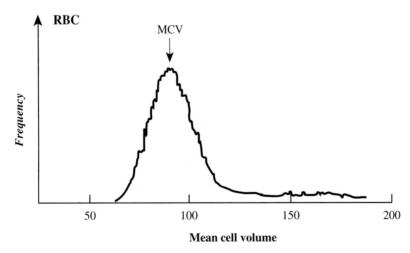

Figure 2–4. **A red blood cell size-distribution curve.** Automated counters display a distribution curve for the red blood cell volume. Direct inspection of the curve offers a sensitive method for detecting small populations of macrocytic or microcytic red blood cells.

deficiency or thalassemia who are unable to synthesize normal amounts of hemoglobin show significant reductions in the MCH.

E. MEAN CORPUSCULAR HEMOGLOBIN CONCENTRATION (MCHC):

The counter also provides a calculated mean corpuscular hemoglobin concentration (MCHC). The normal value of the MCHC is 33 ± 3%. This is the least revealing value provided by the counter. Although it should provide a measurement of the relative concentration of intracellular hemoglobin, it is not very sensitive to disease states where hemoglobin production is defective. This shortcoming is in part due to counter error but also reflects that defects in hemoglobin production are accompanied by a simultaneous reduction in cell size. Thus, empty cells are also small cells. The principal value of the MCHC is to detect patients with hereditary spherocytosis who have very small, condensed spherocytes in circulation. These spherocytes represent cells that because of a membrane defect have lost intracellular fluid. When present in significant numbers, they will cause the MCHC to increase in excess of 36%.

F. RED BLOOD CELL DISTRIBUTION WIDTH (RDW):

In addition to the cell indices, MCV, MCH, and MCHC, automated counters provide an index of the distribution of red blood cell volumes. This is called the red blood cell distribution width (RDW). Counters use two methods to calculate this value. The first is referred to as the RDW-CV. As shown in Figure 2–5, the **RDW-CV** is the ratio of the width of the red blood cell distribution curve at 1 SD divided by the MCV (nor-

mal RDW-CV = 13 ± 1%). Since it is a ratio, changes in either the width or the MCV will influence the result. Microcytosis will tend to magnify any change in the RDW-CV simply by reducing the denominator of the ratio. Conversely, macrocytosis will tend to counterbalance the change in the width of the curve and thereby minimize the change in the RDW-CV. A second method of measuring the RDW, the RDW-SD, is independent of the MCV. The **RDW-SD** is a direct measurement of the red blood cell distribution width taken at the 20% frequency level (normal RDW-SD = 42 ± 5 fL).

Both measurements of the RDW are essentially mathematical representations of anisocytosis (ie, variations in red blood cell size). Increases in the RDW suggest the presence of a mixed population of cells. Double populations of cells, whether microcytic cells mixed with normal cells or macrocytic cells mixed with normal cells, will widen the curve and increase the RDW. The RDW-SD is more sensitive to the appearance of minor populations of macrocytes or microcytes since it is measured lower on the red cell volume distribution curve (Figure 2–5). At the same time, it is overly sensitive to the impact of increased numbers of reticulocytes, which, because of their larger MCV, will broaden the base of the distribution curve. The RDW-CV is less sensitive to the appearance of small populations of microcytes, true macrocytes, or reticulocytes, but better reflects the overall change in size distribution seen with well established macrocytic or microcytic anemias.

G. STAINED BLOOD FILM:

Red blood cell morphology can provide important additional information as to the nature of the anemia.

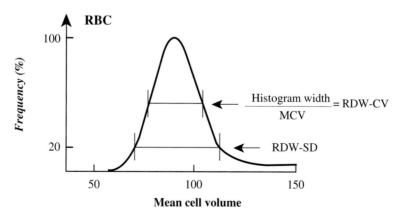

Figure 2–5. **Red blood cell distribution width (RDW).** Automated counters provide measurements of the width of the red blood cell distribution curve. The RDW-CV is calculated from the width of the histogram at 1 SD from the mean divided by the MCV. The normal RDW-CV is 13 ± 1%. The RDW-SD is the arithmetic width of the distribution curve measured at the 20% frequency level. The normal RDW-SD is 42 ± 5 fL.

Blood films are easily prepared using glass slides or a slide spinner (Figure 2–6). The well-dried blood film is then stained with Wright's stain to bring out cytoplasmic and nuclear detail. On inspection, red blood cells should form a single cell layer with most of the cells appearing biconcave, that is, having the distinctive doughnut shape associated with biconcavity (see Figure 1–1). If the film is too thick, cells will overlay each other and appear overly dense. When the film is too thin, as for example at the feathered edge of a hand-prepared blood smear, cells will lose both their biconcavity and round shape. Therefore, it is extremely important that any interpretation of red blood cell morphology be based on inspection of the best area of a well-prepared film. For glass slide films, this is usually close to but not at the feathered end of the film. For spinner films, almost any point on the smear will be representative.

The blood film complements the automated counter measurements of MCV and MCH. As shown in plates 1 and 2 of the color insert, changes in cell diameter, shape, and hemoglobin content can be used to distinguish both microcytic and macrocytic cells from normocytic/normochromic red blood cells. It should be emphasized, however, that the diagnosis of microcytosis or macrocytosis on a blood film involves extrapolation from an observed change in cell diameter to a volume estimate. This is not as sensitive or accurate as the direct measurement of cell volume by an automated counter. Therefore, the counter MCV should be used as the gold standard measurement for average changes in cell volume. At the same time, the stained film provides a more sensitive way to detect small populations of microcytic or macrocytic cells that are missed in the mean cell volume measurement.

The blood film is also used to detect and describe variations in cell size (**anisocytosis**) and shape (**poikilocytosis**). The former complements the automated counter measurement of the RDW. Film morphology provides more information than the RDW, however. It is possible

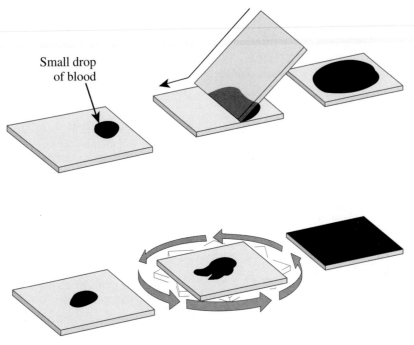

Small drop of blood

Figure 2–6. **Blood film preparation.** Blood films can be prepared by hand or with a slide spinner. If one uses two glass slides and a small drop of anticoagulated blood, it is easy to draw the blood along the length of the slide with a single smooth motion. Spinner films are prepared by putting a drop of blood in the center of a coverslip or glass slide and then rapidly spinning it on a slide spinner apparatus. The centrifugal motion evenly distributes the blood across the surface of the slide. Once the film is completely dry, the slide is stained with Wright's stain. The slide is first flooded with stain for 2–3 minutes and then a buffer solution is added until a green sheen appears on the surface. After another 3–5 minutes, the slide is rinsed with tap water and air dried. To interpret red blood cell morphology, one should select an area on the film where the red blood cells show the typical biconcave, doughnut shape.

to not only grade the degree of anisocytosis on a scale of 0 to 4+ but also comment on the population mix, whether microcytic, macrocytic, or another distinctive red blood cell shape (spherocytes, etc). Poikilocytosis can only be appreciated from the blood film. It is an important finding, because increasing poikilocytosis is associated with defects in red blood cell precursor maturation and certain types of red blood cell destruction. Like anisocytosis, it is graded on a scale of 0 to 4+.

Several unique changes in cell morphology are useful in anemia diagnosis. The first and most important is the **polychromatic macrocyte**, which is a cell that is slightly larger than other red blood cells by 1–2 μm, is grayish-blue in color, and often lacks the normal biconcave shape. These cells represent young reticulocytes (**marrow reticulocytes**) that still contain large amounts of RNA and ribosomes. Their presence on the blood film indicates a shift of marrow reticulocytes out of the marrow into circulation in response to an increased level of erythropoietin stimulation. Polychromasia can be used, therefore, to estimate the adequacy of the erythropoietin response to anemia.

Other distinctive changes in red blood cell morphology are illustrated in plates 1 and 2 of the color insert. Some of these changes, such as cells containing inclusion bodies (nucleated red blood cells, Howell-Jolly bodies, etc), are indicators of abnormalities in marrow production or splenic function. Others such as sickle cells, spherocytes, target cells, and elliptocytes are indicators of a specific disease state. The mechanism behind the appearance of each of these cells is discussed extensively in sections dealing with individual anemic states.

H. RETICULOCYTE COUNT:

The reticulocyte count is an essential component of the CBC and plays a prominent role in initially classifying any anemia. The reticulocyte is a young red blood cell containing residual ribosomal RNA that can be stained with a supravital dye such as acridine orange or new methylene blue. Two methods are used to quantitate the number of reticulocytes in circulation. The first involves mixing and incubating a drop of fresh blood with a few drops of new methylene blue solution and then preparing a spinner smear for counterstaining with Wright's stain. The dye precipitates and stains the RNA, marking the cell as a reticulocyte, and permitting the technician to count the number of reticulocytes versus the number of adult red blood cells. For accuracy, at least 1000 red blood cells should be counted to determine the reticulocyte percentage. Alternatively, a fresh blood sample can be stained with acridine orange and the number of reticulocytes counted using a flow cytometer. By this technique, reticulocytes are identified as cells of slightly larger size that fluoresce because of the RNA binding of the acridine orange.

The normal reticulocyte count for the new methylene blue method is 1% with a range of 0.5–1.7%. The normal value for the flow cytometry method can range from 1% to 2% depending on the cutoff point used to separate reticulocytes from the normal red blood cell population. Even though the standard error of these methods is quite high, the accuracy is good enough for clinical purposes. The main application of the reticulocyte count is to identify patients with major increases in red blood cell production of between three and five times normal. The routine reticulocyte count is accurate enough to identify such patients.

For one to use the reticulocyte count as a measure of red blood cell production, the count needs to be corrected for both changes in hematocrit (red blood cell count) and the effect of erythropoietin on reticulocyte release from the marrow. Most laboratories automatically correct the reticulocyte percent count to an absolute number either by multiplying it against the red blood cell count (normal absolute count = 50,000 reticulocytes/μL) or multiplying it by the fraction of the patient's hematocrit over the normal hematocrit as illustrated in the following formula:

$$\% \text{ reticulocytes} \times \frac{\text{patient Hct}}{45}$$
$$= \text{absolute reticulocyte percentage}$$
or
$$\% \text{ reticulocytes} \times \text{red blood cell count}$$
$$= \text{absolute reticulocyte count}$$

An example for a patient with a reticulocyte count of 6% and a hematocrit of 22% (red cell count of 2.6×10^6) would provide the following results:

$$6\% \times \frac{22}{45} = 3\% \text{ or } 6\% \times 2.6 \times 10^6$$
$$= 156{,}000 \text{ reticulocytes/μL}$$

To obtain the true index of marrow production in a severely anemic patient, a second correction must be made for the release of marrow reticulocytes under stimulation of high levels of erythropoietin. As shown in Figure 2–7, marrow reticulocytes are shifted out of the marrow and into circulation at an earlier stage with increasingly severe anemia. This process has the effect of lengthening the maturation time of reticulocytes in circulation. Whereas normal reticulocytes lose their RNA within 24 hours, a severely anemic patient with a full erythropoietin response will release reticulocytes that take from 2 to 3 days to lose their RNA. This has the effect of raising the reticulocyte count simply because reticulocytes produced on any single day will be

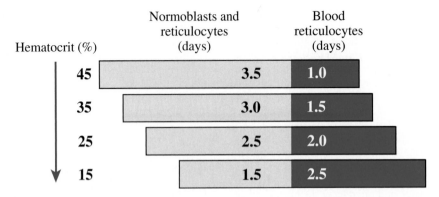

Hematocrit (%)	Normoblasts and reticulocytes (days)	Blood reticulocytes (days)
45	3.5	1.0
35	3.0	1.5
25	2.5	2.0
15	1.5	2.5

Figure 2–7. **Reticulocyte shift.** As anemia worsens and the level of erythropoietin stimulation increases, marrow reticulocytes leave the marrow at an earlier point in their maturation. This prolongs their maturation time in circulation. Whereas the normal reticulocyte matures in less than a day, reticulocytes in anemic patients take from 1.5 to 2.5 days. This must be taken into account when calculating the reticulocyte production index.

counted for 2 or more days. The absolute reticulocyte count can be corrected for shift (**early release**) using a simple formula as follows:

$$\frac{\text{Absolute reticulocyte percentage (or number)}}{2} = \text{reticulocyte production index}$$

When applied to the prior example, results in a patient with an initial reticulocyte count of 6% would be corrected as follows:

$$6\% \times \frac{22}{45} \times \frac{1}{2} = 1.5 \text{ (production index)}$$

or

$$6\% \times 2.6 \times 10^6 \times \frac{1}{2} = \frac{78,000}{50,000} = 1.5$$

The correction for the shift phenomenon should be applied to any patient with anemia and a very high reticulocyte count. To confirm that a high erythropoietin level is causing a shift of marrow reticulocytes into circulation, one can identify polychromatic macrocytes on the stained smear. The correction should not be applied when polychromasia is absent, as observed, for example, with a hypoproliferative anemia secondary to inflammation (the anemia of chronic disease).

The **reticulocyte production index** is an excellent measure of effective red blood cell production. When a patient responds to anemia (hematocrit less than 30%) with an increase in the reticulocyte index to levels greater than 3 times normal, it can be assumed that the patient has normal renal function, a full erythropoietin response, and a normal erythroid marrow. Moreover, it strongly suggests that the anemia is the result of hemolysis or hemorrhage. Diseases that interfere with marrow precursor proliferation or maturation are characterized by lower levels of effective red blood cell production.

Additional evidence of hemolysis is provided by serum bilirubin and lactic dehydrogenase levels (LDH). The indirect (unconjugated) serum bilirubin concentration correlates with the rate of red blood cell turnover. Normally, serum bilirubin is between 0.4 and 1 mg/dL, most of which is indirect bilirubin (70–80%). With hemolysis or severe ineffective erythropoiesis, indirect bilirubin increases to 0.8–3 mg/dL. As long as the patient's liver function is normal, direct or conjugated bilirubin level shows little change.

The serum LDH is also sensitive to increased rates of red blood cell destruction. Red blood cells are rich in LDH, especially LDH 1. Patients with hemolytic anemias show rises in their serum LDH concentrations in excess of 1000 IU/L (normal 300–600 IU/L), without abnormalities in other liver enzymes. With severe hemolysis or marked ineffective erythropoiesis, the LDH level can reach several thousand units.

I. MARROW EXAMINATION:

A sample of marrow can easily be obtained by needle aspirate or biopsy to evaluate overall cellularity, the ratio of erythroid to granulocytic precursors (**E/G ratio**), and cellular morphology. The marrow examination is of greatest value in patients who fail to show an appropriate increase in the reticulocyte production index in response to anemia. In these patients defects in erythroid precursor proliferation or maturation play a major role.

In adults, the marrow aspirate or biopsy is best obtained from the posterior iliac crest (Figure 2–8). The **iliac crest** is identifiable as a palpable bony ridge, approximately 2 cm from the midline at the level of the sacrum. The cortex of the crest is quite thin and easily punctured with a standard aspiration or biopsy needle, using a small amount of local anesthetic to numb the skin and periosteal membrane. The marrow aspirate specimen is used for evaluating cell morphology, whereas needle biopsy is best suited for evaluating overall cellularity and the relationship of marrow structure to hematopoietic cells.

1. Marrow aspirate—The quality of the marrow aspirate specimen is extremely important. Very small amounts of marrow should be aspirated using a 1- to 2-mL syringe and immediately expressed onto a watchglass. Marrow particles can then be harvested with a capillary tube and spread on slides or coverslips. Once air dried, smears are stained with a Wright's-Giemsa stain to bring out the details of nuclear and cytoplasmic structure. The best aspirate specimens show stromal particles surrounded by a field of hematopoietic cells of all types. It should also be possible under oil immersion to identify and classify each cell, whether a myeloid or

erythroid precursor. If cells are sparse or severely distorted, the preparation is not interpretable.

Inspection of a marrow aspirate starts with a low power scan for particle cellularity, and distribution and frequency of megakaryocytes, which because of their large size and multiple nuclei are easily identified. There is no exact way of enumerating megakaryocytes. It should not be difficult, however, to find them in a normal marrow specimen. Inspection of the other cell types is then carried out under oil immersion (100×). Several high-power fields adjacent to a stroma particle should be scanned to estimate the E/G ratio. As long as the patient's white blood cell production is normal, the E/G ratio provides a rough index of red blood cell production.

The red blood cell precursor population is carefully examined for evidence of a maturation abnormality (Figure 2–9). This includes a study of cell size, nuclear morphology, and hemoglobin development. Patients with a megaloblastic marrow (defect in DNA metabolism) show a preponderance of young, large erythroblasts with nuclei containing lacy, poorly staining chromatin. Older precursors show a discrepancy between nuclear maturation and hemoglobin synthesis, where the nucleus appears less mature than it should for the amount of hemoglobin synthesized. Patients with defects in hemoglobin synthesis show normal nuclear maturation but poor cytoplasmic maturation.

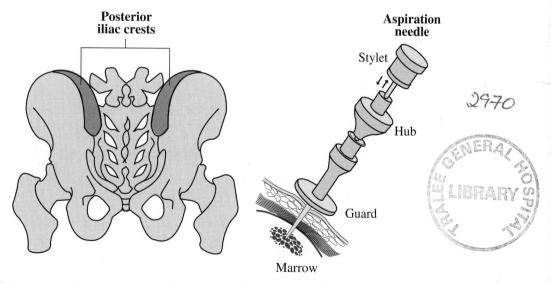

Posterior iliac crests

Aspiration needle

Stylet

Hub

Guard

Marrow

Figure 2–8. Marrow aspiration technique. A marrow aspirate is most easily obtained from the posterior iliac crest, a bony ridge that is usually easily palpable 2 cm from the midline at the level of the sacrum. An inspiration needle with stylet in place is easily pushed through the external cortex of the crest using a slight twisting motion. Once the needle is firmly in the marrow cavity, the stylet is withdrawn and a small (1- to 2-mL) syringe is used to aspirate a few drops of marrow. The marrow is then expelled on a watchglass and particles are harvested to make marrow smears.

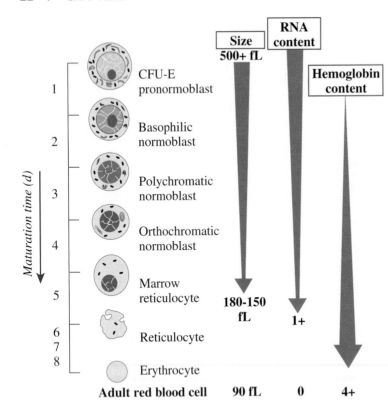

Size
500+ fL

RNA content

Hemoglobin content

CFU-E pronormoblast

Basophilic normoblast

Polychromatic normoblast

Orthochromatic normoblast

Marrow reticulocyte

Reticulocyte

Erythrocyte

Maturation time (d)

1
2
3
4
5
6
7
8

180-150 fL

1+

Adult red blood cell   **90 fL**   **0**   **4+**

Figure 2–9. **Erythroid marrow maturation.** Red blood cell precursor maturation proceeds through a series of morphologically distinct stages over 6–7 days. Identifiable populations in this maturation sequence include pronormoblasts; basophilic, polychromatic, and orthochromatic normoblasts; and the marrow reticulocytes. With development, there is a progressive reduction in cell size, a shrinkage of the cell's nucleus, a loss of cellular mitochondria and RNA, and a dramatic increase in hemoglobin. Specific red blood cell disorders can be identified from disruptions in this normal maturation sequence.

Marrow aspirate particles should also be stained with Prussian blue to evaluate reticuloendothelial cell iron stores and iron deposits in individual red blood cell precursors. Hemosiderin particles within the reticuloendothelial cells of the marrow stroma stain a deep blue color. The greater the amount of iron stores, the more dramatic the staining. Iron stores can be estimated using a scale of 0 to 4+, where the normal adult male with 1000 mg of iron stores will be 3+ and a normal adult female with 200–300 mg of iron stores will be 1+.

Close inspection of individual red blood cell precursors will also reveal a few dustlike iron (ferritin) granules in maturing normoblasts. Up to one-third of red blood cell precursors will contain blue-staining ferritin granules. These cells are referred to as **sideroblasts,** whereas marrow reticulocytes containing iron granules are **siderocytes.** A decrease in the number of sideroblasts and siderocytes is a morphologic indication of iron-deficient erythropoiesis. In contrast, an increase in the number and size increase in iron granules in erythroid precursors suggests a defect in hemoglobin synthesis. Patients with specific disorders of mitochondrial function can exhibit **ringed sideroblasts,** which are distinctive cells with several large granules distributed in a ring

around the nucleus. This condition results from iron loading of the mitochondria that surround the nucleus.

2. Marrow biopsy—If an adequate specimen cannot be obtained by aspiration, a needle biopsy needs to be performed. Needle biopsies are also indicated in patients being evaluated for tumor infiltration of the marrow, fibrosis, or aplasia. The biopsy specimen permits a better evaluation of the marrow structural elements and the relationship of stroma to hematopoietic cells.

Independent of the type of needle used, it is important to obtain a good core of marrow. The specimen is fixed, decalcified, and stained with periodic acid–Schiff and hematoxylin & eosin stains. Other special stains, such as a silver stain for reticulin fibers or a trichrome stain for collagen, can help in diagnosing specific disorders of marrow structure.

As with the aspirate, initial inspection of a biopsy specimen should be carried out under low power to evaluate adequacy of the specimen, general architecture, and overall cellularity. The cellularity of hematopoietic tissue in the central skeleton decreases with age. Two-thirds or more of the marrow space in a young adult is taken up by hematopoietic tissue and one-third is filled with fat cells. This ratio reverses over the next several decades; older individuals have one-half to two-thirds of their marrow space filled with fat cells. The biopsy specimen is also good for evaluating the presence of megakaryocytes. As with the aspirate, the megakaryocytes are easily identified because of their large size and multinuclearity. Finally, needle biopsy is clearly preferred for the detection of structural abnormalities such as myelofibrosis and infiltration of the marrow by malignant cells, especially lymphomas and carcinomas.

J. TESTS OF IRON SUPPLY:

Studies of iron supply, including measurements of serum iron, transferrin iron binding capacity, and serum ferritin level, play an important role in the initial differential diagnosis of an anemia. They are essential companions to the marrow iron stain whenever a marrow aspirate is performed.

1. Serum iron level—The **serum iron (SI)** is a measure of the amount of iron bound to transferrin. A normal individual has an SI of 50–150 µg/dL. The proliferative capacity of the erythroid marrow and its ability to synthesize hemoglobin are functions of the serum iron level. When the SI falls to levels below 50 µg/dL, the erythroid marrow cannot increase production above basal levels and new red blood cells will be poorly hemoglobinized. Levels of marrow production that are three times the basal level or greater require a serum iron in excess of 100 µg/dL.

2. Total iron-binding capacity—The **total iron-binding capacity (TIBC)** is a measure of the amount of iron that can be bound by transferrin. In effect, it is equivalent to measuring the level of transferrin protein. The normal TIBC is 300–360 µg/dL. The importance of the TIBC is twofold. First, the TIBC changes independently of the serum iron in situations of iron deficiency. Although TIBC declines in patients with the anemia of chronic disease (inflammation), it typically increases in excess of 360 mg/dL in patients with severe iron deficiency. The TIBC is also used to calculate a percent saturation of transferrin:

$$\frac{SI}{TIBC} = \% \text{ saturation}$$

A normal individual has a percent saturation of between 20% and 50%. When the percent saturation falls below 10%, the patient usually has absolute iron deficiency. With values between 10% and 20%, it is more likely that the decrease in iron supply is the result of an inflammatory state. Iron overload, especially idiopathic hemochromatosis, is associated with an increased percent saturation, which exceeds 50% and often approaches 90–100%.

3. Serum ferritin level—Ferritin is a spherical protein made up of 24 subunits: L (light), H (heavy), and G (glycosylated). **Serum ferritin** contains mostly L and G subunits, whereas tissue ferritins are largely L and H subunit types. Since the serum ferritin level generally parallels total body storage iron, it is used clinically to evaluate body iron stores. A normal adult male will have a serum ferritin level of between 50 and 150 µg/L, reflecting iron stores of 600–1000 mg. When iron stores are depleted, the serum ferritin falls. Levels below 10–15 µg/L indicate store exhaustion and iron deficiency. With iron overload, the serum ferritin level will exceed 300 µg/L and may reach several thousand micrograms per liter. Liver disease and inflammation disproportionally elevate the serum ferritin, perhaps by the release of tissue ferritins.

4. Serum transferrin-receptor level—Erythroid precursor cells express transferrin-receptors (TfR) on their surface according to their level of maturation and the adequacy of iron supply (see Chapter 5). Measurements of the serum TfR level (normal level = 4–9 µg/L) generally reflect the level of expression of receptors on the cell surface as well as the absolute number of erythroid precursors. Therefore, the serum TfR increases with both iron deficiency (**iron store exhaustion**) and erythroid precursor proliferation. It can be useful in the differential diagnosis of absolute iron deficiency versus the anemia of chronic disease (**inflammatory anemia**), where iron stores are maintained and the anemia is hypoproliferative (Chapters 4 and 5).

K. OTHER LABORATORY MEASUREMENTS:

Several other laboratory tests are used in the diagnosis of specific hematopoietic disorders. A partial list of these assays grouped according to category of disease is provided in Table 2–3. Detailed descriptions of assay methods and test interpretations are provided as a part of the discussion of individual disorders.

APPROACH TO THE PATIENT

The key to any anemia evaluation is the clinician's skill in applying and interpreting the results of these laboratory tests according to the clinical presentation. Often, the workup of the anemia is carried out as a part of the evaluation and management of other illness. This process requires knowledge and understanding of the impact of disease states on red blood cell production and survival. It is also important to complete the basic workup as quickly as possible, since delay can lead to confusion. For example, a patient with a maturation defect secondary to drug effect or vitamin deficiency can show dramatic changes in the CBC, serum iron studies, and marrow morphology within a few days of changes in medication and diet, or the treatment of a second illness.

Table 2–3. **Laboratory assays in the diagnosis of specific red cell disorders.**

Hypoproliferative anemias
Cytometric assay of CD59/CD55 levels (Paroxysmal nocturnal hemoglobinuria)
Chromosomal analysis (Leukemias)
Marrow aspirate/biopsy special status
    Trichrome stain (Myelofibrosis)
    Silver stain for reticulin (Myelofibrosis)
    Peroxidase, esterase, and PAS stains (Acute leukemia)
Maturation disorders
Serum vitamin B_{12} level (Vitamin B_{12} deficiency)
Serum/red blood cell folate levels (Folic acid deficiency)
Urine/serum methylmalonic acid level (B_{12} and folate deficiency)
DU suppression test (B_{12} deficiency)
Hemoglobin electrophoresis (Thalassemia)
Hemoglobin A_2 level (β-thalassemia)
Hemoglobin F level—alkali denaturation (β-thalassemia)
Acid elution slide test for hemoglobin F (Thalassemia versus hereditary persistence of hemoglobin F)
Brilliant cresyl blue stain (Hemoglobin H)
Red blood cell protoporphyrin level (Iron deficiency—lead poisoning)
Hemolytic anemias
Hemoglobin electrophoresis (Hemoglobinopathies)
Coombs test (Autoimmune hemolytic anemia)
Cold agglutinin titer (Autoimmune hemolytic anemia)
Haptoglobin level (Hemolysis)
Serum/urine hemosiderin (Intravascular hemolysis)
Osmotic fragility (Hereditary spherocytosis)
Incubated autohemolysis test (Congenital nonspherocytic hemolytic anemias)
G6PD screen (G6PD deficiency)
Heat/isopropanol denaturation tests (Unstable hemoglobins)
Polycythemia
^{51}Cr—red blood cell mass (Erythrocytosis)
Red blood cell P_{50} (Abnormal hemoglobin)
Red blood cell 2,3-DPG level (Abnormal hemoglobin)
CO level (Carboxyhemoglobinemia)
Serum erythropoietin level

Whenever possible, the battery of routine laboratory tests and the marrow aspirate or biopsy (or both) should be performed on the same day. This procedure will help avoid any misinterpretation of a test result simply because it was drawn at a time when the patient's clinical picture had changed. For example, since the reticulocyte count measures red blood cell production on a daily basis, it will change much more quickly than red blood cell morphology, which takes 2–3 months to turn over completely.

Another important rule is never to assume a diagnostic relationship. Even though the cause of the anemia may be suggested by the clinical presentation, a full laboratory evaluation is always important. Often, the anemia is caused by several contributing factors. For example, the patient with small-bowel disease and malabsorption can present with a combination of deficiencies in iron, folic acid, and vitamin B_{12}, as well as an anemia typical of a chronic inflammatory disease state. The diagnostic challenge is to identify each etiologic component.

Classification of Anemia

Anemia diagnosis can be organized as a three-branch algorithm based on routine laboratory test results. The first step is to categorize the erythropoietic abnormality as one of three functional defects: (1) a failure in red blood cell production, (2) an abnormality in cell maturation, or (3) an increase in cell destruction. This first step relies on the CBC and reticulocyte index. As shown in Figure 2–10, defects in production (hypoproliferative anemias) are characterized by a low reticulocyte index coupled with little or no change in red blood cell morphology. Maturation disorders demonstrate a low reticulocyte production index together with either macrocytic or microcytic red blood cell morphology. Patients with increased red blood cell destruction owing to hemolysis show a compensatory increase in the reticulocyte index to levels greater than three times normal and red blood cell morphology that may or may not be distinctive for the disease process.

This first step in classifying an anemia is important for both diagnosis and management. From the diagnostic viewpoint, each category encompasses a limited number of possibilities (Figure 2–11). This situation makes it possible to organize the rest of the laboratory evaluation around those tests that best discriminate among several diagnostic choices. Management of the patient will also vary according to the functional defect. For example, the need to provide a transfusion for a patient early in the course of the workup will depend on the expected ability of the patient to respond to a specific therapy.

Hypoproliferative Anemias

A **hypoproliferative anemia** (ie, an anemia resulting from a failure in the erythroid marrow production response) can result from damage to the marrow structure or precursor stem cell pool, a lack of stimulation by erythropoietin, or iron deficiency. Patients with these conditions usually present with a normocytic, normochromic anemia of moderate severity. The reticulocyte production index is less than 2 and the marrow

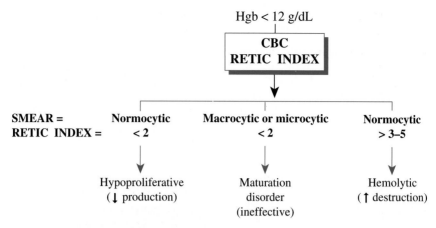

Figure 2–10. **Initial classification of anemia.** The CBC and reticulocyte index is used to classify an anemia as hypoproliferative, a maturation disorder, or a hemorrhagic/hemolytic anemia.

E/G ratio is less than 1:2. Measurements of red blood cell destruction such as the bilirubin and LDH are normal or decreased. In essence, this is the profile of a marrow that has not responded appropriately (increased red cell production) to the patient's anemia.

Most anemias encountered in clinical practice are hypoproliferative. They are most often associated with a chronic illness, especially an inflammatory disorder. Iron deficiency is another prominent cause of hypoproliferative anemia. Therefore, a careful clinical evaluation is required to understand the cause of the anemia and to plan management. A full discussion of marrow damage anemias is covered in Chapter 3, whereas anemias associated with chronic disease are discussed in Chapter 4.

Maturation Defects

Disruption of the erythroid precursor maturation sequence can result from deficiencies in vitamins such as folic acid and vitamin B_{12}, exposure to chemotherapeutic agents, or a preleukemic state. Since these are all defects in nuclear maturation, patients present with

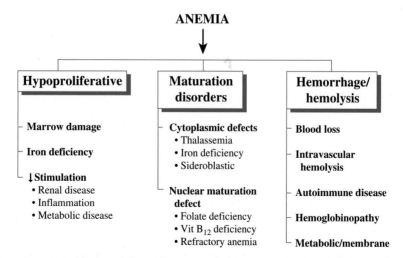

Figure 2–11. **Functional classification of anemia.** Each of the major categories of anemia (hypoproliferative, maturation disorders, and hemorrhage/hemolysis) can be further subclassified according to the functional defect in the several components of normal erythropoiesis.

macrocytic anemias and megaloblastic bone marrow morphology. Defects in hemoglobinization, including severe iron deficiency and inherited defects in globin chain synthesis, the thalassemias, produce a microcytic, hypochromic anemia and markedly ineffective erythropoiesis. An extensive discussion of maturation disorders is provided in Chapter 5 (Iron-Deficiency Anemia), Chapter 6 (Thalassemia), and Chapter 8 (Macrocytic Anemias).

Increased Red Blood Cell Destruction

Blood loss or hemolysis will stimulate a compensatory red blood cell production response. Thus, the increased cell destruction category of anemia is characterized by an increase in the reticulocyte production index to greater than three times normal and a similar increase in the E/G ratio to levels greater than 1:1. The impact of high levels of erythropoietin stimulation in the marrow is also apparent from the appearance of large numbers of polychromatic macrocytes (marrow reticulocytes) on the peripheral blood smear. Other changes in morphology may provide a specific clue as to the cause of a hemolytic anemia. A full discussion of both diagnosis and management of blood loss anemia is provided in Chapter 10. The approach to diagnosis and management of the various hemolytic anemias is discussed in Chapters 7 and 11.

MANAGEMENT GUIDELINES

The management of any anemia must be based on the diagnosis. Therefore, the sooner the workup is complete and the diagnosis confirmed, the better. Shotgun therapy, where several therapeutic agents are given simultaneously, can make accurate diagnosis nearly impossible and can lead to inappropriate maintenance therapy with one or more hematinics. Thus, the clinician should withhold therapy at least until all of the necessary laboratory tests have been obtained.

Therapy should not be delayed, however, if the patient is physiologically unstable. Severe anemia in the elderly patient can lead to confusion, obtundation, heart failure, and organ ischemia. This condition needs to be treated immediately with transfusion of packed red blood cells to stabilize the patient while the anemia workup proceeds. As long as the volume of blood transfused is limited, it will not interfere with the diagnostic workup. However, massive transfusion will obscure the results of key laboratory tests, including the CBC, reticulocyte count, serum iron studies, and marrow morphology.

A wide range of therapies is available for treating various anemias, ranging from red blood cell transfusion and vitamin replacement therapy to bone marrow transplantation. With the availability of recombinant erythropoietin, the anemias associated with renal damage and chronic disease can be effectively treated. The details of specific treatments are covered in the individual chapters on these topics.

BIBLIOGRAPHY

Bessman JD: *Automated Blood Counts and Differentials.* Johns Hopkins University Press, 1986.

Fauci AS et al: *Principles of Internal Medicine,* 14th ed. McGraw-Hill, 1998.

Hillman RS, Finch CA: *Red Cell Manual,* 7th ed. FA Davis, 1997.

Marrow-Damage Anemia

Disruption of the erythroid precursor pool or the structure of the marrow can produce a marrow-damage anemia. The severity of the anemia depends on the nature of the disorder. **Relatively mild marrow-damage anemias** are seen in association with drug toxicity and tumor infiltration. **More severe anemias** are typically seen in patients with acute leukemia and aplastic anemia.

The **prevalence** of marrow-damage anemias in any population is a function of the incidence of various disease states and environmental challenges. Impairment of red blood cell production is anticipated in most patients receiving tumor chemotherapy. In contrast, aplastic anemia characterized by a marked reduction in all hematopoietic precursors is a relatively rare event. Higher rates of aplastic anemia in the developing world are usually a result of the level of exposure to toxic drugs and chemicals in the workplace and environment.

MARROW STRUCTURE

Anatomical Distribution

The capacity of the erythroid marrow to compensate for anemia or hypoxia requires a normal pool of committed stem cells and a nurturing environment. The anatomical distribution of the marrow is illustrated in Figure 3–1. In normal adults, marrow is concentrated in the axial skeleton and proximal portions of the long bones. It can, however, extend out into more peripheral sites in response to long-standing anemia or as a result of myeloproliferative disease. Patients with thalassemia major can show extension of marrow even into the small bones of the hand.

RBC Growth

On a microscopic level, red blood cells grow in clusters within a matrix of reticular cells, reticular fibers, and a network of vascular sinusoids. This framework provides free access to plasma nutrients but holds the cells in place during maturation, allowing only mature cells to escape into the bloodstream. Red blood cell precursors tend to cluster around marrow macrophages, suggesting a nurse cell role for these structural cells. There is evidence for direct reticuloendothelial cell to red blood cell precursor transfer of iron to support hemoglobin synthesis. Other structural cells play an equally impor-

tant role in providing growth factors (interleukin-3 [IL-3], granulocyte macrophage colony stimulating factor [GM-CSF], and stem cell growth factor [SCF]), which are essential to the first steps in cell differentiation and proliferation (Figure 3–2). T cells also influence early stem cell growth. Erythropoietin has its principal effect on committed red blood cell precursors such as the burst forming unit–erythroid (BFU-E) and colony forming unit–erythroid (CFU-E).

Aging Process

Humans are born with a self-replicating stem cell pool that supports all hematopoietic cell lines throughout the natural lifespan. There is no evidence for a failure of red blood cell production as a part of the aging process. Older patients do, however, show a decrease in marrow cellularity. Although the ratio of hematopoietic tissue to fat cells in the younger patient favors hematopoietic tissue, older patients show an increasing number of fat cells. This is not a sign of marrow damage or a failed capacity to respond to anemia or hypoxia. With a sustained stimulus, marrow cellularity can increase to the point of displacing all visible adipose tissue.

Damaging Factors

Both the stem cell pool and marrow structure can be damaged by external factors. Ionizing radiation can result in a loss of stem cells and irreversible damage to the blood supply and suspensary structures of the marrow. Several chemicals and drugs will also cause irreversible loss of replicating stem cells. Finally, the nurturing environment of the marrow can be impaired by overexpansion of a single line of hematopoietic cells, as with a leukemia, or invasion by tumor. These cells compete both for the space and nutrients required for normal red blood cell growth.

CLINICAL FEATURES

Many of the marrow damage anemias can be anticipated from the clinical presentation. **Patients undergoing high-dose multidrug chemotherapy** are expected to develop a marrow damage anemia. The more strenuous the treatment protocol, the more severe the anemia

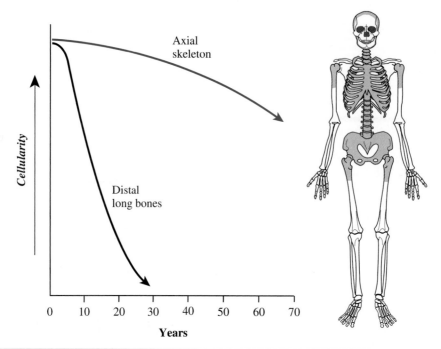

Figure 3–1. Anatomical distribution of the marrow in the adult. At birth, the marrow is widely distributed throughout the skeleton. During childhood and early adult life, marrow in the more distal portions of the long bones is replaced by fat. Active marrow is limited to the axial skeleton and proximal ends of the long bones, as indicated by the shading of the skeleton.

and the more likely there will be an associated leukopenia and thrombocytopenia. If one anticipates both the course and severity of this type of marrow damage anemia, a workup is usually unnecessary and management, whether red blood cell transfusion or treatment with erythropoietin, is easily planned.

In a similar fashion, **marrow damage anemias associated with myeloproliferative disease and widespread invasion of the marrow by tumor** are usually obvious from the patient's clinical picture and the presence of marked abnormalities in other hematopoietic cell lines. The onset can be rapid, as in the patient with acute leukemia. However, even though the anemia may be severe, it usually is overshadowed by defects in the myelocyte and megakaryocyte cell lines. These patients usually present with varying combinations of severe bleeding, acute infection, and symptomatic anemia.

The most characteristic clinical features of a patient with a so-called **idiopathic "aplastic anemia"** are the suddenness of onset and the apparent absence of other illness. Once again, the associated pancytopenia can produce a mixed picture of bleeding, infection, and anemia. However, many patients have variable depressions in their white blood cell and platelet counts, so

the presenting symptoms of anemia may predominate. There is even the rare patient who presents with solitary red blood cell aplasia.

Laboratory Studies

The **complete blood count (CBC), reticulocyte count, serum iron studies, and a well-performed marrow aspirate and biopsy** should make it possible to diagnose a marrow damage anemia. Typical erythropoietic profiles of moderate and severe marrow damage are illustrated in Table 3–1. The CBC and reticulocyte count are characteristic of a hypoproliferative anemia. Red blood cell morphology is normocytic and normochromic, and the reticulocyte index is inappropriately low for the severity of the patient's anemia. A careful inspection of the blood smear may reveal important clues to the presence of marrow structural damage, including the appearance of nucleated red blood cells and abnormal white blood cell precursors.

A. IRON STUDIES:

Iron studies, including the serum iron, total iron-binding capacity (TIBC), and serum ferritin level, pro-

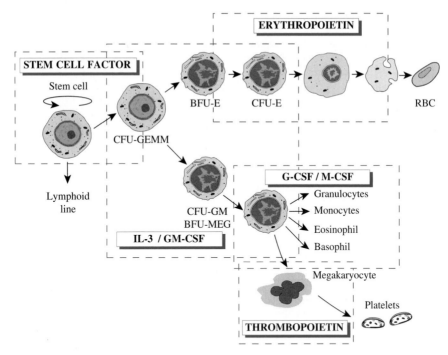

Figure 3–2. **Marrow cell differentiation and proliferation.** A pool of replicating pluripotent stem cells differentiates into the several cell lineages required for erythropoiesis, myelopoiesis, and platelet formation. The most primitive cell in the red blood cell lineage is the blast forming unit–erythroid (BFU-E). Under the influence of erythropoietin, the BFU-E differentiates to the CFU-E and the more mature normoblast series. This process involves both the series of cell divisions and the progressive formation of hemoglobin in the cytoplasm. Growth factors such as IL-3, GM-CSF, G-CSF, and CSF-1 are important first steps in cell differentiation and the proliferation and maturation of myelopoietic cell lines. Thrombopoietin governs the proliferation and maturation of the megakaryocyte cell line.

vide an indirect measure of erythroid marrow cellularity. With severe damage and a marked reduction in red blood cell precursors, iron destined for hemoglobin synthesis accumulates in the plasma and iron storage sites. This situation results in an increase in the serum iron level even to the point of full saturation of the

Table 3–1. Marrow damage anemia erythropoietic profile.

	Moderate	Severe
Red blood cell morphology	Normocytic/normochromic	
Polychromasia	Present	Rare/absent
Nucleated red blood cells	Present with structural damage	
Reticulocyte index	<2	<1
Marrow E/G ratio	<1:3	<1:3
Marrow morphology	Can be diagnostic of disease process	
Serum iron	Normal or slightly increased	Increased
TIBC	Normal	Normal
Percent saturation	30–50	50–100

TIBC. The serum ferritin level also increases, reflecting a rise in reticuloendothelial cell iron stores. Although the serum ferritin level may only be modestly elevated when the patient first presents, it increases to very high levels (greater than 1000 μg/L) when the patient repeatedly receives transfusions.

B. MARROW ASPIRATE AND BIOPSY:

A well-performed marrow aspirate and biopsy are essential for diagnosis. In patients with severe aplastic anemia, advanced myelofibrosis, or marked infiltration of the marrow with tumor, the aspirate can be difficult or impossible to obtain (a "dry tap"). In this circumstance, a **marrow core biopsy** should be performed using a standard marrow biopsy needle. The core sample is used to make touch preparations for cell morphology and, after fixation and sectioning, for study of overall structure and cellularity. In addition to the standard **hematoxylin & eosin** and **periodic acid–Schiff stains** for cell characteristics, special stains such as a **trichrome stain** for collagen tissue and a **silver stain** for reticulin fibers are used to identify marrow structural abnormalities. Patients with myelofibrosis or tumor metastases to marrow can show increasing amounts of collagen and reticulin fibers, even to the point of obliterating the space available for hematopoietic cells.

A **Prussian blue stain** of marrow aspirate and biopsy material is also important. In addition to permitting evaluation of the level of iron stores, it also allows the detection of red blood cell precursors with abnormal amounts of intracellular iron. A marrow damage anemia pattern is seen in some patients with sideroblastic anemias. Likewise, occasional ringed sideroblasts are seen in patients with secondary marrow damage anemias. The amount of iron stored in reticuloendothelial cells is dramatically increased in patients with severe marrow damage anemias who have received many transfusions.

Although marrow biopsy provides an excellent measure of the structure and cellularity of a small area of marrow, it does not provide a sense of total marrow mass and distribution. Radiologic techniques can be used to measure marrow distribution. The **technetium sulfa colloid scan** measures the integrity of the vascular and structural elements of the marrow. In patients with severe fibrosis or widespread invasion of marrow by tumor, the technetium scan will be abnormal, showing either total loss of uptake or a patchy distribution. The presence and distribution of red blood cell precursors can be imaged using ^{111}In. Indium, like iron, is avidly absorbed by red blood cell precursors.

Magnetic resonance imaging (MRI) of the vertebral spine provides qualitative information as to the cellularity of the marrow by discriminating between marrows that are largely replaced by fat cells and those where hematopoietic or tumor tissue is present. In patients with an aplastic or hypoplastic anemia, the characteristic fatty appearance may not be observed when there are excessive marrow iron deposits (**hemosiderosis**) secondary to iron loading or transfusion. MRI is the preferred imaging technique in the evaluation of patients with myeloma, lymphoma, and tumor metastases, where marrow involvement is focal and patchy. It also allows a better assessment of complications of marrow disease, such as compression/pathological fractures, epidural disease with cord compression, and soft tissue/node extension. Finally, serial MRI studies are much more useful in monitoring responses to therapy and disease progression.

C. MISCELLANEOUS STUDIES:

Other studies for evaluating patients with marrow damage anemia include **cytogenetic and phenotypic studies** of cells in circulation and in the marrow. Both techniques are helpful in detecting a malignant cell line and providing supporting evidence for diagnoses such as myelodysplasia, myelofibrosis, and leukemic states. **Measurement of red blood cell hemoglobin F content** has been used in the diagnosis of patients with Fanconi or constitutional anemia.

Characteristically, levels of hemoglobin F increase. Tests that help in the diagnosis of specific disease states include the **CD59/CD55 phenotype assay** for paroxysmal nocturnal hemoglobinuria and **marrow culture studies** to help diagnose immune-related aplastic anemia and Fanconi anemia.

DIAGNOSIS

The approach to diagnosis of any marrow damage anemia depends on the clinical setting. As summarized in Table 3–2, marrow damage anemias predictably result from diseases that have a destructive impact on the marrow, or as a side effect of chemotherapy or radiotherapy. When the primary disease diagnosis is obvious, the workup of the anemia can be truncated. CBC, reticulocyte count, iron studies, and marrow examination are usually all that is required and even this workup is unnecessary when patients are undergoing high-dose chemotherapy.

The diagnostic workup needs to be pursued more aggressively when a patient presents with a **sudden onset of severe anemia or pancytopenia** without clear evidence of other disease. **Severe marrow damage** should be relatively easy to diagnose based on the marked pancytopenia. However, successful management of a patient with an **idiopathic aplastic anemia** depends on rapid and accurate diagnosis of the underlying cause. In some patients, clues to the cause may be provided by the CBC and marrow studies, especially the marrow biopsy, while in others, more elaborate studies of mar-

Table 3–2. **Causes of marrow damage anemias.**

Stem cell damage
 Chemo/radiotherapy
 Chemicals, toxins, heavy metals
 Infections
 Leukemias, lymphomas
 Paroxysmal nocturnal hemoglobinemia
Structural damage
 Metastatic malignancy
 Granulomatous disease
 Radiation
 Gaucher's disease
 Myelofibrosis
Autoimmune disease
 Rheumatologic disorders
 Viral infections
 Graft-versus-host disease
 "Idiopathic" aplastic anemia
 Pure red cell aplasia
Congenital disorders
 Fanconi anemia
 Diamond-Blackfan anemia
 Dyskeratosis congenita

row precursor cytogenetics and growth characteristics may be necessary. In many cases, the nature of the disorder may only become clear with the patient's response to therapy.

Drug & Radiation Damage Anemia

A. DRUG TOXICITY:

Marrow damage anemia is a predictable side effect of chemotherapy. When a single chemotherapeutic drug is given, the resulting anemia is usually mild. However, patients with marrow damage secondary to malignancy can have a significant worsening of an already existing anemia, even to the point of becoming transfusion dependent. **High-dose, multidrug chemotherapy** results in severe pancytopenia that requires both red blood cell and platelet transfusion support. In both situations, the drug effect falls short of irreversibly damaging the marrow stem cells, thereby allowing recovery once the drugs are discontinued. Moreover, growth factors can be used therapeutically to counteract the drug effect and speed recovery.

Several drugs have been associated with the development of severe, often irreversible, **aplastic anemia.** Table 3–3 lists the more common classes of drugs associated with marrow damage. At the same time, the clinician must suspect any drug as a possible cause of marrow damage when a patient lacks other obvious reasons for his or her pancytopenia. Several drugs can be

highlighted for their common association with **severe aplasia**, including chloramphenicol, phenylbutazone, propylthiouracil, and the tricyclic antidepressants. Obviously, the frequency of the association of marrow damage with these drugs will reflect the relative frequency of their use. More important, the marrow damage that results is hard to predict, and can be both severe and irreversible. This situation is especially true with chloramphenicol because irreversible aplastic anemia can appear without warning after only a few doses of the drug. Therefore, even though the actual incidence of fatal aplastic anemia in patients treated with chloramphenicol is less than 1 in 20,000, routine use of the drug is strongly discouraged. The pancytopenia experienced with phenylbutazone, propylthiouracil, and the tricyclic antidepressants has a more gradual onset and is reversible if the drug is immediately withdrawn.

The development of **pancytopenia** secondary to any of the drugs listed in Table 3–3 is best detected with a routine CBC and not the symptoms or signs of anemia, leukopenia, or thrombocytopenia. This is important both diagnostically and therapeutically. Periodic measurements of blood counts during hospitalization or as a part of long-term drug therapy are necessary. Moreover, careful attention needs to be paid to the results. As a rule, drug-induced cytopenias will rapidly reverse if the inciting drug or drugs are quickly removed.

B. RADIATION:

High-energy radiation can also produce a **marrow-damage anemia and pancytopenia.** The effect can be predicted according to the type of radiation, the dose, and the extent of marrow exposure. High-energy radia-

Table 3–3. **Classes of drugs associated with marrow damage.**

Antibiotics (chloramphenicol, penicillin, cephalosporins, sulfonamides, amphotericin B, dapsone, streptomycin)
Antidepressants (lithium, tricyclics)
Antiepileptics (dilantin, carbamazepine, valproic acid, phenobarbital)
Anti-inflammatory drugs (phenylbutazone, nonsteroidals, salicylates, gold salts)
Antiarrhythmics (lidocaine, quinidine, procainamide)
Antithyroid drugs (propylthiouracil)
Diuretics (thiazides, pyrimethamine, furosemide)
Antihypertensives (captopril)
Antiuricemics (allopurinol, colchicine)
Antimalarials (quinacrine, chloroquine)
Hypoglycemics (tolbutamide)
Tranquilizers (prochlorperazine, meprobamate)
Platelet inhibitors (ticlopidine)

tion can be used therapeutically at high doses without the appearance of marrow damage as long as the treatment fields spare major marrow sites. In patients who receive **whole body irradiation,** the effect on the marrow is dose dependent. At doses less than 1 Sv (equivalent to 1 Gy or 100 rads for x- and γ-rays), there will be little effect on the marrow. A reversible fall in the blood counts is seen between 1 and 2.5 Sv (100 and 250 rads). Irreversible loss of stem cells is seen at higher doses. With doses of 5–10 Sv, patients will die of marrow failure if they do not receive a bone marrow transplant. Long-term exposure to low levels of external radiation or ingested radioisotopes can also produce **aplastic anemia,** although the dose relationship is much less predictable.

C. OTHER CHEMICALS:

Several chemicals have also been implicated in causing severe aplastic anemia. **Benzene and chemicals containing benzene derivatives** have been associated both with aplastic anemia and acute myelocytic leukemia. These findings have led to very strict federal regulations limiting occupational exposure to organic solvents containing benzene derivatives. Many other chemicals, insecticides, and heavy metals have also been associated with marrow-damage anemia and pancytopenia. It is essential, therefore, to question a patient with marrow-damage anemia at length regarding occupational chemical exposure.

Marrow-Damage Anemia–Related to Infection

Marrow-damage can result from direct invasion of the marrow structure by an infectious agent or immunosuppression of stem cell growth. **Miliary tuberculosis** is perhaps the best example of the first mechanism. Extensive involvement of the marrow as evidenced by widespread granuloma formation and marrow fibrosis can produce a marrow-damage anemia and in some cases a pancytopenia. Early on, the clinician's index of suspicion must be high to successfully make this diagnosis. The patient can present with little evidence of widespread tuberculosis and on hematologic evaluation may appear to have idiopathic myelofibrosis or a myelodysplastic syndrome. Therefore, a careful search for granulomas in the marrow biopsy specimen, using an acid-fast stain to help identify the organism, is essential.

Aplastic anemia is seen following viral illnesses such as viral hepatitis, Epstein-Barr virus infection, HIV, and rubella. Parvovirus B19 infection can cause an acute, reversible pure red blood cell aplasia in patients with congenital hemolytic anemias (sickle cell anemia, hereditary spherocytosis, etc). In immunocompromised patients who fail to produce neutralizing antibody to parvovirus, a chronic form of red cell aplasia can develop. The most dramatic relationship of viral infection to severe pancytopenia is the fatal aplastic anemia seen during recovery from viral hepatitis. Generally, this occurs in young males who have had an uncomplicated episode of hepatitis, and is most common in low-income populations in Asian countries. Although this anemia was originally associated with non-A and non-B hepatitis, recent studies would appear to exclude hepatitis C as the putative agent. Thus, the responsible agent and the nature of the subsequent immune process that results in marrow stem cell suppression are still unknown.

Malignancy & Marrow Damage

Marrow-damage anemias can result from an infiltration of the marrow by nonhematopoietic tumors or a malignant transformation of marrow stem cells. **Metastatic malignancies** such as prostate and breast carcinoma generally produce a relatively mild anemia without changes in other cell lines. The mechanism involved is a progressive interference with the support structure of the marrow. The tumor occupies the space needed for marrow precursors, stimulates collagen growth, and cuts off normal blood supply. The resultant disorganization is frequently detectable simply by inspecting the blood smear. The appearance of nucleated red blood cells in circulation in a patient with a mild, normocytic, normochromic anemia can be a tip-off to the presence of metastatic tumor within the marrow.

Malignant transformations of hematopoietic stem cells produce severe marrow-damage anemias. This process involves a loss of stem cells committed to differentiation along the erythroid line. The same is true for the other cell lines, which makes the diagnosis relatively easy. Patients presenting with leukemia have characteristic changes both in the number of cells in circulation and in cellular morphology. The examination of the marrow also reveals the nature of the malignant cell line. Although the diagnosis of an acute leukemia is relatively easy, patients with myelodysplasia, myelofibrosis, paroxysmal nocturnal hemoglobinuria, or a sideroblastic anemia can be more of a diagnostic challenge (see Chapter 9).

Aplastic Anemia of Unknown Etiology ("Idiopathic")

An otherwise healthy patient can present with the sudden onset of pancytopenia and a markedly hypoplastic or aplastic ("empty") marrow. In some instances, blood counts will recover spontaneously, suggesting an acute exposure to a drug or chemical agent. In others, spontaneous recovery is much less likely. This is especially true when the pancytopenia is severe, leukocyte counts are < 200/µL, and the marrow cellularity is below 20% of normal. This situation suggests an irreversible loss of stem cells owing to a toxin or an autoimmune disease process. Various studies have reported that 15–50% of patients with aplastic anemia will show clones of paroxysmal nocturnal hemoglobinuria–positive cells at some point in their illness (see Chapter 9). However, the implications of this finding are still unclear.

Patients with an autoimmune process can show increased numbers of activated cytotoxic lymphocytes in circulation. It has also been demonstrated using progenitor assays that T-cell depletion of the cultured marrow will increase the BFU-E and CFU-E numbers in some of these patients. The role of CD8 T-cell–driven direct cytotoxicity and indirect inhibition via γ-interferon and tumor necrosis factor is further supported by the response of these patients to immunosuppressive therapy. However, the T-cell response is usually polyclonal, suggesting a secondary response to an inciting event such as a viral infection or chromosomal translocation with production of an abnormal protein/progenitor cell.

Any patient with **severe "idiopathic" aplastic anemia** needs to be quickly and fully evaluated as a guide to management. When there is no obvious reversible cause for the marrow damage, early bone marrow transplantation or immunosuppressive therapy should be considered. The patient's age and availability of a histocompatible sibling will determine the choice of therapy. Younger patients with a matched donor should receive transplants without delay since the risk of graft-versus-host disease (GVHD) is low and the opportunity for a sustained recovery is high. Older patients and patients who have received multiple blood transfusions are better managed with immunosuppressive therapy.

Constitutional Aplastic Anemia (Fanconi Anemia)

Fanconi anemia is an autosomal recessive disorder that presents as severe pancytopenia during the first 2 decades of life and, in many cases, progresses to acute leukemia. In Western societies, the frequency of the heterozygote state is about 1 in 200 persons, though it may be as high as 1 in 80 in white South Africans. When fully expressed, the disorder is characterized by a triad of aplastic anemia (pancytopenia), multiple physical defects, and chromosomal abnormalities. However, patients can present without the typical physical defects.

The **diagnosis** of Fanconi anemia is confirmed by the demonstration of chromosomal abnormalities in lymphocyte culture. The traditional test uses cross-link-ing agents such as mitomycin C or diepoxybutane as provocative agents in culture to bring out chromosomal abnormalities. **Three Fanconi anemia genes** (FANCA, -C, and-G) have been cloned, each of which encode a different protein, and 5 additional **mutations** (FANCB,-D,-E,-F, and-H) are suggested by complementation studies. Normally, FANCA and FANCC proteins within the cell cytoplasm combine, enter the nucleus, and help mediate chromosomal repair or stabilization. Failure of any of the Fanconi genes interferes with the binding and subsequent translocation of the protein complex to the nucleus, resulting in chromosomal instability. Mutations in the FANCA and-G genes are associated with poor hematologic outcomes.

Dyskeratosis Congenita

Aplastic anemia is seen in at least 50% of patients with **dyskeratosis congenita,** an inherited X-linked, recessive disorder characterized by skin pigmentation, leukoplakia, and nail dystrophy. The mucocutaneous abnormalities generally appear well before puberty, whereas the aplastic anemia occurs late in the second or third decades. Since the clinical presentation can be quite variable, it should be considered in the differential of adult aplastic anemia. **The responsible gene** has been mapped to Xq28 locus. Like Fanconi anemia, the dyskeratosis congenita defect best fits a chromosome instability abnormality, although the patient's lymphocytes do not show sensitivity to mitomycin C or diepoxybutane.

Pure Red Blood Cell Aplasia

Isolated aplasia of erythroid progenitors (producing anemia without leukopenia or thrombocytopenia) can present as a self-limited "aplastic crisis" or as severe irreversible marrow damage anemia. As with pancytopenia, pure red blood cell aplasia can result from exposure to a number of drugs and infections. Short periods of pure red blood cell aplasia have been reported in patients with mycoplasma and parvovirus (HPV B19) infections, mumps, and viral hepatitis. Patients with congenital hemolytic anemias, especially hereditary spherocytosis, appear to be quite sensitive to parvovirus infection. Patients with immunosuppression, especially those infected with HIV-1, may be unable to resolve an HPV B19 infection, resulting in severe, persistent red cell aplasia. In all of these situations, the patient presents with the sudden appearance of anemia without pancytopenia. Inspection of a marrow aspirate shows essentially normal cellularity and morphology except for the absence of red blood cell progenitors.

Prolonged red blood cell aplasia has been associated with several diseases including lupus erythematosus, rheumatoid arthritis, chronic active hepatitis, parvovirus infection, lymphoid malignancies, myelodysplasia, and thymoma. It also occurs without apparent cause, although studies of BFU-E and CFU-E growth characteristics suggest that most patients with pure red cell aplasia have a T-cell- or antibody-mediated inhibition of erythropoiesis. This has been reflected clinically in the success of immunosuppressive therapies. Pure red cell aplasia unresponsive to immunosuppressive therapy is most often the initial presentation of a dysplastic/sideroblastic anemia (see Chapter 9).

The **workup** for a patient with a pure red cell aplasia should include, in addition to a detailed history, physical examination, and routine CBC and blood chemistries, a bone marrow examination, cytogenetics, lymphocyte immunophenotyping or T-cell gene rearrangement studies (or both), and serum analysis for HPV B19. A search should be made for thymic enlargement, which may play an etiologic role in up to 15% of patients. Typically, the thymomas associated with pure red blood cell aplasia remain encapsulated and can be easily resected. Histologically, they are made up of spindle cells with loss of germinal centers and some infiltration with small lymphocytes.

Diamond-Blackfan Anemia

Diamond and Blackfan described a congenital form of pure red blood cell aplasia that appears early in childhood. By 6 months of age, 80% of children are anemic; by 9 months, 90% are affected. The typical erythropoietic profile shows a somewhat macrocytic, normochromic anemia, reticulocytopenia, and an absence of red blood cell progenitors in a marrow with normal white blood cells and platelet production. Serum levels of erythropoietin are increased. Many children have minor physical defects including strabismus and bony abnormalities of fingers and ribs. Disruption of the **ribosomal protein gene**, RPS19, localized to chromosome 19q13.2, has been implicated in a quarter or more of cases, with evidence suggesting two other loci in the remainder.

The nature of the red blood cell defect in Diamond-Blackfan anemia is unclear. Studies suggest that erythroid progenitors are intrinsically abnormal, responding poorly to erythropoietin or SCF, and exhibiting accelerated programmed death. Although the presence of a humoral or cellular inhibitor has not been detected, 70% or more of patients with Diamond-Blackfan anemia will respond clinically to relatively low doses of **prednisone**. Allogeneic bone marrow transplantation has also proved effective in patients with matched donors. **Transfusion** is the mainstay for the others. Overall, life expectancy has improved significantly; patients now live well into their third or fourth

decade. Diamond-Blackfan has been associated with an increased incidence of malignancy, especially acute myeloid leukemia.

DIFFERENTIAL DIAGNOSIS

Severe aplastic anemia is readily detected and easily distinguished from most other forms of hypoproliferative anemia. The one exception is **myelodysplasia** with a severely hypoplastic marrow (see Chapter 9). With this exception, the involvement of all cell lines in the marrow both confirms the diagnosis and often explains the reason for the marrow failure. Iron studies provide another indicator of severe marrow damage. Patients with **aplastic anemia** show an elevation in the serum iron level to full saturation of the TIBC (see Table 3–1). Similarly, the diagnosis of **pure red blood cell aplasia** is relatively straightforward. The striking reticulocytopenia, the virtual absence of red blood cell precursors in an otherwise normal marrow, and the increase in serum iron level are unique and are not mimicked by other forms of anemia.

Less severe marrow damage anemia is not as easily distinguished from other hypoproliferative anemias such as early iron deficiency, the anemias of renal failure and hypothyroidism, and the anemia that develops as a part of an inflammatory disease process. As long as the patient's hemoglobin level is greater than 11 grams per deciliter, changes in red blood cell and marrow morphology may not be diagnostic. The only distinguishing feature is the pattern of iron studies (Table 3–4). Patients with **iron deficiency** or **an inflammatory anemia** can usually be identified on the basis of changes in serum iron, TIBC, and serum ferritin levels. The differential diagnosis of a **hypoproliferative anemia characterized by normal iron studies** is more difficult. Studies of renal function and thyroid function should be performed. In addition, careful examination of the peripheral blood smear and both the marrow aspirate and biopsy specimen are recommended. The appearance in circulation of even a few nucleated red blood cells in a patient with a hypoproliferative anemia can be an early clue to involvement of the marrow with a malignancy. A close examination of the marrow specimens may also reveal the cause of an early marrow-damage anemia. Table 3–5 lists several disease states that are associated with marrow-damage anemia and that can be detected by inspecting the marrow.

THERAPY

The management of a marrow-damage anemia will vary considerably according to the cause of the anemia or pancytopenia, the severity of the damage, and both the patient's age and transfusion history. The impor-

Table 3–4. **Iron studies in hypoproliferative anemias.**

	Iron Deficiency	Inflammation	Renal/Endocrine Disease	Marrow Damage	
				Mild	*Severe*
Serum iron (µg/dL)	<30	<40	Normal	50–150	> 150
TIBC (µg/dL)	>350	>300	Normal	Normal	Normal
Percent saturation (%)	<10	10–20	Normal	30–60	>60
Ferritin (µg/L)	<12	30–300	Normal	30–600	>1000
Marrow iron stores	Absent	Increased	Normal	Increased	Increased

tance of the cause as a predictor of final outcome is obvious. In the patient with a hematologic malignancy, return to normal marrow function will depend on responsiveness of the tumor to chemotherapy. The same is true with marrow damage anemias secondary to a metastatic malignancy. It is **essential to consider drug exposure** as a potential cause of marrow damage, even in patients who have other disease. Although some drugs are known for their propensity to cause damage, virtually every drug must be considered as a possible etiologic agent and, if possible, withdrawn.

Patients who present with a **severe aplastic anemia** need special attention. They should be quickly evaluated to identify any possible reversible cause of the aplasia and to rule out malignant disease. When the marrow is severely hypoplastic or aplastic, the chance of spontaneous recovery is very low. Younger patients should be considered immediately for marrow transplantation. They also need to be protected from exposure to blood-component transfusions if transplantation is to be successful. If possible, transfusions should be withheld until immunosuppressive therapy is begun

in preparation for the transplant to avoid alloimmunization. Finally, both patients with severe aplastic anemia and patients who are at risk for severe marrow damage should be HLA typed. This not only is required for marrow donor selection but it is also important in planning transfusion support. Patients not eligible for transplantation can show a high rate response to immunosuppressive therapy, alone. Unfortunately, up to 40% of patients treated with immunosuppression, who survive 10 years or longer, are at risk for developing a clonal malignancy, paroxysmal nocturnal hemoglobinuria, or myelodysplasia progressing to acute myeloid leukemia.

Transfusion Support

A **relatively mild anemia or pancytopenia** can be observed or, if necessary, treated with one or more hematopoietic growth factors. **More severe marrow damage** will generally require supportive therapy with red blood cell and platelet transfusions to maintain oxygen delivery and prevent bleeding. In the adult pa-

Table 3–5. **Marrow-damage anemias associated with abnormal marrows.**

Disease State	Marrow Morphology
Myelofibrosis	Increased collagen and reticulin fibers
Lymphoid malignancies (CLL, lymphomas, Hodgkin's disease)	Increased numbers of lymphocytes, paratrabecular lymphoid nodules, granulomas, Reed-Sternberg cells
Metastatic malignancies (breast, prostate, lung, etc)	Clusters of tumor cells, fibrosis
Myeloma	Increased plasma cells (> 20% of cells)
Drug/radiation damage	Decreased hematopoietic cells, relative increase in plasma cells, mast cells, and structural cells
Marrow infections (tuberculosis, sarcoidosis, etc)	Granulomas, fibrosis, increased plasma cells

tient with little or no red blood cell production, a hemoglobin level of 7–8 grams per deciliter can be achieved with the transfusion of 1 unit of packed red blood cells every other week. Older patients and patients with cardiovascular disease may require transfusion to a higher hemoglobin level.

Patients with aplastic anemia who require long-term transfusion are at high risk of becoming alloimmunized. Clinically, **alloimmunization** may be suspected when the patient repeatedly has fever and chills during or immediately following a red blood cell or platelet transfusion. Another possible sign of alloimmunization is failure to achieve a significant increase in the platelet count following platelet transfusion. The severity of the febrile reaction often correlates with the number of white blood cells contaminating the unit of red blood cells and can be reduced by transfusing leukopoor red blood cells (Chapter 37).

Another predictable side effect of repeated transfusion is the **accumulation of excessive tissue iron stores.** Patients who have severe marrow damage and an elevated serum iron are at risk for iron toxicity and damage to the anterior pituitary, heart, and liver. Tissue damage correlates with the total body iron burden and is likely once 100 units or more of red blood cells have been transfused. These patients should be considered for iron chelation therapy using subcutaneous or intravenous deferoxamine (see Chapter 12).

Leukopenia to levels as low as 300–500 granulocytes/μL is usually well tolerated. Below this level, patients are at risk for **bacterial infections and sepsis.** Localized infections should be treated with the appropriate antibiotic, whereas septic patients should receive broad-spectrum antibiotic coverage, usually a semisynthetic penicillin or a cephalosporin in combination with an aminoglycoside. Recovery from a transient neutropenia can be accelerated by treatment with granulocyte colony-stimulating factor (G-CSF).

Bleeding complications in patients with aplastic anemia are usually the result of the patient's thrombocytopenia. However, in the septic patient, disseminated intravascular coagulation with decreased levels of coagulation factors must also be considered. Any bleeding episode in a patient with aplastic anemia should be initially treated with platelet transfusions, either random donor or single pheresis donor platelets. A transfusion of 6 units of random platelets or the platelets from a single pheresis donor should raise the 1-hour post-transfusion platelet count by 50,000/μL unless the patient is alloimmunized or actively septic.

Patients receiving repeated transfusions who develop anti-HLA antibodies will, in addition to experiencing fever and chills with transfusion, show poor platelet increments and shortened survivals. When a sensitized patient is experiencing a life-threatening

hemorrhage, repeated platelet transfusions 2, 3, or more times per day may be required to attain hemostasis. The use of HLA-matched platelets may also be required. Therefore, it is important to know the patient's HLA type and to have surveyed the patient's family and siblings for HLA compatible donors. Nonrelated HLA matched donors can be provided as part of a community donor pool.

Prophylactic transfusion of platelets may be necessary in patients with severely impaired platelet production. In patients who are otherwise well, a platelet count of as little as 5–10,000/μL should be enough to maintain hemostasis. In the presence of a disease such as leukemia, spontaneous bleeding can occur whenever the platelet count falls much below 20,000/μL. To maintain hemostasis during a minor surgical procedure, platelet counts in excess of 50,000/μL are usually required. Finally, patients should avoid antiplatelet drugs, especially aspirin.

Hematopoietic Growth Factors

Erythropoietin, G-CSF, and GM-CSF can be used for treating reversible marrow damage anemias and pancytopenia. Patients receiving high-dose multidrug chemotherapy can be treated with erythropoietin to reduce the severity of the anemia and avoid transfusion. G-CSF and GM-CSF will speed the recovery of the granulocyte count in patients receiving ablative chemotherapy for treatment of a hematopoietic malignancy. This application has been of greatest value in patients receiving allogeneic and autologous bone marrow transplants. GM-CSF or G-CSF (given in a dose of 10 μg/kg/day beginning 2–4 days after the reinfusion of the marrow stem cells) has been shown to significantly speed recovery following transplantation, thereby decreasing the incidence of infection and the need for broad-spectrum antibiotic coverage.

The usefulness of growth factors in the treatment of severe aplastic anemia is less certain. Patients with severe marrow damage anemias usually have very high serum erythropoietin levels. Administration of additional exogenous erythropoietin adds little to this natural stimulus and therefore cannot be expected to increase red blood cell production. Limited trials of erythropoietin in the treatment of patients with myelodysplasia have reported the occasional response; trials with very high levels of recombinant erythropoietin have not been carried out.

GM-CSF and G-CSF therapy may hold greater promise for treating the **leukopenia associated with aplastic anemia.** However, the effectiveness would appear to reflect the severity of the marrow damage. Patients with absolute granulocyte counts of less than 200/μL generally fail to respond to either growth factor, whereas 60–70% of patients with counts of

200–1500/μL show excellent responses. The effectiveness of growth factors that act at earlier stages in cell development (IL-3 and SCF) still needs to be studied. Limited trials of IL-3 as a single agent suggest that a few patients may experience increases in leukocytes, red blood cells, and platelets. The true test will require studies of a larger number of patients and using combinations of IL-3 and SCF with erythropoietin, GM-CSF, and G-CSF.

The role of growth factors in the treatment of **constitutional aplastic anemia**, and both **Fanconi anemia** and **Diamond-Blackfan anemia**, still needs to be defined. Trials involving small numbers of patients with Fanconi anemia have shown that the leukopenia and anemia can improve with growth factor therapy. G-CSF, given in a dose of 2.5–5 μg/kg every other day, will return the granulocyte count to the normal range in patients with untreated counts as low as 200–500/μL. However, there is an underlying threat that the evolution to a clonal malignancy may be accelerated. IL-3 and GM-CSF therapy has been used in patients with Diamond-Blackfan anemia who are resistant to prednisone therapy with some success; reticulocyte counts increase and transfusion requirements decrease in some patients.

The use of growth factors in the treatment of **aplastic anemia** is still hampered by a lack of knowledge regarding the most appropriate dose and schedule of administration. Studies of erythropoietin in patients with marrow damage anemia have evaluated doses ranging from 100 to 300 U/kg given subcutaneously 2 to 3 times each week. Very-high-dose regimens have not been attempted. Therefore, it is likely that only those patients with an anemia associated with a failed erythropoietin response will have a chance of responding.

The best dosages and dose schedules for G-CSF and GM-CSF alone and in combination with IL-3, IL-6, IL-11, and SCF are also unclear. Studies of GM-CSF in patients with aplastic anemia have used daily doses of from 4 to 64 μg/kg given subcutaneously. Response to G-CSF appears to require a dose of at least 800–1200 μg/m² per day. For both growth factors, higher doses may increase the rate of response. A clear dose-response relationship has been shown in patients with cyclical neutropenia treated with G-CSF. Trials of IL-3 in patients with aplastic anemia, Fanconi anemia, and Diamond-Blackfan anemia have used doses ranging from 3 to 1000 μg/m², again illustrating the lack of knowledge as to the best dose.

Marrow Transplantation

The recommended treatment for the young patient with a severe aplastic anemia is marrow transplantation. Of course, this therapy requires the availability of a histocompatible family member, either a parent or sibling with a 4-locus HLA match or an identical twin. Transplants with nonidentical or unrelated donors are far less successful and should only be considered in patients who fail immunosuppressive therapy.

The success of a marrow transplant depends on the patient's age, transfusion history, clinical status at the time of transplant, and the cause of the marrow damage (Figure 3–3). A younger patient has a greater chance of success, largely because the incidence of GVHD (the major cause of graft failure) increases with

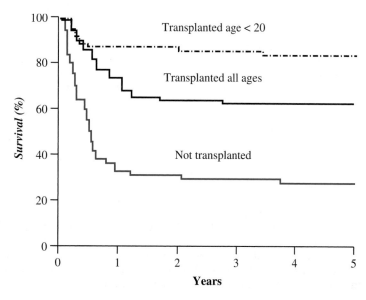

Figure 3–3. **Marrow transplantation in aplastic anemia.** The success of an allogeneic marrow transplant in patients with aplastic anemia depends on the availability of a matched donor, the age of the patient, and the nature of the disease. Young patients who receive transplants early with a well-matched donor have sustained remissions up to 90% of the time. Overall survival for patients of all ages is better than 60%. This rate is in dramatic contrast to patients who do not receive transplants and who did not receive effective immunosuppressive therapy. Their survival over a 5-year period is less than 40%.

age. Although children, teenagers, and young adults can expect a better than 80% chance of long-term survival with good return of marrow function, patients over age 20 will experience significant complications from **GVHD.** Graft rejection is more frequent, and the incidence of post-transplant infections, including interstitial pneumonitis, is much higher. This will be true even if the patient is immunosuppressed both prior to and following transplant.

Transfusions prior to preconditioning immunosuppression increase the chance of graft rejection and GVHD. Even a single blood transfusion can decrease the patient's chance of survival. It is especially important, therefore, to try to avoid multiple transfusions for the few weeks it takes to search the family for a suitable donor. The cause of the disease and the medical condition of the patient at the time of the transplant make a difference. Patients whose transplant course is complicated by infection also do less well. The young patient with severe aplasia of unknown cause who receives a transplant early has the best prognosis. Older patients and patients with less severe hypoplasia are best treated with immunosuppressive therapy initially and should only receive transplants if the response is inadequate.

Patients with **aplastic anemia of unknown cause** must have immunosuppressive therapy prior to transplant not only to guarantee engraftment of the marrow but also to treat an underlying autoimmune disease process. Even in identical twins, a simple infusion of marrow without immunosuppression will not be successful. With the current use of antithymocyte globulin and cyclosporine as pretransplant immunosuppressive therapy and both methotrexate and cyclosporine to manage the patient's GVHD, survivals are now better than 80% at 4 years, including patients up to age 65 years.

Immunosuppression

Immunosuppression alone with combinations of steroids, antithymocyte globulin, and cyclosporine is also effective, especially when the aplasia is caused by an autoimmune disease process. The decision to use an immunosuppressive regimen rather than marrow transplantation will depend on the suspected etiology, the patient's age, the overall clinical condition, and the availability of a marrow donor. An algorithm for selecting therapy is shown in Figure 3–4. Young patients with severe aplastic anemia should receive transplants immediately if a donor is available. Patients who lack a donor, patients over age 40 years, and patients with less severe

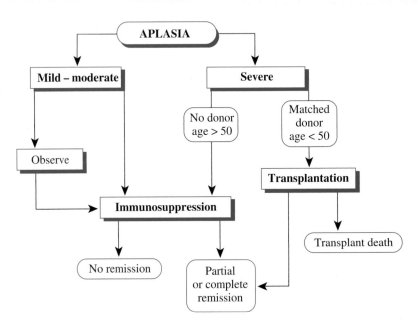

Figure 3–4. **Therapy selection in patients with aplastic anemia.** Management of a patient with aplastic anemia will depend on the patient's age, the severity of the aplasia, and the availability of a matched donor for transplantation. Patients with mild to moderately severe disease may be observed or treated with immunosuppressive therapy. The young patient with severe aplastic disease should receive a transplant without delay if a matched donor is available. Immunosuppressive therapy in older patients and patients who do not have donors can provide a partial remission in 25–85% of patients.

marrow aplasia/hypoplasia are **candidates for immuno-suppression.** With modern regimens that include cyclosporine, overall long-term survival rates are probably comparable to those achievable with transplantation.

Corticosteroids given alone can occasionally result in improved marrow function. This is especially true for patients with pure red cell aplasia. However, both **horse-derived antithymocyte globulin (ATG) or the equivalent rabbit preparation of antilymphocyte globulin (ALG)** in combination with cyclosporine are considered to be more effective immunosuppressive agents. Response rates range from 25–85% of patients with moderate to severe aplastic anemia and survival of responders is 90% at 5 years. Improvement in peripheral blood counts is typically slow, requiring several months of therapy, generally less complete than that seen with marrow transplantation, and patients with very severe aplastic anemia may not survive long enough to benefit from the therapy unless supportive care is excellent. Partial responses are not uncommon (less than half of patients achieve normal blood counts) and as many as 40% of patients relapse a few months to years after successful treatment. However, 50% or more of patients who relapse will respond to additional courses of immunosuppression or, in some cases, maintenance therapy with cyclosporine. **Long-term cyclosporine therapy** is associated with significant adverse effects, including hypertension, hypertrichosis, and nephrotoxicity.

ATG administration is not without its problems. Patients are at risk for an **anaphylactic reaction** to the horse or rabbit proteins in the preparation, and **serum sickness–like reaction** to the ATG/ALG is very common. Patients experience fever, chills, and urticaria with the first infusions and later a flu-like illness with fever, arthralgias, myalgia, a maculopapular rash, and diarrhea. Liver and renal function abnormalities are also common. The severity of these side effects can be in part controlled by the administration of 60–80 mg of methylprednisolone per day in divided doses.

The **mechanism of action of ATG** is not well understood. Although it may decrease subsets of lymphocytes responsible for immune suppression of marrow precursors, it may also stimulate a proliferation of T lymphocytes that produce growth factors such as GM-CSF and IL-3. Clinical trials of ATG and ALG have also reported varied success rates for different lots of material. This has raised questions as to the actual active component of the preparations. It is not simply a matter of decreasing the number of T–suppressor cells, since monoclonal preparations of antihuman T-cell antibodies have little therapeutic effect.

Cyclosporine alone or in combination with ALG and methylprednisolone has also been found to be therapeutically effective. Patients with aplastic anemia treated with the combination of drugs have now been reported to have a 92% survival at 3 years. However, although the early response is better when cyclosporine is used, long-term survival may be no different, and the frequency of the subsequent appearance of a clonal malignancy (eg, acute leukemia, sideroblastic anemia, or paroxysmal nocturnal hemoglobinuria) may be increased. Patients who receive cyclosporine therapy to treat their aplastic anemia are also at greater risk for the development of *Pneumocystis* pneumonia. Finally, clinical trials are currently looking at the effectiveness of cytoxan in combination with cyclosporine and the substitution of a novel immunosuppressive drug, mycophenolate, for cyclosporine. Mycophenolate is cytotoxic for cycling T cells and lacks the renal toxicity of cyclosporine. It may also produce more rapid increases in neutrophil counts.

The choice of therapy for patients with pure red cell aplasia will depend on the diagnosis. Patients with thymomas can respond to surgical resection of the tumor. Patients with chronic parvovirus respond to intravenous immune globulin or ATG. Corticosteroid, by itself, can be effective in many of the patients with an immune component to their disease, whereas most will respond to some combination of prednisone, with ATG, cyclosporine, or Cytoxan. Patients with myelodysplasia are generally refractory to immunosuppressive therapy.

A **therapeutic trial** will usually confirm the diagnosis and is the best approach to management. One choice is a combination of cyclophosphamide or azathioprine (50–100 mg/day escalating to 2.2 mg/kg over 2–3 weeks), together with prednisone 30–60 mg/day. The maximum dose of immunosuppressants is then determined from the impact on the leukocyte and platelet counts. The mean time to remission is 11 weeks, so therapy must be sustained for several months. Up to 60% of patients will respond. ATG and cyclosporine in combination with prednisone have also been used in refractory patients with some success. If a patient fails to respond, a marrow BFU-E culture study can be used to identify those patients who, because they show good BFU-E growth, deserve more aggressive immunosuppressive therapy.

Androgen Therapy

Androgen therapy was used extensively to treat aplastic anemia prior to the advent of marrow transplantation and immunosuppressive therapy. Although most patients do not benefit, an occasional patient will show response, usually limited to the red blood cell line. Androgens can be given orally with some risk for hepatic toxicity (cholestatic jaundice and peliosis hepaticus) or intramuscularly in patients with an adequate platelet count (nandrolone decanoate 2–5 µg/kg/week). The parenteral use of antigens avoids the issue of hepatotoxicity. To achieve any type of therapeutic response, androgens must be given for 4–6 months or longer. Side effects with prolonged therapy include acne, virilization, and hyperlipidemia.

BIBLIOGRAPHY

Clinical Features and Diagnosis

Applebaum FR, Fefer A: The pathogenesis of aplastic anemia. Semin Hematol 1981;18:241.

Barrett J, Saunthararajah Y, Molldrem J: Myelodysplastic syndrome and aplastic anemia: Distinct entities or diseases linked by a common pathophysiology? Semin Hematol 2000;37:15.

Brown KE et al: Hepatitis-associated aplastic anemia. N Engl J Med 1997;336:1059.

Moulopoulus LA, Dimopoulus MA: Magnetic resonance imaging of the bone marrow in hematologic malignancies. Blood 1997;90:2127.

Young NS: Hematopoietic cell destruction by immune mechanisms in acquired aplastic anemia. Semin Hematol 2000;37:3.

Therapy

Charles RJ et al: The pathophysiology of pure red cell aplasia: Implications for therapy. Blood 1996;87:4831.

Crump M et al: Treatment of adults with severe aplastic anemia: Primary therapy with antithymocyte globulin (ATG) and rescue of ATG failures with bone marrow transplantation. Am J Med 1992;92:596.

Doney K et al: Immunosuppressive therapy of aplastic anemia: Results of a prospective, randomized trial of thymocyte globulin (ATG), methylprednisolone, and oxymetholone to ATG, very high-dose methylprednisolone and oxymetholone. Blood 1992;79:2566.

Doney K et al: Primary treatment of acquired aplastic anemia: Outcomes with bone marrow transplantation and immunosuppressive therapy. Ann Intern Med 1997;126:107.

Frickhofen N, Rosenfeld SJ: Immunosuppressive treatment of aplastic anemia with antithymocyte globulin and cyclosporine. Semin Hematol 2000;37:56.

Lieschke GJ, Burgess AW: Granulocyte colony-stimulating factor and granulocyte-macrophage colony-stimulating factor. N Engl J Med 1992;327:28, 99.

Rackoff WR et al: Prolonged administration of granulocyte colony-stimulating factor (filgastrim) to patients with Fanconi anemia: A pilot study. Blood 1996;88:1588.

Welte K et al: Filgastrim (r-metHuG-CSF): The first 10 years. Blood 1996;88:1907.

Anemias Associated with a Reduced Erythropoietin Response

4

Anemia is common in patients with acute and chronic inflammatory disease, renal insufficiency, and hypothyroidism. In each situation, there is an apparent failure in the erythropoietin stimulation of the marrow. Serum erythropoietin levels, although not decreased below basal levels, are not appropriately increased for the severity of the anemia. Marrow cellularity and reticulocyte response are typically hypoproliferative.

The importance of this class of anemias cannot be overemphasized. The clinical incidence of hypoproliferative anemias associated with acute infection or chronic inflammatory disease (the anemia of chronic disease) is far greater than that of other types of anemia. In some cases, appearance of a typical hypoproliferative anemia is the first sign of underlying disease. The pattern of the anemia can also be of considerable value in the diagnosis of the etiology and severity of the disease process. It is important, therefore, that clinicians be skilled in evaluating the patient with a hypoproliferative anemia, even when the anemia is mild.

NORMAL MARROW PROLIFERATION

The **normal proliferative response** of the erythroid marrow to anemia requires an appropriate erythropoietin response, an intact erythroid marrow, and an adequate supply of iron (Figure 4–1). Dedicated peritubular interstitial cells in the kidney are capable of sensing changes in oxygen delivery. A **decrease in hemoglobin level to values less than 12 grams per deciliter** stimulates an increased production of erythropoietin. This process involves recruitment of additional peritubular interstitial cells rather than an upregulation of existing cellular production. The role of the kidney in regulating erythropoietin production is well maintained even with significant renal damage. However, end stage renal disease is uniformly associated with a failure in the erythropoietin response. Since hepatocytes also produce some erythropoietin, anephric patients have measurable serum erythropoietin levels but markedly reduced red blood cell production.

The erythropoietin produced by the kidney travels to the marrow, where it binds to specific receptors (EPOR) on the surface of the burst forming unit–erythroid (BFU-E) and colony forming unit–erythroid (CFU-E) precursors (Figure 4–2). This process initiates a sequence of proliferation and maturation of these committed stem cells to produce new adult red blood cells. The magnitude of the erythropoietin response correlates with the severity of the anemia, and the higher the serum erythropoietin level, the greater the marrow proliferative response. This response can be assessed clinically both from changes in the marrow ratio of erythroid to granu-

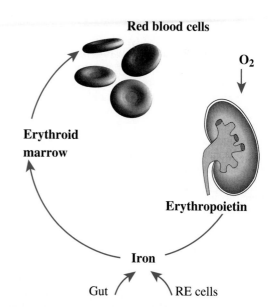

Red blood cells

O_2

Erythroid marrow

Erythropoietin

Iron

Gut   RE cells

Figure 4–1. **Components of the normal marrow proliferative response.** A full response to an anemia requires an appropriate excretion of erythro~~~ the kidney, an adequate supply of iron, and~~ sponsive marrow.

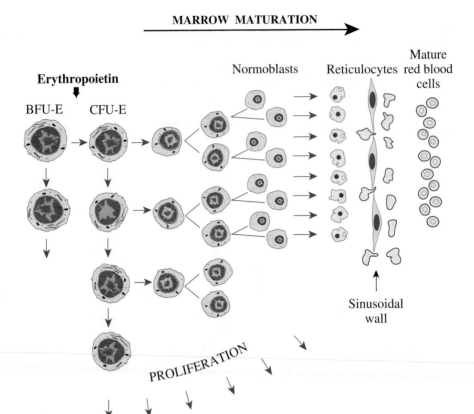

MARROW MATURATION

Erythropoietin

BFU-E   CFU-E

Normoblasts   Reticulocytes   Mature red blood cells

Sinusoidal wall

PROLIFERATION

Figure 4–2. **Erythroid marrow proliferation and maturation.** Erythropoietin stimulates marrow BFU-E and CFU-E to proliferate and differentiate to produce an increasing number of maturing red blood cell precursors. Each committed precursor undergoes four cell divisions, producing 14–16 adult red blood cells. Increased levels of erythropoietin also accelerate normoblast maturation and the release of marrow reticulocytes into circulation.

locytic precursors (E/G ratio) and the reticulocyte response. The normal production response to anemia of increasing severity is discussed in Chapter 2.

The proliferative response also requires an adequate supply of **iron.** Iron required for erythropoiesis is largely provided by the iron recycled from red cell breakdown and reticuloendothelial iron stores. Only a small amount is derived through absorption of food iron. It is transported through the plasma bound to transferrin. The transferrin-iron complex then binds to transferrin receptors on the surface of erythroid precursors. The expression of transferrin receptors and rate of transport of iron into the cell appear to be governed by erythropoietin and a genetically controlled transmembrane protein—HFE (see Chapters 5 and 14). When the amount of iron on transferrin is reduced (a lower than normal serum iron level), both hemoglobin synthesis and the proliferative response of erythroid precursors to erythropoietin are inhibited. Erythropoietin

production, iron supply, and erythroid precursor proliferation are also influenced by cytokines produced during inflammation (tumor necrosis factor [TNF]-α, interleukin [IL]-1, interferon [IFN]-μ, and IFN-α). Direct T-cell suppression of stem cells has been postulated in some cases of hypoplastic anemia.

CLINICAL FEATURES

Hypoproliferative anemias are most often detected as a result of the workup of the patient's primary condition. For example, when a patient is admitted for an acute inflammatory illness such as lobar pneumonia, the complete blood count (CBC) reveals a mild to moderate anemia. The same is true for a patient who is being followed up for progressive **renal failure;** routine CBCs typically show a worsening anemia. Unless the anemia is severe, the patient can be asymptomatic. This situation is not true for **older patients,** in whom even a moderate anemia can exacerbate the symptoms and signs of cardiovascular disease or at least result in fatigue and loss of exercise tolerance.

As a rule, the **severity of the anemia** correlates with the severity of the primary illness. Symptomatic anemia in patients with renal disease is only seen in patients with end stage renal disease. An exception to this observation is in patients with diabetic nephropathy where anemia of moderate severity can occur before significant increases in the blood urea nitrogen (BUN) and creatinine. The anemia that accompanies chronic inflammatory disease, either collagen vascular disease or chronic infections, will correlate with the activity of the inflammatory process. This relationship between illness severity and anemia severity is demonstrated when the patient's primary illness is treated. When a patient with rheumatoid arthritis or polymyalgia rheumatica responds to anti-inflammatory drug therapy, the anemia also improves. Finally, the hypoproliferative anemia seen in patients with hypothyroidism or panhypopituitarism will also correlate best with the severity and duration of the hypometabolic state.

Laboratory Studies

The **CBC, reticulocyte count,** and **serum iron studies,** including a measurement of serum ferritin, should be enough to diagnose this type of anemia. **Typical erythropoietic profiles of anemias** associated with acute and chronic inflammatory disease, renal failure, and hypometabolic states are illustrated in Table 4–1. The CBC and reticulocyte count are characteristic of a hypoproliferative anemia. Red blood cell morphology is normocytic and normochromic and the reticulocyte index is inappropriately low for the severity of the patient's anemia. In patients with severe, chronic inflammatory disorders, a mild microcytic, hypochromic anemia may develop. However, microcytosis is not as marked as that seen in patients with an iron-deficiency anemia of comparable severity.

A. IRON STUDIES:

Iron studies, including **measurements of serum iron, total iron-binding capacity (TIBC), serum ferritin,** and **serum transferrin receptor,** provide important diagnostic information. As illustrated in Table 4–1, patients with renal disease or a hypometabolic state demonstrate essentially normal iron studies. Serum iron, TIBC, and serum ferritin levels are all normal. This may not be true, however, for patients with renal disease who receive chronic dialysis or predialysis patients receiving multiple transfusions. In the former case, repeated hemodialysis can result in a negative iron balance and an iron-deficiency anemia. On the other hand, patients with end stage renal disease who receive chronic transfusions are at risk for iron overload and can show elevated serum ferritin levels.

The diagnostic payoff for iron studies is in the diagnosis of **acute and chronic inflammatory disease anemia** (the anemia of chronic disease). These patients demonstrate a characteristic pattern of low serum iron and low TIBC with a percent saturation between 10% and 20%, coupled with a rising serum ferritin level. This pattern is distinctly different from a true iron-deficiency anemia,

Table 4–1. **Erythropoietic profiles of reduced erythropoietin anemias.**

	Acute and Chronic Inflammatory	Renal Disease	Hypometabolic States
Anemia	Mild	Minor to severe	Mild
MCV (fL)	80–90	90	80–100
Film morphology	Normocytic→microcytic	Normocytic	Variable
Reticulocyte index	< 2	< 2	< 2
Marrow E/G ratio	1:3	1:3	1:3
Serum iron/TIBC	< 5/< 300	Normal	Normal
% Saturation	10–20	Normal	Normal
Marrow iron stores	Increased	Normal	Normal
Serum ferritin	Increased	Normal	Normal
Bilirubin/LDH	Decreased	Decreased	Decreased

where a very low serum iron level is accompanied by a rising TIBC and a very low serum ferritin level (less than 12 μg/L). The relationship of illness severity to anemia is mirrored in the iron studies. The more pronounced the inflammatory component of the patient's illness, the lower the serum iron and TIBC and the higher the serum ferritin level. The latter measurement is also influenced by the level of reticuloendothelial iron stores. Women, with smaller stores, show smaller increases (ferritin levels of 20–200 μg/L), whereas men show a greater rise (ferritin levels of 100–500 μg/L).

The **serum transferrin receptor (serum TfR)** measurement has been popularized as a way to discriminate the anemia of chronic disease from that of iron deficiency. Using the calculated serum TfR/log ferritin ratio, **patients with iron-deficiency anemia** typically have values > 4 (reflecting a rising serum TfR together with a marked fall in the ferritin level), whereas **patients with the anemia of chronic disease** have values < 1 (reflecting a lower serum TfR together with a rising ferritin level). The latter pattern also reflects the hypoproliferative nature of the anemia. In contrast, **patients with severe iron deficiency** will exhibit erythroid marrow expansion and ineffective erythropoiesis, which causes a further rise in the serum TfR level.

B. MARROW AND ERYTHROPOIETIN STUDIES:

The diagnosis of a hypoproliferative anemia that is clearly associated with an inflammatory disorder, renal disease, or an abnormality in thyroid or pituitary function usually does not require a marrow aspirate or biopsy. The combination of normocytic, normochromic morphology, and a lower than predicted reticulocyte response without polychromasia is enough to confirm the hypoproliferative nature of the anemia. Performance of a marrow aspirate merely to assess the E/G ratio is unproductive. Moreover, as long as the patient demonstrates normal leukocyte and platelet counts, it is unlikely that a marrow biopsy specimen will identify a defect in marrow morphology or cellularity.

When a serum ferritin level is unavailable or is in a range that does not support the diagnosis, a marrow aspirate stained with Prussian blue can be used to distinguish true iron deficiency from the anemia of chronic disease. Patients with absolute iron deficiency should have no visible iron stores in reticuloendothelial cells once the percent saturation of transferrin is below 15%. Patients with a low serum iron secondary to inflammatory disease will have normal to increased iron stores on the Prussian blue stain. In patients with chronic inflammatory disease, iron stores often appear increased, with extra large hemosiderin granules in the reticuloendothelial cells.

Direct measurements of the serum erythropoietin level are not helpful in either identifying this class of anemias or in separating individual abnormalities. Although a reduced erythropoietin response is an inherent component of the anemia, the observed range of measured values is quite large. Patients can demonstrate erythropoietin levels that are above basal, although they fall short of the levels achieved by the normal individual responding to a blood loss anemia. This phenomenon is best illustrated by the observed pattern of serum erythropoietin measurements in patients with renal disease (Figure 4–3).

DIAGNOSIS

The approach to diagnosis of a hypoproliferative anemia in a patient with an acute or chronic inflammatory

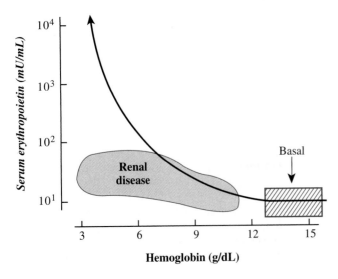

Figure 4–3. **Serum erythropoietin levels in renal disease.** Serum erythropoietin levels in patients with the anemia of end stage renal disease fall well below the levels observed in normal individuals responding to a hemorrhagic anemia.

Table 4–2. Diseases associated with reduced erythropoietin response.

Inflammatory states	Hypometabolic states
Acute and chronic bacterial infections	Protein deprivation
Collagen vascular diseases	Endocrine deficiency states
AIDS	Hypothyroidism
Malignancies	Hypopituitarism
Renal disease	Hyperparathyroidism
Nephritis	
End stage renal disease	

disease, renal damage, or a hypometabolic state depends on the nature and severity of the primary illness and the severity of the anemia (Table 4–2). Since mild to moderate anemia in a patient with progressive renal failure is predictable, there is less need to repeatedly assess the patient for other possible causes of anemia. **For patients with acute or chronic inflammatory disease,** definition of the anemia can be helpful in diagnosing the disorder and assessing its severity. In this case, even a mild anemia should be evaluated with a full panel of studies—CBC, reticulocyte count, and serum iron studies, including a serum ferritin level.

Acute Inflammatory States

Anemia is a common component of acute inflammatory states, especially bacterial infections and collagen vascular disorders. Viral diseases are less likely to produce anemia, or if they do, the anemia is secondary to an autoimmune process or a general failure of stem cells that results in pancytopenia. Parvovirus infection in patients with congenital hemolytic anemias produces a reversible suppression of marrow erythroid precursors without affecting other cell lines (see Chapter 3).

Anemia appears rapidly with the onset of an acute bacterial infection. It is not unusual to see the patient's hemoglobin fall to levels of 10–12 grams per deciliter (hematocrit of 30–36%) within 1 or 2 days after the onset of a bacterial infection, such as acute lobar pneumonia. This initial fall in the hemoglobin level results from a loss of older red blood cells, which are nearing the end of their natural lifespan in circulation. This demonstrates the sensitivity of older cells to changes in the external environment. The release of various cytokines, fever, and local changes in the infected tissue may all play a role in stressing the older red blood cell beyond its metabolic capacity to maintain hemoglobin solubility and cell membrane continuity.

Even though the first step in the evolution of an acute inflammatory anemia is a self-limited hemolytic event, the principal defect is the failure of erythropoietin and erythroid marrow responses. Therefore, the **erythropoietic profile is typically hypoproliferative.** Red blood cell morphology is normocytic and normochromic, the reticulocyte count remains low (a reticulocyte index of less than 2), and there is little or no polychromasia apparent on the blood film. **Iron studies confirm the nature of the anemia.** Within a matter of hours of the onset of an inflammatory condition, serum iron and TIBC fall and the ferritin level begins to rise. Serum transferrin receptor levels remain low, resulting in a low (< 1) serum TfR/log ferritin ratio. This pattern is so distinctive that it is helpful diagnostically, especially if there is some question as to the patient's primary diagnosis (see Table 4–1).

The combination of a subpar erythropoietin response, an inhibition of erythroid precursor proliferation, and a fall in iron supply to the marrow appears to result from the release of several cytokines into circulation. IL-1, **TNF-α, IFN-α, IFN-γ, and neoptrin** all have suppressive effects on erythropoiesis (Figure 4–4). In patients with neoplasms and bacterial infections, TNF-α levels increase dramatically and suppress erythroid progenitor proliferation via the induction of INF-γ from marrow stromal cells. IL-1 plays a similar role in patients with chronic inflammatory states, such as rheumatoid arthritis. IL-1 inhibition of erythroid marrow BFU-E and CFU-E requires the presence of both T lymphocytes and interferon as mediators. Neoptrin may be similar to the interferons by its suppression of erythroid precursors.

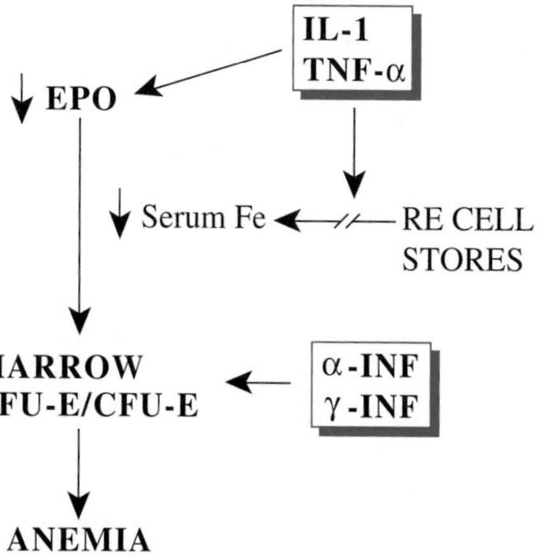

Figure 4–4. Cytokine suppression of erythropoiesis. Bacterial infections and certain neoplasms are associated with increased blood levels of both TNF-α and IFN-γ, which together suppress erythropoietin production, iron release from reticuloendothelial stores, and BFU-E/CFU-E proliferation. In rheumatoid arthritis, IL-1 and the interferons are the principal mediators.

TNF-α and IL-1 suppress the marrow proliferative response by inhibiting erythropoietin production by the kidney and by blocking its action on erythroid precursor cells. This is clinically important because the poor erythropoietin response can be overcome by pharmacological amounts of recombinant erythropoietin. Both these cytokines also reduce iron available for transport to the erythron, blocking the release of iron from reticuloendothelial cells by increasing production of isoferritins and trapping recycled iron in stores. Several anti-inflammatory cytokines (IL-4, IL-10, and IL-13) may also play a role in the retention of iron by the reticuloendothelial cells.

Chronic Inflammatory States: The Anemia of Chronic Disease

Any disease state with a major inflammatory component will be accompanied by a hypoproliferative anemia. Moreover, the erythropoietic profile of that anemia will be typical of an inflammatory cytokine-induced defect (see Table 4–1). However, when an inflammatory state is present for a long period, the **anemia of chronic disease can take on some of the manifestations of iron deficiency.** The smear becomes mildly microcytic (mean cell volume [MCV] 75–85 fL) and hypochromic as the hemoglobin falls to levels below 10 grams per deciliter. At the same time, the reticulocyte response continues to be well below that expected for the severity of the anemia, the E/G ratio does not increase, and the serum iron studies show the typical pattern of low serum iron, low TIBC, and elevated serum ferritin level. Moreover, these patients tend to accumulate iron in their reticuloendothelial stores. Prussian blue stain of the marrow shows an increased amount of iron in reticuloendothelial cells and large hemosiderin granules.

The patient with **active rheumatoid arthritis is a prime example of a chronic inflammatory state** that leads to the anemia of chronic disease. These patients demonstrate a severe anemia; hemoglobin levels range between 8 and 12 grams per deciliter (hematocrits of 25–35%), which correlates best with the serum IL-1 level. Like the anemia of acute infections, the anemia of chronic disease results from a combined suppression of the erythropoietin response, an inhibition of erythropoietin stimulation of erythroid precursors, and an interference with iron supply. The most important component appears to be the interference with erythropoietin stimulation of erythroid precursors. Patients with anemia of chronic disease do have suboptimal but not depressed levels of erythropoietin in circulation and, despite their iron supply abnormalities, do respond to treatment with recombinant erythropoietin. Studies using in vitro culture systems suggest that erythropoietin given in phar-

macological amounts can overcome the IL-1 and interferon inhibition of the erythroid precursors, perhaps by competing for a common binding site.

Unlike adult rheumatoid arthritis, **juvenile chronic arthritis** is associated with a severe microcytic anemia, low serum iron, and elevated ferritin levels. These children demonstrate elevated serum erythropoietins and high serum TfR levels, and they respond well to intravenous iron. The explanation for this would appear to be an excessive production of IL-6 resulting in enhanced ferritin synthesis and liver iron uptake. This results in a severe block in reticuloendothelial iron release without the other components of inflammatory anemia (anemia of chronic disease).

Patients with AIDS demonstrate a hypoproliferative anemia in association with progression of their disease and complicating bacterial infections. Early on, the characteristics of the anemia are those of the anemia of chronic disease, although the severity of the anemia is often made worse by zidovudine therapy, so that the patient becomes transfusion dependent. Later in the course of the disease, HIV involvement of marrow precursor cells can produce a severe marrow damage picture. This process may be recognized from appearance of a marked pancytopenia. Measurement of the serum erythropoietin level may also help distinguish between the 2 types of anemia and has been used as a guide to therapy. Patients with AIDS who have low serum erythropoietin levels typical of a chronic inflammatory anemia (< 500 IU/L) can be expected to respond to treatment with recombinant erythropoietin.

The Anemia of Renal Disease

Severe renal disease is almost always accompanied by a **failure of the normal erythropoietin response.** As with other hypoproliferative anemias, the **erythropoietic profile** is characterized by normocytic, normochromic morphology, a normal MCV, a low reticulocyte count, and an absence of polychromasia on the peripheral blood smear. The severity of the anemia correlates with the severity of the renal failure. Acute loss of renal function as with acute tubular necrosis is associated with the rapid development of a moderately severe anemia, with hemoglobin levels of 7–9 grams per deciliter. **Progressive renal failure** with a BUN in excess of 50 mg/dL and a creatinine above 3 mg/dL is associated with more severe anemia (hemoglobin levels below 7 grams per deciliter). This situation reflects the added impact of marked nitrogen retention on red blood cell survival. Patients with end stage renal disease show significant reductions in red blood cell lifespan that cannot be recognized and compensated for by an increased level of erythropoietin production.

There are clinical situations where the erythropoietin

response and the loss of renal function do not correlate. One example is the patient with **diabetes mellitus,** where the severity of the anemia can be greater than that predicted by measurements of the BUN and creatinine. Patients with diabetes have a moderately severe hypoproliferative anemia relatively early in the evolution of their renal disease. An even more striking dissociation of erythropoietin production from renal function is seen in patients with **hemolytic-uremic syndrome.** They present with severe uremia requiring dialysis but are able to respond to an increased rate of red blood cell destruction with a matched increase in red blood cell production. This situation is one where despite glomerular-tubular damage, peritubular interstitial cells are preserved.

Iron studies are important both in the diagnosis and management of a patient with renal disease anemia. Early in the evolution of the anemia, the serum iron, TIBC, and serum ferritin levels should all be normal (see Table 4–1). This is of value in the differential diagnosis of the renal disease anemia by helping to rule out iron-deficiency anemia or an inflammatory state. Repeated studies are important to patient management. Patients can develop iron deficiency at any time secondary to blood loss, especially if they are receiving chronic hemodialysis. If repeated transfusions are required, they are at risk for progressive iron overload. It is especially essential that the patient's iron status be closely monitored whenever recombinant erythropoietin therapy is used to correct the anemia. The appearance of iron deficiency during the course of erythropoietin therapy is a primary cause of therapeutic failure.

Hypometabolic States

Modest falls in the hemoglobin level are seen with protein starvation and endocrine deficiency states. In both situations, the anemia appears to be secondary to a reduced erythropoietin response that is appropriate for the reduction in tissue metabolism. **Kidney sensor cells,** which measure oxygen delivery according to their metabolic rate, appear to down-regulate erythropoietin production because of their lower oxygen requirement.

A. PROTEIN DEPRIVATION:

The **hypoproliferative anemia of protein deprivation is mild,** a 1–3 grams per deciliter reduction in the hemoglobin level. However, in the markedly marasmic individual, the severity of the anemia may be masked by a simultaneous reduction in the patient's plasma volume and total blood volume. This situation is revealed when the patient is fed. As the production of albumin recovers, the plasma volume expands, which results in a further drop in the hemoglobin level. Poor protein nutrition without calorie deprivation has been considered as a possible cause of mild hypoproliferative anemias in

the elderly. However, it is more likely that the patient has a mild inflammatory or iron-deficiency anemia.

The **erythropoietic profile** of these patients is typical of a hypoproliferative anemia secondary to reduced erythropoietin stimulation. Cell indices and morphology are normal, the reticulocyte count is not increased above basal levels, and polychromasia is absent on the peripheral blood smear. Since prolonged starvation can also result in iron or vitamin deficiencies, the evaluation should include both **iron studies and measurements of folic acid and vitamin B$_{12}$.** Rarely, deficiencies in vitamin B$_6$ and riboflavin can play a role.

B. ENDOCRINE DEFICIENCY STATES:

Testosterone, thyroid hormone, and parathormone all play roles in the regulation of red blood cell production. Testosterone is responsible for the 1–3 grams per deciliter difference in the hemoglobin level between men and women. Anabolic steroids in general are capable of enhancing the erythropoietin stimulation of erythroid precursors. Estrogen administration or castration results in a fall in the hemoglobin level by as much as 2 grams per deciliter.

Hypothyroidism and pituitary deficiency are associated with a modest anemia (hemoglobin levels of 10–12 grams per deciliter). The anemia has all the characteristics of a hypoproliferative anemia secondary to reduced erythropoietin stimulation. The severity of the anemia is usually a good reflection of the severity of the hypometabolic state; the more myxedematous the patient, the lower the hemoglobin level. Iron and folate deficiency can also be present, since patients with markedly hypothyroid conditions demonstrate malabsorption of iron and folic acid as well as a reduced dietary intake. On occasion, one or another of these deficiencies can result in an erythropoietic profile more typical of a nutritional anemia. However, iron and folate therapy will usually not resolve the anemia unless thyroid replacement is also provided.

In patients with **severe pituitary and adrenal insufficiency (Addison's disease),** the severity of the anemia may initially be hidden. This is especially true for patients presenting in Addisonian crisis, when the total blood volume and plasma volume are significantly reduced. This obscures the severity of the anemia until the patient receives volume replacement. The patient with severe Addisonian features may also demonstrate decreased white blood cell counts (3000–5000/μL) and have difficulty mounting a granulocyte response to acute infection.

Patients with **hyperparathyroidism** may exhibit a mild hypoproliferative anemia. The mechanism involved is not well defined. It has been suggested that parathormone may directly inhibit erythroid progenitor proliferation or cause sclerosis of the marrow cavity.

More likely, it relates to the development of renal calcification with an interference in erythropoietin production. The anemia does respond to parathyroidectomy.

DIFFERENTIAL DIAGNOSIS

Differential diagnosis of a hypoproliferative anemia secondary to a poor erythropoietin response can be difficult. The milder the anemia, the harder the task. The anemia is often diagnosed based on the clinical setting. For example, patients with progressive renal disease who present with a mild to moderate anemia and normal iron studies are assumed to have a failure of the kidneys' ability to increase erythropoietin production. There is no direct test to confirm this relationship. **Iron studies and measurements of key vitamins, especially folic acid and vitamin B$_{12}$,** can be invaluable in ruling out a deficiency that will respond to specific therapy. However, iron studies are also useful in detecting the anemia associated with acute and chronic inflammatory disorders.

The differential diagnosis of a mild hypoproliferative anemia in a woman can be even more daunting. Since the range of a normal hemoglobin level in women extends to levels as low as 11 grams per deciliter, it can be difficult to even distinguish an anemic woman from women with normal hemoglobin values.

Pregnancy

The difficulty in diagnosing a hypoproliferative anemia in a woman is worsened by pregnancy. Although the red blood cell mass increases during the second and third trimesters of pregnancy, the plasma volume expands to an even greater extent, which results in a fall in the hemoglobin level. This situation has been referred to as the "physiologic anemia" of pregnancy, even though it is not a true anemia. The woman's oxygen delivery capabilities are actually supernormal.

The physiologic reduction in hemoglobin during pregnancy can mask other types of anemia. Iron and folic acid deficiency are common during pregnancy and can result in hemoglobin falls of 1–3 grams per deciliter without changes in cell morphology. Mild inflammatory conditions and renal damage can also be responsible for a reduced hemoglobin level. As a general rule, a **hemoglobin level below 10 grams per deciliter during pregnancy should be carefully evaluated** for a treatable cause for the anemia. When the hemoglobin level is between 10 and 13 grams per deciliter, it is hard to distinguish true anemia from a physiologic change in the hemoglobin level. Routine prophylaxis with oral iron and folic acid is recommended, therefore, as a preventive measure during pregnancy.

THERAPY

The management of a hypoproliferative anemia will obviously vary according to the patient's primary disorder. There is also the issue of severity. Patients with mild to moderate anemia (hemoglobin levels greater than 9–10 grams per deciliter) tolerate it quite well. Unless they are elderly or have significant cardiovascular disease, they maintain good exercise tolerance and a general sense of well being. Although effective, **transfusion therapy** carries a finite risk of complications, including transmission of infections, alloimmunization, and iron overload. **Growth factor therapy,** although effective in selected situations, is expensive.

When **hypoproliferative anemia is severe,** accurate diagnosis is very important. Even when the anemia is clearly related to a primary disorder such as end stage renal disease, **iron studies** still need to be performed to rule out combination anemias and plan therapy. The presence of iron deficiency in a patient with renal anemia will effectively prevent a response to recombinant erythropoietin. In the case of the anemia of inflammatory disease, the best cure is the effective treatment of the inflammatory condition. With acute bacterial infections, the anemia will resolve spontaneously with effective antibiotic therapy. In the case of chronic inflammatory disorders such as rheumatoid arthritis, treatment with anti-inflammatory drugs will often result in an increase in the hemoglobin level. Recombinant erythropoietin therapy has been approved for use in the treatment of patients with HIV and as an adjunct to chemotherapy in patients with cancer to reduce the transfusion requirement.

Transfusion Support

Severe hypoproliferative anemias that are not expected to respond to either disease-specific therapy or erythropoietin administration will need to be transfused. Amounts of blood required and frequency of transfusion must be determined by trial and error. **Younger patients** will usually tolerate hemoglobin levels of 7–8 grams per deciliter, even though their exercise tolerance is somewhat reduced. **Older patients** will need to be transfused to hemoglobin levels of 10–11 grams per deciliter. Each unit of packed red blood cells should increase the hemoglobin by approximately 1 gram per deciliter (hematocrit by 3–4%). The frequency of transfusion will depend on the patient's own level of red blood cell production. Transfusions can usually be scheduled at intervals of weeks or even months.

When patients receive **multiple transfusions,** they are at risk for alloimmunization and iron overload. However, in contrast to patients with aplastic anemia who have much higher transfusion requirements, sufficient iron overload to produce tissue damage is rarely seen. To avoid the severe fever and chills associated with cytokine release by white cells or an alloimmune reaction or both, patients requiring multiple units of red blood cells over a prolonged period should receive **leukopoor red blood cells** (see Chapter 37).

Erythropoietin Therapy

Recombinant erythropoietin therapy has become the standard treatment in patients with end stage renal disease with severe anemia. It has proved effective in both predialysis and dialysis patients.

A. ANEMIA OF RENAL DISEASE:

Recombinant erythropoietin (Epogen, Procrit) can be administered either intravenously or subcutaneously in doses of 10–300 U/kg 3 times per week. A **typical starting dose** is 50–150 U/kg given 3 times each week. The drug is supplied in single-use vials of 2000, 4000, and 10,000 U of erythropoietin and dosages should be adjusted to use the entire vial and avoid wastage.

At the beginning of therapy, a **CBC must be performed at least once each week** to determine the rate of rise of the hemoglobin (hematocrit). The rise should not exceed 1 gram per deciliter (4% hematocrit rise) over 2 weeks. This procedure will help prevent complications such as exacerbation of the patient's hypertension or induction of seizures. At the same time, an adjustment in hypertensive medications is usually needed during the early treatment phase with erythropoietin.

Once the hemoglobin level approaches 10 grams per deciliter, the dose must be reduced to avoid a rise to levels in excess of 12 grams per deciliter (hematocrit 35%). This will involve frequent follow-up visits with measurements of CBC and serum iron and ferritin levels. The **final maintenance dose for renal patients can vary from as little as 10 U/kg to more than 300 U/kg.** The average maintenance dose is close to 75 U/kg 3 times per week. If a patient does not respond, the dose of erythropoietin should be increased by increments of 25 to 50 U/kg at monthly intervals up to a level of 300 U/kg. Some patients will require both the higher dose and several months of treatment before they will respond.

Iron deficiency, even a relatively poor supply of iron, can block the response. Therefore, **all patients must be evaluated prior to therapy to determine iron store status and then monitored repeatedly** during therapy to detect exhaustion of iron stores. Patients with serum ferritin levels below 200 µg/L (or below 400 µg/L when the percent saturation is less than 20) should be considered for iron loading prior to therapy with 1 or more injections of intravenous iron dextran (InFeD)

(see Chapter 5). Maintenance iron dextran therapy in patients receiving dialysis can reduce the amount of erythropoietin needed by up to 46%, demonstrating the close relationship between iron supply levels and the erythropoietic response. Oral iron therapy with 1 tablet of oral iron 3 to 4 times per day can be used as an alternative, although this may not provide sufficient iron to match the requirements generated by higher-dose erythropoietin therapy.

The National Kidney Foundation has published guidelines for the treatment of the anemia of chronic renal failure. Recommendations regarding iron therapy include the following:

- To achieve target hematocrit levels of 33–36%, **sufficient iron** should be administered to maintain a transferrin saturation > 20% and a ferritin > 200 µg/L.
- **In patients who have a poor response to erythropoietin,** it may be necessary to maintain higher transferrin saturation and ferritin levels (saturations of up to 50% and ferritin levels as high as 400–800 µg/L).
- **Patients receiving hemodialysis** will almost certainly require intravenous iron therapy on a regular basis (50–100 mg once or twice per week) to avoid functional iron deficiency; oral iron will not be sufficient.

Infection with the release of inflammatory cytokines will inhibit red blood cell production, necessitating higher erythropoietin doses to overcome both the inhibition of erythropoietin and the block in iron supply. To help control the high costs of replacement therapy, it may make sense to discontinue erythropoietin during periods of acute inflammatory illness. Oftentimes, the patient's anemia will worsen despite erythropoietin treatment, requiring a reinstitution of periodic red blood cell transfusions. Other factors that may affect the response to erythropoietin in the patient receiving hemodialysis include aluminum toxicity, hyperparathyroidism with marrow fibrosis, carnitine deficiency, and angiotensin enzyme inhibitors.

B. AIDS:

Erythropoietin therapy has been approved for treatment of patients with AIDS, especially those receiving zidovudine (AZT) therapy. Excellent responses are observed in patients who exhibit inflammatory type anemias with low serum erythropoietin levels. Patients with high serum erythropoietin levels (> 500 IU/L) or advanced marrow damage do less well. Erythropoietin therapy will help counteract the erythroid marrow defect induced by AZT.

C. CANCER-RELATED ANEMIA:

Erythropoietin therapy can also reduce transfusion requirements in patients with cancer-related anemia. Up to 50% of patients with myeloma will demonstrate a poor erythropoietin response before chemotherapy or with the onset of advanced disease. Most of these respond to recombinant erythropoietin given in doses of 150–250 IU/kg 3 times a week, or given once a week in larger doses. The same may be true for patients with Hodgkin's and non-Hodgkin's lymphomas. Patients with solid tumors receiving chemotherapy will show a statistically significant change in hematocrit, a decrease in transfusion requirement, and an improved quality of life when treated with 100–150 IU/kg 3 times a week.

D. ALLOGENEIC BONE MARROW TRANSPLANTATION:

Erythropoietin has also been used to speed the recovery of red blood cell production after allogeneic bone marrow transplantation.

BIBLIOGRAPHY

Cazzola M, Mercuriali F, Brugnara C: Use of recombinant erythropoietin outside the setting of uremia. Blood 1997;89:4248.

Cazzola M et al: Defective iron supply for erythropoiesis and adequate endogenous erythropoietin production in the anemia associated with systemic-onset juvenile chronic arthritis. Blood 1996;87:4824.

Krantz SB: Erythropoietin. Blood 1991;77:419.

Lee GR: The anemia of chronic disease. Semin Hematol 1983; 20:61.

Means RT, Krantz SB: Progress in understanding the pathogenesis of the anemia of chronic disease. Blood 1992;80:1639.

Nissenson AR, Miner SD, Wolcott DL: Recombinant human erythropoietin and renal anemia: Molecular biology, clinical efficacy, and nervous system effects. Ann Intern Med 1991; 114:402.

Iron-Deficiency Anemia

Iron deficiency is a leading cause of microcytic anemia in children and adults. When iron supply to erythroid marrow is deficient, red blood cell production is impaired and new cells released into circulation are poorly hemoglobinized. The severity of the anemia and the degree of microcytosis and hypochromia generally reflect the severity and chronicity of the iron-deficiency state.

The **prevalence** of iron deficiency in a population depends on the interaction of several factors, including the adequacy of dietary iron supply and the incidence of disease states accompanied by malabsorption or chronic blood loss. In developing countries, inadequate nutrition is a major factor and iron-deficiency is the principal cause of nutritional anemia. In Europe and the United States, chronic blood loss is more frequently responsible for the iron deficiency.

NORMAL IRON METABOLISM

Iron is an essential component in the synthesis of hemoglobin, myoglobin, and several heme and met-alloflavoprotein enzymes. The **major transport pathways** are illustrated in Figure 5–1.

Iron Loss

Iron is highly conserved in humans. Still, enough is lost to require an absorption of between 1 and 4 mg from the diet each day to maintain normal iron balance. The intestine responds to negative iron balance by increasing the efficiency of transport. At the same time, the intestine can virtually shut off transport once stores of iron exceed metabolic requirements.

Iron Transport

Once absorbed, iron binds to a specific plasma protein, **transferrin,** which transports it to tissues. At any moment, about 3 mg of iron is in circulation bound to transferrin. This pool turns over 10 times each day, with a predominant portion of the iron (ie, 25–30 mg) going to the erythroid marrow. Maturing erythroid precursors express **transferrin receptors** (TfR) on the cell surface that specifically bind the iron-laden transferrin. The avidity of the TfR for iron is in part governed by a genetically controlled transmembrane "hemachromato-sis protein," or **HFE protein.** Aggregate iron-TfR complexes are then incorporated into the erythroid cell in intracytoplasmic vacuoles. The iron is released and the transferrin-TfR complex returns to the cell surface, where the transferrin molecule reenters the plasma. Free intracellular iron travels to the mitochondria for the synthesis of heme or is stored as **ferritin,** a semicrystalline iron-protein aggregate.

The end result of this pathway is incorporation of 80–90% of the iron in the hemoglobin of new erythrocytes that then have a lifespan of 100–120 days. The process of new red cell production is not perfect, and 10–20% of precursor red blood cells are destroyed by marrow reticuloendothelial cells prior to release. In addition, about 1% of the red blood cells in circulation are destroyed each day as they reach the end of their lifespan. Together, **these two processes result in the recovery of 25–30 mg of iron each day** by the reticuloendothelial cells of the marrow and spleen. This iron can then be transported back to the marrow by transferrin for new cell production.

An **iron-transport pathway to parenchymal tissues** is also shown in Figure 5–1. Approximately 6 mg of iron is delivered to other tissues each day, especially the liver, where it is incorporated into ferritin stores or used in iron-containing enzymes. At least 1 mg each day is required to replace the iron lost in cells desquamated from the skin and gastrointestinal and urinary tracts.

Body Iron Content

The impact of these variables on body iron content is summarized in Table 5–1. Normal adult males have a total body iron content of close to 4000 mg, including 500–1000 mg of hepatic and reticuloendothelial iron stores. Because of menstrual blood loss and a lower dietary iron intake, adult women have significantly lower amounts of storage iron (usually less than 200 mg).

Serum Ferritin & Serum TfR Levels

Serum ferritin and serum TfR levels can be used to assess iron availability and store status. Translation of these 2 proteins is highly regulated by cytoplasmic iron-regulatory proteins (**IRP-1 and 2**) and an mRNA, non-

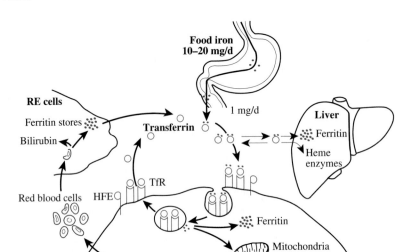

Figure 5-1. **Iron transport pathways.** Iron absorbed from food and iron recovered from senescent red blood cells is transported by transferrin to the marrow and tissues. The iron-laden transferrin binds to transferrin-receptors (TfR) on the surface of erythroid precursors. It is then internalized, at which time the iron is released for use in hemoglobin production. The transferrin-TfR complex is then returned to the surface of the cell and the transferrin is released to complete the cycle. The transmembrane HFE protein (hemochromatosis protein) also plays a role in regulating the uptake of iron by the erythroid precursors by interacting with TfR.

coding iron-responsive element (**IRE**). When iron is scarce, IRP-1 binds to the mRNA IRE and inhibits ferritin synthesis. When abundant, IRP binding is inhibited and ferritin production increases. The opposite is true for TfR; low iron induces receptor expression, whereas high iron allows more rapid mRNA degradation and reduced levels of TfR.

Transferrin-Receptor

Transferrin-receptor is shed from the membrane of red blood cell precursors and other cells during development and circulates as a monomeric fragment bound to transferrin. The serum TfR level will reflect the patient's iron status. Patients with iron deficiency show serum TfR levels of 2 to 4 times normal. This reflects both an increased

expression of the surface receptor and, as the anemia worsens, a proliferation of red cell precursors.

Serum Ferritin Level

The **serum ferritin level** is used to estimate iron store size (Figure 5-2). Each microgram per liter of serum ferritin correlates to 10 mg of tissue stores. Children and menstruating women typically have ferritin levels of 20–50 µg/L (200–500 mg of iron stores), whereas adult men and postmenopausal women have levels of 50–200 µg/L (500–2000 mg of iron stores), depending on their age and level of dietary iron. With iron deficiency, the serum ferritin level falls to levels below 15 µg/L. Iron overload can produce ferritin levels of 300 to more than 1000 µg/L.

Table 5-1. **Body iron content.**

	Adult—Male (80 kg)	Adult—Female (60 kg)
Hemoglobin	2500 mg	1700 mg
Myoglobin and enzymes	500 mg	300 mg
Serum iron	3 mg	3 mg
Iron stores	500–1000 mg	0–200 mg

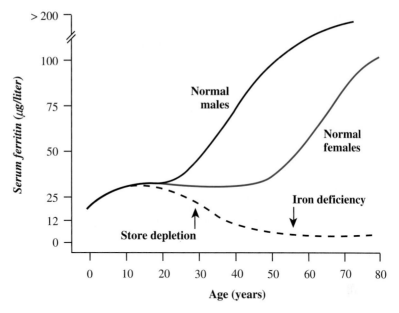

***Figure 5–2.* Serum ferritin levels.** The serum ferritin level correlates with the level of iron stores. Ferritin levels in both sexes are less than 50 µg/L throughout childhood. Adult males and females demonstrate different normal values based on their levels of iron intake and loss. Iron store depletion and iron deficiency are accompanied by a fall in the serum ferritin level to below 15–20 µg/L.

IRON NUTRITION

Iron content of the diet depends on the types of foods eaten and the total daily caloric intake. Meat-derived heme iron is much more available for absorption. Although making up the greater proportion of the daily intake, nonheme vegetable iron is far less bioavailable. Compounds within vegetables, especially phosphates and phytates, inhibit iron absorption to a significant degree. In developed countries, a diet consisting of a balance of meat and vegetable products contains approximately 6 mg of iron per thousand kilocalories. Thus, an adult male ingests between 15 and 20 mg of iron each day, whereas the adult female takes in 10–15 mg.

Adult males and nonmenstruating females with normal dietary habits have little difficulty maintaining normal iron balance. **Menstruating females, rapidly growing infants, children, adolescents, and frequent blood donors** are at some risk and may require supplementation to maintain an adequate iron balance. Iron supplementation is almost always required during **pregnancy.** During the last 2 trimesters, the daily requirement for iron increases to 5–6 mg, a level that cannot be attained by diet alone unless it is especially rich in heme iron.

CLINICAL FEATURES

Clinical states of iron deficiency can be classified as iron-store depletion, iron-deficient erythropoiesis, or iron-deficiency anemia (Table 5–2). In its mildest form, **iron-store depletion** results simply from an imbalance between normal physiologic demands such as rapid growth, menstrual blood loss, and dietary iron intake. **More-severe iron-deficiency with limitation of red blood cell production** is usually the result of blood loss from the gastrointestinal tract or uterus. Less frequently, the cause is malabsorption secondary to small intestinal disease or gastric surgery. **Iron deficiency with marked anemia** and microcytosis is seen in patients with severe malabsorption or chronic blood loss.

Iron-store depletion and iron-deficient erythropoiesis are not associated with any distinctive clinical findings. The **symptoms and signs of severe iron deficiency** are primarily those of severe anemia. Patients complain of fatigue and exercise intolerance, and may show signs of cardiac decompensation. When patients are iron deficient for a prolonged period, they may complain of a sore mouth, difficulty swallowing, or a tendency for their nails to soften and curl, at times producing a characteristic spooning of the nails. **In chil-

Table 5–2. **Causes of iron deficiency.**

Iron-Store Depletion	Iron-Deficient Erythropoiesis	Iron-Deficiency Anemia
Inadequate diet	Excessive menses	Chronic blood loss
Rapid growth	Pregnancy	Varices
Infancy	Acute hemorrhage	Peptic ulcer disease
Adolescence	Malabsorption	Large-bowel tumors
Normal menses	Gastrectomy	Diverticulitis
Blood duration	Regional enteritis	Angiodysplasia
	Inflammation	Intravascular hemolysis
	Acute infections	Hookworm infestation
	Chronic inflammatory states	Severe malabsorption
	Polycythemia vera treated with phlebotomy	Postgastrectomy
		Sprue
		Regional enteritis

dren, iron deficiency has been associated with learning and behavioral problems.

Laboratory Studies

Accurate diagnosis of an iron-deficiency state requires several laboratory tests (Table 5–3). Measurements of the serum iron, transferrin iron-binding capacity, and the serum ferritin level are of greatest importance. Other measurements used include direct inspection of marrow reticuloendothelial iron stores using a marrow aspirate and measurement of the red cell protoporphyrin level.

A. SERUM IRON STUDIES:

The **serum iron** (**SI**) is a direct measure of the amount of iron bound to transferrin. A normal individual has an SI of 50–150 µg/dL. The **total iron-binding capacity** (**TIBC**) is a measure of the amount of iron that can be bound by transferrin and, therefore, is a surrogate

Table 5–3. **Laboratory studies in iron deficiency.**

	Iron-Store Depletion	Iron-Deficient Erythropoiesis	Iron-Deficiency Anemia
Hemoglobin	Normal	Slight decrease	Marked decrease (microcytic/hypochromic)
Iron stores	< 100 mg (0–1+)	0	0
Serum iron (µg/dL)	Normal	<60	<40
TIBC (µg/dL)	360–390	>390	>410
Percent saturation	20–30	<15	< 10
Ferritin (µg/L)	<20	<12	<
Percent sideroblasts	40–60	<10	<10
Red blood cell Protoporphyrin (µg/dL RBC)	30	>100	>200

measure of the serum transferrin level. The normal TIBC is 300–360 µg/dL. Together, the SI and TIBC (transferrin level) are used to calculate the **percent saturation of transferrin with iron** (SI ÷ TIBC = percent saturation). In states of normal iron balance, the percent saturation is between 20% and 50%. When it falls below 20%, the erythroid marrow has difficulty obtaining sufficient iron to support increased levels of erythropoiesis. When the percent saturation exceeds 50–60%, iron delivery to parenchymal tissues increases, resulting in iron loading of hepatocytes, heart muscle, skin, and pituitary gland.

B. SERUM FERRITIN:

The **serum ferritin** is used to evaluate total body iron stores. Normal adult males have serum ferritin levels of 50–200 µg/L. This correlates with the 800–1000 mg or more of tissue iron stores seen in men. As iron stores are depleted, the serum ferritin falls, reaching levels below 15–20 µg/L once stores are exhausted and iron deficient erythropoiesis appears. In iron overload states, serum ferritins can reach levels of several thousand micrograms (Table 5–4).

C. SERUM TRANSFERRIN-RECEPTOR:

An enzyme-linked immunosorbent assay (ELISA) for serum TfR can be used in conjunction with the serum ferritin measurement in diagnosing iron deficiency. Levels of serum TfR (normal = 5–9 µg/L) increase rapidly once stores are exhausted. Iron-deficiency anemia is accompanied by an elevation of transferrin receptor proportional to the severity of the anemia. Serum TfR levels also increase in anemias characterized by erythroid precursor proliferation, whether ineffective or effective, and in some patients with myelo- and lymphoproliferative disease. Patients with inflammatory anemias show near normal serum TfR levels, reflecting their normal to increased reticuloendothelial iron stores and hypoproliferative erythroid marrows. The **serum**

Table 5–4. Measurements of iron stores.

Iron Stores	Serum Ferritin (µg/L)	Marrow Iron Stain (0–4+)
0	< 12	0
1–300 mg	12–20	1+
300–800 mg	20–50	2+
800–1000 mg	50–150	3+
> 1–2 g	150–300	4+
Iron overload	> 500	

TfR/log ferritin ratio is considered by many to be a better discriminator between iron deficiency and inflammation. Low values (< 1) are typical of an inflammatory anemia (anemia of chronic disease); values > 4 suggest iron-deficiency anemia.

D. MARROW IRON STORES:

The amount of iron stores in reticuloendothelial cells can be estimated by inspection of a Prussian blue stain of marrow aspirate particles. A simple scale of 0 to 4+ stores is generally used in reports. This grading system correlates fairly well with the amount of iron available for erythropoiesis (see Table 5–4). At the same time, it does not provide as good a measure of tissue loading as the serum ferritin level. Patients with hereditary hemochromatosis will demonstrate near normal reticuloendothelial stores in the face of marked liver parenchymal cell loading.

The marrow iron stain has also been used to evaluate delivery of iron to erythroid precursors. Normally, 40–60% of developing red blood cell precursors have visible iron granules in their cytoplasm, which represents the excess iron not used for hemoglobin production. These cells are referred to as **sideroblasts.** The number of sideroblasts in marrow decreases rapidly when iron supply to the marrow falls, which provides a sensitive measure of iron-deficient erythropoiesis.

E. RED BLOOD CELL PROTOPORPHYRIN:

A measurement of red blood cell protoporphyrin can also be used to detect early iron-deficient erythropoiesis. Intracellular levels of protoporphyrin will increase even before anemia is present. This process is a result of the imbalance between iron supply and the production of the protoporphyrin by mitochondria. It is especially useful for detection of iron-deficient erythropoiesis in children since the assay requires extremely small amounts of blood. The **average normal red blood cell protoporphyrin** is 30 µg/dL of red blood cells. The level rises quickly to values in excess of 100 µg/dL with iron-deficiency anemia. Increased protoporphyrin levels are also seen in children exposed to lead, which inhibits **heme synthetase,** the enzyme necessary for the final assembly of iron and the protoporphyrin ring required to form heme.

DIAGNOSIS

The diagnosis of an iron-deficiency state is largely a laboratory exercise. As summarized in Table 5–3, iron-store depletion, iron-deficient erythropoiesis, and iron-deficiency anemia can be distinguished from measurements of the hemoglobin, red blood cell morphology, SI, TIBC, serum ferritin, serum TfR, and marrow iron stores.

Iron-Store Depletion

Depletion of iron stores is best assessed using the serum ferritin level or a Prussian blue iron stain of aspirated marrow particles. A serum ferritin of less than 20 µg/L or visible iron stores of 1+ or less (< 200–300 mg) (or both) suggests iron-store depletion. As long as some iron stores are still present, the SI, TIBC, serum TfR, and hemoglobin level should be normal.

Iron-Deficient Erythropoiesis

Iron-deficient erythropoiesis is also **readily diagnosed from the pattern of SI, TIBC, and serum ferritin.** The serum ferritin is less than 15–20 µg/L and the SI falls to levels below 60 µg/dL. This situation is most often accompanied by a rise in the TIBC, which results in a percent saturation of less than 15%. If a marrow aspirate is performed, stainable reticuloendothelial cell iron stores are absent and the number of sideroblasts is reduced.

In the earliest stages of iron-deficient erythropoiesis, the **decrease in iron supply impairs the proliferative capacity of the erythroid marrow.** Clinically, this situation is expressed as a modest fall in the hemoglobin level to as low as 11–12 grams per deciliter. At the same time, there is little or no change in red blood cell morphology and the mean cell volume and mean cell hemoglobin remain normal. It is important that the clinician recognize this fact. With iron-deficient erythropoiesis and early iron-deficiency anemia, red cell morphology/indices are normocytic, normochromic. Microcytosis and hypochromia only appear when the anemia is more severe and has been present for weeks or months.

Iron-Deficiency Anemia

Full-blown iron-deficiency anemia is easy to diagnose. The **SI is very low and the TIBC high,** producing a percent saturation of less than 10% (see Table 5–3). The serum ferritin level is always less than 12 µg/L, the serum TfR level is elevated, and inspection of marrow aspirate particles reveals absent iron stores and sideroblasts. Patients with severe iron deficiency also present with a **moderate to severe anemia and distinctive changes in red blood cell morphology.** Once the hemoglobin falls to below 10 grams per deciliter, erythropoietin stimulation of the marrow results in the production of cells that are morphologically abnormal. Initially, the cells are microcytic without abnormalities in cell shape or hemoglobin content. However, as the anemia worsens, new red blood cells become increasingly microcytic and hypochromic.

The relationship of cell morphology to the severity of the anemia is illustrated in Figure 5–3. While the hemoglobin level is in the range of 9–11 grams per deciliter, the reduction in cell size is roughly equivalent to the loss of cell hemoglobin, so that cells tend to be uniformly microcytic with little or no hypochromia. There are also modest variations in cell size (**anisocytosis**) and cell shape (**poikilocytosis**). As the hemoglobin falls below 9 grams per deciliter, cell morphology becomes increasingly bizarre, with the appearance of many misshapen cells (**poikilocytes**). This situation is a sign of increasing ineffective erythropoiesis in response to high levels of erythropoietin stimulation. Finally, the **presence or absence of cigar- or pencil-shaped red blood cells and target cells** can help in the differential diagnosis of iron deficiency from thalassemia. Cigar cells are only seen with iron-deficiency anemia, whereas target cells are associated with thalassemia.

Determination of the cause of the iron loss is essential to the diagnosis of any iron-deficiency anemia. Because the cause is most often chronic blood loss, symptoms and signs of abnormal bleeding should be sought. If no obvious site of external loss is present, a full evaluation of the gastrointestinal tract for bleeding site is required. Any prolonged delay in working up the patient can result in a missed opportunity to detect a malignancy while it is still at a treatable stage.

The **evaluation of less severe degrees of iron deficiency** depends on the setting. The tenuous nature of iron balance in infants, rapidly growing adolescents, and pregnant women usually makes an exhaustive workup unnecessary. In these situations, a therapeutic trial of iron supplementation is appropriate. However, even the mildest iron deficiency in a male or postmenopausal female should not be dismissed as simple iron imbalance and treated with iron supplements. These patients should always be evaluated for abnormal sites of bleeding.

DIFFERENTIAL DIAGNOSIS

Only a few diseases need to be considered in the differential diagnosis of a microcytic, hypochromic anemia. Congenital defects in globin production (the thalassemias) typically have moderate to severe microcytosis with varying degrees of anemia. An approach to diagnosis of these conditions is discussed in Chapter 6. Unless both conditions are present simultaneously, iron studies and red cell morphology will clearly separate the two.

A more common diagnostic dilemma is **separating iron deficient erythropoiesis secondary to iron loss from that which accompanies acute and chronic inflammation.** As a part of the inflammatory process, the normal recirculation of iron from reticuloendothelial cells to erythroid precursors is disrupted. When the serum iron falls to less than 50 µg/dL, the number of sideroblasts in the marrow declines, and red blood cell

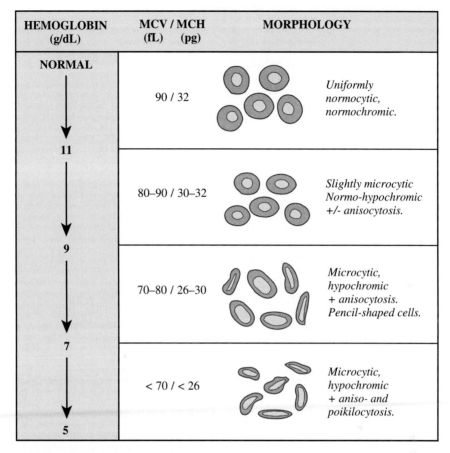

HEMOGLOBIN (g/dL)	MCV / MCH (fL) (pg)	MORPHOLOGY	
NORMAL ↓ 11 ↓ 9 ↓ 7 ↓ 5	90 / 32		*Uniformly normocytic, normochromic.*
	80–90 / 30–32		*Slightly microcytic Normo-hypochromic +/- anisocytosis.*
	70–80 / 26–30		*Microcytic, hypochromic + anisocytosis. Pencil-shaped cells.*
	< 70 / < 26		*Microcytic, hypochromic + aniso- and poikilocytosis.*

Figure 5–3. **Anemia severity and red blood cell morphology.** The appearance of microcytosis and hypochromia in patients with iron deficiency depends on the severity of the anemia. As long as the hemoglobin is above 11–13 grams per deciliter, red blood cells will be normocytic and normochromic. With more severe anemia, new red blood cells will be increasingly microcytic and hypochromic with marked poikilocytosis.

production is suppressed. With an acute inflammatory illness such as a pneumonia or cellulitis, the anemia that results is mild (hemoglobin greater than 10 grams per deciliter) and red blood cell morphology is unaffected. With long-standing, chronic inflammatory illnesses such as rheumatoid arthritis, the defect in iron supply can result in a moderately severe, microcytic/hypochromic anemia.

Iron studies will usually distinguish between true iron deficiency, an inflammatory block in iron delivery (the anemia of chronic disease), and thalassemia (Table 5–5). The pattern of a low serum iron, high TIBC (percent saturation less than 10%), low ferritin level, increased serum TfR/log ferritin ratio, and absent iron stores is unique for true iron deficiency. Although patients with inflammatory anemia also have low serum irons and low percent saturations of transferrin, their

iron stores will still be visible in the marrow and their serum ferritins will be normal or increased. Moreover, the serum TfR/log ferritin ratio will be < 1, not the > fourfold increase seen with true iron deficiency or the ineffective erythropoiesis of thalassemia. Finally, patients with thalassemia minor will have an essentially normal iron profile.

A severe microcytic anemia secondary to poor iron delivery is seen in **children with systemic-onset juvenile chronic arthritis.** This is an example of a marked block in iron supply from reticuloendothelial stores secondary to increased production of IL-6 (see Chapter 4).

Microcytosis can also occur in patients with congenital or acquired defects in mitochondrial function, the so-called sideroblastic anemias. These are uncommon, however, and rarely result in degrees of microcytosis

Table 5–5. Differential diagnosis of microcytic anemia.

	Thalassemia	Iron Deficiency	Chronic Inflammation
SI	Normal/increased	Low	Low
TIBC	Normal	High	Low
Percent saturtion	> 20%	< 10%	10–20%
Ferritin (µg/L)	> 50	< 10	20–200
Serum TfR/log ferritin ratio		> 4	< 1
Iron stores	3–4+	0	1–4+
Transferrin-receptor	Normal/increased	Increased	Normal

and hypochromia that are typical of severe iron deficiency anemia. The characteristics of these diseases are discussed in Chapter 9.

THERAPY

Management of the patient with iron deficiency will depend on the severity of the anemia, the cause of the iron deficiency, and the ability of the patient to tolerate medicinal iron preparations. **With a severe anemia**, immediate red blood cell transfusion may be advisable. This suggestion is especially true for patients who require surgery or are in cardiac failure. The guidelines for transfusion are no different for iron-deficiency states than other types of anemia.

Cause of Iron-Deficient State

It is always important to know the cause of the iron-deficient state. Chronic blood loss needs to be controlled if iron therapy is to be effective. If **significant gastrointestinal malabsorption** is present, the route of iron administration must be modified. The patient should also be questioned regarding any complicating inflammatory illness or a previous history of gastric intolerance to oral iron preparations. **Complicating inflammatory illnesses** will inhibit both iron absorption and the release of iron from reticuloendothelial iron stores. This situation will have the effect of dampening the response to treatment.

Gastrointestinal Intolerance to Oral Iron Preparations

Gastrointestinal intolerance to oral iron preparations can interfere with patient compliance. For maximum effect, **patients must maintain a constant oral intake of iron.** The response of the erythroid marrow correlates with the severity of the anemia (level of erythropoietin stimulation), the structural integrity of the marrow, and

the continuous level of serum iron. Erythropoiesis will be suppressed whenever the SI is below 50 µg/dL. If the SI concentration is kept between 50 and 150 µg/dL, production will increase two- to threefold, resulting in a hemoglobin rise of 0.2–0.5 gram per deciliter per day. In the patient with iron deficiency with a moderately severe anemia, this should result in a 2–3 grams per deciliter rise in hemoglobin within 3–4 weeks. When the anemia is less severe, a hemoglobin greater than 10 grams per deciliter, the response will be slower because of the lower level of erythropoietin stimulation.

Lack of Response to Oral Iron

When the response to oral iron seems to be inadequate, the patient's ability to comply with the regimen should be reviewed and the clinical diagnosis reevaluated. If patient compliance appears to be good, sources of continued bleeding should be looked for and studies performed to detect the presence of inflammatory disease. Oral iron therapy should not be continued beyond 3–4 weeks without evidence of a response. In addition, medicinal iron supplementation should not be routinely prescribed beyond 6 months without a definite reason. There is a small but finite risk of iron overload if the patient has inherited the trait for hemochromatosis.

Oral Iron Preparations

Several oral preparations of iron are available in both tablet and elixir form (Table 5–6). Ferrous sulfate tablets and elixir (Feosol) are the least expensive of the iron preparations and, therefore, preferable. Ferrous fumarate, ferrous gluconate, and polysaccharide-iron complex tablets are equivalent preparations, even though the actual iron contents are somewhat different. Generally, when any of these preparations are given 3 to 4 times a day before meals, between 40 and 60 mg of iron will be absorbed and delivered to the erythroid

Table 5–6. **Oral iron preparations.**

	Tablet (Iron content) (mg)	Elixir (Iron content) (mg)
Ferrous sulfate	325 (65)	300/5 mL (60)
	195 (39)	90/5 mL (18)
Extended release	525 (105)	
Ferrous gluconate	325 (38)	300/5 mL (35)
Ferrous fumarate	325 (107)	100/5 mL (33)
	195 (64)	
Polysaccharide—iron	150 (150)	100/5 mL (100)
	50 (50)	

marrow. This process will support marrow production levels of up to 3 times normal in patients with moderate to severe anemia.

Several other compoundings of iron are available. Enteric-coated and delayed-release preparations hold no great advantage and may actually result in decreased absorption. Some preparations also contain absorption-enhancing substances, including other vitamins, amino acids, and a range of other ingredients. Ascorbic acid is one of the more popular additives. Iron absorption is increased when ascorbic acid is present in amounts of 200 mg or more. At the same time, increased uptake is accompanied by an increase in side effects. All of these preparations are more expensive than ferrous sulfate, while not providing much advantage to the patient.

Dosage Guidelines

Moderate to severe iron deficiency anemia in an adult should be treated with 150–200 mg of elemental iron per day (2–3 mg/kg). For **children** weighing 15–30 kg, the dose should be reduced by half. Smaller children and infants usually can tolerate doses of iron of 5 mg/kg, somewhat larger than the adult dose by weight.

The **patient's compliance is the key** to an effective marrow response to oral iron therapy. A good oral iron regimen requires multiple doses during the day since absorption following each dose is limited to a few hours (Figure 5–4). To achieve a maximum effect, it is also important to ingest the iron medications between meals. This procedure will avoid the inhibiting effect of

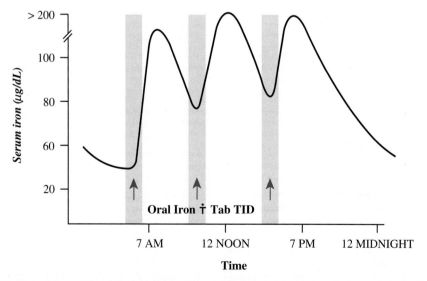

Figure 5–4. **Oral iron absorption.** When medicinal iron is given 3 times a day, each dose raises the SI for several hours. A fourth dose at bedtime can help sustain the SI during nighttime hours.

food substances on iron transport. At the same time, it will tend to increase the gastrointestinal intolerance to the medication. A typical oral iron regimen is 1 tablet of iron 3 or 4 times a day taken prior to meals and at bedtime. The final dose can be very important to maintain an elevated SI during the late evening and night hours. Without it, the SI will fall to levels below 50 μg/dL during the night.

As the hemoglobin level responds to iron therapy, the rate of increase will slow, reflecting a decrease in erythropoietin stimulation as the anemia disappears. Once the hemoglobin rises above 10–12 grams per deciliter, the recovery rate is very much slower, regardless of the level of oral iron intake, and a reduction in the dose can help maintain patient compliance. Finally, at least 6 mo of dietary iron supplementation is required in the normal adult to rebuild reticuloendothelial iron stores.

A. Adjusting Dose for Patient Tolerance:

In all situations, **the dose must be adjusted according to patient tolerance.** With a full treatment dose of 150–200 mg of elemental iron per day (1 iron tablet, 3 or 4 times a day), up to 25% of individuals will complain of some nausea and upper abdominal pain. If a patient experiences gastrointestinal distress, whether abdominal pain, nausea, vomiting, constipation, or diarrhea, the therapeutic dose will need to be reduced. Patient compliance can be increased whenever iron is given over a long period by using a lower dose. Also, higher doses do not have an advantage in patients with mild anemia or where iron is being given to rebuild iron stores.

B. Absorption:

Absorption of iron given in tablet form requires the acid milieu of the stomach to remove the tablet coat. In patients who have had gastric surgery, tablet iron may be poorly absorbed or not absorbed at all. In this situation, therapy with iron elixir should be tried. It may also be necessary to administer the iron with meals to prevent gastric intolerance.

Parenteral Iron Therapy

For those situations where gastrointestinal malabsorption or severe intolerance prevents effective oral iron therapy, parenteral iron can be administered. Two iron dextran preparations are available for use in the United States: INFeD (Schein) and **DexFerrum** (USP/American Regent Laboratories). INFeD is a ferric hydroxide-dextran compound, average molecular weight of 165,000, packaged as a viscous solution containing 50 mg/mL of iron. Two preparations are sold; one containing 0.5% phenol for intramuscular use only and a second that is phenol free for intramuscular or intravenous use. The former

should never be used for intravenous use because it will result in systemic and local reactions.

The **preferred method of administration** of iron dextran injection is by bolus, intravenous injection of 500–2000 mg. The total amount of iron needed by the patient can be calculated as follows:

$$\text{Body weight (kg)} \times 2.3 \times (15 - \text{patient's Hgb in g/dL}) + 500 \text{ mg (for stores)} = \text{total dose (mg)}.$$

An alternative calculation, recommended by the manufacturer, is as follows:

$$[0.476 \times \text{lean body weight (kg)} \times \text{hemoglobin deficit}] + 1 \text{ mL per 5 kg body weight to a maximum of 14 mL (to reconstitute iron stores)} = \text{Total dose in mL of iron dextran solution.}$$

A. Clearance:

Iron dextran given intravenously is rapidly cleared by the reticuloendothelial cell. The iron is then released from the dextran over a period of weeks and transported by transferrin to the erythroid marrow. The rate of release is a function of the particle size of the iron dextran. Some of the particles administered are quite large and slow to dissolve. This situation can result in the accumulation of unused iron dextran particles in the reticuloendothelial cells of patients who receive repeated injections over months or years.

B. Administration and Complications:

When one is administering intravenous iron dextran, great care must be taken to anticipate and **avoid anaphylactic reactions** in patients who are allergic to the dextran portion of the compound. A careful history should be taken to identify those patients who have received dextran in any form previously. The **technique of administration** should involve the initial injection of less than 0.5 mL of the iron dextran compound over 5–10 minutes while the patient is closely observed. The infusion should be stopped immediately if the patient complains of itching, shortness of breath, chest pain, or back pain. The blood pressure should also be monitored over the first hour of administration to detect sudden hypotension. If the initial test dose is well tolerated, the remainder of the dose can be administered slowly. When 500–1000 mg is used on a single occasion, it is best diluted in 250 mL of 0.9% sodium chloride solution and administered over 30–60 minutes.

Iron dextran can be administered by **intramuscular injection.** Five milliliters (250 mg) of iron dextran can be given each time with half of the dose injected in each buttock area. Significant skin staining can occur.

It is also possible to produce sterile abscesses at the site of injections that will take considerable time to resolve. The rate of release of iron from intramuscular iron dextran injection can be slower and less reliable, and the risk of acute anaphylaxis is not avoided. **Late reactions to intramuscular or intravenous iron dextran** include a serum sickness–like reaction with malaise, fever, arthralgias, skin rash, and lymphadenopathy.

BIBLIOGRAPHY

Cook JD, Skikne BS: Iron deficiency: Definition and diagnosis. J Intern Med 1989;226:349.

Cook JD, Skikne BS, Boynes RD: Serum transferrin receptor. Annu Rev Med 1993;44:63.

Finch CA, Huebers H: Perspectives in iron metabolism. N Engl J Med 1982;306:1520.

Guyatt GH et al: Laboratory diagnosis of iron-deficiency anemia: An overview. J Gen Intern Med 1992;7:145.

Hillman RS: Hematopoietic agents: Growth factors, minerals and vitamins. In: *The Pharmacological Basis of Therapeutics,* 10th ed. McGraw-Hill, 2001.

Massey AC: Microcytic anemia: Differential diagnosis and management of iron deficiency anemia. Med Clin North Am 1992;76:549.

Oski FA: Iron deficiency in infancy and childhood. N Engl J Med 1993;329:190.

Thalassemia

In addition to iron deficiency, an inherited defect in globin chain synthesis is the other leading cause of microcytic anemia in children and adults. The frequency and severity of the several types of thalassemia depend on the **racial background** of the population. For example, β-thalassemia is commonly seen in individuals from Africa and the Mediterranean area, whereas α-thalassemia and hemoglobin E disease are common in Southeast Asian populations. For certain subpopulations, the incidence of a microcytic, hypochromic anemia secondary to thalassemia can exceed that due to iron deficiency anemia.

The diagnosis of thalassemia requires an understanding of normal globin chain synthesis, familiarity with the laboratory tests used to identify chain deficiencies, and a careful clinical evaluation of the patient. Because it is easy to confuse microcytosis of iron deficiency with that of thalassemia, **iron studies** need to be performed on all patients. **Accurate diagnosis of the chain synthesis abnormality** is also important for genetic counseling.

NORMAL GLOBIN CHAIN SYNTHESIS

Types of Globin

Globin, the protein portion of the hemoglobin molecule, is a tetramer of two α and two non-α-globin chains (Figure 6–1). The α-globin chains are encoded by two closely linked genes (α_2 and α_1) on chromosome 16. The non-α genes, β, γ, and δ, are encoded by a cluster of genes on chromosome 11. The pairing of these several globin chains produces **three types of hemoglobin:** hemoglobin F ($\alpha_2\gamma_2$), hemoglobin A ($\alpha_2\beta_2$), and hemoglobin A_2 ($\alpha_2\delta_2$). A failure in α-globin chain synthesis can result in hemoglobin H, a tetramer of β-globin chains.

Quantity of Hemoglobin & Diagnosis

Globin gene expression varies with the patient's age. **Throughout fetal life,** red blood cells contain only hemoglobin F (Figure 6–2). During the first several months of life, γ-globin gene expression is suppressed and both β-globin and δ-globin synthesis are activated. In adults, red blood cells contain primarily hemoglobin A (96–97% of the cell's hemoglobin) and only small amounts of hemoglobin A_2 (2.5%) and F (< 1%). The quantity of each hemoglobin type is important in diagnosis of thalassemia. Because gene mutations are associated with a quantitative failure in chain production, diagnosis is based on changes in intracellular levels of the major hemoglobin types.

Globin gene expression in adults can also vary according to the level of erythropoietin stimulation and availability of iron. An upregulation of hemoglobin F production has been observed in sickle cell anemia patients who are treated with hydroxyurea. Increased synthesis of hemoglobin A_2 in β-thalassemia patients is inhibited by iron deficiency. This needs to be taken into account when one is analyzing any abnormal hemoglobin electrophoretic pattern.

CLINICAL FEATURES

Depending on the genetic mutation, thalassemia can present as an incidental laboratory finding in an otherwise asymptomatic patient or as a moderate to severe anemia. One unifying feature is the presence of microcytosis and hypochromia, which reflects the decreased synthesis of globin chains.

Racial Background/Family History

Although the morphologic abnormality is very much the same for the various thalassemias, racial background and family history can help in diagnosis. Patients with the **most severe forms of either α- or β-thalassemia** have parents who are heterozygotes for the globin chain defect and have racial ties to high-prevalence population groups (Figure 6–3). Geographic distribution of the major thalassemias appears to reflect the survival advantage of the mutation in regions with a high incidence of malaria. α-Thalassemia is most common in Southeast Asia and Africa, whereas β-thalassemia has a more worldwide distribution. Various combinations of globin chain defects can be seen with intermarriage.

Classification

Thalassemia patients are classified as having thalassemia major, thalassemia intermedia, or thalassemia minor,

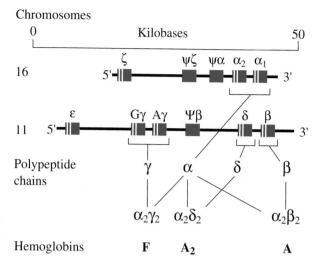

Figure 6-1. Globin genes. Specific genes on chromosomes 16 and 11 control the production of the α-, β-, γ-, and δ-globin chains.

depending on the severity of their anemia (Table 6-1). Worldwide, there are nearly 200 million individuals with thalassemia.

A. THALASSEMIA MINOR:

Most individuals with thalassemia are thalassemia minor patients who are heterozygotes for either an α-globin or β-globin gene mutation. α-Thalassemia trait patients with deletion of two genes, heterozygous β-thalassemia patients, and patients with partial deletions of both the δ- and β-genes, such as hemoglobin Lepore [(δβ)+ thalassemia] and hereditary persistence of fetal hemoglobin [(δβ)0 HPFH], demonstrate microcytosis and hypochromia, which is usually out of proportion to the severity of their anemia. Patients with α-thalassemia (deletion of a single gene), hemoglobin Constant Spring (α^{CS}—a nondeletional form of α-thalassemia), and certain subtypes of β-thalassemia have little or no

hematologic disease. They deserve the title of "silent" carrier state.

B. THALASSEMIA INTERMEDIA:

Thalassemia intermedia patients present with more severe anemia and prominent microcytosis and hypochromia. Not only do they complain of symptoms secondary to their anemia, but they also have related physical abnormalities such as hepatosplenomegaly, cardiomegaly, and on occasion skeletal changes secondary to marrow expansion. These patients have either a milder form of homozygous β+-thalassemia, a combined α- and β-thalassemia defect, β-thalassemia with high levels of hemoglobin F, or (δβ)0-thalassemia.

C. THALASSEMIA MAJOR:

Thalassemia major (Cooley's anemia) patients develop a severe, life-threatening anemia during their first year or

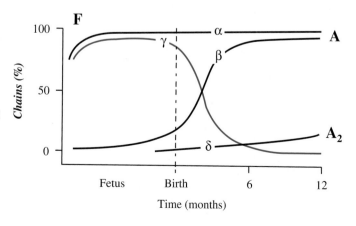

Figure 6-2. Globin chain production and development. Fetal red blood cells contain primarily hemoglobin F ($\alpha_2\gamma_2$). Soon after birth, γ-globin chain synthesis is suppressed and β-globin and δ-globin chain production increase, which results in the appearance of hemoglobins A and A$_2$.

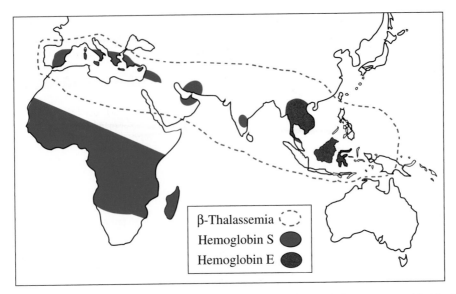

Figure 6–3. **Geographic distribution of hemoglobinopathies.** β-Thalassemia has a near worldwide distribution, as indicated by the dotted line. Hemoglobin S (sickle cell trait and sickle cell anemia) is concentrated in Africa, whereas hemoglobin E and α-thalassemia are most prevalent in Southeast Asia.

two of life. To survive childhood, they require chronic transfusion therapy to correct their anemia and suppress their high level of ineffective erythropoiesis. Otherwise, they either die during childhood or have marked skeletal changes, growth retardation, and failure to reach sexual maturity. The anemia of β-thalassemia major is also associated with a high serum iron (SI) level, saturation of the total iron-binding capacity (TIBC), and a tendency for tissue iron loading. Most patients are homozygous for a β-globin gene deletion, although some are double heterozygotes for β-thalassemia minor and an abnormal hemoglobin such as hemoglobin E ($β^E$).

D. HEMOGLOBIN H DISEASE:

Patients who are double heterozygotes for $α^0$ and $α^+$ or $α^{CS}$ are classified clinically as having hemoglobin H disease. Because of the involvement of three α genes, these patients produce an excess of β-globin chains that combine to form $β_4$ hemoglobin (**hemoglobin H**). Clinically, patients with hemoglobin H disease have characteristics of both thalassemia and a hemolytic anemia. Red blood cell production is not as ineffective as with other forms of thalassemia but hemoglobin H is highly unstable, resulting in increased destruction of circulating red blood cells.

E. HYDROPS FETALIS:

When both parents are $α^0$-thalassemia heterozygotes, there is a chance of producing a fetus with deletion of

all four α-globin genes. This condition, hydrops fetalis, is a lethal defect. The complete absence of α-globin production results in the formation of **hemoglobin Bart's,** which is a poorly functioning hemoglobin made up of four γ-globin chains. The involved fetus has a profound anemia with marked extramedullary hematopoiesis, hepatosplenomegaly, and anasarca. These children die in utero or soon after birth.

Laboratory Studies

The **routine complete blood count (CBC)** and **peripheral blood film** provide the first clues to the presence of a thalassemia (Table 6–2). **Thalassemia minor** patients demonstrate microcytosis (a mean cell volume [MCV] less than 75 fL) and hypochromia with little or no anemia. Because the microcytosis is quite uniform, the red blood cell distribution width (RDW) is not increased. The peripheral blood film is microcytic and hypochromic but shows little anisocytosis, poikilocytosis, or polychromasia. Many red blood cells are targeted. This situation shows that the reduction in intracellular hemoglobin is not always matched by an equal reduction in cell membrane; excess membrane tends to accumulate in the center of the cell, which causes the target shape.

Thalassemia intermedia and thalassemia major patients present with a much more dramatic picture. Their anemia is more severe and the microcytosis and

Table 6–1. Clinical classification of thalassemia.

Clinical Class	Genotype	Severity
Thalassemia minor		
β-thalassemia trait	β/β^0	
α^0-thalassemia trait	$--/\alpha\alpha$	Microcytosis, hypochromia, mild anemia (Hemoglobin 10–14 g/dL)
Hemoglobin Constant Spring	$\alpha^{CS}/\alpha\alpha^{CS}$	
α^+-thalassemia trait	$-\alpha/-\alpha$	
Lepore trait	$\beta/(\delta\beta)^{+Lepore}$	
δβ-thalassemia trait	$\beta/(\delta\beta)^{0\ or\ +}$	
$(\delta\beta)^0$ HPFH homozygotes	$(\delta\beta)^0 HPFH\beta/(\delta\beta)^0 HPFH$	
Thalassemia intermedia		
$\beta^{+Africa}$-thalassemia	$\beta^{+Africa}/\beta^{+Africa}$	
α^+ and β^0-thalassemia double heterozygote	$-\alpha/-\alpha/\beta/\beta^0$	Microcytosis, hypochromia, moderate anemia
β^0-thalassemia major with high hemoglobin F	β^0/β^0 with increased F production	
$(\delta\beta)^{0\ or\ +/Lepore}$ homozygotes	$(\delta\beta)^{0\ or\ +Lepore}/(\delta\beta)^{0\ or\ +Lepore}$	
Thalassemia major		
β^0 thalassemia major	β^0/β^0	Severe microcytosis, hypochromia, and severe anemia (Hemoglobin 3–6 g/dL)
β^0/hemoglobin E disease	β^0/β^E	
Hemoglobin H disease		
α^+ and α^0 double heterozygote	$--/-\alpha$	Microcytosis, hypochromia, moderate anemia with reticulocytosis
α^0 and Constant Spring double heterozygote	$--/\alpha\alpha^{CS}$	

hypochromia are much more pronounced. There is a greater amount of anisocytosis and poikilocytosis on the peripheral film with a concomitant increase in the RDW. Polychromasia and targeting are also much more pronounced.

A. Marrow and Iron Studies:

Although examination of the marrow is usually not required to detect or diagnose thalassemia in a patient, it does provide information regarding the level of ineffective erythropoiesis and complications such as folic acid or iron deficiency. In some populations, the incidence of iron deficiency can compete with that of thalassemia minor, or both defects can be present simultaneously. **Accurate diagnosis of thalassemia minor** in this situation requires measurements of the SI, TIBC, and ferritin level, and at times, a careful inspection of a marrow specimen stained with Prussian blue.

Patients with thalassemia intermedia and thalassemia major show high levels of ineffective erythropoiesis.

This situation results in an erythropoietic profile that is quite distinctive from that of iron deficiency (Table 6–3). The **marrow of the severe thalassemia patient** is very hyperplastic, with the ratio of erythroid to granulocytic precursors (E/G ratio) easily exceeding 1:1 or 2:1. Since most of the proliferating erythroid cells fail to complete maturation and die within the marrow, the reticulocyte index is lower than expected for the degree of erythroid hyperplasia. In addition, measurements of cell turnover including the lactic dehydrogenase (LDH) level and serum indirect bilirubin are both elevated.

Although severe iron deficiency can cause a degree of ineffective erythropoiesis, the **severely iron-deficient marrow** is never as hyperplastic, the E/G ratio does not exceed 1:1, and even though the reticulocyte index is usually low, the serum bilirubin and LDH levels are never increased. The most obvious difference, however, is that patients with thalassemia intermedia and major show a marked tendency to iron loading. They exhibit high SI levels even to full saturation of the TIBC, very

Table 6–2. Blood count patterns in thalassemia.

	Minor	Intermedia	Major
Hemoglobin (g/dL)	10–14	6–10	< 6
MCV (fL)	60–80	50–70	50–60
MCH (pg)	28–32	22–28	16–22
RDW-CV (9–12%)	Normal	Slightly increased	Increased
Film Microcytosis, hypochromia	Mild	Moderate	Severe
Polychromasia	Very little	Moderate	Marked
Anisocytosis	None	Moderate	Marked
Poikilocytosis	None	Moderate	Marked
Targeting	Present	Present	Present

high serum ferritin levels, and increased reticuloendothelial stores on the marrow aspirate. In contrast, iron-deficient patients show low SI levels, low ferritin levels, and absent stores (see Chapter 5 for further discussion).

B. HEMOGLOBIN ANALYSIS AND QUANTITATION:

Definitive diagnosis and classification of thalassemia requires quantitative measurement of cellular hemoglobins, including hemoglobins A, A_2, F, and H. In populations with a high incidence of double heterozygotes for other hemoglobinopathies, tests must be performed to identify other abnormal hemoglobins, including S, C, E, Lepore, and Constant Spring. Clinical laboratories routinely perform hemoglobin electrophoresis to identify these common hemoglobinopathies, as well as quantitative measurements of both hemoglobin A_2 and F to help diagnose β-thalassemia. A qualitative measure of red blood cell hemoglobin H is possible using the

Table 6–3. Erythropoietic profiles of thalassemia and iron deficiency.

	Thalassemia	Iron Deficiency
Anemia	Minor to severe	Minor to severe
MCV (fL)	< 70	< 80
Film morphology	Microcytic, hypochromic with prominent targeting	Normal to microcytic, hypochromic with pencil forms, no targeting
Reticulocyte index	< 2	< 2
Marrow E/G ratio	> 2:1	1:1–1:3
Serum iron/TIBC	Increased/normal	Very low/increased
Percent saturation	> 50	< 10
Marrow iron stores	Increased	Absent
Serum ferritin (μg/L)	> 100	< 12
Bilirubin/LDH	Increased	Normal

supravital stain, **brilliant cresyl blue.** Quantitation is possible by **starch gel electrophoresis.**

1. Electrophoresis techniques—Electrophoresis techniques commonly used in diagnosing hemoglobinopathies are cellulose acetate, starch, and agar gel with either an alkaline or acid buffer. **Cellulose acetate electrophoresis** with an alkaline buffer is used to initially screen blood samples for common hemoglobinopathies such as S and C. This method can also be used to quantitate hemoglobin A_2. **Citrate agar electrophoresis** with an acid buffer is used to confirm the results of a cellulose acetate study. It is especially valuable in separating hemoglobin C from hemoglobins A and S in infants. Electrophoresis of globin chains after separation from their heme groups using both **citrate agar and cellulose acetate** makes it possible to separate many of the hemoglobin subtypes without expensive structural analysis.

2. Test for quantitating the amount of hemoglobin F—The clinical laboratory also offers a test for quantitating the amount of hemoglobin F (the **alkaline denaturation test for hemoglobin F**). This test takes advantage of the greater resistance of hemoglobin F to denaturation by strong alkali. The same principle has been used to assess amounts of hemoglobin F in individual red blood cells. The acid elution slide test for hemoglobin F (**Kleihauer-Betke acid elution test**) uses a citric acid-phosphate buffer to elute the hemoglobin A from the cells. The hemoglobin F remains behind and

can then be stained with hematoxylin & eosin. Normal quantities of these hemoglobins and the most common patterns for both the β- and α-thalassemias are summarized in Tables 6–4 and 6–5.

3. β-Thalassemia minor—Patients with β-thalassemia minor due to either a gene deletion ($β^0$) or mutation ($β^+$) can be identified from the slight elevation in fetal hemoglobin and an increase in the hemoglobin A_2 level to between 4% and 7%. Confusion can arise if the patient is iron deficient because this will lower the hemoglobin A_2 level to normal. It is essential, therefore, that iron studies be run simultaneously to exclude this possibility.

4. β-Thalassemia intermedia or β-Thalassemia major—Patients with β-thalassemia intermedia or β-thalassemia major are easily identified from their severe microcytosis and hypochromia and markedly increased levels of hemoglobin F on electrophoresis. Hemoglobin A_2 levels are variable and can be reduced, normal, or slightly increased. β-Thalassemia can present as a double heterozygote with α-thalassemia or another β-hemoglobinopathy gene, such as hemoglobin S, C, or E. The most important clinically is the sickle/thalassemia combination. This situation is suggested by microcytosis, hypochromia, and some targeting in a patient who otherwise presents with sickle cell anemia. The electrophoresis pattern should make it possible to accurately diagnose this genetic defect (Table 6–6). If the patient has a mutational defect ($β^+$), the quantity of

Table 6–4. Hemoglobin patterns in β-thalassemia variants.

	Hemoglobin (%)				
	A	*F*	*A₂*	*Lepore*	*S*
Normal	97	< 1	2–3	0	0
β-Thalassemia minor					
Trait β/β$^{0 \text{ or } +}$	90–95	1–5	4–7[a]	—	—
Lepore trait β/(δβ)$^{+Lepore}$	80	1–5	2–3	15	—
β-Thalassemia intermedia					
β$^{+Africa}$/β$^{+Africa}$	30–50	50–70	0–5	—	—
β-Thalassemia major					
β^0/β^0	0	95–100	0–5	—	—
(δβ)$^{+Lepore}$/(δβ)$^{+Lepore}$	0	80	0	20	—

[a] Iron deficiency can lower the hemoglobin A_2 level to normal.

Table 6–5. Hemoglobin patterns in α-thalassemia variants.

	Hemoglobin (%)			
	A	**H(β₄)**	**Bart's (γ₄) (at birth only)**	**Constant Spring**
Normal	97	0	0	0
α⁺-Thalassemia silent –α/αα	98–100	0	(0–2)	0
α⁰-thalassemia trait –α/–α(homozygous α⁺)	85–95	Red blood cell inclusions	(5–15)	5
or				
––/αα (heterozygous α⁰) ααᶜˢ/ααᶜˢ	85–95	0	(5–15)	5
Hemoglobin H disease ––/–α(α⁰/α⁺) ––/ααᶜˢ (α⁰/αᶜˢ)	70–95 60–90	5–30 5–30	trace trace	trace 5–10
Hydrops fetalis ––/––(α⁰/α⁰)	0	5–10	90–95	0

hemoglobin S will be greater than hemoglobin A. This is distinctly different from the pattern seen with hemoglobin S trait where the quantity of hemoglobin A (60–70%) always exceeds hemoglobin S (30–40%). It can be more difficult to discriminate the patient with a deletion defect (β⁰) where no hemoglobin A is produced. However, β⁰/βˢ patients show a significant mi-

crocytosis and hypochromia, which are not explained by iron deficiency and are not typical of sickle cell anemia.

5. α-Thalassemia—The most common hemoglobin patterns for α-thalassemia are summarized in Table 6–5. When only one of the four α-globin chain genes is de-

Table 6–6. Hemoglobin patterns in combined hemoglobinopathies.

	Hemoglobin (%)			
	A	**F**	**A₂**	**E/S/C**
Normal	97	< 1	2–3	0
Hemoglobin E				E
Trait β/βᴱ	60–65	1–2	2–3	30–35
Homozygous βᴱ/βᴱ	0	0	5	95
E/β Thal βᴱ/β⁰	0	45	1–5	40–50
Hemoglobin S				S
Trait β/βˢ	60–70	1–2	2–3	30–40
Homozygous βˢ/βˢ	0	5–30	—	70–95
S/β Thal βˢ/β⁰	0	5–15	—	80–90
βˢ/β⁺	20–30	5–15	—	50–70
Hemoglobin C				C
Trait β/βᶜ	55–65		3–5	30–40
Homozygous βᶜ/βᶜ	0	5–10	—	90–95
C/B Thal βᶜ/β⁰	0	5–10	—	90–95
βᶜ/β⁺	20–30	5–10	—	60–75

fective, the patient has little clinical disease and the condition can only be detected at birth from presence of a small amount of Bart's hemoglobin, a hemoglobin made up of four γ-globin chains. Heterozygous α^0 and homozygous α^+ patients show microcytosis, hypochromia, and a mild anemia, suggesting thalassemia minor. In contrast to those with β-thalassemia minor, however, they have normal hemoglobin F and A_2 levels. Hemoglobin H inclusions can be detected in occasional red blood cells using the brilliant cresyl blue stain but not on electrophoresis. Definitive diagnosis of α-thalassemia minor requires electrophoresis at birth when from 5% to 15% Bart's hemoglobin is present. Patients who are double heterozygotes for hemoglobin Constant Spring also have up to 15% Bart's hemoglobin at birth and approximately 5% hemoglobin Constant Spring as adults.

6. Hemoglobin H disease and hydrops fetalis— **Hemoglobin H disease** is produced when a patient is a double heterozygote for α^0 and α^+ or α^0 and hemoglobin Constant Spring. In both situations, only one α gene is truly operating. In the adult, hemoglobin H disease is detected using starch gel electrophoresis where from 5% to 30% of hemoglobin H is present with small amounts of both Bart's hemoglobin and hemoglobin Constant Spring. Finally, a deletion of all four α-globin chain genes results in the condition called **hydrops fetalis,** where only Bart's and hemoglobin H are produced. This is not compatible with life and results either in fetal wastage or death soon after delivery.

7. Hemoglobin E (β^E)/thalassemia—Hemoglobin E (β^E)/thalassemia is an important double heterozygote, especially in Southeast Asia. Hemoglobin E can be combined with either β- or α-thalassemia and, depending on the type of thalassemia gene, will have a variable clinical presentation. The hemoglobin pattern of patients with hemoglobin β^E/β^0-thalassemia shows hemoglobins E, F, and A_2 but not hemoglobin A.

C. MOLECULAR DIAGNOSIS:

Detection of the actual mutation responsible for the thalassemia is now possible using polymerase chain reaction (PCR) together with primer-specific probes complementary to the most common mutations. More than 200 different mutations have been described in patients with β-thalassemia, but fewer than 10 mutations are responsible for the majority of cases. When one of these common mutations is not detected the gene defect can be determined by direct sequencing.

Most β-thalassemias are due to a point mutation involving one or several nucleotides that then interferes with the coding of the gene; rarely is there gross dele-

tion of the β-gene. Other mutations result in abnormal splicing or a defect in RNA processing. The location of the gene mutation determines hematological phenotype, whether β^0, β^+, or a complex thalassemia such as $(\delta\beta)^{0 \text{ or } +}$-thalassemia, where there is a partial deletion of both the δ- and β-gene. Mutations in or near to the promoter sequences and in the 5' untranslated regions of the gene interfere with transcription and usually result in mild (β^+)-thalassemia. Mutations that interfere with translation of the globin chain tend to produce severe (β^0)-thalassemia. Molecular diagnosis has also helped identify compound heterozygotes with more severe disease.

DIAGNOSIS

Initial detection and diagnosis of a thalassemia depends to a large extent on the severity of the gene defect. **Silent carrier states,** by definition, cause no clinical illness and will not be picked up by screening programs. These individuals can only be detected as a part of a family analysis. **Thalassemia minor patients** will be identified during screening programs, as a part of routine health maintenance, or less frequently, because of a clinical symptom or sign relating to their hematologic defect. In contrast, **patients with thalassemia intermedia or thalassemia major** require medical attention because of their anemia. β-Thalassemia major is often identified early in childhood because of the severe anemia, if not at birth, as a result of prenatal screening of the parents.

Initial Detection

Stepwise diagnostic strategies for detecting and diagnosing thalassemias have been developed by national screening programs. Figure 6–4 gives an example of one such algorithm. Another entry point to the diagnosis of thalassemia is the **detection of some combination of anemia, microcytosis, and hypochromia on the routine CBC.** Since these patients are at equal or greater risk for an iron deficiency state, testing for iron deficiency with measurements of SI, TIBC, serum ferritin, and red blood cell protoporphyrin can be highly productive. At the same time, however, it is expensive. As an alternative, young patients who are at little or no risk of pathologic blood loss can be treated with oral iron therapy for 2–3 months followed by a repeated CBC. Correction of the anemia and microcytosis will rule against but not necessarily rule out thalassemia.

A. THALASSEMIA MINOR VERSUS IRON DEFICIENCY:

Some simple hematologic observations can help discriminate between thalassemia minor and iron deficiency.

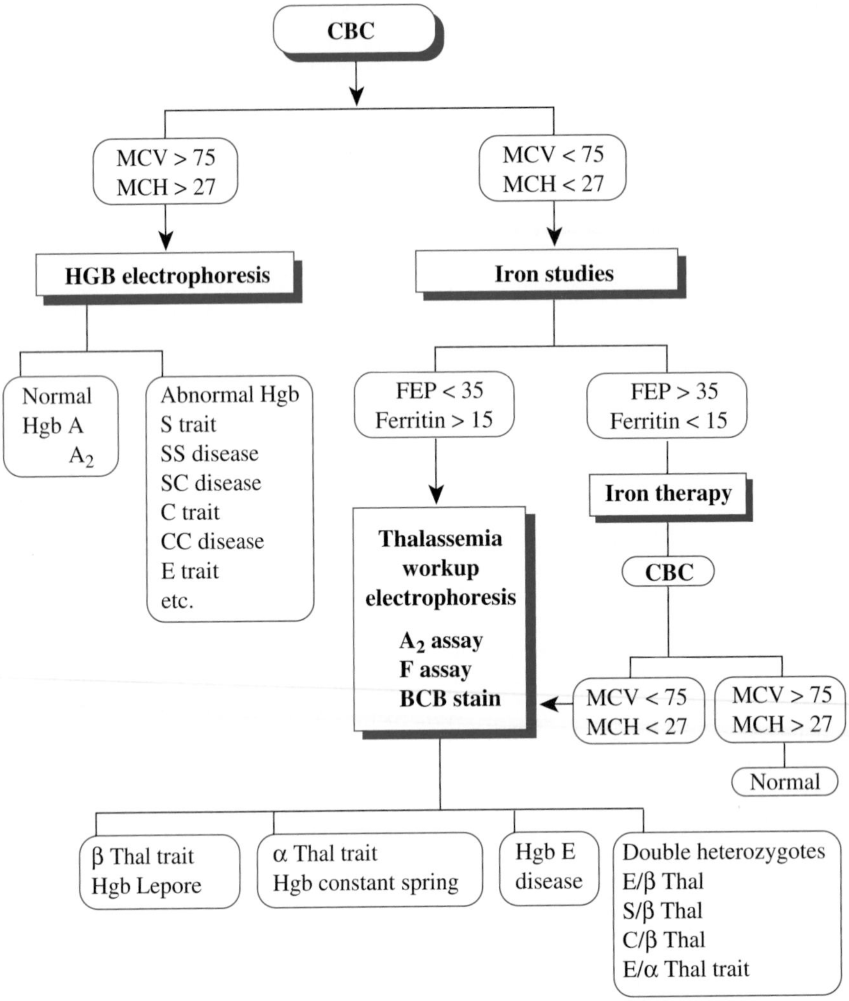

Figure 6–4. **Stepwise approach to the diagnosis of the thalassemias.** The CBC, free erythrocyte protoporphyria (FEP), hemoglobin electrophoresis, and measurements of iron supply can be used to separate patients with iron deficiency anemia from those with hemoglobinopathies.

The first is the **degree of microcytosis versus the severity of the anemia.** As a rule, **thalassemia minor patients** have more severe microcytosis (MCV below 75 fL), at a time when there is little or no anemia. In addition, they usually have a normal RDW, which indicates a uniform population of microcytic cells. The **iron deficient patient** is just the opposite. Microcytosis is not seen until the hemoglobin falls below 10–11 grams per deciliter for some period of time. An exception is the **patient with polycythemia vera** where the increased drive for red blood cell production will result in prominent microcytosis even while the hemoglobin/hematocrit is normal or increased. In addition, the RDW in iron-deficient patients is usually increased, indicating a mixed population of microcytic and normocytic cells.

Inspection of the film provides additional clues. **Patients with α- and β-thalassemia minor** show a uniform population of microcytic, hypochromic cells with frequent target cells. In contrast, **iron deficiency anemia patients** show a mixed population of small and normal-sized cells (**anisocytosis**) with variable hypochromia. More important, targeting is not a common feature of iron deficiency; instead, these patients will show occasional pencil-shaped red blood cells.

B. COMBINATION ANEMIAS:

Since populations at risk for thalassemia are also at risk for iron deficiency, combination anemias are clearly possible. The patient who presents with a hematocrit below 35% with an MCV less than 70 fL, an RDW that is above normal, and a film showing anisocytosis, poikilocytosis, and target cells must be considered for a combined abnormality. The situation can be made more complicated by the presence of other disease. For example, a **vitamin deficiency state or liver disease,** both of which are common in populations at risk for thalassemia, can affect all elements of the CBC, including the severity of the anemia, the MCV, RDW, and film morphology.

Prenatal Diagnosis

For high-risk populations, **prospective screening programs** have been established to identify young individuals at risk for transmitting a thalassemia gene to their children. The more frequent the expression of an abnormal gene(s), the more likely that couples will be at risk of producing a child with double heterozygous or homozygous thalassemia. Screening should be provided by a well-organized, skilled professional group that not only can accurately diagnose the genetic defect but also has experience in counseling affected individuals.

Another approach is to screen mothers at the time of their **first prenatal visit.** If the mother is a thalassemia carrier, the father should also be evaluated. When there is a risk of the child being a homozygote or double heterozygote (ie, having thalassemia major or intermedia), prenatal diagnosis is possible using the techniques of fetal blood sampling or chorionic villus biopsy. The latter can be performed as early as the ninth week of gestation and diagnosis made by direct analysis of fetal DNA. Testing methods are still in evolution. DNA analysis using restriction fragment length polymorphism (RFLP) analysis or PCR with oligonucleotide probes to compare fetal and parental DNA are now in use.

Prenatal diagnosis is essential for the pregnant woman who has already had an affected child, especially a child with β-thalassemia intermedia or major, or homozygous α^0 (hydrops fetalis). When both parents are carriers of a severe form of thalassemia (β^0 or α^0), accurate prenatal diagnosis makes it possible to offer a therapeutic abortion during the first trimester.

DIFFERENTIAL DIAGNOSIS

The differential diagnosis of the various thalassemias can appear to be a daunting task. Despite the large number of genetic defects and combinations of defects, however, individual thalassemias present as one of only a half a dozen clinical vignettes. This fact is of great value not only in selecting and interpreting the necessary laboratory tests but also in organizing the differential diagnosis and treatment plan.

Silent Carrier States

Thalassemia in these patients is rarely detected since they have no hematologic disease; their CBC and blood film are normal. The existence of thalassemia can be discovered during a family study initiated because of disease in a sibling or offspring. The most common silent carrier states are β^+-thalassemia minor, $\alpha^{0 \text{ or } +}$-thalassemia single-gene defects, and heterozygous hemoglobin Constant Spring.

Microcytosis With Little or No Anemia

These patients present with a normal to slightly reduced hemoglobin level, a definite microcytosis (MCV below 75 fL), and hypochromia. They are not clinically symptomatic and not at risk for iron overload. In fact, they run a greater risk of iron deficiency, which can make diagnosis difficult. All patients who present with what appears to be thalassemia minor should be tested for iron deficiency with an SI, TIBC, and serum ferritin level.

A. MOST COMMON GENOTYPES:

The most common genotypes responsible for thalassemia minor include heterozygous β^0-thalassemia, $(\delta\beta)^{0 \text{ or } + \text{ (Lepore)}}$-thalassemia, $(\delta\beta)^0$ HPFH, homozygous α^+-thalassemia, and heterozygous α^0-thalassemia (see Table 6–1). As long as the patient is not iron deficient, patients with β-thalassemia minor will show an increased level of hemoglobin A_2 (4–7%), with a slight increase in hemoglobin F. Patients with $(\delta\beta)^0$-thalassemia, patients with hemoglobin Lepore trait, and $\alpha\beta$ compound heterozygotes will show normal hemoglobin A_2 and F levels. Patients with $(\delta\beta)^0$ HPFH show levels of hemoglobin F that approach 100%. Patients with α^0- and α^+-thalassemia demonstrate small amounts of Bart's hemoglobin at birth and occasional hemoglobin H red blood cell inclusions on blood films stained with crystal violet. Finally, patients with homozygous hemoglobin Constant Spring show small amounts of Bart's hemoglobin at birth and up to 5% hemoglobin Constant Spring as adults.

B. α-THALASSEMIAS:

α-Thalassemias, both α^0 and α^+, are most common in Asian populations. This situation sets the stage for the inheritance of a double gene defect to produce a more severe form of α-thalassemia, either hemoglobin H disease or hydrops fetalis. In Africa, the α^0 genotype is very rare. Thus, only heterozygous and homozygous forms of

α^+ are observed in blacks. The first of these is a silent carrier state, whereas the homozygotes show clinical manifestations of thalassemia minor. Hemoglobin H disease and hydrops fetalis are less common in blacks. They do occur in Mediterranean and Arabian populations secondary to nondeletion mutations of the α gene.

Moderate Anemia With Marked Microcytosis

These patients present with a definite anemia and marked microcytosis (MCV less than 70 fL) and hypochromia on the blood film. They commonly seek medical attention because of symptoms and signs related to their anemia. Splenomegaly, skeletal changes secondary to marrow expansion, and cardiomegaly are usually present, and patients are at risk for iron overload. This situation can worsen if the patient requires chronic blood transfusions.

This hematologic picture is typical of patients with thalassemia intermedia (see Table 6–1). Principal causes genetically are homozygous β-thalassemia of the $\beta^{+\ Africa}$ subtype, coinheritance of α- and β-thalassemia, compound heterozygosity for two mild β-globin gene mutations, or homozygous β-thalassemia with variably increased hemoglobin F production. Rarely, a mutation at the third exon of the β-globin gene will result in an intermedia phenotype despite a β-trait genotype.

Severe Anemia & Microcytosis

During the first year or two of life, these patients present with a severe, life-threatening anemia, marked microcytosis (MCV less than 60 fL), and hypochromia with pronounced targeting on the blood film. Symptoms and signs of anemia are striking. Children require long-term transfusion to function. They also manifest marked splenomegaly, skeletal changes secondary to marrow expansion, growth and sexual retardation, and aggressive iron loading even without transfusion. Without treatment, affected children will die of heart failure during the first two decades of life.

This presentation is typical of patients with thalassemia major. Principal genetic mutations responsible are homozygous deletion (β^0) and nondeletion (β^+) forms of β-thalassemia, and the compound heterozygote for β-thalassemia and hemoglobin E (β^E). Hemoglobin electrophoresis patterns show mostly hemoglobin F with little or no hemoglobin A.

Hemolytic Anemia & Microcytosis

These patients present with mild to moderate anemia (hemoglobin 7–10 grams per deciliter), an elevated reticulocyte count, and microcytosis and hypochromia with targeting on the blood film. Their erythropoietic profile is more typical of a hemolytic anemia than the ineffective erythropoiesis seen with thalassemia intermedia or major. Moreover, their clinical course is characteristic of hemolysis. Most patients have splenomegaly and exhibit reticulocytopenic crises in response to infections and exposure to oxidant drugs.

This clinical pattern is typical of patients with hemoglobin H disease secondary to deletion of 3 α-globin genes—the double heterozygote for α^0 and α^+ and the compound heterozygote α^0 and hemoglobin Constant Spring. The **definitive test for hemoglobin H disease** is demonstration of excess hemoglobin H by starch gel electrophoresis or supravital stain of blood with brilliant crystal blue (or both). Depending on severity of the illness and whether the patient has had a splenectomy, 5–30% of the hemoglobin on electrophoresis will be hemoglobin H (β_4). If blood is tested at birth, red blood cells will contain up to 40% Bart's hemoglobin. Patients with α^0/hemoglobin Constant Spring show 5–10% hemoglobin Constant Spring on electrophoresis in addition to the hemoglobin H.

The **supravital stain film** shows a mix of heavily stained reticulocytes and cells with a fine, lightly stained, granular inclusion pattern. The latter are the cells that contain hemoglobin H. If the patient has a functional spleen, only a small number of circulating cells will have hemoglobin H inclusions. After splenectomy, virtually all cells will be filled with inclusions, reflecting the loss of the pitting function of the spleen.

Lethal Defect

Asian couples who are carriers for α^0 are at risk for producing a fetus that is homozygous for α^0. This lethal defect results in death in utero or shortly after birth. The fetuses have a characteristic appearance with marked anasarca, hepatosplenomegaly, and extramedullary hematopoiesis. On hemoglobin electrophoresis, only Bart's hemoglobin can be detected.

Compound Hemoglobinopathies

Both α- and β-thalassemia can present as a double heterozygote with another β-globin hemoglobinopathy gene. Most common combinations are with hemoglobin S, C, and E. The clinical presentation combines aspects of both gene defects. The incidence of the various combinations is geographically quite different. Combinations of hemoglobin E with thalassemia, as well as homozygous E disease, which clinically resembles thalassemia minor, are limited to Southeast Asia. Hemoglobin S and C/thalassemia have a more worldwide distribution.

A. HEMOGLOBIN E/β-THALASSEMIA:

Hemoglobin E results from a β-**globin chain defect** (substitution of lysine for glutamic acid at position 26), which interferes with mRNA processing and the synthesis of β^E-globin chains. Moreover, the β^E hemoglobin is unstable, which further contributes to production of microcytosis and hypochromia. Both heterozygous and homozygous forms of hemoglobin E disease show microcytosis (MCV less than 75 fL) and hypochromia with prominent targeting on the blood film. Heterozygotes are not anemic and the homozygous state is associated with a mild anemia similar to that observed with β-thalassemia minor. The **incidence** of hemoglobin E disease in Southeast Asian populations is extremely high. A 30–40% gene frequency for hemoglobin E has been reported for the Khmer populations in Cambodia and Thailand, and the double heterozygote—hemoglobin E/β-thalassemia is the most frequent serious hemoglobinopathy in the world.

Patients with hemoglobin E/β-thalassemia can have **clinical features** of severe β-thalassemia major or much milder disease, resembling thalassemia minor or intermedia. In part, this reflects genetic factors such as the nature of the β-thalassemia mutation, level of hemoglobin F, and coinheritance of α-thalassemia. The latter can result in a much milder phenotype. Environmental factors, such as exposure to infections, may also play a role. **Children with severe disease** usually require chronic transfusion and are at risk for iron loading. The severity of the clinical condition clearly separates hemoglobin E/β-thalassemia from homozygous hemoglobin E disease. Hemoglobin electrophoresis will also separate the conditions (see Table 6–6).

B. Hemoglobin S/Thalassemia:

The double heterozygote, hemoglobin S (β^S)- and β-thalassemia, is most commonly seen in African and Mediterranean populations. These patients present with the symptoms and signs of sickle cell anemia, including typically painful, vasoocclusive crises. In contrast to those with homozygous S sickle cell anemia, most patients have splenomegaly. Otherwise, their symptoms, signs, and clinical course are the same.

The **erythropoietic profile** shows features of both gene defects. Patients are moderately to severely anemic, microcytic (MCV less than 65 fL), and hypochromic with prominent poikilocytosis and targeting. Sickle cells may be seen, but are rare in patients with intact spleens. Following splenectomy, sickle cell forms are common. The **hemoglobin electrophoresis pattern** also reflects the double gene defect (see Table 6–6). Patients with a β-globin chain deletion defect can have a pattern identical to that of homozygous SS disease; patients with hemoglobin β^S/β^+-thalassemia can show small amounts of hemoglobin A, increased amounts of hemoglobin F, and up to 7% hemoglobin A_2.

Hemoglobin S can also be inherited together with $(\delta\beta)^0$-thalassemia or hemoglobin Lepore $(\delta\beta)^{+Lepore}$-thal-

assemia, resulting in a moderately severe hemolytic anemia with splenomegaly. The patient's CBC is microcytic and hypochromic with prominent targeting on the blood film. These patients tend to have milder disease with few if any painful vasoocclusive events, perhaps because of increased amounts of hemoglobins Lepore and F. **Patients with hemoglobin β^S/$(\delta\beta)$-thalassemia** present with a much milder disease. They are not anemic and do not have vasoocclusive events. Their CBCs do show microcytosis, hypochromia, targeting, and occasional sickle cells. Here again, concentrations of hemoglobin F from 20% to 40% appear to be protective.

C. Hemoglobin C/Thalassemia:

In Mediterranean and African populations, hemoglobin C can be inherited as a double heterozygote with β-thalassemia. Hemoglobin β^C/β^0-thalassemia is associated with a moderately severe hemolytic anemia, splenomegaly, and a microcytic, hypochromic red blood cell population. In blacks, hemoglobin C is often associated with the β^+-thalassemia gene producing a milder disease. In both situations, the peripheral blood film shows close to 100% targeting of red blood cells.

THERAPY

Management of a patient with thalassemia varies according to the severity of the anemia. **Heterozygote patients with α- and β-thalassemia** are not clinically symptomatic, have only a mild anemia, and are not at risk for iron overload. They should be reassured of the benign nature of the inherited defect, and when appropriate, counseled regarding the risks of transmitting the defect with childbearing. **Thalassemia minor patients** should not receive long-term iron therapy and do not require folic acid supplementation.

Patients with thalassemia intermedia or major who are homozygotes or double heterozygotes for α- or β-thalassemia will require almost continuous medical attention beginning early in childhood. Principal management issues include transfusion support, the prevention of iron overload, and the management of hypersplenism. Thalassemia major patients represent the greatest challenge. **Children with the homozygous, deletional form of β-thalassemia** (β^0/β^0) present during the first year of life with severe, life-threatening anemia. Their survival depends on a carefully orchestrated program of transfusion support and iron chelation therapy to prevent iron overload and tissue toxicity.

Transfusion Therapy

The decision to initiate a program of chronic transfusion will depend on the type of gene defect and the severity of the anemia. In general, **children with β-thalassemia major and hemoglobins of less than 6–7 grams per deciliter** should receive chronic transfusions. It is important to start early before the child has a chance to develop splenomegaly and hypersplenism, or exhibit skeletal changes and growth retardation. It is also important to establish a reliable, routine transfusion schedule that maintains hemoglobin levels of 9–10 grams per deciliter. Below this level, the marrow will be stimulated to maintain a high level of ineffective erythropoiesis. This will lead to expansion of the marrow cavity, causing skeletal changes and increasing the splenomegaly and hypersplenism. Metabolic requirements of the expanded marrow will also result in growth retardation. Erythropoiesis will be suppressed when the hemoglobin is kept close to 10 grams per deciliter. Transfusion to levels higher than 10 grams per deciliter increases the risk of organ damage from iron loading.

A. REDUCING RISKS OF TRANSFUSION:

Care should always be taken to reduce potential risks of transfusion. Early in life, children should be immunized for hepatitis B. They should also be monitored for the development of minor blood group antibodies and should receive only leukopoor packed red blood cells. If over time, a patient does develop HLA alloantibodies and exhibits febrile reactions with transfusion, he or she can be premedicated with acetaminophen (Tylenol) and diphenhydramine (Benadryl).

B. TRANSFUSION REQUIREMENTS:

Transfusion requirements will obviously vary according to the patient's age and physical size. As a general rule, it should be possible to maintain hemoglobin levels of 10 grams per deciliter with a transfusion of 12–15 mL/kg of packed red blood cells every 3–4 weeks. This requirement can increase if the patient develops significant red blood cell antibodies or hypersplenism. The latter is signaled by the development of increasing splenomegaly, splenic discomfort, and on occasion, infarction. When the yearly red blood cell transfusion requirement exceeds 250–300 mL/kg, hypersplenism is almost certainly present and a therapeutic splenectomy should be considered. If performed, both pneumococcal and *Haemophilus influenzae* type B vaccine should be given prior to surgery.

Iron Chelation Therapy

Severe iron overload is another major threat to the survival of the thalassemia major patient. Iron absorption is increased in all thalassemic patients with high levels of ineffective erythropoiesis, so they are at risk for iron overload even without transfusion. Abnormal iron absorption can increase body iron from 2–5 grams each year, depending on the severity of the anemia and ineffective erythropoiesis. Chronic transfusion therapy only worsens the situation. Therefore, such patients must be considered as early candidates for iron chelation therapy with deferoxamine (DF).

A. THERAPY IN CHILDREN:

Children with thalassemia major should begin therapy at the earliest possible age and certainly by the time they have accumulated more than 7 grams of excess iron. In young children, a serum ferritin level much greater than 1000 μg/L or 1 year of regular transfusions (or both) can be used as surrogate indicators to initiate chelation therapy.

B. MONITORING IRON CONCENTRATION:

Correlation of ferritin levels with tissue iron loading is less than precise. Severe ineffective erythropoiesis, hepatic damage, ascorbate deficiency, and inflammation can all interfere with the serum ferritin/iron overload relationship. Therefore, liver biopsy with quantitative measurement of hepatic iron concentration is the gold standard. Normal individuals have hepatic iron concentrations of approximately 1–2 mg/g dry weight tissue, whereas heterozygotes for the hemachromatosis gene show levels of 3–7 mg. Concentrations exceeding 15 mg/g dry weight tissue are associated with progressive organ damage and early death.

C. TREATMENT WITH DEFEROXAMINE:

The most reliable therapy for the control of iron overload is the subcutaneous or intravenous administration of the iron chelator DF. DF can be administered at the time of red blood cell transfusions and subcutaneously during sleep hours using a syringe pump. Using a dose of 25–50 mg/kg of DF infused over 12 hours each day, it should be possible to maintain a negative iron balance despite the high level of iron absorption and red blood cell transfusions. In adults with severe iron overload and life-threatening cardiac disease, DF can be administered as a continuous intravenous infusion through a central venous catheter in doses of 40–100 mg/kg/day. This will more rapidly unload iron from tissues and improve cardiac function. It is especially of value for the rapid and sustained reversal of life-threatening cardiac arrhythmias.

Survival can be correlated with the hepatic iron concentration or the patient's mean ferritin level. If periodic ferritin levels fall below 2500 μg/L, children can expect a better than 90% survival at 15 years. When most values fall above 2500 μg/L, only 20% of children will survive 15 years without cardiac disease. Repeated liver biopsy can be used to give a definitive measure of iron control. Follow-up liver biopsy can be important in children who receive treatment at an early age with a lower dose of DF, 25 mg/kg/day, to guarantee effective therapy as they grow. The therapeutic goal is to keep the hepatic iron concentration between 3 and 7 mg/g dry weight tissue.

DF therapy is not without its **complications.** Some children may be unable to tolerate the drug because of local skin reactions. Other children are at risk for the development of neurotoxic side effects, including changes in visual acuity with central scotomata and impaired color vision, as well as the appearance of a high-frequency auditory sensory deficit. These abnormalities are dose-related, most often seen in patients receiving more than 50 mg/kg/day of DF, and can be reversed by reducing the dose. Since the chance for DF toxicity increases as the iron burden falls, a useful rule of thumb is to **keep the ratio of the daily DF (in mg/kg) dose to the serum ferritin level (in μg/L) below 0.025.** It is also important to monitor the patient very closely with **periodic audiometry and eye examinations.**

D. Treatment With Deferipone:

Treatment with deferipone, an oral chelating preparation, does not control iron accumulation as well as DF therapy. Most patients will demonstrate a rise in their serum ferritin to levels greater than 2500 μg/L while receiving therapy. In patients treated with deferipone for 2–6 years, more than 50% accumulated 15 grams or more of hepatic iron and were at risk, therefore, for cardiac disease. In addition, adverse effects including arthralgias, joint effusions, nausea, zinc deficiency, reversible granulocytopenia, and aplastic anemia have been observed, requiring careful monitoring of therapy.

Augmentation of Fetal Hemoglobin Production

It is well recognized that coinheritance of hereditary persistence of fetal hemoglobin with homozygous β-thalassemia results in milder disease. This has led to studies of several agents that have been used in the treatment of sickle cell anemia, including 5-azacytidine, hydroxyurea, erythropoietin, and butyric acid compounds. Although some of these agents seem capable of increasing hemoglobin F production in the patient with thalassemia, none have as yet shown clear clinical efficacy.

Bone Marrow Transplantation

More than 1000 children and adults with thalassemia major have now received bone marrow transplants from HLA-identical siblings that have led to reversal of the genetic disorder. Children who undergo the procedure at an early age before iron overload and organ damage become problems do the best, with disease-free survivals of better than 90%. Overall survival falls to 60–70% and disease-free survival falls to 50% in older patients with disease-related complications, especially chronic active hepatitis. Marrow rejection and nonrejection mortality are both increased in these patients.

The procedure can result in a stable mixed chimerism. Clearly, the future of transplantation will involve transduction of globin encoding genes into the patient's own hematopoietic stem cells. Early clinical trials of this approach are now under way.

CLINICAL COURSE

Without long-term transfusion and iron chelation therapy, **children with thalassemia major** will not survive much past the second decade of life. In addition, they will exhibit major growth and sexual retardation. Complications from iron overloading include cardiac, hepatic, and endocrine abnormalities. Iron loading of myocardial muscle cells results first in diastolic and then systolic dysfunction, and life-threatening atrial and ventricular arrhythmias. Often arrhythmias are preceded by an episode of pericarditis. When a child has poorly controlled anemia and does not receive any iron chelation therapy, death will occur at an early age. **When patients with less severe thalassemia develop heart failure** during middle age, they should be aggressively treated with iron chelation therapy at a maximum dose. This procedure can result in an improvement in cardiac function.

As with hereditary hemachromatosis, iron overload in thalassemia can result in **cirrhosis and diabetes** (see Chapter 14). This situation can be prevented by effective iron chelation therapy during childhood. **Other endocrine abnormalities** include a marked failure of sexual development secondary to iron damage to the anterior pituitary. Children will fail to enter puberty and will have low levels of luteinizing and follicle-stimulating hormones. Once this occurs, it is irreversible by chelation therapy, and either testosterone or estrogen supplementation will be required to achieve sexual maturation. Finally, a few patients may present with **hypoparathyroidism,** characterized by tetany, hypocalcemia, and hyperphosphatemia.

The **survival potential** of well-treated thalassemic individuals is quite good. Patients should be followed up in a clinic experienced in the rigors of both transfusion and iron chelation therapy. Successful treatment and survival will depend on the patient's ability to comply with the treatment schedule. A few thalassemia major patients have been treated definitively by **allogeneic marrow transplantation.** There is, however, a significant risk of death as a part of the transplantation procedure, and patients are at risk for graft-versus-host disease.

BIBLIOGRAPHY

Angelucci E: Needle liver biopsy in thalassaemia: Analyses of diagnostic accuracy and safety in 1184 consecutive biopsies. Br J Haematol 1989;73:403.

Brittenham GM et al: Hepatic iron stores and plasma ferritin concentration in patients with sickle cell anemia and thalassemia major. Am J Hematol 1993;42:81.

Bunn HF, Forget BG: *Hemoglobin: Molecular, Genetic and Clinical Aspects.* WB Saunders, 1986.

Cao A et al: Molecular diagnosis and carrier screening for β-thalassemia. JAMA 1997;278:1273.

Cazzola M et al: Relationship between transfusion regimen and suppression of erythropoiesis in beta thalassemia major. Br J Haematol 1995;89:473.

Davis BA, Porter JB: Long-term outcome of continuous 24-h deferoxamine infusion via indwelling intravenous catheters in high-risk β-thalassemia. Blood 2000;95:1229.

Ehlers KH et al: Prolonged survival in patients with beta-thalassemia major treated with deferoxamine. J Pediatr 1991; 118:540.

Embury SH: Advances in the prenatal and molecular diagnosis of the hemoglobinopathies and thalassemias. Hemoglobin 1995;19:237.

Lucarelli G et al: Bone marrow transplantation in adult thalassemic patients. Blood 1999;93:1164.

Olivieri NF: The β-thalassemias. N Engl J Med 1999;341:99.

Olivieri NF, Brittenham GM: Iron-chelating therapy and the treatment of thalassemia. Blood 1997;89:739.

Hemoglobinopathies

7

Inherited defects in globin struct... form twisted
African, Indian, Asian, and ... ...d blood cell,
Most of these invo... ...ubstitutions
in one of th... ...tion of the
fect ca... ...moglobin-
mia. Si... ...ve now
valine fo... ...inically
chain, is... ...ts that
has a worl... ...finity
and it was... ...t of-
a molecular... ...ges
  Managem... ...ane-
depends not o... ...amino acid
der but also on... ...unique structural
sion of the defe... ...morphologically. The most
screening and g... ...t of these are hemoglobins S and C.
any increased pre...

NORMAL GLOB...

The globin portion o... ...e can be
defined according to c... α-globin and β-,
γ-, or δ-globin chains, ...no acid sequence of the
individual chains, and the three-dimensional structure
of the folded molecule. As discussed in Chapter 6, **genetic defects** resulting in impaired globin chain synthesis produce microcytic, hypochromic anemias and distinctive changes in pairing of the several globin chains. In contrast, **amino acid substitutions** in either the α-globin or β-globin chains can disrupt the molecular structure and function of hemoglobin.

Normal globin is made up of two α-globin chains, each with 141 amino acids, and two β-globin chains, each with 146 amino acids. The four polypeptide chains form a helical structure with hydrophobic pockets holding four heme groups. A central cavity between the two β-globin chains houses 2,3-diphosphoglycerate (2,3-DPG) (Figure 7–1). This complex structure is essential to hemoglobin function.

Even a single amino acid substitution can interfere with the helical structure and make the globin unstable. The most common clinical example of this is sickle cell disease (hemoglobin S-β^S). Replacement of glutamic acid with valine at position 6 on the β-globin gene results in a dramatic change in the solubility. Deoxy-

CLINICAL FEATURES

The clinical presentation of a hemoglobinopathy is a function of the severity of the genetic defect and its impact on hemoglobin structure and function. Heterozygote patients tend to have little or no clinical disease and are most often identified by routine screening. In contrast, some heterozygote and most homozygote patients present with a moderate to severe hemolytic anemia, or, in case of the high oxygen–affinity hemoglobins, erythrocytosis (see Chapter 12). The most common of the hemoglobinopathies (hemoglobins S, C, D, and E), when present in their homozygote form or as a compound heterozygote, result in severe disease (Table 7–1).

Sickle Cell Anemia

Sickle cell anemia, the homozygous form of hemoglobin S disease ($\beta^S\beta^S$), presents early in life with a severe hemolytic anemia and vasoocclusive disease involving the marrow, spleen, kidney, and central nervous system (CNS). **Involved children** first complain of recurrent painful crises characterized as deep-seated bone and joint pain that may or may not be associated with other intercurrent illness. When frequent, these painful episodes are devastating, and over time, patients be-

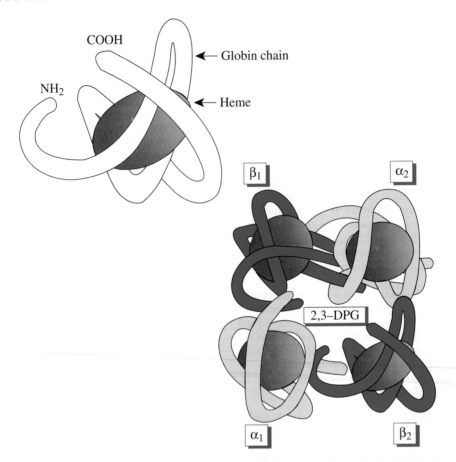

Figure 7–1. **Hemoglobin structure.** Each hemoglobin molecule is composed of 2 α-globin (light shading) and 2 β-globin chains (dark shading), each of which contains a single heme group in a hydrophobic pocket. A central cavity between the 2 β-globin chains houses a molecule of 2,3-DPG. This is important for the respiratory function of hemoglobin.

Table 7–1. Common hemoglobinopathies.

Severe anemia/disease
  Hemoglobin S/S (sickle cell anemia)
  Hemoglobin S/C
  S/β⁰-thalassemia
  Hemoglobin S/E
Mild anemia/disease
  S/β⁺-thalassemia
  Hemoglobin C/C
  Hemoglobin S/Lepore
  Hemoglobin S/D
  Hemoglobin S/O—Arab
Minimal anemia/no disease
  Hemoglobin S trait
  Hemoglobin C trait
  Hemoglobin D trait

come disabled and dependent on pain medications. Organ damage starts early in childhood. Splenic infarction with loss of splenic function occurs in the first decade of life. The renal medulla is another prime target. The concentrating ability of the kidney is invariably lost, and patients can experience episodes of gross hematuria. Sickle cell anemia patients are at risk for death from a CNS thrombosis or overwhelming sepsis. Loss of splenic function and the recurrent infarction of marrow and bone set the stage for infections with organisms such as *Streptococcus pneumoniae, Haemophilus,* and salmonella.

Adult sickle cell anemia patients who have recurrent vasoocclusive crises can develop significant bone and joint disease, including aseptic necrosis of the femur and humerus heads, muscle wasting, and flexion contractures of major joints. During the second and third decades of life, damage to the pulmonary vasculature can result in pulmonary hypertension, cardiac failure, and death. When patients receive long-term transfusion therapy, crises can be prevented but only at the risk of progressive iron overload.

Compound Hemoglobinopathies

Compound hemoglobinopathies such as SC disease or the combination of hemoglobin S with either α- or β-thalassemia vary in their presentation. **Hemoglobin SC disease patients** tend to have less difficulty with painful crises and do not have infarction of their spleens. At the same time, they do have problems with gross hematuria, aseptic necrosis, and in women, increased maternal or fetal death with pregnancy. **Hemoglobin S/thalassemia patients** usually present with a variable anemia and can experience vasoocclusive crises, but often have milder forms of vascular disease. The severity of the clinical picture in these patients in large part depends on the level of hemoglobin F in red blood cells.

Hemoglobin C Disease & the Unstable Hemoglobinopathies

Homozygous hemoglobin C disease and hemoglobinopathies associated with an unstable hemoglobin molecule generally present with a well-compensated hemolytic anemia. Although they do not have vasoocclusive disease, patients are subject to hemolytic crises where an increased rate of red blood cell destruction, secondary to intercurrent illness or drug ingestion, produces a sudden worsening of their anemia. They also exhibit the symptoms and signs associated with continuous high levels of red blood cell turnover, including jaundice, splenomegaly, and an increased risk of gallstone formation.

Several **amino acid substitutions** of the globin chain result in a change in hemoglobin-oxygen affinity.

When the oxygen affinity is reduced, patients generally have a well-compensated hemolytic anemia. The shift in the hemoglobin-oxygen dissociation curve maintains tissue oxygen delivery despite the hemoglobin level. In contrast, patients with high oxygen–affinity hemoglobinopathies present with erythrocytosis (see Chapter 12).

Laboratory Studies

The complete blood count (CBC) and hemoglobin electrophoresis are the key tests for detecting and diagnosing common hemoglobinopathies. The characteristic erythropoietic profile for these patients is shown in Table 7–2. Most hemoglobinopathies are associated with a lifelong hemolytic anemia. This situation is readily apparent when the reticulocyte index increases to greater than three to five times normal when patients are otherwise healthy and in a well-compensated state. Other signs of increased level of hemoglobin turnover include high lactic dehydrogenase (LDH) and indirect bilirubin levels. Patients with moderately severe hemolytic anemias, a reticulocyte index greater than three times normal, will demonstrate LDH levels of greater than 1000 IU and indirect bilirubins of 1–3 mg/dL.

A. RED BLOOD CELL INDICES AND MORPHOLOGY:

Red blood cell indices and film morphology can provide important clues to the cause of the anemia. Although most hemoglobinopathies present with a normocytic, normochromic anemia, sickle cell anemia patients with large numbers of sickle cells in circulation can show a slight reduction in the mean cell volume (MCV). Combinations of hemoglobin S or C with thalassemia or hemoglobin E will have more marked microcytosis with concomitant reductions of the MCV to levels below 70 fL (see Chapter 6). To complicate the situation, all hemolytic anemia patients are at risk for

Table 7–2. Hemoglobinopathy erythropoietic profile.

Red blood cell morphology	Normocytic, normochromic to slightly microcytic (MCV 80–90 fL), abnormal cell shapes (sickle cells, target cells, etc)
Polychromasia	Present to prominent
Nucleated red blood cells	Present after splenic infarction
Reticulocyte index	> 3–5
Marrow E/G ratio	> 1:1
Bilirubin/LDH	Increased
Serum iron/TIBC	Normal to increased/normal
Serum ferritin	> 100 µg/L

development of **folic acid deficiency,** since their folate requirements are increased. When present, this situation will result in megaloblastic erythropoiesis and the production of macrocytic red blood cells. When severe, the MCV will increase. A more sensitive measure of folate deficiency is the detection of occasional macroovalocytes or multilobed polymorphonuclear leukocytes on the peripheral film.

Cell morphology can make the diagnosis. With homozygous hemoglobin S disease, sickle forms are usually present on a Wright's stained film. The classic sickle cell looks like a crescent moon or banana. Other shapes include fragments of cells and partially distorted cells with sharp pointed extensions. The distinctive sickle shape is the result of the tendency for hemoglobin S to form rigid, crystallike structures within the cell. Other morphologic features of hemoglobinopathies include targeting, the presence of intracellular inclusions of precipitated hemoglobin (**Heinz bodies**), and, in homozygous hemoglobin C disease, the formation of a blocklike crystal in the center of the red blood cell. Prominent targeting is most common in patients with hemoglobin C and SC disease and those with S or C/β-thalassemia.

B. Hemoglobin Electrophoresis:

Definitive diagnosis of a hemoglobinopathy is usually possible by **cellulose acetate hemoglobin electrophoresis.** When performed at an alkaline pH, hemoglobin S migrates more slowly than hemoglobins A and F (Figure 7–2). Moreover, hemoglobin C migrates even more slowly, permitting the separation of the more common hemoglobinopathies including hemoglobin S, hemoglobin C, and combinations of hemoglobins S and C with β-thalassemia. Sickle cell anemia can also be detected at birth using agar gel electrophoresis at an acid pH (**acid citrate agar electrophoresis**). This permits the separation of small amounts of hemoglobin S and A from the predominant hemoglobin F of the fetal red blood cell. Prenatal diagnosis in families where both parents carry sickle cell trait is possible using the technique of **chorionic villus biopsy** with restriction fragment length polymorphism/Southern blot analysis or polymerase chain reaction amplification of genomic DNA and oligonucleotide probes.

Hemoglobinopathies resulting in unstable hemoglobins present with evidence of increased hemolysis, including an elevated reticulocyte index, high LDH level, and an increase in the indirect bilirubin level with clinical jaundice. Hemoglobin levels may be decreased, normal, or increased according to the oxygen affinity characteristics of the abnormal hemoglobin. Red blood cell morphology can be either normocytic and normochromic or show slight hypochromia, and aniso-

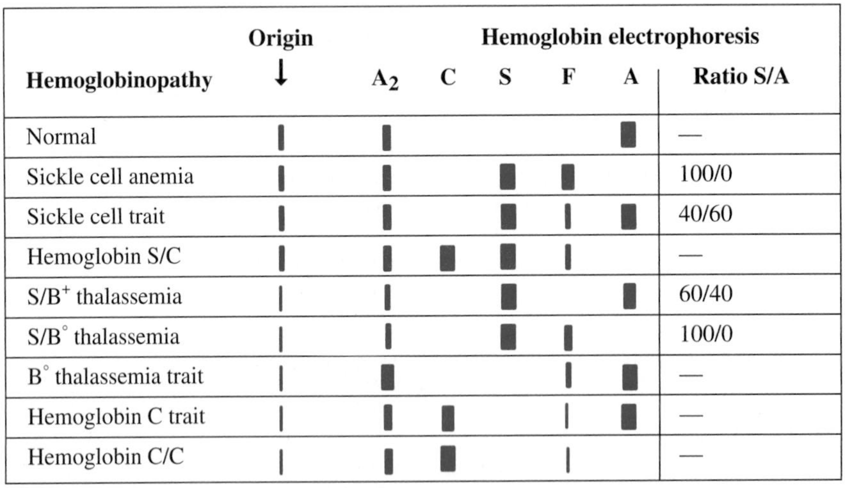

Hemoglobinopathy	Origin ↓	A₂	C	S	F	A	Ratio S/A
Normal							—
Sickle cell anemia							100/0
Sickle cell trait							40/60
Hemoglobin S/C							—
S/B⁺ thalassemia							60/40
S/B° thalassemia							100/0
B° thalassemia trait							—
Hemoglobin C trait							—
Hemoglobin C/C							—

Figure 7–2. Cellulose acetate hemoglobin electrophoresis at an alkaline pH. Cellulose acetate electrophoresis is used clinically to separate the more common hemoglobinopathies. **Top:** The normal hemoglobin pattern. More than 97% of the hemoglobin in normal individuals is hemoglobin A, with very small amounts of hemoglobin A₂ (2–3%) and F (trace). Hemoglobins S and C migrate more slowly than hemoglobin A and are clearly separated by this technique. Patients with β-thalassemia trait show an increase in hemoglobin A₂; double heterozygotes for hemoglobin S and β-thalassemia show variable amounts of hemoglobin F. The ratio of hemoglobin S/A is important in distinguishing sickle cell trait from hemoglobin S/β⁺-thalassemia.

and poikilocytosis, secondary to intracellular hemoglobin denaturation and pitting of red blood cell inclusion bodies by the spleen. Diagnosis depends on demonstrating hemoglobin instability and defining its oxygen-carrying characteristics.

C. ISOPROPANOL STABILITY TEST:

The **isopropanol stability test** is performed by adding fresh red blood cell hemolysate to a 17% buffered solution of isopropanol kept at 37°C. The mixture is then observed at frequent intervals for the appearance of a flocculent precipitate. Unstable hemoglobins will usually precipitate within the first 5–20 minutes, whereas normal hemoglobin is stable for 40–60 minutes.

D. HEAT STABILITY TEST:

The **heat stability test** is performed by mixing 3 mL of a fresh hemolysate of washed red blood cells with 3 mL of tris buffer, followed by heating in a water bath of 50°C for 2 hours. Normal hemoglobin is stable at this temperature, whereas unstable hemoglobins will precipitate. This result can be detected by centrifuging the sample after 2 hours and measuring the hemoglobin level in the supernatant.

E. DETECTION OF INTRACELLULAR INCLUSION BODIES:

Two stains, brilliant cresyl blue and methyl violet, can be used to identify intracellular inclusions of denatured hemoglobin. When fresh whole blood is incubated with **brilliant cresyl blue,** unstable hemoglobins precipitate, resulting in a diffuse cobblestone-type stippling of red blood cells. The **methyl violet stain** does not by itself denature hemoglobin. It can be used, however, to detect free-form hemoglobin inclusions (Heinz bodies) in circulating red blood cells. This test works best in patients who lack splenic function, where Heinz bodies accumulate in red blood cells, appearing as a few to many small, violet-colored inclusions. They are seen not only with unstable hemoglobins but also in patients with α- and β-thalassemia and G6PD deficiency.

DIAGNOSIS

Diagnosis of a hemoglobinopathy involves both accurate identification of a specific gene defect and assessment of the patient's clinical status. The first step may be possible simply from the clinical presentation, as with sickle cell anemia. However, other hemoglobinopathies may only be diagnosed after a careful laboratory evaluation. As for assessment of the patient's overall clinical status, this involves a broader evaluation of both the erythropoietic profile and functional status of various organ systems.

Hemoglobin S Disease

Diagnosis of homozygous sickle cell disease in a child of appropriate racial background is usually not difficult. Detection and diagnosis of the hemoglobin S heterozygote and the patient with a compound hemoglobinopathy are greater challenges.

A. SICKLE CELL TRAIT:

Sickle cell trait, the heterozygous form of hemoglobin S ($\beta\beta^S$), is not associated with anemia or clinical disease. It is, however, a very common genetic abnormality; some 7–8% of American blacks carry the trait. The frequency of sickle cell trait in certain African countries can be even higher, and the chance of forming a compound heterozygote with thalassemia is greatly increased. This situation is thought to reflect a survival advantage that sickle hemoglobin imparts in those regions where there is a high incidence of malaria. The protective role of hemoglobin S is further demonstrated by the observation that the same β-globin chain position 6 Glu to Val mutation has originated in four different locations in Africa.

Overall clinical health of the individual is not affected by the inheritance of a single sickle gene (Table 7–3). Lifespan is normal and these individuals do not have painful crises or organ damage. The **only abnormality that has been associated with sickle cell trait** is the occurrence of self-limited episodes of painless hematuria in up to 3% of patients. There have also been a few case reports of sickle crisis and sudden death with severe exertion and dehydration, or exposure to very low oxygen tensions.

The routine CBC is normal and sickle cells are not observed in the peripheral blood film. Furthermore, the lifespan of the red blood cells is not significantly shortened, so there is no evidence of a hemolytic anemia and the reticulocyte index, LDH, and indirect bilirubin levels all are normal. The hemoglobin electrophoresis pattern is diagnostic; 40–45% of the hemoglobin in red blood cells migrates as hemoglobin S (Figure 7–2 and Table 7–3).

B. SICKLE CELL ANEMIA:

Sickle cell anemia, the homozygous form of hemoglobin S disease ($\beta^S\beta^S$), is easier to diagnose. It is largely limited to black populations and occurs in families where both parents are heterozygotes for hemoglobin S. It almost always causes clinical disease as the child approaches 6 months of age, because for the first 6–12 weeks of life, severe intravascular sickling is prevented by high levels of fetal hemoglobin.

1. Classic symptoms and signs—As described in the section on clinical presentation, classic symptoms and signs of sickle cell anemia include recurrent, painful

Table 7–3. Clinical features of sickle hemoglobinopathies.

	Clinical Abnormalities	CBC/HGB Electrophoresis
Sickle trait	None, rare painless hematuria	Hgb: normal Hgb S/A 40/60
Sickle cell anemia	Vasoocclusive crises with infarction of spleen, marrow, kidney, etc Aseptic necrosis of bone Gallstones Priapism Ankle ulcers	Hgb: 7–10 g/dL MCV: 80–100 fL Hgb S/A: 100/0 Hgb F: 2–25%
S/β^0-Thalassemia	Vasoocclusive crises Aseptic necrosis of bone	Hgb: 7–10 g/dL MCV: 60–80 fL Hgb S/A: 100/0 Hgb F: 1–10%
S/β^+-Thalassemia	Rare vasocclusive disease or aseptic necrosis	Hgb: 10–14 g/dL MCV: 70–80 fL Hgb S/A: 60/40
Hemoglobin S/C	Rare vasoocclusive disease or aseptic necrosis; painless hematuria more common	Hgb: 10–14 g/dL MCV: 80–100 fL Hgb S/A: 50/0 Hgb C: 50%

crises secondary to intravascular sickling, small-vessel occlusion, and tissue infarction. The organs that are at greatest risk for infarction include marrow, kidney, spleen, lung, and brain. **Young children** can present with acute dactylitis secondary to marrow necrosis in the small bones of the hands and feet. **Older children** complain of recurrent episodes of joint or bone pain, and abdominal pain secondary to splenic infarction. Pneumococcal sepsis is a leading cause of death in children with sickle cell anemia, because of the loss of spleen function. Damage to vital organs including lung, heart, and brain increases as the child grows older. In **untreated patients,** there is a constant risk of vascular occlusion, with death occurring from either a stroke or major cardiopulmonary damage before the fourth decade. Risk of stroke in untreated children is on the order of 10% per year. This can be reduced to less than 1% by chronic transfusion therapy. This observation has led to the recommendation that all children with homozygous sickle cell disease, between 2 and 16 years of age, be screened every 6 months by **transcranial doppler,** with the clinician looking for elevated blood flow velocity in the middle cerebral or internal carotid arteries.

2. Severity—The severity of sickle cell anemia is a function of several variables including the concentra-

tion of hemoglobin S, the degree of hemoglobin deoxygenation, the intracellular hemoglobin concentration, and the level of hemoglobin F. Homozygous $\beta^S\beta^S$ cells also show a **tendency to become dehydrated** secondary to an increased rate of potassium-chloride cotransport out of the cell and an activation of the calcium dependent (**Gardos**) **potassium export channel** when the red cell membrane is distorted. This hastens the polymerization process. It also plays a role in the formation of target cells in patients with SC and CC disease.

Whole blood viscosity and blood flow through the tissue microcirculation correlate with the degree of deoxygenation and formation of irreversibly sickled cells. Oxygenated sickle blood has a viscosity of 1.5 times normal, rising to 10 times normal with deoxygenation. In part, the increase in viscosity is compensated for by the patient's anemia. However, with deoxygenation blood flow is strikingly diminished, especially at the level of the small arterioles. Any rise in the patient's hematocrit, as with marked dehydration, will further increase viscosity and contribute to the severity of the disease.

The **frequency and severity of vasoocclusive events** also reflects the tendency of sickle cells to adhere to the endothelium. Sickle cells express several adhesion receptors including CD36, $\alpha_4\beta_1$ integrin, sulfated gly-colipid, and the Lutheran blood group antigen. Cytokine-induced endothelial vascular adhesion molecule-1 (VCAM-1) and $\alpha_v\beta_3$ integrin that binds von Willebrand factor and thrombospondin help mediate sickle cell adherence. Red cell binding to endothelial cells, together with platelet adhesion and white cell activation/adhesion, contributes to the severity of the occlusive event. With progression of the disease, tissue damage leads to disrupted blood flow and an even greater opportunity for marked hemoglobin S polymerization and sickle cell adherence. Finally, the intracellular concentration of hemoglobin F, by physically inhibiting polymer formation, plays a major role in determining the severity of disease.

Sickle cell anemia patients also show **signs of a severe hemolytic anemia.** Their LDH and indirect bilirubin levels are increased and they may be clinically jaundiced. They are at risk for sudden and repeated aplastic crises where a self-limited failure of stem cells precipitates a major worsening of their anemia. Parvovirus infection can be one cause of aplastic crisis; another is major damage to the kidney with loss of erythropoietin stimulation. Expansion of erythroid marrow can be impressive. Active marrow may be detected in distal bones, at times accompanied by thinning of the bony cortex and remodeling of the bone, especially the skull. Frontal bossing is a sign of severe sickle cell anemia in the child or adolescent. Thinning of the bony cortex of long bones is also seen.

3. Complications—Slight to moderate **growth retardation** with delayed puberty may be observed. This condition may be related to zinc deficiency. However, sickle cell anemia patients will attain normal physical size and sexual maturation by age 18 to 21. Women have no difficulty bearing children, although the number and severity of **crises can increase during pregnancy.** With puberty, young men often have recurrent episodes of **priapism.**

Other complications of sickle cell anemia include proliferative retinopathy, gallstones, aseptic necrosis of the femoral and humeral heads, leg ulcers, renal insufficiency, and acute chest syndrome. A **proliferative retinopathy** usually appears later in life, whereas most sickle cell anemia patients will develop bilirubin pigment **gallstones** by the second or third decade. Poorly healing **leg ulcers** secondary to infarction of the subcutaneous fat and skin over the malleoli appear in the second and third decades.

Aseptic necrosis of the femoral or humeral heads can produce a crippling arthritis requiring prosthetic surgery. Furthermore, aseptic necrosis is associated with pulmonary fat embolism and is a risk factor for the development of a salmonella or *Staphylococcus aureus* os-

teomyelitis. **Renal insufficiency,** which leads to renal failure, may be seen later in life. **Acute chest syndrome** is a life-threatening complication in adult sickle cell patients. It presents with symptoms of fever, cough, and chest pain, usually without evidence of a viral or bacterial infection. Chest x-ray shows multilobe infiltrates that reflect widespread thrombosis/fat embolism on autopsy. This can lead to marked hypoxia, respiratory failure, and death. **Multi-organ damage** and "**watershed**" **strokes,** often associated with sudden increases in hematocrit and whole blood viscosity, are also life-threatening complications.

4. Overall course of the disease—The overall course of the patient's disease is marked by the frequency of vasoocclusive events, the severity of the anemia, and the presence of other abnormal hemoglobins (Figure 7–3). Hemoglobins C and D can actually increase disease severity, while high levels of intracellular hemoglobin F are associated with milder disease. Sickle cell patients from the Middle East and West Africa who have a strong hereditary persistence of hemoglobin F production have very mild disease. A decrease in the hemoglobin concentration in the red blood cell secondary to iron deficiency or combined inheritance of thalassemia can also significantly reduce the sickling tendency and the frequency of vasoocclusive crises.

C. HEMOGLOBIN SC DISEASE:

Hemoglobin SC disease ($\beta^S\beta^C$) is less common than SS disease. Clinically, it can present with the same manifestations as sickle cell anemia, although frequency and severity of the vasoocclusive manifestations are somewhat less. In contrast to sickle cell anemia, splenic infarction is uncommon and most adult patients with SC disease have an easily palpable, enlarged spleen. Damage to other organs, including renal medullary infarction, CNS thrombosis, and cardiopulmonary thrombosis, is less common. Hemoglobin SC patients present more frequently with gross hematuria, and the rate of spontaneous abortion in women with SC disease is very high.

The **laboratory diagnosis** of SC disease is easy. Patients show a mild to moderate hemolytic anemia, prominent red blood cell targeting on the peripheral blood film, hemoglobin C crystal formation in some red blood cells, a tendency to form spherocytes with a slight rise in the mean corpuscular hemoglobin concentration (MCHC), but an absence of true sickle cells. The hemoglobin electrophoresis pattern is diagnostic (see Figure 7–2 and Table 7–3).

D. HEMOGLOBIN S/β-THALASSEMIA:

The combined inheritance of hemoglobin S and β-thalassemia is another common disorder in black and

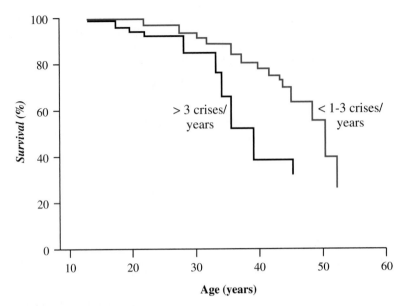

***Figure 7–3.* Survival of sickle cell anemia patients.** The overall survival of patients with sickle cell anemia correlates with the severity of their disease state, especially the number of crises per year. Patients who experience between one and three crises per year have a median survival of nearly 50 years, whereas patients with more than three crises per year will experience fatal complications during the fourth and fifth decades of life.

Mediterranean populations. **When S hemoglobin is combined with β$^{+Africa}$-thalassemia,** the patient's disease is mild and resembles that of sickle cell trait. Patients can demonstrate a mild to moderate hemolytic anemia and splenomegaly. On hemoglobin electrophoresis, they show a reduction in hemoglobin A production, which results in a hemoglobin S to A ratio of 60%/40% or higher depending on the level of production of hemoglobins F and A$_2$. The preponderance of S hemoglobin clearly distinguishes patients with S/β$^+$-thalassemia from those with heterozygous S (sickle cell trait) (see Figure 7–2 and Table 7–3).

The **combination of hemoglobin S with β^0-thalassemia** in Mediterranean populations results in more severe disease. These patients present with most or all of the symptoms of sickle cell anemia, although they do not infarct their spleens. The severity of the vasoocclusive manifestations of hemoglobin S/β^0-thalassemia depends on the level of hemoglobin F in red blood cells. When F levels are greater than 10–15% and evenly distributed throughout the red blood cell population, the patient manifests much less severe disease. When hemoglobin F production is low, the clinical picture, blood film findings, and hemoglobin electrophoresis pattern mimic SS disease.

E. Other Double Heterozygotes:

Hemoglobins D, O-Arab, and Lepore are other β-globin chain defects that are commonly inherited together with hemoglobin S. Hemoglobin SD disease and S/O-Arab disease produce clinical manifestations similar to but milder than those of sickle cell anemia. Hemoglobin S/Lepore also results in milder disease.

Hemoglobin C Disease

Hemoglobin C production results from the substitution of lysine for glutamic acid at the sixth position of the β-globin chain. Hemoglobin C tends to form intracellular blocklike crystals, which increase the rigidity of the red blood cell, shorten its lifespan, and cause fragmentation and formation of spherocytes in circulation.

Patients with homozygous hemoglobin C disease (β^{C}β^C) have a mild to moderate hemolytic anemia, hemoglobin levels of 8–12 grams per deciliter, and obvious splenomegaly. They do not have the vasoocclusive problems of the sickle cell anemia patient. The diagnosis may be apparent from the blood film based on the prominent targeting that accompanies both homozygous (80–90% of red blood cells) and heterozygous

(20–50% of red blood cells) C disease and the presence of blocklike crystals of hemoglobin C. **Patients with C trait** ($\beta\beta^C$) demonstrate a normal erythropoietic profile other than the presence of targeting on the blood film.

Hemoglobin D Disease

Hemoglobin D (β^D) production results from the substitution of glutamine for glutamic acid at position 121 on the β-globin chain. Hemoglobin D disease is most prevalent in India. Heterozygotes are not anemic, whereas homozygotes demonstrate a mild hemolytic anemia. Laboratory diagnosis requires electrophoresis on acid citrate agar, since hemoglobin D comigrates with S on cellulose acetate electrophoresis at an alkaline pH.

The Unstable Hemoglobins

Mutations in the amino acid sequence of the globin chains can also produce unstable hemoglobins that tend to denature and form insoluble precipitates in the cell, so-called **Heinz bodies.** Other unstable hemoglobins have an increased tendency to form methemoglobin. In both situations, the loss of soluble, functional hemoglobin results in a chronic hemolytic anemia. Often, the mutation also changes the oxygen affinity of the abnormal hemoglobin. When the oxygen affinity is decreased, the patient's anemia is compensated for by increased delivery of oxygen to tissues. When it is increased, the patient can present with an abnormally high hemoglobin level (see Chapter 12).

Although many unstable hemoglobins have now been described, the clinical frequency of patients with disease is very low. Most of the unstable hemoglobins represent **defects of the α-globin chain** and are inherited as autosomal dominant traits. Two relatively prevalent β-globin chain mutants are hemoglobins Zurich and Köln. Those patients that do come to medical attention usually have a well-compensated hemolytic anemia, characterized by a normal or slightly decreased hemoglobin level and a high reticulocyte index. The MCH may be decreased and inspection of the film may show hypochromia, and mild aniso- and poikilocytosis. Basophilic stippling and occasional Heinz bodies may be observed, but generally they are not impressive unless the patient has had a splenectomy. Episodes of increased hemolysis can occur with exposure to oxidant drugs or illness, similar to those seen with G6PD deficiency and other hemolytic anemias.

Laboratory confirmation of an unstable hemoglobin involves using both the isopropanol and heat stability tests and the brilliant cresyl blue and methyl violet stains. Although these tests have the ability to uncover an unstable hemoglobin, they do not define the specific genetic defect. This process requires hemoglobin electrophoresis, globin chain purification, peptide analysis, and gene sequencing.

THERAPY

The management of a patient with a hemoglobinopathy varies greatly according to the genetic defect. Patients with **homozygous S disease or one of the combinations** of hemoglobin S and another β-globin chain defect present the greatest challenge. The patients who are **heterozygous for one of the hemoglobinopathies** generally do not have significant clinical disease. Effective screening and accurate diagnosis of the heterozygous individual is essential, however, for appropriate counseling and prenatal diagnosis. **Patients at risk because of racial background** should be routinely screened with a CBC and cellulose acetate hemoglobin electrophoresis. This battery of tests will detect most high-risk hemoglobinopathies. Furthermore, if a heterozygous individual plans to bear children, it is essential that the mate be screened both for counseling and to guide the use of prenatal diagnostic techniques.

Prenatal diagnosis makes it possible to anticipate the birth of homozygous and compound heterozygous children, thereby permitting parents to make an early decision regarding abortion. Accurate diagnosis of fetal hemoglobin SS disease is now possible using fetal DNA from amniotic fluid or chorionic villus biopsy and a specific restriction enzyme that recognizes the A to T base switch responsible for the Glu to Val substitution.

Sickle Cell Anemia

Management of the sickle cell anemia patient begins in the first year of life. Continuous, unbroken medical follow-up is essential, and a full range of health care and social support services needs to be provided. Several medical issues will need to be addressed during the lifespan of the patient. These issues include the recurrent, painful sickle crises, the severe hemolytic anemia, organ damage from vasoocclusive disease, priapism in teenage males, the tendency to form pigment gallstones, the poorly healing leg ulcers, the danger of overwhelming sepsis due to hyposplenism, and the tendency for patients to become disabled and narcotic dependent.

A. PAINFUL SICKLE CRISES:

The pain and pain crises experienced by sickle cell patients can vary considerably. Children are at risk for vasoocclusive infarction of marrow, spleen, and renal medullary tissue. They present with recurrent episodes of extremity and abdominal pain that may or may not be precipitated by other illness. Unless very severe, **crises** can usually be managed at home with varying combinations of pain medications such as nonsteroidal analgesics, acetaminophen, and, if necessary, oral narcotics. A high level of **fluid intake must be maintained and the CBC monitored** for evidence of acute infection or sudden worsening of the patient's anemia. As the child grows older, and splenic function is lost, there is an **increased risk of life-threatening sepsis** with organisms such as *S pneumoniae* and *H influenzae,* and osteomyelitis secondary to infection with salmonella.

The **severely ill child may need to be admitted to the hospital** to receive parenteral fluid therapy, higher-dose narcotic analgesia, and, if necessary, red blood cell transfusion to correct a worsening anemia. Although a vasoocclusive crisis that is well established cannot be reversed, red blood cell transfusions will decrease the tendency to further vessel occlusion by diluting the number of sickle cells in circulation. Long-term prophylactic cell transfusion can be used to decrease the frequency of painful crises in patients who have frequent crises or life-threatening vasoocclusive episodes.

Teenage and adult patients develop their own characteristic pattern of recurrent painful crises. One-third or more report relatively infrequent episodes of slight to moderate aching pain in bones and joints, requiring nothing more than a few days of nonnarcotic analgesia. Others have frequent, severe crises presenting as incapacitating pain of large joints, especially the wrists, ankles, knees, hips, and shoulder joints. These crises are only occasionally associated with other illness. The inciting event can be completely unknown or may relate to small changes in routine activity, diet, or fluid intake. Survival correlates with the frequency of crises (see Figure 7–3). Patients who have three or more crises each year have a significantly shortened life span.

A **severe crisis in the adult** is a devastating illness. It can be difficult to control pain despite the use of large amounts of narcotics, and patients will generally require hospitalization for fluid management. Because sickle cell anemia patients are unable to adequately concentrate their urine owing to renal medullary damage, they need to be aggressively hydrated with a mix of D5W and D1/2 NS. An adequate regimen of pain medication is also essential. Patients should have a **fixed-schedule narcotic regimen,** either meperidine or morphine at a dosage that will relieve their pain. Younger patients often require higher doses. Continuous intravenous morphine or patient-controlled analgesia are the preferred routes of administration as long as limits are set for total narcotic dosage.

The total dose of narcotic needed to control the pain can be quite high. It is important, therefore, to **closely monitor the patient for side effects.** In the case of meperidine, the accumulation of the toxic metabolite nor-meperidine, which has a half-life of 18 hours, can produce marked anxiety, tremors, myoclonus, and seizures. Accumulation of the morphine-6-glucuronide metabolite in patients receiving high-dose morphine therapy is associated with marked sedation and respiratory depression.

There is **little risk for narcotic abuse when patients are managed well.** Poor control of pain during a crisis, inadequate follow-up, and overuse of emergency rooms by the sickle cell patient can lead to addictive behavior. When painful crises occur at frequent intervals, sickle cell anemia is a debilitating illness that interferes with every aspect of normal living. Patients are chronically ill, unable to work or go to school, and in need of long-term support. The sickle cell anemia patient has every reason to be angry and depressed and to feel poorly served by the medical system. This situation needs to be recognized in the long-term care of the patient. Painful episodes, and even mild ones, must be taken seriously. The patient needs to be trained on how to use pain medications, emphasizing dosing at frequent, fixed intervals rather than as needed. In addition, the tendency to have depression should be recognized and treated with appropriate use of antidepressants and social support.

B. PREVENTION OF PAINFUL CRISES:

It has been well recognized that the frequency and severity of painful crises can be reduced by **decreasing the relative amount of sickle hemoglobin** in circulation. This process is possible either by diluting the number of sickle cells in circulation by transfusion of normal red blood cells or reducing the amount of intracellular sickle cell hemoglobin by increasing hemoglobin F production. Iron deficiency may also reduce the frequency of sickle crises by reducing intracellular hemoglobin S concentration. It is difficult, however, to induce iron deficiency in a sickle cell anemia patient. Attempts at phlebotomy are frustrated by the severity of the patient's anemia.

1. Transfusion therapy—When transfused with normal red blood cells sufficient to reduce the number of sickle cells by one-third or more, most patients will experience a reduction in the frequency of painful crises. At least two units of packed red blood cells must be transfused every 2 weeks in the adult patient. If larger amounts of red blood cells are given to increase the hemoglobin to levels greater than 10–11 grams per deciliter, the patient's erythropoietin response will be suppressed, and new sickle red blood cell production will decrease, as illustrated by the reticulocyte index.

It is possible to hypertransfuse a patient and virtually shut off hemoglobin S production. This approach, however, increases the exposure of the patient to transfused blood with its associated complications. Therefore, **hypertransfusion** is only indicated for the severely ill patient who does not respond to smaller amounts of blood. For **patients undergoing general anesthesia,** transfusion to a hematocrit of 30% is sufficient to prevent perioperative complications. Recent clinical trials have demonstrated the efficacy of repeated transfusion in reducing risk of recurrent stroke in children with sickle cell anemia. **Prophylactic transfusion is now recommended in children** with transcranial doppler blood flow velocities of greater than 200 cm/second in the middle cerebral or internal carotid arteries. Sufficient red cell transfusions need to be given to reduce the S hemoglobin to 30% of the total hemoglobin concentration. **Other indications for acute and long-term transfusion** are listed in Table 7–4.

Complications of transfusion therapy include formation of alloantibodies to minor blood group antigens, acute or delayed hemolytic transfusion reactions, and, with chronic transfusion, iron overload. **Alloantibody formation** to red blood cell antigens is a difficult problem. For whatever reason, up to 30% of sickle cell anemia patients will form alloantibodies, making crossmatching of future transfusions increasingly difficult. Therefore, it is important that all transfused units be matched for minor blood groups such as C, c, E, e, and Kell. Moreover, if the pool of donors used for transfusion is kept relatively small, it can help avoid antibody formation.

Hemolytic transfusion reactions can be acute or delayed and are of particular concern. With acute hemolysis, patients will complain of back, flank, or chest pain (or all of these) and will develop fever and malaise. Transfusion-induced hemolysis may also precipitate a typical vasoocclusive crisis. At the same time, reticulocytopenia and a fall in the hematocrit to levels below that present prior to transfusion may be the first and only clue to an acute or delayed hemolytic reaction. While formation of alloantibodies often explains the reaction, the mechanism behind some of these events remains unclear.

Every unit of packed red blood cells contains 200 mg of iron. Even a minimum transfusion regimen of one unit every 2 weeks contributes an excess load of iron of nearly 5 grams each year. This places the patient at **risk for tissue iron overload** and damage (see Chapter 14). If **long-term transfusion therapy is used in a young patient,** it is essential that the patient be considered for long-term deferoxamine (DF) therapy. As long as the patient can comply with the rigors of DF therapy, the risk of iron overload can be greatly diminished.

2. Induction of hemoglobin F—The observation that high levels of intracellular hemoglobin F in sickle cell anemia patients are associated with milder disease has led to attempts to induce hemoglobin F production with drugs. Clinical trials using a daily dose of hydroxyurea have demonstrated the ability to increase hemoglobin F levels from 1.5–16 fold (2–20%). Both the number of F cells and the intracellular level of F are increased. The response correlates both with the patient's initial hemoglobin F level and the maximally tolerated hydroxyurea dosage. **Hydroxyurea can be given without apparent toxicity for relatively long periods.** However, depending on the dose, patients will develop a significant macrocytosis, usually without becoming more anemic, and a slight to moderate leukopenia, thrombocytopenia, or both.

Even patients who realize relatively small increases in hemoglobin F (5–10%) appear to benefit from ther-

Table 7–4. Indications for transfusion.

Acute Transfusion	Long-term Transfusion
Acute, increasingly severe anemia Aplastic crisis Inflammatory illness Hemolytic event	Recurrent acute chest syndrome Pulmonary hypertension Congestive heart failure Chronic lung disease with hypoxia
Acute chest syndrome	Recurrent stroke
Acute stroke/TIA	Abnormal transcranial doppler
Multiorgan failure	Severe, recurrent pain crises
General anesthesia	
Severe, prolonged pain crisis	

apy. In fact, correlation of the frequency of vasoocclusive crises with the rise in hemoglobin F has only been documented during the first few months of therapy. Sustained improvement correlates better with reduction in the neutrophil, monocyte, and reticulocyte counts, perhaps by reducing binding of these cells to the endothelium and their role in inflammation. **Hydroxyurea has effects outside of the increase in hemoglobin F,** including reductions in sickle cell and endothelial adhesion receptors and other changes in the coagulation system. What role these changes play is also unclear.

Several **clinical trials of hydroxyurea** have now reported significant decreases in the number of sickle crises and complications, together with increases in body weight, well-being, and function. In a pediatric clinical trial (age range 2–22 years), a dose of 20 mg/kg/day for 6 months produced hemoglobin F increases of 5–22% and a major decrease in the number of hospitalizations. These children showed little change in their other blood count parameters. A 1-year trial of doses up to 30 mg/kg/day in 52 children, aged 5–15 years, has confirmed the safety of the drug. Blood count changes were mild and readily reversible, and there was no impact on growth rate.

In **adult patients,** therapy should begin with a daily dose of 500 mg of hydroxyurea (10–15 mg/kg/day). After 6–8 weeks of therapy, the dose can be increased to 1000 mg/day if the patient's blood counts are stable. Most patients will tolerate hydroxyurea doses of 1000–2000 mg/day (20–30 mg/kg/day), although up to 10% will not tolerate a dose of even 10 mg/day. Blood counts need to be checked frequently, every 2 weeks until the dose is stabilized, and then every 6–8 weeks for the duration of therapy. Up to 20% of patients will fail to respond to even high doses of hydroxyurea.

Small numbers of **patients have now received hydroxyurea for 5 or more years** without evidence of secondary malignancy, myelodysplasia, or marrow chromosomal abnormalities. Much longer-term experience with chronic hydroxyurea therapy is necessary; however, before its effectiveness can be compared with possible long-term complications. There is still no firm evidence that hydroxyurea will prevent or reverse organ damage over time.

Arginine butyrate and other short-chain fatty acids are also capable of inducing fetal hemoglobin production. In fact, in a study of pulse arginine butyrate, given intravenously for 4 days every 2–3 weeks, the increase in fetal hemoglobin was even more dramatic than that seen with hydroxyurea. A rise in the total hemoglobin levels was also observed. Further clinical trials are needed to determine the overall effectiveness of this agent in changing the course of the disease.

3. Reduction in intracellular hemoglobin concentration—Hemoglobin SS polymerization is highly dependent on the intracellular hemoglobin concentration. Therefore, a sustained reduction in MCHC will, theoretically, decrease the chance of a sickle crisis. Currently, clinical trials are studying the ability of clotrimazole, an antifungal drug, to inhibit calcium-dependent (Gardos channel) potassium efflux and prevent cell water losses. Another trial involves oral magnesium (Mg) supplementation with Mg picolate which, by increasing intracellular red cell Mg, appears to inhibit the K-Cl cotransport system. Future therapies may well combine hydroxyurea with clotrimazole, Mg, or both.

4. Bone marrow (stem cell) transplantation—A small number of children (less than 16 years of age) with severe sickle cell disease including recurrent painful crises, acute chest syndrome, and stroke have successfully received **transplants with allografts from HLA-identical siblings** (A/A or A/S hemoglobin patterns). The patients were initially treated with a combination of busulfan, Cytoxan, and antithymocyte globulin. Most had stable engraftment of donor cells with improvement in clinical status. Since the availability of a normal HLA-matched related donor is so low, future trials may look at the use of unrelated cord-blood stem cells.

Additional therapeutic strategies will involve altering the interaction between sickle cells and endothelial cells. The sickled red cell has an increased tendency to adhere to the endothelium and by way of its effect on the hemostatic system create a hypercoaguable state. However, the pathophysiology of these interactions is extremely complex and will need to be better understood before a successful therapy can be designed.

Management of Other Complications

Most sickle cell anemia patients form **pigment gallstones** and are at **risk for cholecystitis and cholangitis.** Cholecystectomy is indicated at an early age in patients who are symptomatic. To prevent a sickle crisis in the perioperative period, patients should be transfused to a hemoglobin of 10–11 grams per deciliter and a hemoglobin S/A ratio of 60/40 or lower. In addition, laparoscopic cholecystectomy is associated with less postoperative morbidity and a shorter length of stay. **Aseptic necrosis of the femoral and humeral heads** is another common complication. It can usually be managed conservatively with pain medications, although severe bony destruction can require the placement of an orthopedic prosthesis.

Acute chest syndrome in adults can rapidly proceed to respiratory failure and death in up to 5% of patients. It should, therefore, be aggressively treated with exchange transfusion and antibiotics. About one-third of adults dying of acute chest syndrome are bacteremic. Anticoagulation therapy may also be considered in patients with signs of **marked pulmonary thrombosis/fat embolism.** Recent studies of acute chest syndrome have shown a pathologic expression of **VCAM-1,** suggesting a possible therapeutic role for inhibitors of VCAM-1 such as dexamethasone and nitrous oxide.

Priapism in teenage males can usually be managed with pain medications alone or in combination with nifedipine, given in repeated dosages of 10 mg. Priapism that lasts for more than a day can be treated by penile aspiration and epinephrine irrigation of the corpora cavernosa. **Leg ulcers,** which usually appear in the third or fourth decades, are very difficult to treat. Meticulous local care to prevent superinfection and the application of an Unna boot (zinc oxide, impregnated bandage) can provide protection and encourage healing. Patients will also need to decrease their activity level and keep their legs elevated. Blood transfusion, even hypertransfusion, will not speed healing.

Women with sickle cell anemia can undergo **pregnancy** without an increase in the frequency of crises or complications. Spontaneous abortion is rare. However, women of SS phenotype tend to have low birth weight infants. An increase in number and severity of crises during the third trimester and the induction of premature labor put both mother and child at risk. **Transfusion therapy can be quite effective in the third trimester** to prevent painful crises and life-threatening vasoocclusive events during labor.

Similarly, **prophylactic red blood cell transfusion** can be used when patients undergo **major surgery** to prevent a perioperative crisis. As a rule, 30% or more of the circulating red blood cells need to be normal cells containing hemoglobin A to prevent a vasoocclusive event. The decision to transfuse prophylactically is a clinical one. There is no protocol regarding which surgical procedures or which patients require this therapy.

Sickle cell anemia patients are at risk for overwhelming **sepsis** with organisms such as *S pneumoniae* and *H influenzae.* They should receive polyvalent pneumococcal vaccine early in childhood with a booster at age 10, and should be carefully instructed regarding their response to sudden fever. Young children should also receive prophylactic oral penicillin at 125 mg twice a day. Adult sickle cell anemia patients who have repeated infarctions of marrow and demonstrate aseptic necrosis of the femoral or humeral heads are at risk for developing **salmonella osteomyelitis.** This needs to be considered in any patient who complains of chronic, localized bone pain or manifests a fever of unknown origin.

A. ROUTINE HEALTH MAINTENANCE:

Sickle cell anemia patients should be routinely monitored for progression of their disease. **Periodic CBCs** are very important. Each patient will demonstrate an erythropoietic profile that is normal for their compensated state. Severity of their anemia can vary according to the **level of intracellular hemoglobin F.** The higher the hemoglobin F level, the less severe the anemia based on the reduced tendency to form irreversibly sickled cells that are rapidly destroyed. The likelihood of the patient experiencing painful crises also correlates with the hemoglobin F level.

Any **sudden change in the patient's hemoglobin level,** whether a decrease or increase, can trigger a major vasoocclusive event. A fall in the hemoglobin level can result from a sudden increase in the rate of hemolysis, a decrease in erythropoietin production, or appearance of a maturation defect secondary to folic acid deficiency. The latter should be anticipated and the diet of a sickle cell anemia patient should always be supplemented with 1–2 mg of folic acid taken orally daily. Increased rates of red blood cell destruction are seen with any intercurrent illness and as a part of organ infarction, whereas falls in red blood cell production occur with inflammatory diseases and renal damage. Sickle cell anemia patients are also at risk for self-limited failure of stem cell proliferation secondary to parvovirus infection.

A **full evaluation of the erythropoietic profile** should be performed whenever a patient presents with a vasoocclusive crisis and a fall in hemoglobin level or reticulocyte index. Renal function studies are important to look for a failure in erythropoietin stimulation. A marrow aspirate and measurements of iron and folic acid supply will uncover reversible defects in red blood cell progenitor proliferation and maturation. A worsening anemia secondary to chronic inflammatory disease or renal damage will increase risk for severe vasoocclusive crises. This situation is also true for patients who develop severe cardiopulmonary disease and hypoxia. In these situations, long-term transfusion therapy may be the only way to maintain a patient's functional status.

Compound Hemoglobinopathies

Management of a patient with a compound hemoglobinopathy will depend largely on the incidence of vasoocclusive disease. **Patients with hemoglobin S/β⁰-thalassemia** follow a clinical course similar to that of sickle cell anemia. They have frequent painful crises and have a very high incidence of aseptic necrosis of the femoral and humeral heads. In contrast, **patients with S/β⁺-thalassemia** have much milder disease (see Table 7–3). **Patients with hemoglobin S/C disease** tend to have fewer vasoocclusive crises and a milder hemolytic anemia. At the same time, they should be followed up closely for complications such as gross hematuria and, in women with S/C disease, spontaneous abortion and complications with delivery.

The Unstable Hemoglobins

Patients with unstable hemoglobins tend to have well-compensated hemolytic anemias or tendency to erythrocytosis. Those patients with hemolytic anemia should **receive 1–2 mg oral folic acid daily.** Otherwise, they require little in the way of therapy unless they present with a sudden fall in their hemoglobin level. As with other compensated hemolytic anemias, they are at risk for increased hemolysis secondary to intercurrent illness or drug ingestion and reversible red blood cell aplasia secondary to parvovirus infection.

BIBLIOGRAPHY

Hemoglobin Structure and Function

Bunn HF, Forget BG: *Hemoglobin: Molecular, Genetic and Clinical Aspects.* WB Saunders, 1986.

Hebbel RP: Adhesive interactions of sickle erythrocytes with endothelium. J Clin Invest 1997;99:2561.

Little JA et al: Metabolic persistence of fetal hemoglobin. Blood 1995;85:1712.

Clinical Features

Nagel RL: Severity, pathobiology, epistatic effects and genetic markers in sickle cell anemia. Semin Hematol 1991;28:180.

Petz LD et al: The sickle cell hemolytic transfusion reaction syndrome. Transfusion 1997;37:382.

Reed W et al: Acute anemic events in sickle cell disease. Transfusion 2000;40:267.

Vichinsky EP et al: Acute chest syndrome in sickle cell disease: Clinical presentation and course. Blood 1997;89:1787.

Therapy

Atweh GF et al: Sustained induction of fetal hemoglobin by pulse butyrate therapy in sickle cell disease. Blood 1999;93:1790.

Brugnara C et al: Therapy with clotrimazole induces inhibition of the Gardos channel and reduction of erythrocyte dehydration in patients with sickle cell disease. J Clin Invest 1996; 97:1227.

Bunn HF: Pathogenesis and treatment of sickle cell disease. N Engl J Med 1997;337:762.

Charache S et al: Effect of hydroxyurea on the frequency of painful crises in sickle cell anemia. N Engl J Med 1995;332:1317.

Charache S et al: Hydroxyurea: Effects on hemoglobin F production in patients with sickle cell anemia. Blood 1992;79:2555.

Ferster A et al: Hydroxyurea for treatment of severe sickle cell anemia: A pediatric clinical trial. Blood 1996;88:1960.

Haberken CM et al: Cholecystectomy in sickle cell anemia patients: Perioperative outcome of 364 cases from the National Preoperative Transfusion Study. Blood 1997;89:1533.

Kinney TR et al: Safety of hydroxyurea in children with sickle cell anemia: Results of the HUG-KIDS study, a phase I/II trial. Blood 1999;94:1550.

Rodgers GP: Recent approaches to the treatment of sickle cell disease. JAMA 1991;265:2097.

Sickle Cell Disease: Screening, Diagnosis, Management, and Counseling in Newborns and Infants. Agency for Health Care Policy and Research, Public #93-0562, 93-0563, and 93-0564.

Steinberg MH: Management of sickle cell disease. N Engl J Med 1999;340:1021.

Walters MC et al: Bone marrow transplantation for sickle cell disease. N Engl J Med 1996;335:369.

Wayne AS, Kevy SV, Nathan DG: Transfusion management of sickle cell disease. Blood 1993;81:1109.

Macrocytic Anemias

Folic acid and vitamin B$_{12}$ deficiency are primary causes of macrocytic anemia in adults. Both vitamins are essential for normal DNA synthesis, and high turnover tissues such as marrow are especially sensitive to any deficiency state. The marrow becomes megaloblastic; marrow precursors appear much larger than normal and are unable to complete cell division. This results in ineffective erythropoiesis, release of macrocytic red blood cells into circulation, and worsening anemia. The severity of the anemia and the degree of macrocytosis depends on severity and duration of the deficient state.

Prevalence of folic acid deficiency depends on the frequency of diseases associated with a decreased dietary intake of folic acid, malabsorption, or an increased requirement. Alcoholism is a common cause of folic acid deficiency in Western societies because of the poor dietary habits of the alcoholic and alcohol's interference with folate metabolism. In developing countries, tropical and nontropical sprue are more common etiologies. **Vitamin B$_{12}$ deficiency** can result from an autoimmune process or several disorders of the gastrointestinal tract.

NORMAL FOLIC ACID & VITAMIN B$_{12}$ METABOLISM

Major metabolic pathways of folic acid and vitamin B$_{12}$ are illustrated in Figure 8–1. These two vitamins are closely linked in the support of DNA synthesis. Within the cell, vitamin B$_{12}$ is present in two forms. As deoxyadenosyl B$_{12}$, it supports conversion of l-methylmalonyl-CoA to succinyl-CoA. It also accepts a methyl group from methyltetrahydrofolate to support synthesis of methionine. The transfer of a methyl group from methyltetrahydrofolate provides the tetrahydrofolate necessary for synthesis of various folate coenzymes needed for purine and glycine synthesis and for conversion of deoxyuridylate to thymidylate for DNA synthesis.

A lack of either vitamin interferes with **DNA synthesis.** When methyltetrahydrofolate is in short supply, tetrahydrofolate cannot be generated to support other folate coenzymes. When vitamin B$_{12}$ is lacking, there is no acceptor for the methyl group from methyltetrahy-

drofolate. This situation creates a "methylfolate trap" and reduced availability of tetrahydrofolate to support DNA synthesis.

Absorption & Distribution of Vitamin B$_{12}$

Pathways of absorption and distribution of vitamin B$_{12}$ to tissues are shown in Figure 8–2. Food B$_{12}$ is initially bound to a salivary binding protein (an R-protein) until it reaches the small bowel, where pancreatic proteases release the vitamin for subsequent binding to the glycoprotein, intrinsic factor. The **B$_{12}$-intrinsic factor (cobalamin-IF) complex** then binds to a receptor on ileal mucosal cells and is transported across the gut wall to circulation. In the absence of intrinsic factor, vitamin B$_{12}$ absorption virtually ceases. Several transcobalamin proteins in circulation are capable of binding free B$_{12}$. However, **transcobalamin II** is the principal transport protein for delivery of B$_{12}$ to tissues and liver. From 1–10 mg of vitamin B$_{12}$ accumulate in liver stores in a normal adult on an adequate diet. Daily turnover of vitamin B$_{12}$ reflects tissue requirements and size of body stores and can range from as little as 0.5 to as much as 8 µg per day.

Absorption & Distribution of Folic Acid

Dietary folic acid follows a similar pathway (Figure 8–3). An essential step in absorption is hydrolysis of folate polyglutamates present in food to methyltetrahydrofolate monoglutamate. This process depends on a carboxypeptidase located on the mucosal cell membrane and a dihydrofolate reductase enzyme in mucosal cells. Most absorption occurs in the proximal portion of the small intestine. The methyltetrahydrofolate is then rapidly transported to tissues to enter the intracellular metabolic cycle required for purine and pyrimidine metabolism and DNA synthesis. Although there are proteins in plasma that bind folate, their primary affinity appears to be for nonmethylated congeners that are not essential for transport to tissues.

Both methylated and nonmethylated congeners of folate are absorbed by the **liver,** where they are stored as methyltetrahydrofolate polyglutamate. Depending on the level of folate in the diet, the liver can contain sev-

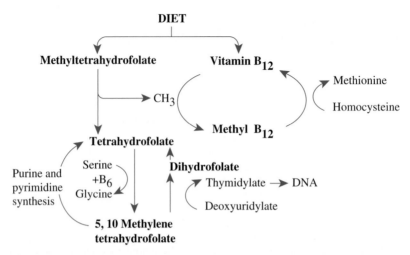

Figure 8–1. Metabolic pathways of folic acid and vitamin B$_{12}$. An adequate supply of both methyltetrahydrofolate and vitamin B$_{12}$ are required for normal DNA synthesis. Methyltetrahydrofolate donates a methyl group to vitamin B$_{12}$ in support of methionine metabolism. This generates the tetrahydrofolate needed for purine and pyrimidine synthesis and the production of thymidylate for DNA synthesis.

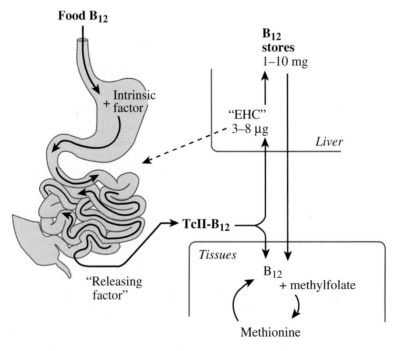

Figure 8–2. Vitamin B$_{12}$ absorption and transport to tissues. Dietary vitamin B$_{12}$ is sequentially bound to R-protein and intrinsic factor in preparation for binding to receptors on ileal mucosal cells. It is then transported on TC II to liver and tissues.

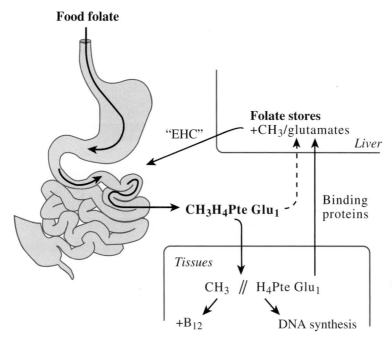

Figure 8–3. Folic acid absorption and transport. Folate polyglutamates in food are hydrolyzed, reduced, and methylated to form methyltetrahydrofolate monoglutamate. This is then transported to tissues where it participates actively as a methyl donor and as substrate for both purine and pyrimidine metabolism and DNA synthesis. Liver folate stores play an important role in providing a constant supply of folate through the enterohepatic cycle for reabsorption.

eral milligrams of folate stores. The liver also plays an essential role in providing a constant supply of folate to tissues. It maintains an active transport of methyltetrahydrofolate into bile for reabsorption by the gut. This enterohepatic cycle of folate is important for maintaining folate hemostasis. Any interference with the ability of the liver to store and release folate into bile or with the reabsorption of folate returned to the gut will rapidly disrupt folate supply to tissues.

FOLATE & VITAMIN B_{12} NUTRITION

Most foods, especially leafy vegetables, are rich in folate. However, excessive cooking and food processing can significantly reduce folate content, so that a Western diet may provide as little as 50–100 μg per day. This amount barely meets the minimum daily requirement of an adult and may be insufficient during pregnancy or for patients with high rates of cell turnover (hemolytic anemias). Chronic alcoholics, whose principal source of calories is derived from their alcohol intake, are at great risk of developing folate deficiency.

Dietary supply of vitamin B_{12} is derived largely from meat and meat by-products; vegetables are essentially free of the vitamin. Usually, the daily requirement of 3–5 μg is easily supplied by a Western diet. Only strict vegetarians are at risk for a true dietary deficiency state.

CLINICAL FEATURES

Symptoms and signs of a **severe vitamin B_{12} deficiency** include those of **marked anemia** and **neuropathy.** Most often, patients complain of the gradual onset of fatigue, exercise intolerance, and progressive cardiac decompensation. The latter is associated with a severe anemia (a hematocrit less than 15–20%). Vitamin B_{12} deficiency also has an impact on the central nervous system. Patients develop a demyelinating lesion of the neurons of the spinal column and cerebral cortex. This condition results in paresthesias of the hands and feet, unsteadiness of gait, and eventually memory loss and personality changes. The most distinctive characteristics of the neuropathy are the dorsal column and corticospinal tract lesions (subacute combined degeneration of the spinal cord), which result in a loss of vibration and position sense and the development of an unsteady gait and a positive Romberg test. Neuropathy may be present without anemia. It is important therefore to consider vitamin B_{12} deficiency as a possible cause of a peripheral neuropathy, dementia, or a psychiatric disorder.

Other symptoms and signs of vitamin B_{12} deficiency include complaints of a **sore mouth and loss of taste,** in addition to **atrophy of the mucosa of the tongue.** The tongue appears smooth, red, and shiny on physical examination. In addition, patients who develop pernicious anemia often have **vitiligo** and are prematurely gray. Several **disorders of the gastrointestinal tract** can result in vitamin B_{12} deficiency. The most common causes in the United States include pernicious anemia associated with antibodies to parietal cells, intrinsic factor, or the cobalamin-IF complex; gastrectomy, gastric bypass, or bowel resection; bacterial overgrowth of the small intestine; and pancreatic insufficiency.

Patients with folic acid deficiency anemia often go undiagnosed, especially alcoholics who have a very poor diet and maintain blood alcohol levels above 100 mg/dL for extended periods. At this level of alcohol intake, the enterohepatic cycle of folate supply to the intestine and tissues is impaired, setting the stage for a folate deficiency anemia. However, unless anemia is severe, the patient is relatively insensitive to its symptoms when compared to the other problems associated with alcoholism. Diagnosis is also made difficult by rapid return of intracellular folate metabolism to normal once alcohol ingestion ceases. Within hours of alcohol withdrawal and resumption of a normal diet, the serum folate returns to normal and the megaloblastic defect begins to resolve. Therefore, clinicians must be highly suspicious of the possibility of folate deficiency in alcoholics and perform the workup while the patient is still inebriated.

Folate deficiency during pregnancy is associated with a high incidence of fetal developmental abnormalities, especially neural tube defects. **Peripheral neuropathies** and **neuropsychiatric disorders** (dementia, psychosis, and depression) in adult patients who are folate deficient and have normal vitamin B_{12} levels may also be observed. **Subacute degeneration of the cord,** usually associated with vitamin B_{12} deficiency, has been reported in the occasional patient with folate deficiency. The difference in incidence may have more to do with the duration of the deficiency state than the vitamin involved.

Laboratory Studies

Accurate diagnosis of folic acid or vitamin B_{12} deficiency requires several laboratory studies (Table 8–1). **Serum folate and serum cobalamin levels** provide the most sensitive measure of ongoing supply of these vitamins to tissues. **Other tests,** including measurement of

Table 8–1. Laboratory studies in the diagnosis of macrocytic anemias.

Screening tests
  Complete blood count/reticulocyte index
  Marrow aspirate
  Iron studies—SI, TIBC, serum ferritin level
  Multilobed polymorphonuclear leukocyte count
  Serum/urine methylmalonic acid and homocysteine levels
Vitamin B_{12} deficiency
  Serum cobalamin (vitamin B_{12}) level
  Transcobalamin protein levels
  Serum antiparietal cell and anti-intrinsic factor antibody
    assays
  Schilling test
  DU suppression test
Folic acid deficiency
  Serum and red blood cell folate levels

plasma transcobalamin protein and transcobalamin saturation, serum methylmalonic acid level, and red blood cell folate level, can help when the diagnosis is unclear. Measurements of antiparietal cell and anti-intrinsic factor antibodies and the absorption of radiolabeled vitamin B_{12} (Schilling test) are used to determine the pathophysiology of a malabsorption defect.

A. SERUM AND RED BLOOD CELL FOLATE LEVELS:

The **serum folate level** is measured by isotope dilution assay. The amount of vitamin in serum is determined by its ability to compete with a known amount of radiolabeled vitamin for a binding protein. A milk protein binder is commonly used in the folate assay. Normal serum folate levels range from 5 to 30 ng/mL. The level needs to be greater than 4 ng/mL to sustain normal DNA synthesis.

The serum folate level is exquisitely sensitive to the intake of dietary folate. Even in chronic alcoholics, the level will quickly return to normal when alcohol is withdrawn and food intake resumes or when a folate supplement is provided. In this circumstance, it is still possible to detect a folate-deficient state by assaying **red blood cell folate** that reflects the state of folate supply when the red blood cells were first produced. However, intracellular folate is stored as folate polyglutamate, which must first be hydrolyzed to the monoglutamate prior to assay. This preparation step is difficult to standardize, making the measurement less reliable. In addition, the red blood cell folate level will only be abnormal if the patient has been folate deficient for some period and has not received a transfusion. A falsely low level is also seen in 50–60% of patients with primary vitamin B_{12} deficiency.

B. SERUM COBALAMIN (VITAMIN B₁₂) LEVEL:

The serum cobalamin level is also measured by isotope dilution assay, using purified intrinsic factor as the binding protein. A significant error can be introduced if R-proteins are used as the binder or the intrinsic factor preparation contains significant amounts of R-proteins. R-proteins are less specific than intrinsic factor; they bind inactive cobalamin analogues as well as true cobalamin. In the past, this made several of the radioisotope dilution assay kits unreliable because they falsely elevated vitamin levels. **Normal serum cobalamin levels** range from 200 to 500 pg/mL. Levels below 100 pg/mL are clearly deficient, whereas levels between 100 and 200 pg/mL may or may not be associated with abnormal DNA synthesis or neurologic dysfunction.

Misleading cobalamin levels are seen in certain clinical settings. Falsely low measurements have been reported with normal pregnancy, oral contraceptive use, multiple myeloma, transcobalamin I deficiency, and the presence of a second isotope in the serum. Patients who are folic acid–deficient and people taking large doses of ascorbic acid can have low serum cobalamin levels because of interference with vitamin B_{12} absorption and metabolism. Conversely, normal or elevated cobalamin levels are seen in patients with megaloblastic anemia secondary to nitrous oxide exposure, inborn errors of cobalamin metabolism, isolated transcobalamin II deficiency, and high levels of plasma transcobalamin I and III secondary to severe liver disease or a myeloproliferative disorder.

C. METHYLMALONIC ACID AND HOMOCYSTEINE LEVELS:

l-Malonylmutase and methionine synthetase are cobalamin-dependent enzymes. Early in development of vitamin B_{12} deficiency, even before obvious changes in marrow or red blood cell morphology, serum homocysteine and serum and urine methylmalonic acid will increase. Using a capillary gas chromatography–mass spectrometry method, measurements of serum methylmalonic acid and total homocysteine show elevated levels of one or both substances in 95% of cobalamin-deficient patients. Although homocysteine elevations occur with both cobalamin and folic acid deficiency, less than 2% of folate deficient patients will have an elevation of serum methylmalonic acid. The **normal range for serum methylmalonic acid** is 73–271 nM/L (19–76 ng/mL), whereas the **normal serum total homocysteine** ranges from 5.4 to 16.2 nM/L. Vitamin B_{12}–deficient patients have elevations of methylmalonic acid of from 2 to 100 times the upper limit of normal, and homocysteine elevations of 2–20 times normal. Folate-deficient patients typically have normal methylmalonate levels and elevations of homocysteine of 2–10 times normal.

D. SERUM VITAMIN B₁₂ BINDING PROTEINS:

Transcobalamin II (TC II) is the primary plasma-binding protein responsible for the transport of vitamin B_{12} to tissues. Cobalamin absorbed from food or given parenterally is avidly bound to TC II in gastrointestinal mucosal cells and serum. The cobalamin-TC II complex gains access to cells by binding to a specific membrane receptor that is then internalized and delivered to a lysozyme for digestion and release of free cobalamin. The turnover of cobalamin-TC II complex in plasma is very rapid, in contrast to the slower turnover of cobalamin and cobalamin analogues bound to transcobalamin I.

The level of **cobalamin-TC II complex (holoTC II)** may be the most sensitive measure of early negative vitamin B_{12} balance. Normal individuals have holoTC II levels greater than 50 pg/mL, whereas negative vitamin B_{12} balance is associated with values below 40 pg/mL.

E. TESTS OF VITAMIN-DEFICIENT ERYTHROPOIESIS:

From a morphologic standpoint, the earliest sign of vitamin B_{12} or folic acid deficiency is the appearance in circulation of **hypersegmented polymorphonuclear leukocytes,** which are leukocytes with five or more segmented lobes. In part, sensitivity of the leukocyte to vitamin deficiency reflects the more rapid turnover of this cellular population. Red blood cell morphology changes come on more slowly. At first, a few macroovalocytes can be detected on the peripheral film; later on, as the anemia worsens, the mean cell volume (MCV) becomes elevated.

Patients with severe anemia, macrocytosis, and a megaloblastic marrow will manifest **severe ineffective erythropoiesis** (Table 8–2). This condition is characterized by marked poikilocytosis on the peripheral blood film, an increase in the serum lactic dehydrogenase (LDH) level, and an increase in the serum iron level to the point of full saturation of the total iron-binding capacity (TIBC). There is also an obvious mismatch between the increased ratio of erythroid to granulocytic precursors (E/G ratio) and reduced production of new red blood cells, as measured by the reticulocyte production index.

F. ANTIPARIETAL CELL AND ANTI-INTRINSIC FACTOR ANTIBODY:

Autoantibodies against parietal cells, intrinsic factor, and cobalamin-intrinsic factor complex can be detected in the sera of most patients with pernicious anemia. **Antiparietal cell antibody** appears to be the most sensitive and specific for atrophic gastritis leading to vitamin B_{12} malabsorption. **Antibodies against intrinsic factor and cobalamin intrinsic factor complex** are seen in 60–70% of pernicious anemia patients. These

Table 8–2. Erythropoietic profile of severe macrocytic anemia.

Anemia	Severe (Hgb < 8–10 g/dL)
MCV (fL)	110–140
Film morphology	Macrocytic, normochromic
Reticulocyte index	< 1
Marrow E/G ratio Morphology	> 1:1 Megaloblastic
Serum iron/TIBC	Increased/normal
% Saturation	> 50
Marrow iron stores	Increased
Serum ferritin	Increased
Bilirubin/LDH	Increased/increased

patients can also exhibit antibodies against thyroid epithelium, renal collecting duct cells, and lymphocytes.

G. SCHILLING TEST:

The **Schilling test** is used to define the nature of a vitamin B_{12} malabsorption defect, not to diagnose vitamin B_{12} deficiency. The test involves oral administration of 0.5 μc (0.5–2.0 μg) of radiolabeled cyanocobalamin while the patient is fasting, followed by measurements of appearance of radioactivity in serum and urine. For the urine test of absorption, 1 mg of nonradioactive cyanocobalamin must be given intramuscularly (IM) 2 hours after the ingestion of the isotope to saturate the serum-binding proteins and flush the radioactive cobalamin into the urine. A 24-hour complete urine collection is essential. Normal subjects should excrete 7% or more of the ingested isotope in the first 24 hours after the flushing dose.

To determine whether vitamin B_{12} malabsorption is related to a lack of intrinsic factor or an interference with intestinal absorption of the cobalamin-intrinsic factor complex, the Schilling test is repeated with the simultaneous ingestion of 60 mg of purified, hog intrinsic factor. This should correct malabsorption secondary to intrinsic factor deficiency but not the malabsorption owing to small-bowel disease. To avoid a false-positive result, the Schilling test should be performed some days or weeks after vitamin therapy is initiated.

Accuracy of the Schilling test requires cooperation by the patient. Inadequate flushing with nonradioactive vitamin B_{12} or an incomplete urine collection

will lead to false-positive results. In addition, if the intrinsic factor preparation used in the second part of the Schilling test is not fully active, confusion can arise as to the cause of the vitamin B_{12} malabsorption. Finally, use of crystalline cyanocobalamin in the test will not detect those patients who malabsorb food cobalamin secondary to hypo- or achlorhydria. Acid gastric juice containing pepsin is essential to normal absorption of food cobalamin.

DIAGNOSIS

As with iron deficiency, diagnosis of vitamin B_{12} or folic acid deficiency relies heavily on laboratory tests. The concept of stages of deficiency including store depletion, abnormal DNA synthesis without anemia, and a fully developed deficiency state with a macrocytic anemia also applies to vitamin B_{12} and folic acid deficiency. However, unlike iron deficiency, available laboratory methods do not provide as clear-cut a definition of each state.

Vitamin B_{12} & Folic Acid Store Depletion

Accurate measurement of liver stores of either vitamin B_{12} or folic acid would require a direct assay of liver tissue. There are no indirect measures of the quantity of stores of these vitamins similar to the serum ferritin level in iron metabolism. An exception to this statement is the use of the holoTC II level as an indicator of negative vitamin B_{12} balance. When vitamin B_{12} intake is inadequate, the **holoTC II level** falls below 40 pg/mL, indicating that the rate of intake is insufficient to match the rate of vitamin B_{12} clearance from the TC II protein. However, this still does not provide a quantitative measure of store depletion.

Once vitamin stores are exhausted, serum cobalamin and folic acid levels measured in the fasting state will indicate inadequate tissue supply. **Serum cobalamin** falls to levels below 200 pg/mL and the **serum folate** to less than 4 ng/mL. This decrease reflects the fact that liver stores must be present to support normal serum vitamin levels in the fasting state. To make this interpretation with any certainty, however, other causes of false elevations or depressions of the vitamin levels must be excluded.

Abnormal DNA Synthesis Without Anemia

A significant defect in DNA synthesis can be present without appearance of a macrocytic anemia. Clinically, some patients with vitamin B_{12} deficiency will develop a neuropathy without hematologic changes. Therefore, it can be important to identify the earliest signs of abnormal DNA synthesis. The best tests for this are measurements of serum methylmalonic acid and total homocysteine. Both metabolites increase early in development of a deficiency, even though sensitivity of the tests will be lower than that reported for a full-blown deficiency state.

In the research setting, the deoxyuridine (DU) suppression test can be used to directly test the DNA synthesis of marrow precursors. This method measures the ability of the cells to convert radiolabeled deoxyuridine monophosphate to thymidylate. Because this reaction requires adequate levels of both vitamin B_{12} and folic acid, the DU suppression test can be made even more specific by testing the effect of adding each vitamin to the reaction mixture. An abnormal DU suppression test that is corrected by the addition of cobalamin but not methyltetrahydrofolate is a sensitive measure of early vitamin B_{12} deficiency. However, this sophisticated radioisotope technique is not available in most clinical laboratories.

Vitamin B_{12}– & Folic Acid–Deficiency Anemia

A full-blown macrocytic anemia secondary to vitamin B_{12} or folate deficiency is relatively easy to diagnose (see Table 8–2). With moderate to severe anemia, the MCV increases to values in excess of 110 fL and the peripheral blood film shows a marked distortion of morphology with macroovalocytes, aniso- and poikilocytosis, and multilobed polymorphonuclear leukocytes. As the anemia worsens, the hematocrit can fall to levels below 15–20% (hemoglobin 6 grams per deciliter or less), and both leukopenia and thrombocytopenia can develop.

Distortions of marrow morphology are equally impressive. The marrow is strikingly megaloblastic with a shift in the E/G ratio to 1:1 or greater. Most of the erythroid marrow proliferation is limited to the earliest precursors (ie, the basophilic and polychromatophilic normoblasts). This is, in fact, a demonstration of the

ineffective erythropoiesis that accompanies megaloblastosis. Erythroid precursors are arrested in S phase, cannot go through cell division, and die within marrow. This is reflected by a mismatch between the E/G ratio of 1:1 (greater than three times normal) and a reticulocyte production index of less than 1. Other laboratory signs of the ineffectiveness of erythropoiesis include elevations in serum LDH level and an increase in the serum iron to full saturation of the TIBC. There may also be a modest increase in the indirect bilirubin level.

Serum vitamin levels should confirm the diagnosis (Table 8–3). The patient with a pure vitamin B_{12} deficiency and a well-developed macrocytic anemia will almost certainly have a serum cobalamin level below 100 pg/mL. At the same time, the serum folate level will be normal or increased. Patients with severe liver disease or myeloproliferative disorders who have very high levels of transcobalamin I/III are exceptions to this rule.

The diagnosis of a macrocytic anemia secondary to folic acid deficiency can be more difficult. This diagnosis is especially true for the alcoholic patient where there is a close relationship between the patient's diet, level of alcohol ingestion, and serum folate level. Alcohol has a dramatic and rapid effect on the serum folate level. At blood alcohol levels of 100 mg/dL or higher, release of folate from hepatic stores to recycle through the enterohepatic pathway for tissue supply is impaired. In the patient who has little or no dietary intake of folate, this results in a rapid fall in the serum folate level to values below 4 ng/mL. Thus, an acute alcoholic can show low serum folate levels within a matter of a few days of a drinking binge, even though liver folate stores are not exhausted.

This phenomenon is easily detected if a serum folate level is drawn while the patient is still inebriated. However, a delay of a day or two following withdrawal of alcohol and placing the patient on a normal diet will result in a rise in the serum folate to normal levels. Delays of several days or a week can result in an even

Table 8–3. Test of vitamin B_{12} folic acid deficiency.

	Vitamin B_{12} Deficiency	Folic Acid Deficiency
Serum B_{12} (normal > 200 pg/mL)	< 100	> 200
Serum folate level (normal > 4 ng/mL)	>4	< 3
Serum methylmalonic acid (normal < 270 nM/L)	2–100 × normal	Normal
Serum homocysteine (normal < 16 nM/L)	2–20 × normal	2–10 × normal

more confusing picture. By this time, the patient's abnormal marrow morphology will have disappeared. Moreover, the anemic patient will mount a reticulocyte response suggesting either a hemolytic anemia or a recovery from a bleeding episode. In this situation, the only clue to a prior deficiency in folic acid will be the occasional macroovalocyte on the peripheral blood film and a lower than normal red blood cell folate level.

Approach to diagnosis is also influenced by the **severity of the anemia.** If the patient requires immediate treatment, it is essential that all necessary laboratory studies be drawn prior to transfusion or vitamin administration. The tests should include a CBC, reticulocyte count, marrow aspirate for morphology and assessment of iron stores, serum cobalamin and folate levels, and serum iron, TIBC, and ferritin levels. This battery of tests should make it possible to confirm the defect in cell maturation, distinguish vitamin B_{12} from folic acid deficiency, and provide an assessment of iron stores. The latter is especially important in planning therapy. Patients with small-bowel malabsorption can present with a single deficiency of vitamin B_{12}, folic acid, or iron or any combination of the three. Moreover, it is not uncommon that therapy with vitamin B_{12} and folic acid, alone or in combination, will uncover an iron deficiency state.

In patients with less-marked anemias, **vitamin B_{12} and folic acid therapy can be used diagnostically.** This therapy is most applicable for patients with vitamin B_{12} deficiency owing to an autoimmune process (pernicious anemia), where folic acid and iron deficiency are unlikely. To perform a therapeutic trial, the patient is given 1–10 μg vitamin B_{12} parenterally each day for 10–14 days. The response to therapy can be measured in several ways. As shown in Figure 8–4, the LDH level and elevated serum iron level fall rapidly over the first 2–3 days as the patient's erythropoiesis becomes effective. This decrease is followed on days 3–5 with an increase in the reticulocyte count. Recovery of the hematocrit is much slower and takes several weeks. Although a response to small amounts of vitamin B_{12} strongly suggests a vitamin B_{12} deficiency state, it is not absolute proof; serum vitamin levels are still important to confirm the diagnosis.

DIFFERENTIAL DIAGNOSIS

The differential diagnosis of a vitamin deficiency state involves not just identifying whether it is vitamin B_{12} or folic acid deficiency but also the cause of the vitamin deficiency. There is also the task of distinguishing the macrocytic anemia associated with vitamin B_{12} and folic acid deficiency from the macrocytosis observed in patients with dysplastic anemias, liver disease, hemolysis, and exposure to chemotherapeutic agents.

Macrocytosis

Macrocytosis, an MCV greater than 100 fL, is seen in several clinical settings (Table 8–4). In patients with a hemorrhagic or hemolytic anemia, where there is a high level of stimulation of the marrow by erythropoietin,

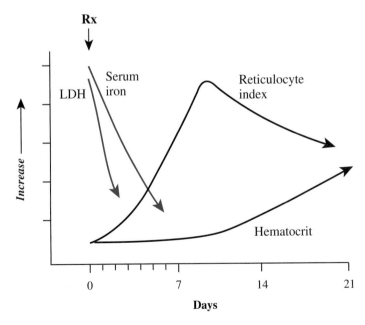

Figure 8–4. Therapeutic response to vitamin B_{12} or folic acid. The first sign of an effective response to one or the other vitamin is a fall in serum iron and LDH levels. This reflects a correction of the patient's ineffective erythropoiesis. On or about day 3, the reticulocyte index increases, peaking by the eighth day. The subsequent level of red blood cell production and rate of hematocrit rise will reflect the severity of the patient's anemia, adequacy of iron supply, and presence of other complicating illness.

Table 8–4. Causes of macrocytosis.

	MCV (fL)	Morphology
Normal	90	Normocytic
Reticulocytosis	90–110	Polychromasia (shift reticulocytes)
Liver disease	95–110	Uniform macrocytosis, targeting
Megaloblastic anemia	100–130	Macroovalocytosis, marked poikilocytosis
Cell counter artifact	100–130	Red blood cell agglutination or marked leukocytosis

the release of marrow reticulocytes with an MCV in excess of 140 fL will increase the MCV. The higher the reticulocyte count, the greater the increase in MCV. Patients with reticulocyte counts greater than 20% can have MCVs in excess of 110–120 fL, and the red blood cell–volume histogram will show the double population of very large reticulocytes and normal mature red blood cells. **Uniform macrocytosis of a moderate degree** is observed in patients with hypothyroidism and liver disease. In the latter case, it may represent an accumulation of excess membrane secondary to disturbed cholesterol metabolism and is usually accompanied by the appearance of target cells in circulation.

More severe macrocytosis with poikilocytosis on film and megaloblastic marrow morphology is seen not only in vitamin deficiency patients but also with myelodysplasia and in patients receiving chemotherapeutic agents such as hydroxyurea and methotrexate. Just as with the vitamin deficiency states, these patients have a true nuclear maturation defect. Their marrow morphology is abnormal and they exhibit varying degrees of ineffective erythropoiesis. Abnormalities in white blood cell and platelet components of the blood count are also common.

Macrocytosis can be an **artifact of the automated cell counter technique.** Patients with cold agglutinins or marked elevations of their white blood cell count may be reported to have an MCV in excess of 110 fL. In the first case, it is related to clumping of red blood cells in the counter, whereas with marked leukocytosis white blood cells are being counted as red blood cells. Modest increases in the MCV can also be seen in **patients with hyperglycemia.** This condition is an artifact of the dilution step when the cells are prepared for counting. Because of the high intracellular glucose content, cells swell rapidly when they are placed in the isosmotic diluent.

Causes of Vitamin B$_{12}$ Deficiency

Evaluation of a patient with a low serum cobalamin level requires consideration of several possible causes (Table 8–5). Dietary history may suggest **poor intake of vitamin B$_{12}$.** However, only the strictest of vegetarians are at risk for developing a deficiency state. Infants born to vegetarian mothers are at risk for **cobalamin deficiency.** It is much more likely, however, that the patient has an **impairment in vitamin B$_{12}$ absorption,** either intrinsic factor deficiency or a defect in small-bowel absorption. Rarely, the abnormality is one of **impaired metabolism.** TC II deficiency and congenital defects in DNA metabolism are detected soon after birth, at a time when vitamin B$_{12}$ availability and small-bowel function are usually not an issue. The impairment of vitamin B$_{12}$ metabolism by nitrous oxide inac-

Table 8–5. Causes of vitamin B$_{12}$ deficiency.

Congenital defects
 Intrinsic factor deficiency
 TC II deficiency
 Immerslund-Grasbeck disease
 Juvenile pernicious anemia

Poor vitamin B$_{12}$ intake (vegans)
Malabsorption
 Intrinsic factor deficiency
  Autoimmune—antiparietal cell/anti-intrinsic factor
   antibody (pernicious anemia)
  Gastric surgery
 Pancreatic insufficiency
 Small intestine absorption defect
  Crohn's disease
  Sprue
  Lymphoma
  Diverticulosis or blind loop with bacterial overgrowth
  Fish tapeworm
  Ileal resection
  Zollinger-Ellison syndrome
  AIDS

Vitamin B$_{12}$ destruction
 Nitrous oxide exposure

tivation of methionine synthase is also suggested by the patient's clinical history. It occurs following exposure to high levels of nitrous oxide anesthesia for several hours or with repeated low-level exposures over a long time in at-risk individuals, such as dentists.

A **full evaluation of vitamin B$_{12}$ absorption** includes a careful review of the clinical history and an evaluation of small-bowel anatomy and function. Patients with ileitis, ileal resection, small-bowel dysfunction secondary to diverticulitis and bacterial overgrowth, fistula formation, or sprue may be recognized from the clinical presentation with the help of radiologic and endoscopic studies. Patients with nontropical sprue may be diagnosed by biopsy of the small bowel. Presence of one of these conditions obviously sets the stage for vitamin B$_{12}$ malabsorption. To confirm this, a Schilling test first without and then with intrinsic factor needs to be performed. Any of the defects in vitamin B$_{12}$ transport or absorption secondary to small-bowel disease will show abnormal absorption of crystalline B$_{12}$ in both parts of the study. Intrinsic factor does not correct the absorption defect.

The patient with intrinsic factor deficiency can be diagnosed using a combination of laboratory studies and the Schilling test. The patient presenting with a macrocytic anemia, a serum cobalamin level less than 100 pg/mL, and a positive antiparietal cell or anti-intrinsic factor antibody is almost certainly an example of vitamin B$_{12}$ deficiency secondary to an intrinsic factor defect. This is a relatively common diagnosis that is most frequently detected in adult patients in their later years. Intrinsic factor deficiency is seen in children who are born with an intrinsic factor production defect. Adults who have gastrectomies where a major portion of the fundus of the stomach is removed or a gastric bypass operation will predictably develop vitamin B$_{12}$ de-

ficiency secondary to intrinsic factor lack, usually within 2–4 years if they do not receive parenteral vitamin B$_{12}$ on a regular basis.

Causes of Folic Acid Deficiency

The causes of folic acid deficiency are listed in Table 8–6. **Poor dietary intake coupled with alcohol ingestion** is an obvious cause of folic acid deficiency in the adult population. Obviously, the history and physical examination are important in identifying the alcoholism and the level of dietary intake. Accurate diagnosis of alcohol-related folic acid deficiency requires an immediate workup of the patient, at a time when the impact of alcohol on folate metabolism is still operative.

There are clinical settings where even a normal diet will not maintain folate requirements. **Patients with high levels of cell turnover** (eg, hemolytic anemias, psoriasis, and exfoliative dermatitis) can develop folic acid deficiency even while on a normal diet. This is also true for **normal pregnancy.** Prophylactic supplementation with folic acid is recommended for these situations.

As with vitamin B$_{12}$ deficiency, **disease of the small intestines** can result in folic acid malabsorption. Patients with sprue (especially tropical sprue), bacterial overgrowth, and short bowel syndrome are at risk for developing a macrocytic anemia due to folic acid deficiency. In the case of tropical sprue, folate deficiency is thought to play an integral role in the disease process. Treatment with folate is therapeutic for this condition.

Finally, several **drugs have an antifolate action.** Methotrexate, triamterene, and sulfamethoxazole with trimethoprim (Bactrim) are competitive inhibitors of methyl folate and DNA metabolism. Methotrexate

Table 8–6. Causes of folic acid deficiency.

Poor folic acid intake	Increased requirement
Dietary lack/alcoholism	Hemolytic anemias
Goat's milk anemia	Exfoliative dermatitis/psoriasis
Parenteral nutrition	Pregnancy
Malabsorption	**Metabolic inhibition**
Sprue (nontropical and tropical)	Dihydrofolate reductase inhibitors (methotrexate, trimethoprim, etc)
Lymphoma	Alcohol
Small-bowel resection	Vitamin C deficiency
Crohn's disease	
Anticonvulsant drugs	
Loss/destruction	
Hemodialysis	
Tropical sprue	

given in therapeutic amounts is the strongest of these agents and with long-term therapy can be expected to produce macrocytosis and a pancytopenia. Anticonvulsants (phenytoin, primidone, and phenobarbital) appear to be weak inhibitors of folic acid absorption. These drugs can cause macrocytosis and anemia when given in high doses to children.

THERAPY

General Guidelines

Folic acid and vitamin B_{12} are available in their purified forms for oral and parenteral use and are incorporated in several multivitamin preparations sold as nutritional supplements. The selection of preparation, dose, and treatment schedule must be appropriate to the clinical setting. Misdiagnosis can result in a treatment failure and worsening of the patient's clinical condition. This fact is of special importance in the patient with vitamin B_{12} deficiency because a delay in therapy or mistreatment with folic acid may result in irreversible neurologic damage. Therefore, both the nature and cause of the deficiency state must be well defined as a foundation for planning management.

A. SEVERE, LIFE-THREATENING ANEMIA:

The treatment of a patient with a severe macrocytic anemia will need to **proceed prior to completing the diagnostic workup.** Once appropriate laboratory studies, including serum cobalamin, folate, methylmalonic acid, and homocysteine levels, are drawn, the patient should receive full therapeutic doses of both vitamin B_{12} and folic acid, using the parenteral route to avoid the issue of malabsorption. Furthermore, this treatment should be continued with daily administration of both vitamins until a response is evident or the diagnosis is clear. If the patient is unstable from a cardiovascular standpoint, he or she should receive a transfusion with packed red blood cells. This must be done with caution, however, since patients with vitamin B_{12} deficiency are usually older and have marginal cardiovascular compensation. Any sudden increase in blood volume as with a rapid red blood cell transfusion can induce a fatal arrhythmia or acute congestive heart failure. Therefore, packed red blood cells should be infused slowly and carefully with concomitant use of a diuretic or simultaneous phlebotomy to avoid increasing the blood volume.

Treatment with both vitamin B_{12} and folic acid does not interfere with the subsequent evaluation of the patient for malabsorption. Radiologic and functional studies of the small bowel can still be performed once the anemia is corrected. This includes the use of the Schilling test to distinguish intrinsic factor deficiency from an abnormality in small intestinal absorption.

B. ASYMPTOMATIC DEFICIENCY STATES:

Whenever possible, therapy should be targeted to the specific deficiency state. In the patient with a **mild to moderate macrocytic anemia,** this will mean a delay until a full hematologic workup can be performed and the serum cobalamin and folate levels are measured. If the patient presents with **neurologic disease and no anemia,** measurements of serum methylmalonic acid and homocysteine can suggest the diagnosis. It is these settings where a therapeutic trial with a specific vitamin can also help confirm the deficiency state. For the **vitamin B_{12}–deficient patient,** a therapeutic trial can be performed using 1–10 μg of vitamin B_{12} given IM daily for 10 days while monitoring changes in the methylmalonic acid level, or when anemia is present, the serum iron, LDH, reticulocyte count, and over several weeks, the hematocrit and MCV. Similarly, a therapeutic trial can be performed using 50–100 μg of folic acid given parenterally on a daily schedule for 10–14 days to confirm an isolated **folic acid–deficiency** state. This low level of folic acid will not run the risk of either inducing a hematologic response or worsening the neurologic signs in a vitamin B_{12}–deficient patient. Also, it will not correct the high serum methylmalonic acid level of vitamin B_{12} deficiency.

As a practical point, therapeutic trials with small amounts of either vitamin B_{12} or folic acid are difficult to perform and often hard to interpret because other disease states can interfere with the response. If the patient is iron deficient or has an inflammatory illness, the lack of iron substrate and suppression of erythropoietin will dampen the reticulocyte and hematocrit responses. In addition, a therapeutic trial with low doses of vitamin B_{12} will delay the performance of a Schilling test since the performance of this test includes administering a flushing dose of 1000 μg of nonisotopic vitamin B_{12}. In effect, the flushing dose is therapeutic.

C. VITAMIN PROPHYLAXIS:

There are clinical situations where vitamin B_{12} or folic acid therapy should be given prophylactically. These situations include conditions where the rate of use of either vitamin exceeds the dietary supply, and disease states where malabsorption can be anticipated. For example, patients who have had a gastrectomy will exhibit vitamin B_{12} malabsorption and should, therefore, receive long-term vitamin prophylaxis. Normal pregnancy is an example of an imbalance between folate needs for fetal growth and folate supply in the diet. All pregnant women should receive supplementation with a multivitamin that contains folic acid.

Vitamin B_{12} Preparations

Vitamin B_{12} is available in its pure form, **cyanocobalamin,** in concentrations of 30, 100, and 1000 μg/mL for IM or deep subcutaneous injection. The dose administered will depend on the management plan. A dose of 1–10 μg IM daily is typically used in therapeutic trials where the purpose is to confirm vitamin B_{12} deficiency or distinguish vitamin B_{12} deficiency from folic acid deficiency. When a diagnosis of vitamin B_{12} is established, the patient with a **severe macrocytic anemia** should be treated with at least 100 μg of cyanocobalamin daily for at least 2 weeks. This regimen will guarantee a maximum therapeutic response and encourage rebuilding of liver vitamin B_{12} stores. Subsequently, patients should receive 100–1000 μg of cyanocobalamin once a month for the rest of their lives. This situation will maintain their balance unless there is a high level of cell turnover. If this is true, twice-monthly injections are advised. Patients with a **vitamin B_{12} deficient neuropathy** should be treated more aggressively with weekly or biweekly injections for several months to encourage maximum recovery.

Administration of more than 100 μg of cyanocobalamin in any single injection exceeds the binding capacity of TC II and results in a rapid clearance of most of the excess vitamin B_{12} into urine. Therefore, there is no advantage to using a dose of 1000 μg of cyanocobalamin. At the same time, cyanocobalamin is very cheap and the higher dose is harmless.

Several vitamin preparations that contain vitamin B_{12} are marketed as **nutritional supplements.** Some of these contain not only cyanocobalamin but also intrinsic factor concentrate prepared from animal stomachs. Theoretically, the latter should provide an effective oral medication for the treatment of patients with poor absorption secondary to intrinsic factor deficiency. However, its effectiveness cannot be assumed. Patients can develop refractoriness to these preparations perhaps because of the appearance of an antibody against the animal protein. Oral maintenance therapy is possible using very high doses of vitamin B_{12} on the rationale that a small amount of it will leak across the intestine. Although this does work, patients will need to be monitored closely for any clinical evidence of recurrence of their deficiency. The cost of this increased level of observation can cancel any advantage of oral over parenteral therapy.

Multivitamin preparations containing small amounts of vitamin B_{12} are marketed as **over-the-counter medications.** Some of these contain as much as 80 μg of cyanocobalamin combined with 500–1000 μg of folic acid, ascorbic acid, and iron. They are very useful as nutritional supplements in patients who are on an inadequate diet or have an increased requirement.

Folic Acid Preparations

Pharmaceutical preparations of folic acid include **pteroylglutamic acid folate congener** (folic acid, folvite), and **5-formyltetrahydrofolate congener** (folinic acid, leucovorin, citrovorum factor). Both are formulated for either oral or parenteral administration. Folic acid tablets (**folvite**) contain 0.1, 0.4, 0.8, or 1 mg of pteroylglutamic acid, whereas folic acid for injection contains 5 mg/mL. Pteroylglutamic acid must first be reduced and methylated by either intestinal mucosal cells or hepatocytes before it participates in cellular DNA metabolism.

Folinic acid tablets (leucovorin) contain 5, 10, 15, or 25 mg of 5-formyltetrahydrofolate. The principal application of folinic acid is to circumvent the inhibition of dihydrofolate reductase by the chemotherapeutic agent, methotrexate. Leucovorin will also correct the defect in thymidylate production both in patients who lack methyltetrahydrofolate and those who are vitamin B_{12} deficient. It should be avoided when treating vitamin B_{12}–deficient patients because it can correct the hematologic abnormality while allowing the neurologic findings to progress.

The approach to folic acid therapy will vary according to the management plan. If a **therapeutic trial** is attempted, the patient should be given a daily parenteral injection of 50–100 μg of folic acid (folvite). This treatment will require a meticulous dilution of the 5 mg/mL commercial preparation in order to avoid a high dose that might give a partial response in the vitamin B_{12}–deficient patient. It is also important to recognize the difficulties associated with a therapeutic trial of folic acid. Patients with alcohol-induced defects in folate metabolism often demonstrate a spontaneous recovery of their hematologic abnormality with alcohol abstention. This reflects the reversal of the alcohol-induced defect in liver folate–store metabolism. Patients with folic acid deficiency can also demonstrate a combined defect in vitamin B_{12} and iron metabolism. In this situation, a therapeutic trial with a single vitamin will not give an interpretable response.

Patients with **severe macrocytic anemias** are best treated with a combination of 100 μg of cyanocobalamin IM and either oral or parenteral doses of 1–5 mg of folic acid. Generally, oral doses of folic acid are adequately absorbed, even in patients with known defects in small intestinal absorption. It is a water-soluble vitamin that can cross the mucosal barrier by passive diffusion when given in large doses. Therefore, it is common practice to treat patients with oral folic acid in daily doses of 1–5 mg regardless of the cause of the deficiency state.

Prophylactic administration of folic acid in patients with poor diets or high levels of cell turnover will vary according to the individual clinical situation. Multivitamin preparations containing as much as 1 mg of folic acid are used in pregnancy and as a supplement for nursing mothers because as much as 50 μg of folate is secreted each day in the breast milk. Patients with hemolytic anemias or exfoliative dermatitis are usually given a higher dose (1 or 2 mg of folic acid orally each day). Like vitamin B_{12}, the safety range of folic acid is very large and no side effects are seen even with doses exceeding 20 mg per day. However, there have been reports of an increase in the frequency of seizures in children who receive large amounts of folic acid to prevent the antimetabolite effect of antiepileptic medications.

The **long-term management** of any patient with a vitamin B_{12}– or folic acid–deficiency state requires periodic reevaluation to guarantee therapeutic effectiveness. Since the deficiencies are most often the result of an underlying defect in absorption, patients may need to maintain their vitamin therapy for the rest of their lives or at least until the absorption defect has been cured. There is also a constant risk that multiple vitamin and mineral deficiencies will occur. This risk is most typical of the patient with sprue or widespread intestinal disease from other causes where the patient is at risk for folic acid, vitamin B_{12}, and iron deficiency. Less commonly, vitamin C deficiency can play a role. The patient with scurvy can exhibit a macrocytic/megaloblastic anemia secondary to a defect in intracellular folate metabolism resulting from low cellular vitamin C levels.

Periodic evaluations of patients receiving maintenance vitamin therapy should include a careful history and physical to look for reappearance or progression of the patient's neuropathy, a complete blood count, iron studies, and measurements of serum cobalamin and folate levels.

BIBLIOGRAPHY

Allen RH et al: Diagnosis of cobalamin deficiency: I. Usefulness of serum methylmalonic acid and total homocysteine concentrations. Am J Hematol 1990;34:90.

Chanarin I et al: Cobalamin and folate: Recent developments. J Clin Pathol 1992;45:277.

Cooper BA, Rosenblatt DS: Inherited defects of vitamin B_{12} metabolism. Ann Rev Nutr 1987;7:291.

Green R, Miller JW: Folate deficiency beyond megaloblastic anemia: Hyperhomocysteinemia and other manifestations of dysfunctional folate status. Semin Hematol 1999;36:47.

Hillman RS: Hematopoietic agents: Growth factors, minerals and vitamins. In: *The Pharmacological Basis of Therapeutics,* 10th ed. McGraw-Hill, 2001.

Lederle FA: Oral cobalamin for pernicious anemia: Medicine's best kept secret? JAMA 1991;265:94.

Lindenbaum J et al: Diagnosis of cobalamin deficiency: II. Relative sensitivities of serum cobalamin, methylmalonic acid and homocysteine concentrations. Am J Hematol 1990;34:99.

Stabler SP et al: Clinical spectrum and diagnosis of cobalamin deficiency. Blood 1990;76:871.

Toh BH, vanDriel IR, Gleeson PA: Mechanisms of disease: Pernicious anemia. N Engl J Med 1997;337:1441.

The Dysplastic and Sideroblastic Anemias

The dysplastic and sideroblastic anemias are primary stem cell disorders, many of which eventually evolve to acute leukemia. Recognition and differential diagnosis of these disorders revolves around characteristic changes in film and marrow morphology. The **dysplastic anemias** present with varying combinations of anemia, leukopenia, and thrombocytopenia together with macrocytosis, distorted marrow precursor maturation, and ineffective erythropoiesis. **Sideroblastic anemias** are defined by the distinctive appearance of ringed sideroblasts on the Prussian blue stain of the marrow. Although the incidence of these disorders is low, only 1:100,000 population, they do represent a diagnostic and therapeutic challenge.

NORMAL BLOOD FILM & MARROW MORPHOLOGY

Morphology of the marrow aspirate and peripheral film provides a sensitive measure of precursor proliferation, maturation, and adult cell production. **Marrow biopsy** is used to estimate overall cellularity. Normal aging is associated with a gradual increase in the ratio of fat cells to hematopoietic cells. Although less than one-third of the biopsy comprises of fat cells in a young adult, 50% or more of the marrow in an elderly patient will be fat. Reversal of the ratio suggests hematopoietic cell hyperplasia.

Marrow **cellularity and distribution** can also be assessed using a ^{99}technetium or ^{111}indium scan or magnetic resonance image. **Indium,** like iron, is preferentially taken up by erythroid precursors, whereas **technetium** measures the reticuloendothelial portion of the marrow. In normal adults, activity is limited to the axial skeleton and proximal portions of the long bones. In patients with dysplastic syndromes, marrow can expand into shafts of long bones, skull, and on occasion, extramedullary sites.

A **marrow aspirate stained with Wright's-Giemsa** provides a vivid display of the proliferation and maturation of each cell line. The **E/G ratio** is an estimate of the relative numbers of erythroid to myeloid precur-

sors. It is very useful for detecting a marked decrease or increase in the proliferation of one cell line as long as the others are normal. It is less useful when a disorder of the marrow involves all cell lines.

Individual cell morphology is also important. Distribution of cells in a marrow aspirate is not random. By scanning a number of fields using high power, however, it is possible to estimate numbers of the most distinctive cell types (Table 9–1). For example, about 25% of all the cells in a normal marrow are **mature granulocytes** that comprise the marrow granulocyte reserve pool. Another 25% or more are **developing myelocytes** and monocytes that may be distinguished by their size, nuclear shape, and cytoplasmic granulation. Maturing myelocytes can be subdivided into promyelocytes, myelocytes, and metamyelocytes (bands) according to their nucleus and content of primary and secondary granules. **Erythroid progenitors** are readily identified from a condensation of the nucleus and a cytoplasm that contains hemoglobin, not granules. Together, these three components make up 80% or more of the cells observed in a normal marrow.

Several minor cell populations may also be identified, including megakaryocytes, lymphocytes, plasma cells, undifferentiated blasts, and mast cells. The **number and morphologic characteristics of megakaryocytes** are best evaluated using low-power magnification. In a cellular marrow, it should not be difficult to identify megakaryocytes based on their large size and multinuclearity. Because they make up less than 1% of a normal marrow, it is difficult to accurately estimate their level of proliferation. Still, increases in the number of megakaryocytes in patients with immune thrombocytopenia can usually be appreciated. Moreover, distortions in individual cell morphology, as for example a decrease in nuclear ploidy typical of a dysplastic marrow, are easily appreciated.

The **number of lymphocytes** in a marrow aspirate can vary. Normal marrow contains focal areas of lymphocyte hyperplasia and when one of these areas is sampled, 20% or more of the cells in an aspirate can be lymphocytes. Moreover, they may appear in an irregu-

Table 9–1. Marrow cell types.

Type	Percentage (%)
Erythroid progenitors	20–25
Myeloblasts	< 2
Promyelocytes	5
Myelocytes	10–15
Metamyelocytes (bands)	10–20
Mature granulocytes	20–30
Lymphocytes	5–15
Plasma cells	5

lar distribution; some high-power fields will show mostly lymphocytes, whereas others very few. Each of the other cell lines including primitive blasts, plasma cells, and mast cells should not exceed 5% of the total population. **Mast cells** are integral to the structure of the marrow stroma. Because of this fact, they are best viewed by low-power inspection of stromal particles.

Individual cell morphology provides important information regarding such **defects in cell maturation** as size of the cell; size and shape of the nucleus; ratio of the nucleus to the cytoplasm; presence, number, and size of the nucleoli; and presence of cytoplasmic granules. **Leukemias** can be recognized morphologically both by proliferation of primitive, poorly differentiated cells and by disruption of individual cell morphology. Increases in cell and nuclear size, presence of one or several large nucleoli in the nucleus, and proliferation without maturation are all **signs of malignancy. Dysplastic and sideroblastic anemias** are identified based on unique distortions in precursor maturation. Cells appear megaloblastic with a predominance of younger forms (**maturation arrest**), and many of the mature cells contain distorted nuclei. **Sideroblastic anemias** are distinguished by the characteristic appearance of excess cytoplasmic iron granules in a perinuclear distribution.

CLINICAL FEATURES

The initial presentation of the dysplastic and sideroblastic anemias follows a bimodal age distribution. The rare infant or child who presents with a refractory anemia may be found to have marked erythroid precursor multinuclearity (**congenital dyserythropoietic anemia**) or prominent ringed sideroblasts on iron stain (**hereditary sideroblastic anemia**). More often, however, de novo dysplastic and sideroblastic anemias are disorders of the elderly, usually men in the fifth, sixth, or seventh decade

of life. The incidence of secondary myelodysplasia leading to acute myeloid leukemia (AML) has been reported to be as high as 3–7% in lymphoma patients exposed to multiple courses of chemotherapy and autologous bone marrow transplantation. The use of alkylating agents in patients with ovarian cancer, lung cancer, and multiple myeloma is also associated with a higher incidence of myelodysplasia.

Presenting symptoms and signs of these disorders are a function of the severity of the anemia or pancytopenia. The patient may complain of nothing more than weakness or easy fatigability. **Severe anemia** can provoke congestive heart failure. A **tendency to easy bruising** may signal thrombocytopenia, and **recurrent infections** may reflect a significant leukopenia. If the patient is not symptomatic, the disorder is first detected from a routine complete blood count (CBC). Patients typically show varying combinations of pancytopenia and abnormal cell morphology.

The onset is usually so gradual that patients will have difficulty identifying a starting point for the illness. A few patients will present with an immune-mediated disease such as skin vasculitis, temporal arteritis, or polymyalgia rheumatica. Since the **initial symptoms and signs are nonspecific,** a broad search should be made for an inciting cause or clues that suggest another type of anemia or pancytopenia. Dysplastic refractory anemias can be seen in younger patients as a result of exposure to radiation, cytotoxic drugs, or toxic chemicals. Patients exposed to alcohol, lead, and certain antibiotics such as chloramphenicol and isoniazid can present as having a sideroblastic anemia. It is important not to miss these reversible conditions.

Laboratory Studies

Routine CBC, blood film, and marrow aspirate and biopsy are the key studies used in diagnosing and classifying the dysplastic syndromes. Most patients are anemic on presentation. With time, most patients also develop leukopenia and thrombocytopenia. The severity of the anemia can vary from very mild to so severe that the patient requires blood transfusion.

A. PERIPHERAL BLOOD FILM MORPHOLOGY:

Peripheral blood film morphology may also be helpful. Patients can present with a macrocytic, normocytic, or slightly microcytic anemia with varying degrees of anisocytosis and poikilocytosis. Teardrop forms and nucleated red blood cells may be present, especially if the patient has a severely dysplastic or fibrotic marrow with extramedullary hematopoiesis. Both the granulocytes and platelets can be morphologically abnormal. Granulocytes with bilobed nuclei (**Pelger-Huët anomaly**) may be observed and platelets can be pale and poorly granulated. With progression of the disease to acute leukemia, the number of granulocytes and platelets falls even further and abnormal blasts appear in circulation.

B. Marrow Aspirate and Biopsy:

A good marrow aspirate and biopsy are essential. **Marrow cellularity** is usually increased, although it can be irregularly distributed in the medullary cavity and separated by areas of excess fat or fibrous tissue. Often this situation is associated with expansion of actively proliferating marrow into the shafts of long bones or extramedullary sites. Some patients will present with a normocellular or even hypocellular marrow. This can present a diagnostic dilemma if the hypoplasia is severe enough to suggest aplastic anemia. A careful inspection of the blood smear and marrow aspirate may help distinguish the two conditions. Presence of agranular neutrophils on smear and marrow megakaryocytes with from one to three separate nuclei (**pawn-ball nuclei**) suggest myelodysplasia. Abnormalities in red cell morphology are not helpful in the differential diagnosis.

Marrow aspirate morphology will usually reveal disturbances in **cell proliferation and maturation.** If the patient has a macrocytic anemia, the erythroid marrow is usually hyperplastic, megaloblastic, and ineffective (Table 9–2). Megakaryocyte and white cell morphology may also be abnormal. The number of megakaryocytes may be increased, with individual cells that are smaller than normal with decreased ploidy. Similarly, myelocytic maturation may be abnormal, with an apparent maturation arrest and poor granulation of mature granulocytes. Finally, an iron stain of the marrow aspirate is important to look for abnormal sideroblasts, especially ringed sideroblasts.

C. Chromosomal Analysis:

Chromosomal analysis can help both in diagnosis and prognosis because up to 80% of patients with dysplastic anemias will demonstrate a chromosomal abnormality

Table 9–3. Chromosomal abnormalities in dysplastic anemias.

Partial or full deletions (60–70% of cases)	Numeric abnormalities
Chromosome 5:5q minus syndrome	Monosomy 5, 7
	Trisomy 8
Chromosome 20	**Structural defects**
Loss of Y chromosome	Nonspecific defects, 1, 3, 6, and 17

(Table 9–3). Deletions of chromosomes 5, 7, and 20, and trisomies of 8 and 21, are the most common abnormalities and are diagnostic for myelodysplasia. Patients with a deletion of the long arm of chromosome 5 (5q minus syndrome), seen in 15% of de novo myelodysplasia and 50% of secondary dysplasias, represent a subgroup with a relatively good prognosis. Several genes are lost in the 5q deletion, including IL-3, 4, 5, and 9; granulocyte macrophage colony stimulating factor; c-fms; PDGF-receptor; IRF-1; EGR-1; Flt-4; and CD14. Point mutations that activate the *ras* proto-oncogene and multiple chromosome abnormalities, involving chromosomes 5 and 7, predict a worse outcome. A number of patients will also have a positive sugar water or Ham-acid hemolysis test or, preferably, a flow cytometric assay showing GPI anchored protein deficiencies (CD59-/CD55- red cells or CD16-/CD66b- granulocytes) indicative of paroxysmal nocturnal hemoglobinuria.

DIAGNOSIS

Classifications of dysplastic and sideroblastic anemias have been developed based on marrow and peripheral blood morphology, number of cytopenias, percentage of marrow blasts, and marrow cytogenetics. The **FAB ("French-American-British") classification** emphasizes

Table 9–2. Dysplastic anemias erythropoietic profile.

	Dysplastic	Sideroblastic
Red blood cell morphology	Mixed macro-, normo-, microcytic; moderate aniso- and poikilocytosis	
Reticulocyte index	< 2	
Marrow E/G ratio	> 1:1 to hypoplastic	
Marrow morphology	Megaloblastic to normoblastic Ringed sideroblasts	
Serum iron/TIBC	Normal/normal	Increased/normal
Serum ferritin	Normal	

the predominant cell line involved, number of blasts, and presence or absence of ringed sideroblasts. Major categories include refractory anemia (RA), refractory anemia with ringed sideroblasts (RARS), refractory anemia with excess blasts (RAEB), refractory anemia with excess blasts in transformation (RAEB-T), and chronic myelomonocytic leukemia (CMML). Recently, the RAEB-T subclassification has been dropped since it appears to be of little value in predicting response to therapy and survival. A new international scoring system for predicting outcome in myelodysplasia patients focuses on age and gender, marrow blast percentages, number of cytopenias, and cytogenetics. It can help identify higher-risk individuals in each of the FAB subgroups. It does not change the fact that all of these conditions are clonal malignancies with varying potential for evolution to acute leukemia.

Refractory Anemia (RA)

RA patients generally present with a mild to moderately severe anemia or pancytopenia and a hyperplastic marrow. Variable macrocytosis, mild to moderate aniso- and poikilocytosis, and abnormal maturation of marrow precursors help define the condition. At the same time, many of the features of the other dysplastic and sideroblastic disorders are not present. Less than 5% of the marrow cells are blasts and there are no ringed sideroblasts. Cytogenetic studies may or may not demonstrate a specific chromosomal defect. Research studies of mutations of the *ras* oncogene have shown point mutations in less than 10% of RA patients. These data are in contrast to the higher incidence in RAEB and CMML.

Since distinctive clinical and laboratory findings are less prominent in RA, **it is important to exclude reversible marrow damage anemia or pancytopenia.** Any history of exposure to radiation, drugs, or toxic chemicals is important. If the patient is young, has a significant exposure history, and demonstrates a somewhat hypoplastic marrow without morphologic or cytogenetic abnormalities, marrow damage is likely (see Chapter 3). Of course, these same exposures can incite a preleukemic condition, presenting as RA. Similar to idiopathic aplastic anemia, there is now evidence that T-cell-mediated suppression of marrow progenitors is an important component in the clinical picture in RA. However, the CD8 T-cell expansion is usually a secondary polyclonal response to one or more progenitor cell mutations, not a primary autoimmune disorder.

Refractory Anemia With Ringed Sideroblasts (RARS)

RARS is most often seen in older males. It usually appears in the fifth or sixth decade of life and follows a long, indolent course. Since the initial anemia is mild and the clinical findings are nonspecific, diagnosis is frequently delayed. Many patients will give a history of several years of treatment with various hematinic agents, including vitamin B_{12}, folic acid, vitamin B_6, and even iron, without noticeable effect. Over time, with RARS patients demonstrate a worsening anemia, increasing macrocytosis, aniso- and poikilocytosis, and both granulocytopenia and thrombocytopenia. Other morphologic clues include appearance on the blood film of small numbers of hypochromic cells and on occasion, heavily stippled red blood cells. The stippling tends to be coarser than that seen with lead poisoning and represents fragments of iron-encrusted mitochondria.

Definitive diagnosis is made from the marrow morphology. Typically, RARS patients have hyperplastic erythroid marrows that are somewhat megaloblastic with variable ineffective erythropoiesis. Often, many late erythroid marrow precursors show distorted, lobated nuclei with heavy stippling of the cytoplasm. The more hyperplastic the marrow, the easier it is to find abnormal late forms (**orthochromatic normoblasts**). These patients also show large numbers of **ringed sideroblasts** on the Prussian blue stain, that is, erythroid precursors that show a ring or collar of large, blue-staining granules immediately surrounding the nucleus. These can be demonstrated by electron microscopy to be iron-encrusted mitochondria and fragments of mitochondria. By light microscopy, their size and position readily distinguish them from cytoplasmic ferritin granules.

The frequency of ringed sideroblasts and the severity of the erythroid hyperplasia can vary widely. In some patients, most late erythroid precursors contain excess iron granules. More often, however, ringed sideroblasts represent a minor proportion of the developing erythroblasts. The latter is more typical of patients who demonstrate less erythroid hyperplasia or appear to have a relatively hypoplastic marrow. Whether this represents a difference in mechanism of disease or simply reflects a stage in the evolution of RARS is unclear. Patients with less proliferative marrows, few blasts, and few ringed sideroblasts may demonstrate a more prolonged, indolent clinical course.

Patients with RARS with **severe ineffective erythropoiesis** typically have high serum iron and serum ferritin levels. They are at risk for tissue iron loading with potential damage to liver and myocardium. This process can be made significantly worse if the patient requires long-term transfusion therapy or is a heterozygote for idiopathic hemachromatosis (see Chapter 14). Patients with RARS show less than 5% blasts on mar-

Table 9–4. Causes of sideroblastic anemia.

Hereditary (X-linked)
Acquired
  RARS
  Erythroleukemia
  Alcohol/folate/vitamin B_6 deficiency
  Copper deficiency
  Drugs: isoniazid, pyrazinamide, chloramphenicol, cycloserine,
    azathioprine, D-penicillamine
  Heavy metals: lead, zinc, arsenic
  Chronic inflammatory conditions

row examination and, like patients with RA, have a low potential for conversion to leukemia.

Idiopathic acquired RARS must always be distinguished from other causes of sideroblastic anemia (Table 9–4). Mitochondrial function can be impaired by several antibiotics and heavy metals (Figure 9–1). Isoniazid, pyrazinamide, cycloserine, azathioprine, d-penicillamine, and alcohol impair the vitamin B_6–dependent initial step in porphyrin production. Lead has a wider inhibitory effect. Patients with neoplasms or inflammatory disorders can occasionally present with a hypoproliferative anemia and occasional ringed sideroblasts. These appear to relate to the primary disease process and cannot be explained by drug effect or the appearance of true RARS. The potential interaction of heterozygosity for idiopathic hemachromatosis has not been well defined.

Refractory Anemia With Excess Blasts (RAEB)

Patients with either RAEB generally present with pancytopenia or severe anemia and granulocytopenia. Unlike RA and RARS, the blood film shows varying numbers of myeloblasts and bilobed granulocytes (**Pelger- Huët anomaly**). Diagnosis is made from marrow morphology. Cellularity of the marrow can vary from hyperplastic to hypoplastic with a patchy distribution on biopsy. On examination of the marrow aspirate, 5–20% of the cells are primitive blasts, either undifferentiated (**Type I myeloblasts**) or cells containing a few azurophilic granules (**Type II myeloblasts**). In addition, the number of monocytes and monocyte precursors may be increased, especially in patients with granulocytopenia. Finally, many of these patients show an increased number of small megakaryocytes with reduced ploidy.

The original classification of dysplastic anemias recognized a subset of patients with **RAEB-T** (**refractory anemia with excess blasts in transformation**). These patients were defined as having similar morphologic abnormalities but the number of blasts in peripheral blood is increased to more than 5% and the number of Types I and II myeloblasts in marrow is more than 20%. Since this distinction adds little in the way of understanding the etiology of the disease or planning therapy, it has been dropped. However, as a rule, the greater the number of the blasts, the more disturbed the morphology, and the more severe the patient's cytopenias, the more likely the patient will demonstrate multiple chromosomal abnormalities and a worse prognosis.

More attention is now being given to **chromosomal**

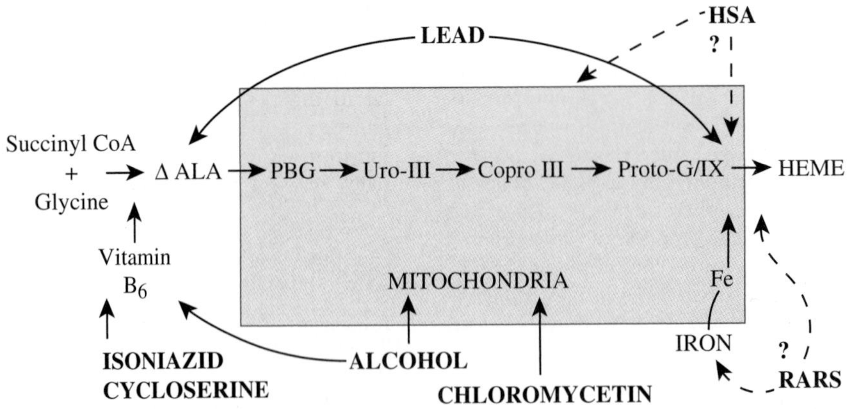

Figure 9–1. **Impairment of mitochondrial function and porphyrin synthesis.** Several drugs and heavy metals can interfere with several steps in porphyrin metabolism necessary to produce ringed sideroblasts. RARS and hereditary sideroblastic anemia (HSA) appear to interfere with the final heme synthetase step, possibly in conjunction with an inherited tendency to iron overload.

abnormalities associated with myelodysplasia, especially the most common defects—5q minus syndrome (a deletion in the long arm of chromosome 5) and monosomy 7. **5q minus syndrome** is most often seen in older women, is associated with marked dyserythropoiesis, and has a somewhat better prognosis. **Monosomy 7** appears to occur more frequently in patients with secondary myelodysplasia and carries a worse prognosis. It more rapidly evolves into acute myelogenous leukemia.

Chronic Myelomonocytic Leukemia (CMML)

Patients with CMML present with a blood picture that resembles RAEB, although their monocyte count is usually greater than $1000/\mu L$, and the marrow shows an increased number of monocytic precursors. Marrow blast count is less than 20%, and megakaryocyte maturation is usually normal. Chromosomal abnormalities are seen in up to 50% of CMML patients.

Dysplastic syndromes may be associated with several other abnormal laboratory findings. In the red blood cell area, patients usually show increased levels of hemoglobin F and less commonly, an altered globin chain synthetic rate that results in production of hemoglobin H. Patients can also demonstrate abnormalities of the red blood cell membrane such as changes in blood group antigens and the appearance of a membrane defect resembling paroxysmal nocturnal hemoglobinuria (PNH).

Both granulocyte and platelet function defects may be detected, leading to an increased susceptibility to infection and abnormal bleeding. In CMML patients, the blood and urinary lysozyme levels are usually increased, and the leukocyte alkaline phosphatase can be decreased in up to 20% of cases. Finally, some patients with RAEB and CMML will show fibrosis on marrow biopsy.

DIFFERENTIAL DIAGNOSIS

With the diversity of clinical and laboratory findings in dysplastic and sideroblastic anemias, it is not surprising that other disorders share features with these conditions. PNH, myelofibrosis (myeloid metaplasia), DeGuglielmo's anemia, and rare benign conditions such as congenital dyserythropoietic anemia (CDA) and hereditary sideroblastic anemia (HSA) all need to be considered in the differential diagnosis.

Paroxysmal Nocturnal Hemoglobinuria (PNH)

PNH is a clonal disorder of hematopoietic cells caused by a somatic mutation of the *pig*-A gene on the short arm of the X chromosome. More than 170 mutations in the *pig*-A gene have been reported. Some result in inactivation of the gene and a complete failure in the production of the GPI anchor protein—glycosylphosphatidylinositol glycan (**PNH III**)—while others result in a partial deficiency of the GPI anchor protein (**PNH II**). In both cases, binding of several other proteins is disturbed, including the amount of **protectin (CD59)** on the cell membrane. The loss of CD59, which normally regulates the assembly of the C9 attack complex, appears to play a key role in both red cell hemolysis and the hypercoagulable state seen in PNH patients. The phenotype of the disease is in part influenced by the nature of the mutation, with PNH III cells being more susceptible to hemolysis. However, it is also clear that both PNH II and PNH III clones can exist side by side in the same patient.

A. PRESENTATION AND COMPLICATIONS:

Patients with PNH present either with a **hemolytic anemia** with intravascular hemolysis and episodes of nocturnal hemoglobinuria or with a **pancytopenia** with a dysplastic or aplastic marrow morphology. Hemolytic disease is more often associated with a large, dominant clone of PNH cells, while aplastic and dysplastic individuals usually have few GPI-negative cells in circulation. One conclusion drawn from this observation is that marrow damage (bone marrow failure) somehow induces the PNH somatic mutation as a secondary manifestation of the disease, not that the mutation is the primary cause of the dysplastic or aplastic anemia.

Patients with PNH are also at **increased risk for venous thrombosis,** owing to complement-driven activation of platelets lacking CD59 and also, perhaps, impaired fibrinolysis. Thrombosis of hepatic veins (**Budd-Chiari syndrome**) or the portal, splenic, or mesenteric veins is a common manifestation of the hypercoagulable state and can lead to death or a clinical picture similar to that of disseminated intravascular coagulation. Patients with chronic hemolysis are at risk for developing **iron deficiency secondary to urine iron loss.** Finally, severe thrombocytopenia and granulocytopenia can lead to **major bleeding or infection.**

PNH can present anytime from the second to eighth decades of life. The diagnosis should be considered as a **part of the differential diagnosis of an anemia,** especially when accompanied by other cytopenias, a history of passing dark urine, iron deficiency without an obvious cause, or signs or symptoms suggesting venous thrombosis. Recurrent attacks of abdominal pain may indicate intra-abdominal thrombotic disease. PNH tends to be a chronic disorder; median survival after diagnosis is 8–10 years. Up to 15% of patients will demonstrate a spontaneous remission, whereas many die of either uncontrolled hemorrhage or thrombosis. Patients presenting with a marrow picture of aplasia or dysplasia frequently go undiagnosed if no one thinks to order a flow cytometric assay of cell surface CD59/CD55 levels.

B. DIAGNOSTIC TESTS:

Historically, the **sugar water test** was used as a convenient screening test for PNH. It is performed by adding a small amount of the patient's red blood cells to an isotonic sucrose solution laced with fresh complement. More than 5% lysis of cells suggests PNH, whereas less than 5% lysis may be seen in patients with megaloblastic and autoimmune hemolytic anemias. A somewhat more definitive test is the **Ham-acid hemolysis test,** which detects sensitivity of the PNH red blood cells to fresh complement and acidification. However, now that flow cytometry is available in most laboratories, a **cytometric assay of red cell CD59/CD55 levels** is clearly preferred. It is more sensitive and specific and can identify small subpopulations of abnormal cells. Two other GPI-anchored proteins, **CD16 and 66b, can also be measured** on granulocytes in patients with equivocal red cell results to further increase the sensitivity of the test.

All cell lines, including granulocytes and platelets, are involved in PNH and are susceptible to lysis. Although this may be responsible in part for the pancytopenia, many patients present with a hypocellular, even aplastic, marrow. In these patients, **marrow culture studies** demonstrate a reduced number of all progenitor lines, similar to the findings in marrow damage/aplastic anemia. The presence of GPI-negative cells is most often seen with T-cell-mediated marrow failure. It has now been reported that 15–50% of patients with idiopathic aplasia or myelodysplasia will demonstrate a PNH clone. Patients with marrow failure after chemotherapy, transplantation, immunotherapy, or secondary to large granular lymphocytosis (T-cell lymphoma) rarely have GPI-negative cells detected.

Myelofibrosis (Myeloid Metaplasia)

Myelofibrosis is another clonal malignancy that shares many of the features of the dysplastic anemias (see Chapter 18). Patients usually present later in life with a gradual onset of anemia, pancytopenia, and impressive splenomegaly. The dominant feature of the disorder is **progressive fibrosis of the marrow cavity** that results in dramatic expansion of extramedullary hemopoiesis in spleen and liver. The basis for this severe marrow fibrosis appears to be release of fibroblastic growth factors from an abnormal megakaryocyte line. Fibroblasts themselves do not share the chromosomal abnormalities observed in the hematopoietic cells.

Several **clinical features help distinguish myelofibrosis** from other dysplastic anemias. The blood film typically shows a combination of teardrop-shaped red blood cells and nucleated red blood cells. When extramedullary hematopoiesis is advanced, normal and abnormal myelocytes, a few blasts, and Pelger-Huët cells may be observed in circulation. The platelet count may be decreased, normal, or increased. In the latter case, it can reach levels in excess of 1 million/μL with the appearance in circulation of giant platelets and fragments of megakaryocytes.

A. DIAGNOSTIC TESTS:

Definitive diagnosis is made from the **marrow examination.** Often as not, attempts to aspirate marrow are unsuccessful and a biopsy is needed to demonstrate the fibrotic lesion. The marrow cavity can be virtually obliterated by dense collagenous tissue or demonstrate a patchy involvement with alternating areas of hyperplastic marrow. A **silver stain of the marrow biopsy** will highlight the fibrotic abnormality. Typically, myelofibrosis patients show a marked increase in reticulin fibers in the fibrous portions of the marrow. Granulocyte and megakaryocyte hyperplasia with abnormal maturation may also be observed.

B. CAUSES OF MYELOFIBROSIS:

The more abnormal the appearance of the hematopoietic cells, the more likely the patient will demonstrate a **chromosomal abnormality.** This abnormality includes deletions and translocations of chromosomes 1, 5, 7, 8, 9, and 20. Myelofibrosis can also occur secondary to infiltration of the marrow by **metastatic carcinoma** or as a result of **infections with mycobacteria.** The latter should always be considered in the differential diagnosis of myelofibrosis or myelodysplasia because failure to treat it can result in the patient's death.

DeGuglielmo's Syndrome (Erythroleukemia)

DeGuglielmo's anemia has been separately described as a **clonal malignancy that rapidly progresses to erythroleukemia.** At the same time, it shares features with RARS and RAEB. Some patients will present with a slightly macrocytic anemia, pancytopenia, and a hyperplastic marrow. With time, the pancytopenia worsens and the patient takes on characteristics of an acute leukemia of the erythroid line.

Common features of DeGuglielmo's anemia include red blood cell macrocytosis, marked aniso- and poikilocytosis, siderocytes and nucleated red blood cells on the peripheral blood film, and appearance of ringed sideroblasts in the marrow of some patients. **Distinguishing features** for the condition include appearance of late erythroid precursors with multiple nuclei, nuclear budding, and cloverleaf-shaped nuclei. Some of the late precursors also show a heavy cytoplasmic stippling, reminiscent of RARS. A unique finding, however, is the dramatic appearance of the periodic acid–Schiff (PAS) stain. The cytoplasm of mature red blood cell precursors is filled with large PAS-positive granules. Finally, close examination of the reticuloendothelial portion of the marrow aspirate may reveal erythrophagocytosis.

Congenital Dysplastic & Sideroblastic Anemias

Inherited defects in precursor maturation can result in a lifelong anemia with features similar to those of acquired dysplastic and sideroblastic anemia. Congenital dyserythropoietic anemias are a group of disorders **characterized by the striking multinuclearity of erythroid precursors. Hereditary sideroblastic anemia** is defined by the presence of ringed sideroblasts in marrow and a defect in hemoglobin production.

A. CONGENITAL DYSERYTHROPOIETIC ANEMIA (CDA):

Patients with CDA are usually diagnosed during childhood, although when anemia is mild they may escape detection until well into adult life. They present with a slightly macrocytic anemia with aniso- and poikilocytosis, a low reticulocyte index, and an otherwise normal CBC. The finding that leads to diagnosis is **marked dysmorphology of the erythroid marrow** (Table 9–5).

CDA is classified according to unique distortions of the nuclei of erythroid precursors. **CDA Type I** is characterized by megaloblastic erythroid hyperplasia with ineffective erythropoiesis, binucleate erythroblasts, and prominent intranuclear chromatin bridging. **CDA Type II** is characterized by more prominent binuclearity, karyorrhexis, and lobulation of the nuclei of the late erythroid precursors. In addition, these patients have a positive Ham-acid hemolysis test. Because of the latter finding, Type II CDA is also referred to as **HEMPAS (hereditary erythroblastic multinuclearity associated**

with a positive acidified serum test). **CDA Type III** is distinguished by the appearance of extremely large late erythroid precursors with up to 12 nuclei per cell. **CDA Type IV** has morphologic characteristics of Type II CDA but a negative acid hemolysis test.

Chromosome studies of CDA patients have failed to show an abnormality that would explain the defect in nuclear maturation. These conditions do not evolve into leukemia and, depending on the severity of the anemia, the prognosis is quite good. As with other conditions characterized by abnormal precursor maturation with ineffective erythropoiesis, **iron overload** can be a significant complication. This situation is worsened if the patient requires long-term transfusion.

B. HEREDITARY SIDEROBLASTIC ANEMIA (HSA):

Patients with HSA usually present during infancy or childhood with a severe microcytic, hypochromic anemia. The defect is usually X-linked, so males present with the most severe form of the disease. It is caused by a mutation of the erythroid-specific δ-aminolevulinic acid synthase enzyme at Xp11.21. Carrier females may be identified because of a dimorphic blood film with even proportions of microcytic, hypochromic, and normal red blood cells. The **diagnostic finding** is the presence of classic ringed sideroblasts on Prussian blue stain.

THERAPY

The most important principles in managing the dysplastic and sideroblastic anemias are to **provide maximum support and encouragement** to the patient over the prolonged course of their disease and to **avoid potentially harmful treatments in early stages** of the disease. The **classification of dysplastic anemias** provides guidance as to the patient's prognosis (Figure 9–2).

Prognosis & Survival

Patients with RA and RARS and less severe anemia are slow to evolve to more severe disease or to acute

Table 9–5. Profiles of congenital dyserythropoietic anemias.

Type	MCV (fL)	Marrow Morphology
CDA I	95–110	Megaloblastic with binucleate erythroblasts and chromatin bridging
CDA II HEMPAS	90	Normoblastic with marked binucleate erythroblasts; *positive* acid hemolysis test
CDA III	90–100	Giant, multinucleate erythroblasts
CDA IV	80–90	Normoblastic with marked bi- or multinucleate erythroblasts; *negative* acid hemolysis test

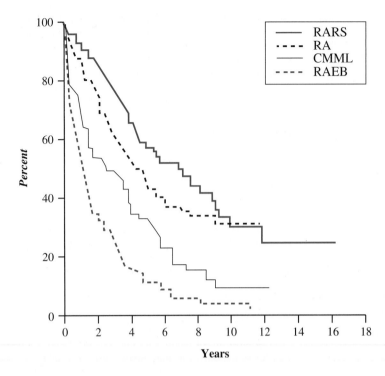

Figure 9–2. **Patient survival according to the classification of the dysplastic anemias.** Patients with RARS or RA have significantly better survivals when compared with patients with RAEB or CMML.

leukemia. Patients with RA and RARS have median survivals in excess of 36–72 months, and less than 10% become leukemic, whereas **patients with RAEB** have median survivals of 5–15 months with better than a 50% chance of transformation to acute myelogenous leukemia.

The international prognostic scoring system classifies myelodysplastic anemias into one low-risk category, two intermediate-risk (INT-1 and INT-2) categories, and one high-risk category. By weighting the impact of age, abnormal cytogenetics, cytopenias, and blast number, it is somewhat more accurate in its prediction of survival. **Patients with normal karyotypes or deletions of only 20q, 5q, or the Y chromosome** do much better than those with **multiple abnormalities** involving chromosomes 5 and 7 (median survival greater than 12 months with single chromosome abnormalities as compared with survivals of less than 6 months with multiple abnormalities). Younger patients with fewer cytopenias and lower blast counts also do better. Overall, **low-risk patients** have median survivals of almost 6 years, as compared with 3.5 years for those with INT-1, 1.2 years for those with INT-2, and 0.4 years for high-risk patients.

Patients at Risk for Iron Overload

Patients with sideroblastic or dysplastic anemias with marked ineffective erythropoiesis and a high transfu-sion requirement are at great risk for iron overload. This needs to be considered early in the course of their management and they need to be followed up closely over time. Repeated iron studies are an essential component of patient management. Treatment with deferoxamine can prevent organ damage and, on occasion, by reducing the patient's iron load, improve hematopoiesis (Chapter 14).

Patients With PNH

Management of patients with PNH will vary according to the nature of the clinical presentation. When hemolysis is the dominant feature, folic acid and iron supplementation are needed to sustain red blood cell production levels. Iron therapy can worsen the patient's episodes of PNH by increasing the daily production of PNH cells. This should not, however, be taken as a reason to stop therapy. Long-term anticoagulation should be considered in all PNH patients, especially those with thrombotic disease, unless there is a major contraindication such as severe thrombocytopenia. Platelet and red blood cell transfusions will be necessary in patients with marked marrow dysplasia or aplasia. Young patients with PNH and severe disease are candidates for allogeneic bone marrow transplantation. Immunosuppressive therapy has had limited success but may improve the cytopenias.

Blood Component Therapy

As patients become more severely anemic or pancytopenic, they need to be supported with red blood cell and platelet transfusions. Red blood cell transfusions should not be initiated until the patient is symptomatic. In an otherwise healthy individual, this will mean a hemoglobin level of 8 grams per deciliter or less. Elderly patients with cardiovascular disease may need to receive transfusions at an earlier stage, however. With time, patients usually become very good judges of their own transfusion needs, decreasing the need for frequent hemoglobin measurements.

Once transfusion therapy is initiated, it is likely that patients will become **transfusion dependent.** Moreover, it can be anticipated that the transfusion requirement will gradually increase. This tendency is accelerated in patients who develop red blood cell antibodies or splenomegaly (**hypersplenism**). Long-term transfusion therapy also runs the risk of stimulating HLA alloantibodies. It is advisable, therefore, to **use leukofiltered red blood cells** for transfusion. Certainly, any patient who experiences chills and fever with transfusions should only receive leukopoor red blood cells.

A. IRON OVERLOAD:

Patients who have a tendency toward iron overload will be at a greater risk for iron toxicity when they receive transfusions over a long period. The **rate of iron accumulation** is easily calculated from the transfusion record; each 200-mL unit of packed red blood cells contributes approximately 200 mg of excess iron. **Long-term chelation therapy with deferoxamine** should be considered for younger patients with RA and RARS. Not only will this decrease the rate of iron loading, but in the case of RARS, chelation therapy may also improve red blood cell production.

B. PLATELET TRANSFUSION:

Prophylactic platelet transfusions should not be routinely used because of the risk of HLA alloimmunization and platelet refractoriness. If possible, platelet transfusions should only be used to prepare a patient for a surgical procedure or treat an acute hemorrhage. Usually, the patients can tolerate platelet counts as low as 5–10,000/µL without spontaneous bleeding. They should be advised, however, to avoid aspirin and nonsteroidal anti-inflammatory agents that can inhibit platelet function.

C. INFECTIONS:

Life-threatening infections are uncommon in dysplastic and sideroblastic anemia patients unless the absolute granulocyte count falls below 300–500/µL. Localized infections should be treated promptly with the appropriate antibiotic, since these patients often lack granulocyte reserves and can develop leukopenia with uncontrolled infections. Dysplastic anemia patients do appear to be a greater risk for reactivation of mycobacterial infections. Any patient who presents with sustained fever, malaise, a worsening pancytopenia, and abnormal liver chemistries should be evaluated for a systemic mycobacterial or fungal infection.

Vitamin Therapy

Although many of the dysplastic anemias present with a macrocytic anemia and megaloblastic marrow, treatment with either vitamin B_{12} or folic acid is ineffective. Patients with hereditary, x-linked, sideroblastic anemia often respond to **pyridoxine therapy** and should be tried on a regimen of 50 mg/day pyridoxine orally for 2–3 months to document response. The rare patient with RARS may respond to vitamin B_6 (pyridoxine) given in doses of 50 mg or more per day by mouth. Parenterally administered **pyridoxal-5-phosphate** has also been reported to partially correct the sideroblastic anemia in some patients. This has not been accepted as standard therapy, however. Other hematinics are not indicated. Certainly, iron should not be administered to patients with a sideroblastic anemia or ineffective erythropoiesis where there is a tendency to iron overload. Androgens, steroids, and immunosuppressive therapy have also been of little value.

Chemotherapy & Bone Marrow Transplantation

Cytotoxic chemotherapy has been used in **younger patients with RAEB** with approximately the same response as seen in AML (excluding acute promyelocytic leukemia). Therefore, as the patient takes on more features of acute leukemia, it makes sense to attempt a regimen similar to that used in treating AML, a two- or three-drug regimen containing a cell-cycle–specific agent. **Elderly patients** do not do well with these regimens. They tolerate less drug, develop marked marrow hypoplasia, and fail to enter a sustained remission. **Patients with complex chromosomal abnormalities or monosomy 7** also do less well; fewer than 50% will achieve a complete remission. Even with the best candidate, event-free survival at 2–3 years is less than 30%.

Allogeneic bone marrow transplantation may work in patients with RAEB. The largest series of some 66 patients reported a 24% 5-year disease-free survival rate regardless of their pretransplant chemotherapy history. A recent report of allogeneic and syngeneic transplantation in older patients (ages 55–66) with RA and RAEB showed even better success rates, 30–60% estimated 3-year survivals according to the extent of cytogenetic abnormalities. It would appear that marrow transplantation can be carried out successfully even when the patient's marrow is quite fibrotic.

Low-dose treatment with **cytarabine** has been used to encourage differentiation of malignant cell lines and thereby inhibit both the proliferation of blasts and the suppression of normal cell maturation. Cytarabine, given in dosages of 20 mg/m^2/day in single or divided subcutaneous or intravenous doses over 14–21 days, can result in a partial remission in up to 40% of patients. This therapy can improve the peripheral blood counts and reduce both red blood cell and platelet transfusion requirements. Usually, the response lasts for only a few months and overall survival is unaffected. Some trials have used several cycles of low-dose cytarabine with some success. The retinoid, **13-*cis*-retinoic acid,** can also induce cell differentiation in dysplastic anemia patients. An oral, daily dose of 20 mg or 100 mg/m^2 is well tolerated and may produce some improvement in the blood picture in up to 30% of patients. Side effects include stomatitis, cheilitis, arthralgias, headache, thrombocytopenia, and hepatotoxicity. Overall, the survival does not appear to be improved.

Immunosuppressive Therapy

T-cell-mediated suppression of marrow progenitor cells has been implicated as a mechanism contributing to pancytopenia in dysplastic anemias. A limited number of trials of ATG and cyclosporine have shown responses in a third or more of patients, with the highest response rate in RA patients. Patients with severely hypoplastic marrows have also shown a better response rate, perhaps raising the question of whether they represent a form of severe aplastic anemia (see Chapter 3). Response criteria were transfusion-independence, increases in neutrophil and platelet counts, and progression-free survival. There is concern that immunosuppressive therapy will accelerate progression of patients to RAEB and acute leukemia.

Hematopoietic Growth Factors

Most patients with dysplastic and sideroblastic anemias can be expected to have very high levels of endogenous erythropoietin. This assumption can be confirmed by **measurements of plasma erythropoietin level.** A few patients (10–15%) do appear to have a suboptimal erythropoietin response, however, and will respond to standard doses of 150–300 U/kg of recombinant erythropoietin given subcutaneously three times a week. Routine therapeutic trials with erythropoietin are to be discouraged, simply on the basis of expense. If erythropoietin is used, it should be in patients who have low serum erythropoietin levels.

Granulocyte colony-stimulating factors (both G-CSF and GM-CSF) are effective in stimulating granulocyte production. When given in dosages of 1–3 μg/kg/day, per day, G-CSF will increase the granulocyte count in 40–50% of patients. Similarly, GM-CSF given in dosages of 3 μg/kg/day per day will increase the granulocyte count to a level of 5–10,000/μL in most leukopenic patients. This increase can be useful in managing pancytopenic patients with acute infection.

Long-term administration of these growth factors raises concern that they may actually speed the progression to acute leukemia. A single multicenter trial of G-CSF versus observation did not show a significant increase in rate of progression to AML in 102 RAEB/RAEB-T patients. Trials using combinations of growth factors (erythropoietin plus G-CSF, GM-CSF, or interleukin-3 [IL-3], or IL-3 plus GM-CSF) have shown somewhat better neutrophil and red blood cell responses, although at a cost of increased side effects when IL-3 is included.

BIBLIOGRAPHY

Dysplastic and Sideroblastic Syndromes

Bottomley SS: The spectrum and role of iron overload in sideroblastic anemia. Ann NY Acad Sci 1988;526:331.

Bottomley SS, Muller-Eberhard U: Pathophysiology of heme synthesis. Semin Hematol 1988;25:282.

Doll DC, List AF: Myelodysplastic syndromes. West J Med 1989;151:161.

Estey E et al: Effect of diagnosis (refractory anemia with excess blasts, refractory anemia with excess blasts in transformation, or acute myeloid leukemia [AML]) on outcome of AML-type chemotherapy. Blood 1997;90:2969.

Foucar K et al: Myelodysplastic syndromes: A clinical and pathologic analysis of 109 cases. Cancer 1985;56:553.

Greenberg P et al: International scoring system for evaluating prognosis in myelodysplastic syndromes. Blood 1997;89:2079.

Kouides PA, Bennett JM: Morphology and classification of myelodysplastic syndromes. Hematol Oncol Clin North Am 1992;6:485.

Paroxysmal Nocturnal Hemoglobinuria

Dunn DE et al: Paroxysmal nocturnal hemoglobinuria cells in patients with bone marrow failure syndromes. Ann Intern Med 1999;131:401.

Hall SE, Rosse WF: The use of monoclonal antibodies and flow cytometry in the diagnosis of paroxysmal nocturnal hemoglobinuria. Blood 1996;87:532.

Hillmen P et al: Natural history of paroxysmal nocturnal hemoglobinuria. N Engl J Med 1995;333:1253.

Luzzatto L: Paroxysmal murine hemoglobinuria(?): A model for human PNH. Blood 1999;94:2941.

Rosse WF, Ware RE: The molecular basis of paroxysmal nocturnal hemoglobinuria. Blood 1995;86:3277.

Therapy

Anderson JE et al: Stem cell transplantation for secondary acute leukemia: Evaluation of transplantation as initial therapy of following induction chemotherapy. Blood 1997;89:2578.

Deeg HJ et al: Allogeneic and syngeneic transplantation for myelodysplastic syndrome in patients 55 to 66 years of age. Blood 2000;95:1188.

Janasova A et al: Cyclosporine A therapy in hypoplastic MDS patients and certain refractory anemias without hypoplastic bone marrow. Br J Haematol 1998;100:304.

Kizaki M, Koeffler HP: Differentiation-inducing agents in the treatment of myelodysplastic syndromes. Semin Oncol 1992;19:95.

Mogl P: Management of patients with myelodysplastic syndromes. Mayo Clin Proc 1991;66:485.

Molldrem JJ et al: Antithymocyte globulin for patients with myelodysplastic syndrome. Br J Haematol 1997;99:699.

Blood Loss Anemia

Acute blood loss has a direct impact on the integrity of the blood volume and oxygen supply to tissues. Sudden, severe hemorrhage can induce hypovolemic shock, cardiovascular failure, and death. When blood loss is more gradual, the hemoglobin level can fall to a point where oxygen delivery to vital organs is compromised. Chronic blood loss will deplete iron stores and produce an iron deficiency anemia. Therefore, diagnosis and management of a blood loss anemia must take into account the reason behind the loss, the rate and amount of blood loss, and the capacity of the patient to compensate for both volume losses and anemia.

NORMAL RESPONSE TO BLOOD LOSS

Compensation for acute hemorrhage involves both a well-defined cardiovascular response to hypovolemia and the erythropoietic response to a reduction in red blood cell mass.

Cardiovascular Response

Blood volume **losses of up to 20% of the total blood volume** are readily tolerated by a normal individual (Table 10–1). This is accomplished by redistribution of blood flow, principally a contraction of the venous blood pool by reflex venospasm. Pain, fever, or a vasovagal response can interfere with this normal compensatory mechanism. An obvious example of this is the vasovagal syncope reaction to a painful injury or the anxiety initiated by acute blood loss.

When acute blood loss exceeds 20% of the total blood volume (more than 1000 mL in a 70-kg adult with an estimated blood volume of 5000 mL), venospasm alone will not compensate for the reduction in blood volume. These individuals will want to remain supine and may demonstrate a postural drop in blood pressure on sitting or standing. They will also become tachycardic with exercise. Once blood loss exceeds 30% of the blood volume (1500 mL), postural hypotension is clearly present and patients may faint if they stand up. Hypovolemic shock starts once blood loss exceeds 40% of the total blood volume (2000 mL).

When blood loss is gradual, compensation is provided by expansion of plasma volume. The ability to acutely mobilize **albumin,** the principal oncotic protein of plasma, from extravascular sites is limited, however. New production of albumin is a relatively slow process, so full restoration of an acute volume loss of 1000–1500 mL can take 20–60 hours. At the same time, normal individuals easily tolerate chronic blood losses of 1000 mL or more per week, producing sufficient albumin to replace their plasma losses. Albumin production is well maintained even when nutrition intake is temporarily restricted.

Erythroid Marrow Response

As discussed in Chapter 1, the normal erythroid marrow rapidly increases red blood cell production in response to anemia or hypoxia. The **capacity of marrow to respond** depends on the level of erythropoietin stimulation, the presence of a normal complement of erythroid precursors in a normal marrow structure, and an adequate supply of iron. The erythropoietin response is a function of anemia severity. Once the hemoglobin falls to levels below 11 grams per deciliter, the normal kidney secretes increasing amounts of erythropoietin. This response occurs within a matter of hours. At the same time, marrow expansion, which leads to an increase in the reticulocyte count and a rise in the total number of circulating red blood cells, takes days to weeks.

The **pattern of response to a sudden reduction in hematocrit** is summarized in Table 10–2. During the first 2 days, initial evidence of an increased level of erythropoietin stimulation is the appearance in circulation of **polychromatic macrocytes (shift cells).** These are marrow reticulocytes that are released 1–2 days early under the stimulation of a high level of erythropoietin. Although appearance of these young reticulocytes will raise the percent reticulocyte count, the actual **index of production** (absolute reticulocyte count corrected for the early release of marrow reticulocytes) will not have increased (see Chapter 2). Furthermore, if the marrow is examined, the ratio of erythroid to granulocytic precursors (E/G ratio) is still 1:3. Overall, the erythropoietic profile during the first 1–2 days after an acute hemorrhage fits the description of a hypoproliferative anemia.

Table 10–1. Symptoms and signs of blood volume losses in the adult.

Percent Lost	Volume Lost (mL)[a]	Symptoms	Signs
< 20	< 1000	+/– Anxiety	+/– Vasovagal reaction
20–30	1000–1500	Anxiety, exercise intolerance, may faint on standing	Orthostatic hypotension, exertional tachycardia
30–40	1500–2000	Syncope when sits or stands	Orthostatic, anxious, tachycardic at rest
> 40	> 2000	Anxious, restless, often confused, may be short of breath	Hypovolemic shock, fall in supine blood pressure, tachycardic with cool, clammy skin

[a] Calculated for a 70-kg adult with a blood volume of 5000 mL.

A definite **increase in erythroid marrow response** should be detectable during the next several days. Initially, by days 3–6 the marrow E/G ratio increases to levels of 1:1 (a threefold expansion of erythroid precursors), followed by an increase in the reticulocyte index. An **apparent imbalance** between the level of proliferation of the marrow and the reticulocyte response should not be interpreted as ineffective erythropoiesis. Rather, it reflects the fact that the erythropoietic response has not yet reached steady state. By days 7–10, the reticulocyte production response should reach a level of at least three times basal. Now, the marrow E/G ratio of 1:1 and the reticulocyte production index of three times normal are in balance. This process depends, however, on the level of iron supply. When reticuloendothelial iron stores are depleted, red blood cell production may never reach three times basal and certainly cannot be sustained at that level without iron supplementation.

Red Blood Cell Oxygen Delivery

Although the marrow response to a blood loss anemia is slow, circulating red blood cells are able to quickly compensate by increasing their transfer of oxygen to tissues. This is a two-step process. When acute hemorrhage reduces the number of red blood cells or the blood flow to a tissue (or both), the red blood cells perfusing the tissue respond to the more acidic environment with an instantaneous shift in the hemoglobin-oxygen dissociation curve to the right, which is known as the **Bohr effect.** In effect, it facilitates transfer of oxygen to tissues. Over the next several hours, this phenomenon leads to an **increased production of 2,3-diphosphoglycerate** in the red blood cell. This process maintains the higher level of oxygen delivery. Together, these mechanisms can maintain relatively normal levels of oxygen delivery to key organs with only half the normal number of circulating red blood cells.

CLINICAL FEATURES

Clinical presentation of a blood loss anemia will vary according to the site and severity of blood loss. Massive hemorrhage from the gastrointestinal tract or an external trauma site will be immediately obvious. The rate and magnitude of the blood loss may also be apparent. Slower bleeding internally can be harder to diagnose. In the case of gastrointestinal blood loss, patients may only present once they have developed an iron deficiency anemia. With bleeding into tissues or a closed cavity, however, the presenting anemia may mimic acute hemolysis. Therefore, severity of the bleed, rate and site of the bleed, and capacity of the patient to respond are all integral in defining the clinical presentation.

Table 10–2. Erythropoietic response to acute hemorrhage.

Days after Bleed	1–2	3–6	7–10
Marrow reticulocyte shift (polychromasia)	+	++	+++
Reticulocyte production index (times normal)	1	1–2	> 2–3
E/G ratio	1:3	1:1	> 1:1

Large Volume Blood Loss

Sudden loss of a large volume of blood has an immediate impact on the patient's cardiovascular status. Relatively healthy, young to middle-aged individuals can tolerate acute volume **losses of up to 30% of their blood volume** with few symptoms other than mild postural hypotension (see Table 10–1). This situation may not be true, however, for elderly individuals or patients with complicating illness. Fever, severe pain, and exposure can all interfere with the reflex mechanisms that compensate for modest volume losses. Once an acute loss of blood **exceeds 30% of the patient's blood volume,** postural hypotension worsens and symptoms and signs of hypovolemic shock appear, including a rapid, thready pulse; cool, clammy skin; air hunger; and confusion. **When blood loss approaches 50% of blood volume,** heart failure and death are imminent unless volume expanders are administered immediately.

The impact on the blood volume overshadows the effect of acute blood loss on red blood cell mass. Even as a patient approaches death from hypovolemia and cardiovascular shock, **depletion of red blood cell mass** is still less than 50%. This level of red blood cell loss would not be life-threatening, however, in a normal individual with a normal blood volume and cardiovascular system. Oxygen delivery to tissues will remain close to normal because of the shift in the hemoglobin-oxygen dissociation curve. When red blood cell loss is combined with blood volume loss, however, tissue perfusion fails and severe tissue hypoxia appears as a major component of hypovolemic shock.

Important features in the clinical presentation include the cause, location, magnitude, and duration of the blood loss. External trauma can result in either arterial or venous hemorrhage and produce hypovolemic shock within a matter of minutes. Large volume bleeding from the gastrointestinal tract is seen with esophageal varices, esophageal tears, or ulcer-induced arterial bleeds. A less obvious presentation is a major bleed into a closed cavity or tissue. Patients who fracture their hip or pelvis can lose 1–2 liters of blood into the thigh and pelvic area. Bleeds into the pleural and peritoneal cavities can easily exceed 30% of the patient's blood volume and result in the rapid onset of hypovolemic shock.

Lower Volume, Slower Blood Loss

When the amount of blood loss is less and the rate slower, the **plasma volume expands to maintain a relatively normal total blood volume.** A normal individual can usually keep up with rates of 200–300 mL of whole blood loss per day without experiencing symptoms or signs of hypovolemia. This level may not suffice for the patients with liver disease or a chronic debilitating illness that interferes with their ability to produce new oncotic protein. These patients will exhibit a combination of postural hypotension and congestive heart failure. Severe right heart failure with marked edema and ascites can be anticipated in these patients if their albumin production is significantly impaired.

In the absence of hypovolemia, patients with ongoing, gradual losses of blood will present with the **symptoms and signs of anemia.** These signs will vary depending on the rate of onset, the severity of the anemia, and the patient's age. Younger, healthy individuals will tolerate moderately severe anemias with little complications other than a loss in stamina and some increase in heart rate and dyspnea with exercise. Older individuals become symptomatic with even mild anemias (hemoglobins of 10–11 grams per deciliter). They are also at risk for the early onset of heart failure if they have coexisting cardiovascular disease.

Once the hemoglobin level falls below 8–9 grams per deciliter, most patients will report palpitations, shortness of breath, and easy fatigability with exertion. They may also report difficulty with concentration, sleep disturbance, and pounding headaches. Clinical signs of a **worsening anemia** include tachycardia, signs of an increased cardiac stroke volume, and a loss of skin and mucous membrane color. On physical examination of the heart, the apical impulse is more forceful and flow murmurs secondary to increased blood turbulence can be heard as mid- or holosystolic murmurs at the apex and along the left sternal border.

Small Volume, Chronic Blood Loss

Loss of small volumes of blood (less than 100 mL per day) is **easily compensated by albumin production and plasma volume restoration.** In addition, anemia develops over weeks, permitting maximum compensation by the shift of the oxygen dissociation curve, production of new red blood cells by erythroid marrow, and, when anemia is severe, changes in cardiac output and blood flow. Because of this, patients may not be symptomatic enough to seek medical attention. This will delay the diagnosis and lead to the appearance of an iron deficiency anemia.

The slower and more protracted the bleeding, the more likely the patient will **present with symptoms and signs of iron deficiency,** which include a general loss of stamina and well-being, cardiovascular symptoms and signs of severe anemia, sore mouth and difficulty swallowing, and a softening and spooning of the fingernails. Children often develop **pica,** an unusual appetite for ice or dirt.

Chronic blood loss leading to iron deficiency is usually caused by gastrointestinal blood loss. However, some patients may present with a defect in iron absorption, secondary to small-bowel disease, such as nontropical sprue or extensive Crohn's disease. Patients who have had a Billroth II operation with vagotomy for ulcer disease can also exhibit food iron malabsorption. In developing countries, hookworm infestation is a frequent cause of chronic blood loss leading to severe iron deficiency. Less frequently, patients can present with a blood loss anemia secondary to hemoglobinuria (paroxysmal nocturnal hemoglobinuria), pulmonary hemosiderosis, or a self-induced blood loss.

Perisurgical Blood Loss

Blood losses can usually be predicted according to the surgical procedure. Unanticipated excessive bleeding can, however, result in a large volume loss picture, requiring both **plasma volume and red cell mass support.** With massive blood losses, **platelet and coagulation factor replacement** will be necessary to guarantee hemostasis. In order to minimize the patient's exposure to homologous blood, patients should not be overtransfused. It is preferable to leave the physiologically stable patient with a significant postoperative anemia, hematocrit in the 20–30% range. This will not interfere with recovery and wound healing.

In the case of a significant preoperative anemia (hematocrit less than 36%), small body size predicting a small blood volume, or an expected blood loss of more than 1000 mL, consideration should be given to **autologous blood storage, perioperative erythropoietin therapy, or both.** When these therapies are used in combination, it is possible to avoid homologous blood transfusion in many patients undergoing elective noncardiac procedures with predictable major blood losses.

Laboratory Studies

Laboratory findings will also vary according to the size and rate of blood loss. The behavior of the complete blood count (CBC) is a good example. Although it would seem to make sense that the hemoglobin level (hematocrit) would provide a good measure of red blood cell loss, it is not necessarily the case. Hemoglobin and hematocrit measurements are volume ratios where the quantity of red blood cells depends on the volume of diluent plasma. Immediately after an acute, severe hemorrhage, there will be little change in the hemoglobin (hematocrit) until the plasma volume has time to expand (Figure 10–1). Without fluid administration, this process takes more than 24 hours. If a volume expander is given, the change in hemoglobin level correlates as much with the volume transfused as with the volume of blood lost.

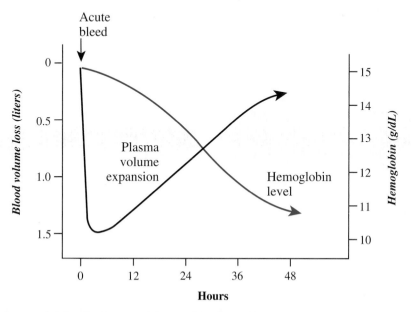

Figure 10–1. Changes in blood volume and hemoglobin level after an acute bleed. The compensatory expansion of the plasma volume following an acute bleed can take more than 48 hours if a volume expander is not administered. The hemoglobin level will reflect this delay in volume expansion. It will not reach its lowest point until full plasma volume expansion has occurred.

Severe hemorrhage may be accompanied by other changes in the CBC. The granulocyte count can increase dramatically to levels of 20,000/μL or higher, and immature white cell forms can appear in circulation. This situation reflects a demargination of granulocytes secondary to the patient's catecholamine response and a release of granulocytes from the marrow storage pool. With **hypovolemic shock and hypoxia,** very immature cells, including metamyelocytes, myelocytes, and nucleated red blood cells, can also appear in circulation. A rise in the platelet count to levels exceeding 1 million per microliter can also occur in the days after a severe hemorrhage. The explanation for this rise in platelet count is unclear.

A. FINDINGS IN THE DAYS AFTER BLOOD LOSS:

In the days following a significant blood loss, laboratory studies will demonstrate a normal erythroid marrow compensatory response to anemia. The first surge of erythropoietin will within a matter of hours cause marrow reticulocytes to enter circulation. This shift phenomenon can be appreciated from the appearance of polychromatic macrocytes on the peripheral film. Changes in the marrow E/G ratio and reticulocyte index will then follow the predictable, normal response pattern to anemia (see Table 10–2). Laboratory studies during the first week after hemorrhage must be interpreted against this template of the "normal" erythropoietic response.

B. FINDINGS AFTER THE FIRST WEEK:

After the first 7–10 days, the **reticulocyte count** should provide a good measure of effective red blood cell production. This count requires calculating the **reticulocyte index,** which is the percent count corrected for anemia and shift (Chapter 2). With an acute, self-limited blood loss, recovery of the **hemoglobin (hematocrit)** over the next several weeks can also be used to estimate effective red blood cell production. The change in the hemoglobin level is much slower than the reticulocyte production index, however, and full recovery can take many weeks.

Laboratory testing is of greatest value during **recovery. Serial measurements of reticulocyte count** in the weeks following a hemorrhage provide an important indicator of the effectiveness of the marrow's response. Given an adequate supply of reticuloendothelial iron stores, a normal adult should increase his or her reticulocyte production index to two to three times basal after 7–10 days and sustain this production level over the next several weeks. If the reticulocyte index falls back toward the basal level, iron studies should be performed to look for the emergence of iron deficiency or an inflammatory suppression of both the erythropoietin response and iron supply.

DIAGNOSIS

Types of Bleeding

When patients present with **severe, ongoing hemorrhage,** the diagnosis can be made at the bedside, and the location and rate of the bleeding can help predict the magnitude of the red blood cell loss. If symptoms and signs of hypovolemia are present, the patient will almost certainly develop a relatively severe blood loss anemia. Patients presenting with **less severe, slower bleeding** are a greater diagnostic challenge. Most of these patients will have a gastrointestinal abnormality and will follow a clinical course typical for their disease. The timing and location of the bleed will determine the patient's presenting symptoms, physical signs, and laboratory findings. For example, patients with advanced cirrhosis have episodic, large volume bleeds from varices, accompanied by sudden, dramatic hematemesis and melena. Patients with gastritis or peptic ulcer disease present in a similar fashion or with melena alone.

Bleeding from the small or large intestine may only be evidenced by routine Hemoccult screening. When the amount of blood lost exceeds 50–100 mL per day, patients will report black, often foul-smelling stools. If the loss into the small intestine is greater than 200 mL per day, the blood will act as a laxative, resulting in multiple black to maroon-colored, loose stools. The more rapid the bleeding, the greater chance the patient will exhibit symptoms and signs of hypovolemia.

Physical examination and laboratory findings in **patients with slower bleeds** will depend on the clinical course of the illness. Many patients will bleed for some period before seeking medical attention and will have had time to respond with an expansion of their plasma volume. It should be possible, therefore, to detect many symptoms and signs of anemia. Laboratory studies such as the hemoglobin (hematocrit) should provide a fair measure of anemia severity, whereas the reticulocyte count and red blood cell indices provide a sense of the level of effective red blood cell production and adequacy of iron supply.

Timing of the Bleeding Episode

Interpretation of any set of laboratory studies depends on the timing of the bleeding episode. If a patient presents soon after the bleeding begins, laboratory studies must be interpreted according to the template of the normal erythropoietic response to acute anemia or hypoxia. In contrast, when patients present with a more protracted course of bleeding, it may be assumed that the erythroid marrow has had an opportunity to respond. In this situation, studies of red blood cell production and iron supply are important to look for the appearance of iron deficiency.

Chronic, low-grade blood loss can go undetected for long periods, until the patient presents with symptoms and signs of anemia and iron deficiency. The more severe the anemia, the easier the laboratory diagnosis of iron deficiency. Normal adult males will exhaust their iron stores when more than 1000 mL of red blood cells are lost. The young to middle-aged adult female can become iron deficient with losses of as little as 200–300 mL of red blood cells. Once stores are exhausted, the serum iron falls to below 30 µg/dL and the serum ferritin to below 20 µg/L. In addition, the erythroid marrow begins to produce microcytic, hypochromic red blood cells.

Iron Deficiency

As described in Chapter 5, the pattern of laboratory findings in **iron deficiency** varies according to the severity and duration of the anemia. As long as the hemoglobin level is greater than 10 grams per deciliter, patients will exhibit a normocytic or slightly microcytic anemia with a low reticulocyte production index. At lower hemoglobin levels, microcytosis and hypochromia become more pronounced. Initially, the cell distribution curve and blood film show a mixed population of microcytic and normocytic cells while the mean cell volume (MCV) is still normal. This situation reflects the initial mixing of newly produced microcytic cells with existing normocytic cells. After some weeks or months, the entire circulating population becomes microcytic with a fall in the MCV and mean cell hemoglobin. The red blood cell distribution width (RDW) can also give a sense of the evolution of the film morphology from normocytic to microcytic. Both RDW-CV and RDW-SD will increase as greater numbers of small cells are mixed with the normal population.

THERAPY

Management of a patient with a blood loss anemia requires not only good clinical decision making but also appropriate use of volume expanders, blood components, and iron supplements. **First steps in stabilizing a severely hemorrhaging patient** are the essential components of first aid. Most important, any obvious bleeding sites should be controlled. If available, **military antishock trousers (MAST)** can be applied to redistribute intravascular volume and maintain the patient's blood pressure until adequate fluids are administered. The MAST suit can provide an autotransfusion of 600–1500 mL of blood by compressing the lower extremities and abdomen. It can also tamponade arterial or venous bleeders in the lower extremities of a trauma victim.

The next important step is to establish reliable intravenous access and begin an aggressive program of **fluid and volume expander administration.** Choice of volume expanders will depend on the type and severity of the bleeding, symptoms and signs of hypovolemia, and patient age. There is also the issue of what products are readily accessible. Electrolyte solutions and purified colloid preparations are immediately available, whereas the administration of red blood cells, platelets, and fresh frozen plasma will involve some delay.

Electrolyte Solutions

Two standard electrolyte solutions, **Ringer's lactate** and **normal saline,** can be used as volume expanders. Although they lack oncotic protein, they will expand the intravascular volume if given in sufficient quantities. To attain an intravascular volume expansion of 1 liter, 3–4 liters must be infused at a rapid rate, since electrolyte solutions immediately equilibrate with the extravascular space, which is about twice the size of the intravascular space. In a life-threatening situation, volumes of 8 or more liters of electrolyte can be safely administered to younger patients. However, older patients and patients with cardiovascular disease can have difficulty tolerating this much fluid. They almost certainly will develop subcutaneous edema and may experience pulmonary edema or, even worse, acute respiratory distress syndrome (ARDS). The latter is most commonly seen in patients who are also septic or have experienced a severe crush injury.

There are **limits to how long a patient can be sustained on electrolyte solutions solely.** When 6 or more liters of fluid are required in the first 1–2 hours, it is unlikely the patient can be maintained without the infusion of a colloid solution and red blood cells. Older patients should be considered for colloid and red blood cells at an even earlier stage to prevent cardiovascular decompensation.

Colloid Solutions

Several colloid solutions are available that provide reliable volume expansion for volume infused. These include 5% albumin solution, purified plasma protein fraction, and hydroxyethyl starch solution (Table 10–3). For management of an acute, severe hemorrhage, these products are interchangeable. When large volumes are required, protein-containing products are preferred.

A. PROTEIN SOLUTIONS:

Albusimol, a purified preparation of 5% albumin in isotonic saline, is a hepatitis-free, HIV-free, extremely reliable volume expander. It can be stored at room tem-

Table 10–3. Volume expanders.

Product	Advantages	Disadvantages
Electrolyte solution (saline, Ringer's lactate)	Readily available, inexpensive	Need to give large volumes; can induce congestive failure
Protein solutions (PPF, Albumisol)	Volume-for-volume expansion, no side reactions	Expensive; may be in short supply, hyponatremia
Hydroxyethyl starch solution	Volume-for-volume expansion, less expensive	Can inhibit platelet function
Fresh frozen plasma	Contains coagulation factors	Allergic reactions; expensive

perature for long periods and infused at rapid rates without allergic reactions. In a hypovolemic patient, it gives volume-for-volume expansion. Moreover, because human albumin is the primary oncotic protein in plasma, volume expansion is sustained for several days until the patient's own albumin production can compensate. This product is also quite safe if excess volumes are given. As long as cardiac and renal functions are relatively normal, patients will compensate with a salt and water diuresis, even raising serum albumin concentrations to supernormal levels.

Plasma protein fraction (PPF) (**Plasmanate**) is a popular alternative to 5% albumin solution. PPF contains a mixture of albumin (4 grams per deciliter) and other globulins (1 gram per deciliter). The protein fraction is prepared as a sodium acetate precipitate of human plasma proteins. Because of this, the protein is resuspended in a solution that may vary from isotonic to hypotonic with sodium levels of 140–110 mEq/L and very low chloride levels. Because of this, the patient should be followed up for hyponatremia if large volumes are administered (more than 2–3 L). Otherwise, PPF is also hepatitis- and HIV-free and gives predictable volume expansion.

B. HYDROXYETHYL STARCH SOLUTION (HETASTARCH, HESPAN):

Hydroxyethyl starch solution is another popular alternative. It is made up as a 6% solution in isotonic saline, which will give volume-for-volume intravascular expansion. It is much less expensive than either 5% albumin solution or PPF, and it has a stable shelf life. Its **use is limited,** however, by its more rapid removal from circulation and its tendency to inhibit platelet function. It is usually recommended that infusions of hydroxyethyl starch solution be limited to 1–2 liters.

When massive transfusion is needed to save an exsanguinating patient, volume expanders will need to be accompanied by transfusions of red blood cells, platelets, and fresh frozen plasma. Hypovolemic shock

and hypoxia, which lead to lactic acidosis, ARDS, and brain damage, are still the principal issues. They need to be dealt with by very aggressive administration of volume expanders and packed red blood cells. It is also important to anticipate the diluting effect of electrolyte and colloid solutions on the levels of plasma coagulation factors and platelets. When the volume of blood lost exceeds the patient's blood volume (more than 5 liters), a mix of colloid expander, fresh frozen plasma, packed red blood cells, and platelets must be administered. The patient's bleeding can be worsened if this therapy is not implemented.

C. FRESH FROZEN PLASMA (FFP):

Fresh frozen plasma is essentially frozen normal human plasma, prepared as a part of routine fractionation of whole blood. Each unit of FFP contains approximately 200 mL of plasma with levels of coagulation factors, including fibrinogen, prothrombin, and factors XI, IX, VIII, X, V, and VII, which approach those found in fresh plasma. When administered to a patient with a plasma volume of approximately 3 liters, each unit will increase individual factor levels by only 5–7%. In order to make a significant impact on the coagulation profile of a massively bleeding patient, at least 4–6 units of FFP must be given. This infusion will temporarily provide a level of 30% or more of the coagulation factors needed for normal hemostasis.

FFP is also a protein-containing volume expander, similar to 5% albumin solution or PPF. However, it is not as trouble-free as the other two solutions. **FFP can induce an IgE immune-mediated allergic reaction** in sensitive patients. In addition, when large volumes of FFP are administered, there is a significant risk in up to 10% of patients of inducing an **acute sensitivity reaction** characterized by widespread urticaria, generalized subcutaneous edema, and acute bronchospasm. On occasion, an allergic reaction is severe enough to actually reduce the plasma volume at a time when the need for volume expansion is critical. It is essential, therefore, that patients receiving FFP be watched for symptoms and signs of a hypersensitivity reaction, including a worsening of the patient's hypotension.

Treatment of pooled human plasma by a solvent-detergent process can inactivate viruses with lipid envelopes (hepatitis B and C, and HIV) without major depletion of coagulation factors. The product is, however, still theoretically capable of transmitting nonenvelope viruses (hepatitis A, parvovirus B19, and TTV, a novel DNA virus, recently detected in blood donors).

Red Blood Cell Transfusion

A major loss of red blood cells with severe hemorrhage needs to be treated by transfusion of packed red blood cells. A unit of packed red blood cells contains approximately 200 mL of red blood cells suspended in 50–75 mL of plasma. Depending on method of preparation, a unit can also contain nonviable platelets and granulocytes and viable lymphocytes.

A. FILTRATION OF RED BLOOD CELLS:

In some blood centers, red blood cell units are filtered prior to storage. This filtration removes most but not all of the granulocytes and platelets. When available, leukofiltered red blood cells do have an advantage of reducing the frequency of acute febrile reactions secondary to cytokines, or alloantibodies to white blood cell HLA antigens, or both (see Chapter 37).

B. SEVERITY AND RATE OF BLOOD LOSS:

The need to transfuse red blood cells will depend on severity and rate of blood loss. Usually, it is not as urgent as the need to treat the patient's hypovolemia. As long as adequate amounts of volume expanders are administered, the patient will tolerate up to 50% loss of circulating red blood cells. This may not be true, however, for elderly patients or patients with cardiovascular disease. The decision to transfuse should be based on the bedside evaluation of the patient's clinical status with emphasis on cardiovascular compensation, mentation, age, and complicating illness. When blood loss is massive, red blood cell transfusion should be initiated as soon as possible as a part of blood volume support.

C. BLOOD TYPING:

If red blood cell transfusion can be delayed for 30 minutes or more, the patient's ABO blood type should be determined and the patient's plasma screened for anti-red blood cell antibodies. ABO typing takes only a few moments. With this information, type-specific red blood cells can be transfused with little or no risk of a transfusion reaction. The only faster way of providing a compatible red blood cell transfusion is to administer Type O (Rh neg) red blood cells. **Type O red blood cells** lack both A and B substance and are, therefore, universally accepted by patients regardless of blood type. At the same time, the supply of O negative blood is quite limited; only 7% of donors are O, Rh negative. Most major trauma centers are unable to supply enough of this product to handle a patient with a massive hemorrhage.

When using type-specific blood, the **patient's Rh status may not be known or may have to be ignored.** For men and women who have passed the childbearing age, a transfusion of Rh positive red blood cells to an Rh negative recipient is of little consequence. If the patient is free of Rh antibody, there is less than a one in five chance of sensitizing a patient and even then this will not result in a significant hematologic abnormality. If necessary, the chance of immunization can be eliminated by the administration of **anti-D antibody** (**RhoGAM**) for up to 3 days following the red blood cell transfusions. This has the effect of suppressing the immune response. When a young Rh negative woman receives a unit of Rh positive red blood cells, she should be treated with RhoGAM. The amount required is considerable, 20 mg of anti-D per milliliter of transfused red blood cells.

D. VOLUME EXPANDERS:

Each unit of red blood cells should increase the hemoglobin level by approximately 1 gram per deciliter (hematocrit increase of 3–4%). Although very little plasma is infused with each unit, there can be a significant volume expansion effect when several units of red blood cells are transfused. This should be recognized when calculating the amount of volume expander administered so as not to induce congestive failure. If a patient has received a large amount of volume expander, especially electrolyte solution, and is stable, the rate of red blood cell transfusion should be slowed and the patient treated with a diuretic.

D. ALLERGIC REACTIONS:

Like FFP, rapid transfusion of several units of packed red blood cells can induce an immune-mediated allergic reaction. Appearance of urticaria, bronchospasm, or a sudden fall in blood pressure suggests an IgE-related reaction, whereas chills, fever, or both are usually caused by cytokines that accumulate during storage or, rarely, bacterial contamination. Prestorage leukoreduction of red cell units may be effective in reducing the level of leukocyte-derived cytokines and the incidence and severity of febrile reactions to transfusion. Transfusions of red blood cells also run the risk of transmitting blood-borne infections.

Platelet Transfusions

Thrombocytopenia is a problem in patients who receive massive transfusions of volume expanders and packed red blood cells. It is good practice, therefore, to closely monitor the platelet count and to prophylactically administer platelets in severely hemorrhaging patients. As a simple rule, a six-pack of platelets (the platelets from six random donors) should be administered with every five units of packed red blood cells. This treatment should prevent thrombocytopenia and avoid the question of whether the patient has sufficient platelets to guarantee hemostasis. If a complicating illness that might contribute to platelet consumption is present, frequent platelet counts should be obtained to confirm the adequacy of platelet transfusion support.

Iron Therapy

Iron plays a key role in the erythroid marrow response to a blood loss anemia. A normal adult male with 1000 mg of reticuloendothelial stores can acutely increase red blood cell production to two to three times normal. This production level cannot be sustained, however, if the blood loss exceeds the amount of stored iron. At this point, the patient must receive iron therapy.

A. DOSAGE GUIDELINES:

Detailed guidelines of oral and parenteral iron therapy are presented in Chapter 5. As a rule, oral iron therapy should be used whenever possible. Adult patients with an acute, self-limited hemorrhage can be treated with one tablet of a standard oral iron preparation three to four times each day, preferably given between meals to increase absorption. Iron therapy should be initiated as soon as possible after the patient is stabilized and should be maintained for 3–6 months. This treatment plan will give time both to repair the anemia and to rebuild reticuloendothelial iron stores.

B. RESPONSE TO ORAL IRON THERAPY:

Response to oral iron therapy will be influenced by such factors as the severity of the anemia, patient compliance, intestinal absorption, and any complicating illnesses that suppress the erythropoietin response. Red blood cell production levels as high as three times normal can be observed in patients with significant anemia (a hemoglobin level less than 10 grams per deciliter) who faithfully take their oral iron and do not have a complicating illness. Renal disease or an inflammatory illness can dampen the erythropoietin response to anemia. Breaks in the oral iron regimen will also interfere with the marrow's response. To maintain a constant supply of iron to erythroid precursors, the doses of oral iron must be taken at even intervals throughout the day.

If the patient has a **less severe anemia** (a hemoglobin level greater than 10 grams per deciliter) because of a more modest bleeding episode or as a result of trans-fusion, oral iron therapy should be modified to encourage gastrointestinal tolerance and patient compliance. Otherwise, the patient will not cooperate with the prolonged course of iron therapy, which is required for the reconstitution of iron stores.

C. IRON DEXTRAN THERAPY:

Patients with malabsorption or a marked intolerance to oral iron will not be amenable to oral iron therapy. Their anemia can obviously be corrected with red blood cell transfusions. They will need to receive parenteral iron, however, to correct their iron balance and rebuild stores. Iron can be given intravenously or intramuscularly as **iron dextran complex.** Detailed instructions for the administration of iron dextran are presented in Chapter 5. When iron dextran is used to treat a patient who is recovering from a blood loss anemia, it is best given as a single, total dose infused intravenously.

Iron dextran can also be of value in treating patients with **chronic blood loss.** Hereditary hemorrhagic telangiectasia is perhaps the best example of a clinical condition where a relentless, daily loss of blood from the gastrointestinal tract can overwhelm the normal routes of iron supply. Reticuloendothelial stores are quickly exhausted and even maximum iron absorption on a full oral regimen cannot match cell losses of 50 mL or more of red blood cells each day. As these patients become severely anemic, they develop a severe iron deficiency anemia with marked microcytosis and hypochromia. They can also exhibit signs of tissue iron deficiency.

Acute, severe episodes of bleeding in patients with **hereditary hemorrhagic telangiectasia** should be treated with red blood cell transfusions, just like any acute blood loss anemia. To counteract the slower, daily loss of blood in these individuals, attempts should be made to provide maximum iron therapy. Not only should the patients receive a constant regimen of oral iron but they should also receive periodic intravenous injections of iron dextran, according to the rate of blood loss. The combination of oral iron and iron dextran can be quite effective (Figure 10–2). In severely anemic patients with hereditary telangiectasia, red blood cell production levels of up to five to six times normal may be achieved for several weeks following an intravenous injection of 1000 mg of iron dextran.

To maintain erythroid marrow production at its maximum level over a prolonged period, the iron dextran **injections must be given every 3–4 weeks.** Otherwise, the level of red blood cell production will fall gradually back to basal level as the release of iron from the iron dextran complex slows. Larger complex particles in the preparation are only slowly dissolved by the reticuloendothelial cell. In fact, the release from some particles can fall behind the rate of the patient's blood

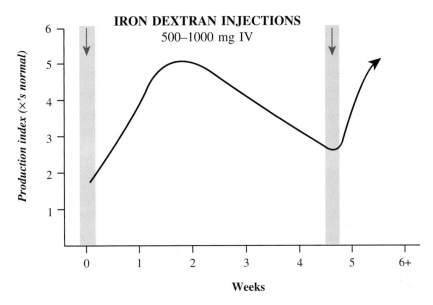

Figure 10–2. Marrow production levels following iron dextran injection. Patients with severe anemia and chronic blood loss can be treated with a combination of oral iron and intermittent intravenous injections of iron dextran. Each bolus of intravenous iron will increase red blood cell production to as high as five to six times normal for several weeks.

loss, so that microcytosis and hypochromia will appear despite the presence of visible iron dextran particles within marrow reticuloendothelial cells. This phenomenon needs to be recognized in the laboratory evaluation of anemia in patients with hereditary hemorrhagic telangiectasia who receive long-term iron dextran therapy. They may present with characteristic findings of an iron deficiency anemia but have easily visible or even increased iron stores of their marrows on the Prussian blue stain.

Perisurgical Blood Loss Management

Elective surgery patients undergoing major noncardiac procedures are candidates for autologous blood storage, perisurgical recombinant erythropoietin therapy, acute normovolemic hemodilution, and blood salvage, alone or in combination. Patients who are moderately anemic (hemoglobins between 10 and 13 grams per deciliter) or of small body size can also benefit, even when the anticipated surgical blood loss is not above 1000 mL.

Together, these several techniques should make it possible to avoid, if not significantly reduce, exposure to homologous blood transfusion. Benefits are considerable. Allogeneic blood transfusion is associated with a demonstrable decrease in cellular immunity, and the postoperative infection rate in patients receiving transfusions has been reported to increase 7- to 10-fold. Furthermore, the postoperative length of stay and hospital

charges can be correlated with the number of homologous units transfused, a relationship that is not seen in a comparable group of patients given autologous blood or erythropoietin.

A. AUTOLOGOUS BLOOD STORAGE:

The amount of blood that can be deposited for subsequent transfusion (autologous donation) will depend on the patient's initial hematocrit and marrow production response. As long as the hemoglobin is above 13 grams per deciliter, the **average-sized patient should be able to donate 3–4 units of red cells.** Smaller patients with hemoglobins below 13 grams per deciliter will require simultaneous erythropoietin therapy to reach more than two units without causing the hematocrit to fall below 33%.

Autologous blood storage is notoriously **expensive.** When blood is stored for surgical procedures with a low risk of major hemorrhage (hysterectomy, transurethral prostatectomy, normal vaginal delivery, etc), up to 90% of the units collected will be discarded. Even with higher-risk procedures, 50% or more of the units will go unused.

There is also the issue of **postoperative anemia,** which can be made worse by autologous donation. Together these drawbacks tend to discourage its use.

The **marrow response to erythropoietin** correlates with the dose and the duration of treatment. When given in a dose of 100–150 IU/kg (approximately

10,000 units) subcutaneously twice a week for 3 weeks, patients will produce 300–400 mL of red blood cells, the equivalent of one and a half to two units of packed red cells. This will usually guarantee storage of up to four autologous units. In addition, they will enter surgery with a higher than normal reticulocyte count. Much higher erythropoietin doses will result in greater production but at considerable financial cost.

An adequate **iron supply** is very important. Patients must be maintained on oral iron, one tab of feosol three times a day (200 mg of elemental iron a day), or receive intravenous iron as iron dextran (1000 mg single infusion) or iron saccharate (200 mg at the time of each autologous donation).

B. PERISURGICAL RECOMBINANT ERYTHROPOIETIN THERAPY:

Perisurgical erythropoietin therapy without autologous donation can also help decrease homologous (allogeneic) blood exposure. Dosing studies have looked at a number of regimens, including daily 100–300 IU/kg injections for 10 days preop to 4 days postoperatively to once or twice a week injections of 600 IU/kg subcutaneously. Aggressive iron supplementation is again key to the patient's response. This therapy will generally produce a 1–2 grams per deciliter rise in the hemoglobin level (3–6% rise in hematocrit), the equivalent of a one- to two-unit packed red cell transfusion. When continued postoperatively, erythropoietin therapy will also accelerate the rate of recovery of the hemoglobin level.

C. ACUTE NORMOVOLEMIC HEMODILUTION:

In selected settings, acute normovolemic hemodilution can help decrease the need for homologous blood. Normovolemic hemodilution follows the same principle as autologous blood storage. Whole blood is removed using standard blood storage bags just prior to surgery and replaced with crystalloid/colloid to maintain normovolemia. It can then be reinfused during or after the procedure to treat major blood losses. Advantages in-

clude the elimination of testing requirements, less preop planning, and a lower cost. Candidates for this approach include patients without symptomatic cardiovascular disease who are expected to experience a blood volume loss in excess of 20% of their blood volume.

D. BLOOD SALVAGE:

Intraoperative blood salvage provides another method for reducing exposure to homologous blood. It is most effective in orthopedic and vascular surgery patients where blood can be scavenged from a relatively sterile field. Cell-washing devices can handle blood losses equivalent to 10 units/hour of stored blood. This can be lifesaving in patients with massive blood losses associated with vascular procedures. Blood can also be recovered postoperatively from surgical drains and reinfused. The blood collected is, however, partially hemolyzed and contains activated platelets as well as cytokines released from fragmented cells.

BIBLIOGRAPHY

Adamson J: Perisurgical use of epoietin alfa in orthopedic surgery patients. Semin Hematol 1996;33:55(suppl 2).

Beutler E et al: *Hematology,* 6th ed. McGraw-Hill, 2001.

Blumberg N: Allogeneic transfusion and infection: Economic and clinical implications. Semin Hematol 1997;34:34.

Cazzola M, Mercuriali F, Brugnara C: Use of recombinant erythropoietin outside the setting of uremia. Blood 1997;89:4248.

Goldberg MA: Perioperative epoietin alfa increases red blood cell mass and reduces exposure to transfusions: Results of randomized clinical trials. Semin Hematol 1997;34:41.

Goodnough LT et al: Transfusion medicine: Blood conservation. N Engl J Med 1999;340:525.

Hillman RS, Finch CA: *Red Cell Manual,* 7th ed. FA Davis, 1997.

Maier RV, Carrico CJ: Developments in the resuscitation of critically ill surgical patients. Adv Surg 1986;19:271.

Thompson JF: Interoperative blood salvage. Haematol Rev 1992;7:55.

Weiskopf RB: Mathematical analysis of isovolemic hemodilution indicates that it can decrease the need for allogeneic blood transfusion. Transfusion 1995;35:37.

Hemolytic Anemias

The distinguishing feature of all hemolytic anemias is the **increased rate of adult red blood cell destruction.** Clinical presentation will vary according to the disease process. Some hemolytic anemias present as acute, self-limited episodes of red blood cell destruction, others as chronic, well-compensated hemolytic states. Signs and symptoms of hemolysis will also differ according to the mechanism of red blood cell destruction. Sudden, intravascular hemolysis results in hemoglobinemia and hemoglobinuria, whereas destruction limited to the extravascular monocyte-macrophage system may only be apparent from a fall in hemoglobin level and a rise in the serum bilirubin and lactic dehydrogenase (LDH) levels. Chronic, well-compensated hemolytic anemias are easily detected from the red blood cell production response (ie, increase in the reticulocyte index).

Red blood cell hemolysis can result because of environmental factors or an inherent defect in red blood cell structure or function. Even normal red blood cells can fall victim to environmental challenges such as mechanical trauma, infection, or autoimmune attack. Patients who inherit defects in membrane structure, hemoglobin stability, or metabolic function demonstrate both spontaneous shortening of red blood cell lifespan and a greater sensitivity to environmental factors.

NORMAL RED BLOOD CELL TURNOVER

Red blood cells are extremely pliable, resilient cells that survive for 100 or more days in circulation. Their capacity to survive is a tribute to the strength of the membrane and the metabolic pathways that supply the high-energy phosphate needed to maintain the membrane and keep hemoglobin in a soluble, reduced state (see Chapter 1). As red blood cells become older, however, metabolic pathways decay, oxidized hemoglobin accumulates, and oxidized phospholipids, especially phosphatidylserine, appear on the surface of the cell. A concomitant loss of flexibility interferes with the cell's ability to move through the microvasculature and initiates the process of removal by the monocyte-macrophage system via the CD36 receptor.

Role of the Spleen

The spleen plays a major role in red blood cell destruction (Figure 11–1). The structure of the spleen is a testing ground of cell flexibility and viability. Blood is delivered by terminal arterioles to the splenic red blood cell pulp, where the volume of plasma is reduced and the cell is subjected to a relatively hypoxic environment. This situation tests the metabolic pathways and, in older or diseased cells, results in a further loss of pliability. To escape and reenter circulation, the red blood cell must then squeeze through a 2- to 5-μm opening in the sinusoidal wall. In effect, this traps rigid cells and leads to phagocytosis and destruction by reticuloendothelial cells lining the sinusoids.

The uniform quality of red blood cell morphology on the blood film is a tribute to splenic function. The trapping-filtering mechanism of the spleen efficiently removes red blood cell inclusions including residual iron granules, nuclear remnants (**Howell-Jolly bodies**), and any denatured hemoglobin (**Heinz bodies**). Spleen reticuloendothelial cells also display receptors for the Fc fragment of immunoglobulin and the C3b component of complement. In patients with autoimmune hemolytic anemias, the spleen is the principal site of red blood cell destruction.

Pathways of Red Blood Cell Destruction

The pathways of red blood cell destruction effectively recover heme iron for new red blood cell production. This process is true whether the red blood cells break down in circulation (**intravascular destruction**) or by the normal reticuloendothelial cell pathway (**extravascular destruction**). Destruction of senescent cells is largely limited to the **extravascular pathway** (Figure 11–2). Red blood cells are phagocytized by reticuloendothelial cells, the membrane is disrupted, and hemoglobin is broken down by lysozymal enzymes. Iron recovered from heme is then stored or transported back to the marrow for new red blood cell production. Amino acids are also recovered. At the same time, the protoporphyrin ring is metabolized to the tetrapyrrol (**bilirubin**) with the release of carbon monoxide. Bilirubin is subsequently transported to the liver, where it is conjugated and excreted into bile.

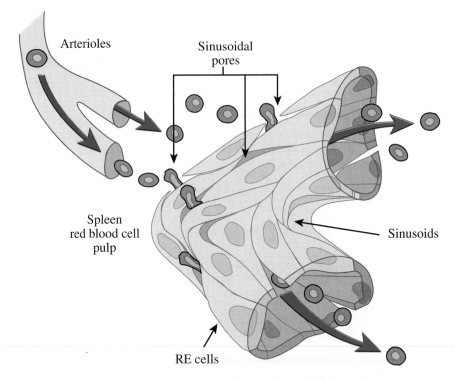

Figure 11–1. **Splenic function.** The anatomic structure of the spleen is ideal for testing the metabolic machinery and pliability of the red blood cells. Within the splenic pulp, red blood cells are concentrated and their intracellular metabolic pathways stressed. Following this, red blood cells must pass through 2- to 5-μm pores to enter the sinusoidal system. Unusually rigid cells or a cell containing inclusion bodies will be unable to pass this test and will be destroyed by sinusoidal reticuloendothelial cells.

Intravascular red blood cell destruction follows a different pathway. Free hemoglobin either dissociates into α-β dimers that bind to haptoglobin or is oxidized to methemoglobin that then dissociates to release the heme group for binding with albumin and hemopexin. The binding step prevents immediate loss of the heme group by glomerular filtration and allows clearance by hepatocytes. The liver then breaks down the heme group to recover iron and produce bilirubin.

The **final common pathway** for both extravascular and intravascular red blood cell destruction is the conjugation of bilirubin by the hepatocyte, its excretion in bile, and the subsequent conversion by gut bacteria to urobilinogen and urobilin. These end products are excreted in both stool and urine.

Clinical Measurements of Red Blood Cell Destruction

The rate of red blood cell destruction can be assessed from measurements of several steps in the process. The most important clinical measurements are listed in Table 11–1. The **reticulocyte production index** provides an indirect measure of red blood cell destruction. When the reticulocyte index is greater than three times normal in a patient with a stable or falling hematocrit, the **destruction index** (the absolute number of red blood cells destroyed) can be assumed to be three times normal or higher. **Direct measurements of red blood cell lifespan** are possible using a ^{51}Cr red blood cell survival. **LDH and indirect bilirubin measurements** provide a qualitative measure of cell turnover. From a research standpoint, ferrokinetics, carbon monoxide excretion, and urobilinogen excretion have been employed to quantitate red blood cell destruction.

Hemolysis & Abnormal Red Blood Cells

Very high levels of hemolysis can overwhelm the extravascular and intravascular pathways for heme iron recovery. There is a limit to the capacity of the reticu-

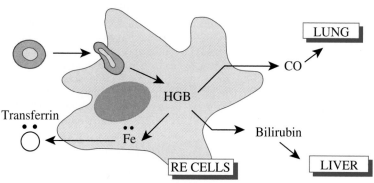

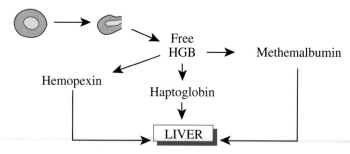

Figure 11–2. **Pathways of red blood cell destruction.** Red blood cell destruction can follow an extravascular or intravascular route. With extravascular destruction, red blood cells are phagocytized by reticuloendothelial cells, the membrane structure is broken down, and the hemoglobin is reduced to its essential components. Iron is recovered for transport by transferrin back to erythroid marrow. The porphyrin ring is broken, and a molecule of carbon monoxide is released. The remaining portion of the porphyrin ring is then transported as bilirubin to the liver for conjugation and excretion in bile. With intravascular red blood cell destruction, free hemoglobin binds either to haptoglobin or hemopexin or is converted to methemalbumin. These proteins are cleared by the liver, where the heme is broken down to recover iron and produce bilirubin.

loendothelial system to clear abnormal red blood cells. When this capacity is exceeded, morphologically abnormal red blood cells appear in circulation. Depending on the cause of disease, these abnormal cells include

Table 11–1. Measurements of red blood cell destruction.

Indirect Measurements	Direct Measurements
Changes in hematocrit	^{51}Cr red blood cell survival
Reticulocyte production index	Ferrokinetics
Serum lactic dehydrogenase (LDH)	CO excretion
	Urobilinogen excretion
Serum indirect bilirubin	

microspherocytes, "bite" cells, fragmented red blood cells, and red blood cells with abnormal inclusion bodies. Presence of these cells in circulation suggests that either the capacity of the spleen is overwhelmed or splenic function is reduced as part of the disease process. Even normal subjects who have had a splenectomy will demonstrate abnormal forms. An overtaxed monocyte-macrophage system will also leak free hemoglobin back into circulation, resulting in a fall in serum haptoglobin level.

Haptoglobin & Hemopexin Clearance Pathways

Intravascular hemolysis easily overwhelms haptoglobin and hemopexin clearance pathways. When hemoglobin binds to either haptoglobin or hemopexin, the complex is quickly cleared by the hepatocyte. The amount of hemoglobin that can be bound and removed depends on the rate of new haptoglobin and hemopexin production. Generally, intravascular lysis of more than 20–40 mL of red blood cells per day will effectively deplete both systems; haptoglobin levels will fall to undetectable levels (Figure 11–3). Once this occurs, free hemoglobin will be detected in both the patient's serum and urine, and methemalbumin levels will rise.

Recovery After an Intravascular Hemolytic Event

It is also important to recognize the pattern of recovery following an intravascular hemolytic event. As shown in Figure 11–3, following a self-limited intravascular hemolytic event, serum hemoglobin levels will drop rapidly as free hemoglobin is cleared into urine. Hemoglobinuria will also be relatively short lived. Haptoglobin levels then rise gradually over the next 24–72 hours. At the same time, methemalbumin levels in plasma will stay elevated for 5–10 days and patients will continue to shed tubular cells containing hemosiderin granules into urine for 1 week or more.

CLINICAL FEATURES

Most hemolytic anemias are associated with few specific symptoms or signs. **When anemia is severe,** patients will complain of increasing fatigue or exercise in-

tolerance and may develop congestive heart failure. This is really no different from the clinical presentation seen with any severe anemia. In contrast, **acute intravascular hemolysis** may be associated with fever, chills, and severe lower back pain. This is most often seen in patients who receive incompatible or infected blood products. A severe intravascular hemolytic event with lysis of more than 20–40 mL of red blood cells will produce noticeable hemoglobinuria.

Since many hemolytic anemias are related to another disease state, a careful history and physical examination are always necessary. A search should be made for any evidence of autoimmune disease. Racial and family background are important. It is also important to try to document the chronicity of the anemia. Patients with congenital hemolytic anemias are frequently aware of other involved members in their family and the results of past blood counts.

Laboratory Studies

Diagnosis of a hemolytic anemia depends heavily on the laboratory. Any workup begins with several screening tests to classify the patient's disorder. This then provides a guide to the application of a larger number of specific tests of cell structure and function.

A. THE COMPLETE BLOOD COUNT:

A complete blood count (CBC) with inspection of the film and measurement of the reticulocyte count is extremely valuable in both detecting a hemolytic anemia

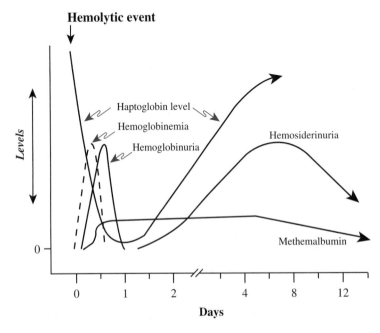

Figure 11–3. **Measurements of acute intravascular hemolysis.** Following an acute hemolytic event, measurements of plasma and urine hemoglobin, serum haptoglobin, serum methemalbumin, and urine hemosiderin follow a characteristic pattern. Hemoglobinemia, hemoglobinuria, methemalbuminemia, and a fall in the serum haptoglobin level are all present during the first 24 hours. If hemolysis does not continue, the patient will demonstrate a gradual return of the serum haptoglobin to normal and the appearance of hemosiderin in the urine for up to 7–10 days. Methemalbumin may be detectable for more than 1 week.

and pointing the way to diagnosis. An **acute hemolytic event** may only be heralded by a sudden fall in the patient's hemoglobin/hematocrit. **Chronic hemolytic states** are more easily detected. These patients have a moderate to severe anemia, a reticulocyte production index of greater than three times normal, and, in most cases, some abnormality of red blood cell morphology.

Most hemolytic anemias are normocytic, normochromic, although the presence of large numbers of microspherocytes on the blood film is accompanied by a rise in the mean corpuscular hemoglobin concentration (MCHC). Very high reticulocyte counts with marked polychromasia may be associated with a rise in the mean cell volume (MCV) to levels between 100 and 110 fL. An MCV greater than 110 fL is seen when the uncorrected reticulocyte count exceeds 25–30%. This situation simply reflects the fact that when large numbers of marrow reticulocytes are added to the circulating normocytic red blood cell population, the MCV will rise. It will also be reflected in an increase in the red blood cell distribution width. The full **erythropoietic profile of a chronic hemolytic anemia** is shown in Table 11–2. The marrow ratio of erythroid to granulocytic precursors (E/G ratio) is increased; red blood cell precursor morphology is usually normoblastic unless the patient becomes folic acid deficient. Iron studies demonstrate a normal serum iron and total iron-binding capacity and a normal or slightly elevated ferritin level. Iron stores on the Prussian blue stain of the marrow are normal to somewhat increased. In patients with very high levels of red blood cell turnover, reticuloendothelial cells are filled with a finely granular, dustlike hemosiderin, which may reflect the rapid turnover of storage iron.

The **indirect bilirubin** and **serum LDH levels** are the most clinically useful measures of total red blood cell destruction. This includes the serum LDH, indirect bilirubin, and observation of changes in the hemoglobin/hematocrit over time. With significant hemolysis, the serum LDH level will quickly rise to levels in excess

of 1000 IU. Levels of 5000 IU/mL or higher are not unusual. The indirect bilirubin level will increase to levels of 1–3 mg/dL in patients with significant hemolysis. Chronic elevations of the indirect bilirubin are also seen in patients with inherited defects in bilirubin conjugation (Crigler-Najjar and Gilbert's disease).

B. DETECTION OF INTRAVASCULAR HEMOLYSIS:

The laboratory profile after an acute intravascular hemolytic event will vary according to the time elapsed. Acute hemolysis is associated with hemoglobinemia, hemoglobinuria, methemalbuminemia, and a rapid depletion of the serum haptoglobin level. Intravascular hemolysis several days prior to evaluation may be detected by measurements of serum methemalbumin level and urine hemosiderin (see Figure 11–3).

1. Plasma hemoglobin level—Intravascular lysis of even small amounts of red blood cells (10–20 mL of packed red blood cells) will impart a pink tint to plasma for a few hours; more severe hemolysis will make plasma look like rosé or red wine. The amount of hemoglobin in plasma can be quantitated. A venous sample should be collected carefully using heparin or ethylenediaminetetraacetic acid (EDTA) as an anticoagulant and be immediately centrifuged, and the color of the plasma should be observed. Quantitation of the plasma hemoglobin is performed using a dye such as benzidine or ortholidine, both of which turn blue in the presence of hemoglobin and hydrogen peroxide. A **plasma hemoglobin level of 50 mg/dL or higher** suggests intervascular hemolysis. It is at this point that the plasma first becomes pinkish. Once the level exceeds 150–200 mg/dL, plasma will be bright red and there will be accompanying hemoglobinuria.

Plasma hemoglobin levels below 50 mg/dL cannot be accurately measured and may be the result of phlebotomy-induced hemolysis. The Hemastix test used for detecting hematuria should never be used to screen for hemoglobinemia. It is much too sensitive and will invariably give a positive result, even in normal subjects.

2. Urine hemoglobin—Hemoglobinuria is suggested when the urine is red or brownish in color after centrifugation to remove intact red blood cells. A qualitative measurement is possible using the Hemastix. The Hemastix reaction does not distinguish hemoglobinuria from myoglobinuria, however. If the plasma hemoglobin level is elevated, it can be assumed that the pigment in urine is hemoglobin. If this is not the case, the two pigments must be separated using electrophoresis or differential solubility in ammonium sulfate.

3. Urine hemosiderin—Urine hemoglobin is reabsorbed by renal tubular cells and broken down to form hemosiderin. Following an intravascular hemolytic

Table 11–2. Chronic hemolytic anemia erythropoietic profile.

Red blood cell morphology	Normocytic/nor-mochromic—abnormalities in red blood cell shape
Polychromasia	Present
Reticulocyte index	> 3–5
Marrow E/G ratio	> 1:1
Marrow morphology	Normoblastic
Serum iron/TIBC	Normal/Normal
Serum bilirubin (mg/dL)	1–3
LDH (IU/mL)	> 1000

event, patients will shed tubular cells containing visible hemosiderin granules for several days to a week or more. This can be detected by performing a Prussian blue stain on the spun sediment of a random urine. A true positive should have distinct, blue granules within intact tubular cells. Free iron outside of cells may be nothing more than contaminant dirt.

4. Serum haptoglobin—Haptoglobin is an α_2-globulin that binds in an equal molar ratio to free hemoglobin. The complex is then cleared from circulation by the liver. Both intravascular and severe extravascular hemolysis are associated with a depletion of the serum haptoglobin level. Normal serum haptoglobin is 50–200 mg/dL or higher in patients with inflammatory illness.

The serum haptoglobin level is easily quantitated by standard turbidometric methods and is provided as a routine part of a serum protein profile. The pattern of behavior of the serum haptoglobin level after a hemolytic event is illustrated in Figure 11–3. It is possible to see a normal haptoglobin level immediately after the initiation of an intravascular hemolytic event, simply because the haptoglobin-hemoglobin complex has not yet been cleared from circulation. Conversely, abnormally low or absent haptoglobin levels are seen in patients with liver failure and individuals with the genetic absence of the protein or a defect in binding sites on the molecule.

5. Methemalbumin—Following an intravascular hemolytic event of sufficient severity to deplete serum haptoglobin, increased amounts of methemalbumin may be detectable in plasma for several days (see Figure 11–3). When present in large amounts, methemalbumin can be measured using a spectrophotometer from its absorption band at 624 μ. A more sensitive and quantitative measurement is possible using Schumm's test.

C. DETECTION OF EXTRAVASCULAR HEMOLYSIS:

Several laboratory methods are used to detect and diagnose abnormalities of red blood cell membrane, hemoglobin, or intracellular metabolism that lead to an increased rate of extravascular hemolysis (Table 11–3). Some of these are provided as routine clinical tests, whereas others require the expertise of a special hematology laboratory.

1. Tests of hemoglobin stability—Many of the inherited hemoglobinopathies are associated with an increased rate of cell destruction. As discussed in Chapter 7, common hemoglobinopathies such as hemoglobin S, C, SC, and compound heterozygotes with thalassemia can be screened for and diagnosed using routine hemoglobin electrophoresis. In addition, the supravital stains, brilliant cresyl blue and crystal violet, can be used to detect intracellular inclusion bodies (**Heinz**

Table 11–3. Laboratory methods in the diagnosis of extravascular hemolysis.

Tests of hemoglobin stability
  Hemoglobin electrophoresis
  Heinz body stains
  Isopropanol and heat denaturation tests
Tests of membrane structure
  Osmotic fragility
  Autohemolysis test
Tests of metabolic machinery
  Autohemolysis test
  G6PD screen/quantitative assay
  GSH assay
  Specific enzyme assays (eg, pyruvate kinase)
Tests of immune destruction
  Direct and indirect antiglobulin tests (Coombs' test or DAT)
  Cold agglutinin titer
  Complement levels
  Donath-Landsteiner test for PCH

bodies) in patients with unstable hemoglobins or thalassemia. The isopropanol and heat denaturation tests are used to detect the patient with an unstable hemoglobin.

2. Tests of membrane structure—The osmotic fragility and incubated autohemolysis tests are used to confirm the presence of the membrane structural defect seen in patients with hereditary spherocytosis. The **osmotic fragility test** involves subjecting the patient's red blood cells to an increasingly hypotonic environment (Figure 11–4). Fresh normal red blood cells are resistant to hemolysis. This situation is also true for fresh cells from patients with hereditary spherocytosis. Once the cells are incubated for 24 hours, however, the fragility of spherocytic red blood cells is far greater than that observed for normal red blood cells.

The **autohemolysis test** can help in diagnosing atypical cases of hereditary spherocytosis. This test is performed by incubating defibrinated whole blood with and without the addition of glucose for 48 hours, followed by the measurement of the plasma hemoglobin level (see Figure 11–4). Normal red blood cells show 2% lysis without glucose and even less when glucose is added to the incubated specimen. Hereditary spherocytosis patients show marked hemolysis without glucose, which is largely corrected when glucose is added. Intracellular enzyme defects also give abnormal test results for both the osmotic fragility and incubation hemolysis test. The hemolysis is less correctable by the addition of glucose, however.

3. Tests of metabolic machinery—Although the osmotic fragility and incubated autohemolysis tests do

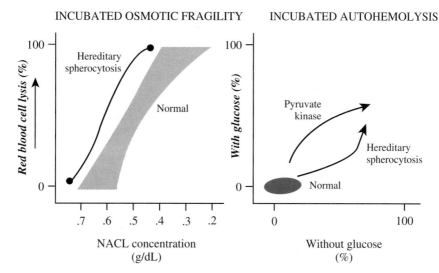

INCUBATED OSMOTIC FRAGILITY   INCUBATED AUTOHEMOLYSIS

Figure 11–4. Incubated osmotic fragility and autohemolysis tests. Defects in red blood cell membrane structure (eg, hereditary spherocytosis) and intracellular metabolism (eg, enzymopathies) can be detected and classified using the incubated osmotic fragility and autohemolysis tests. Hereditary spherocytosis patients show a much greater tendency to cell lysis as the cells are suspended in solutions of decreasing salt concentration. This is enhanced by incubating the blood sample for 24 hours. The incubated autohemolysis test can distinguish between hereditary spherocytosis and pyruvate kinase deficiency based on sensitivity to lysis with and without glucose in the medium.

provide a screening method for detecting defects in one of the metabolic pathways, they do not identify the specific enzyme defect. To look at individual enzymes, assays for **glucose-6-phosphate dehydrogenase (G6PD)** and **glutathione reductase (GSH)** are the most useful, simply because of the prevalence of these gene defects.

a. G6PD dye decolorization screening test—A simplified G6PD dye decolorization screening test can be used to detect deficient patients who are at risk of hemolysis. A small amount of patient blood is added to a solution containing G6PD, nicotinamide adenine dinucleotide phosphate (NADP), and oxidized glutathione incubated for 5–10 minutes at room temperature and then spotted on filter paper. Once dry, the spot is observed for decolorization. A false test result can occur in patients with the A-variant of G6PD deficiency following an acute hemolytic event. This result reflects loss of older, deficient cells and the appearance in circulation of a population of young reticulocytes with normal or increased levels of G6PD activity. The severe deficiency seen in Mediterranean type of G6PD deficiency will always show a positive test regardless of a high level of reticulocytosis. Since G6PD deficiency is sex-linked, women who are heterozygotes will have only moderately reduced levels of the enzyme. A quantitative G6PD assay needs to be used to detect the enzyme deficiency in these individuals.

b. Test for GSH deficiency—GSH deficiency can also result in acute, drug-induced hemolysis and rarely in a chronic hemolytic anemia. A quantitative assay of GSH is possible by measuring the rate of reduction of oxidized glutathione. Severe enzyme deficiency (less than 5% normal activity) is associated with hemolytic events. Riboflavin is an essential cofactor in this reaction, and riboflavin deficiency should be tested for by adding riboflavin to the reaction mixture.

c. Tests for less common enzyme defects—Less common enzyme defects in the anaerobic pathway (eg, glucose phosphate isomerase, phosphofructokinase deficiency, hexokinase deficiency, etc) present as nonspherocytic hemolytic anemias. Some of these are picked up with the incubated autohemolysis screening test. Definitive diagnosis requires a direct assay of enzyme activity by a special hematology laboratory.

4. Tests of immune destruction—Diagnosis of an autoimmune hemolytic anemia depends on the laboratory detection of abnormal autoantibodies capable of red blood cell destruction. The **direct antiglobulin test (DAT)** and **cold agglutinin titer test** are routinely used to screen for presence of an autoimmune hemolytic anemia. A more detailed characterization of the class of immunoglobulin involved, its specificity for red blood cell membrane antigens, and the involvement of complement in the hemolytic process are also important in guiding the diagnosis and management of the individual patient.

a. Polyspecific DAT—Measurement of abnormal amounts of immunoglobulin on the surface of red blood cells is possible using a polyspecific DAT (Figure 11–5). The DAT is also referred to as the **Coombs' test** and has been employed for decades in blood banks as a method in crossmatching. When applied to the diagnosis of autoimmune hemolytic anemia, the polyspecific DAT will detect significant amounts of IgG and C3 on the red blood cell membrane. It is also possible to detect whether one or both are present using monospecific anti-IgG and anti-C3 serum. An antiserum for IgM is not available.

To perform a DAT, polyspecific or monospecific antiglobulin serum is added to washed red blood cells. After brief centrifugation, the specimen is examined for agglutination as cells are gently resuspended. The degree of agglutination can be graded on a scale of from 0 to 4+. The strength of agglutination correlates with the amount of antibody on the red blood cell surface. Patients can have an autoimmune hemolytic anemia with a negative DAT when the number of molecules of autoantibody on the red blood cell surface is relatively low.

The DAT technique can also be used to **detect free antibody in the patient's serum (Indirect Coombs' test)**. This technique is performed by incubating patient serum with washed normal red blood cells, followed by the standard polyspecific antiglobulin test. In the patient with a severe autoimmune hemolytic anemia (where there is excess antibody in serum), this test can be strongly positive. The ability to detect free antibody can also be employed to determine the specificity of the antibody to red blood cell antigens. Many IgG autoantibodies have specificity for the Rh antigens (C, c, D, d, E, e). Less commonly, the autoantibody will have specificity to a minor blood group antigen.

b. Cold agglutinin titer test—Patients who appear to have an autoimmune hemolytic anemia with a positive anti-C3 and negative anti-IgG DAT should be screened for the presence of an IgM cold agglutinin. To measure the titer of the cold agglutinin, patient red blood cells are suspended in serially diluted patient serum followed by incubation at 48°C for at least 2 hours or even better, overnight, to encourage agglutination. Titers of 1:256 or higher are associated with hemolytic anemia. Patients with severe cold agglutinin disease can demonstrate titers in excess of 1:10,000. The temperature specificity of the agglutinin can also be measured. As the titer increases in patients with severe cold agglutinin disease, the activity of the antibody at higher temperatures will also increase, even to where agglutination is observed at 30°C to 37°C.

Measurements of serum complement levels can also help in diagnosing a cold agglutinin hemolytic anemia. Red blood cell destruction by IgM cold agglutinins requires the binding of complement to the cell membrane, thereby depleting serum complement levels. An assay of serum complement levels can, therefore, provide indirect evidence of an IgM antibody. IgM cold agglutinins in patients with infectious mononucleosis demonstrate specificity for i antigen. This situation is easily tested for by reacting the patient's serum with cord blood cells (fetal red blood cells) that express large amounts of i antigen.

c. Donath-Landsteiner test—Paroxysmal cold hemoglobinuria (PCH) is a rare form of autoimmune hemolytic anemia that is associated with a unique autoantibody. The Donath-Landsteiner test for PCH involves incubating red blood cells with the patient's serum first in the cold and then at 37°C with added fresh complement. When the antibody is present, there

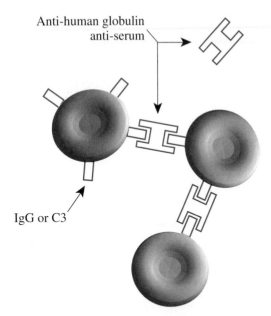

Anti-human globulin anti-serum

IgG or C3

Figure 11–5. **The direct antiglobulin test (DAT or Coombs' test).** The DAT is performed by incubating patient's red blood cells with a polyspecific or monospecific antihuman globulin antiserum. The antiglobulin interacts with surface IgG or C3 and promotes red blood cell agglutination. This is routinely measured by assessing the tendency to agglutinate after gentle centrifugation. A quantitative measure of red blood cell surface antibody is possible using radiolabeled antiglobulin reagents.

is visible hemolysis once the cells are brought back to 37°C. The antibody also demonstrates anti-P specificity.

DIAGNOSIS

The approach to diagnosis of a hemolytic anemia has to match the clinical presentation. Key observations in planning the workup include whether the anemia is acute or chronic and whether the hemolysis is intravascular or extravascular in nature. Therefore, the first step in diagnosis is to try to determine from the clinical setting, the patient's medical history, and routine clinical and laboratory studies the answers to the following questions:

- Is the patient experiencing an acute hemolytic episode? or Is there evidence for a long-standing, compensated hemolytic anemia?
- If the anemia is acute, is the hemolysis occurring intravascularly or extravascularly?

Acute Intravascular Hemolysis

When there is evidence of an intravascular hemolytic event, the **history and examination of the patient usually suggests the cause** (Table 11–4). For example, when a red blood cell transfusion results in severe back pain and hemoglobinuria, there is a good chance the patient has received an ABO mismatched transfusion (usually when a unit of Type A blood is given to a Type O recipient) or infected blood. Other causes for acute intravascular hemolysis include severe thermal burns; snake bites; acute infections with *Clostridium perfringens*, falciparum malaria, or *Bartonella;* and the appearance of a high titer cold agglutinin. Low grade, chronic intravascular hemolysis is seen in patients with mechanical heart valves or paroxysmal nocturnal hemoglobinuria (PNH).

Speed is essential in diagnosis and management of these patients. Both plasma and urine should be examined immediately to document the intravascular nature of the hemolysis. Any obvious cause must also be identified without delay. For example, when a patient is receiving an ABO incompatible unit of blood, the transfusion must be stopped immediately and diuresis with fluids and mannitol initiated without delay. Similarly, patients with clostridial or malarial infections will only survive if appropriate therapy is begun without delay.

When a hemolytic event is less severe, it will often escape detection for several days. In this situation, measurements of serum haptoglobin, methemalbumin, and urine hemosiderin will need to be used to confirm the intravascular nature of the hemolysis and provide information as to the rate and course of the process (see Figure 11–3). A self-limited hemolytic episode can be retrospectively diagnosed from the pattern of recovery of the serum haptoglobin level and the urine hemosiderin. The CBC and peripheral blood film can also provide important information. For example, in patients with mechanical heart valves, widespread malignancy, or chronic disseminated intravascular coagulation (DIC), presence of fragmented red blood cells in circulation suggests ongoing hemolysis. As the patient improves, these cells tend to disappear.

Acute Extravascular Hemolysis

A sudden fall in hemoglobin level without evidence of bleeding or intravascular hemolysis (hemoglobinemia or hemoglobinuria) suggests an **acute extravascular hemolytic event.** Once again, the clinical setting will provide valuable information as to the potential cause (Table 11–5). Acute extravascular hemolysis is frequently seen in association with drug therapy in both normal individuals and patients with enzyme deficiencies, patients with autoimmune diseases, and after certain viral and bacterial infections. Patients who have a chronic, well-compensated hemolytic anemia can also demonstrate dramatic falls in their hemoglobin (hematocrit) secondary to an increased rate of red blood cell destruction or a sudden failure in red blood cell production. The relationship of the sudden hemolysis to the chronic hemolytic state may not be apparent if the patient has not been previously diagnosed.

To diagnose an acute, extravascular hemolytic event, clinicians must have a high level of suspicion; otherwise, the event can go undetected for several days. This delay can make diagnosis much more difficult. It is also important to methodically consider and test for more common causes of extravascular hemolysis, especially infections, drugs, and autoimmune disease. Other conditions that must be considered in differential diagnosis are fragmentation hemolysis secondary to malignancy, hemolytic uremic syndrome, and thrombotic thrombocytopenic purpura (see Chapter 34). In preg-

Table 11–4. Causes of intravascular hemolysis.

Blood transfusion	Bartonellosis
ABO mismatched transfusion	*Mycoplasma pneumoniae*
Infected blood	**Mechanical heart valves**
Thermal burns	**Paroxysmal hemoglobinuria**
Snake bites	PNH
Bacterial/parasitic infections	PCH
Clostridial sepsis	
Malaria	

Table 11–5. Causes of extravascular hemolysis.

Bacterial and viral infections Malaria *Mycoplasma pneumoniae* Infectious mononucleosis **Drug-induced hemolysis** G6PD/GSH deficiency Autoimmune drug reactions Strong oxidant drugs/chemicals **Autoimmune hemolysis** Warm-reacting (IgG) AIHA Cold-reacting (IgM) AIHA	**Hemoglobinopathies (Chapters 7 and 8)** **Membrane structural defect** Hereditary spherocytosis Hereditary elliptocytosis Acanthocytosis **Environmental disorders** Malignancy/DIC TTP/HUS Eclampsia or pre-eclampsia

nant women, acute hemolysis may be observed late in the third trimester in association with eclampsia or preeclampsia.

A. BACTERIAL AND VIRAL INFECTIONS:

Extravascular hemolysis can occur with several bacterial and viral infections. Mild, self-limited destruction of older red blood cells in circulation is typical of almost all bacterial infections (see Chapter 4). This is not associated with ongoing hemolysis; septic patients typically present with a hypoproliferative anemia.

More severe hemolysis is seen in patients with malaria, bartonellosis, clostridial sepsis, and Epstein-Barr (EBV) and mycoplasma infections. The severity of the hemolysis in malaria patients depends on the organism involved. Most **patients with vivax and falciparum malaria** have relatively mild, extravascular hemolysis. However, up to 20% of patients with falciparum malaria can have severe intravascular hemolysis (black water fever). **Clostridial sepsis** can also be associated with severe, life-threatening intravascular hemolysis. A self-limited, usually mild hemolytic event is often seen during the convalescent phase of *Mycoplasma pneumoniae.* It is associated with appearance of a high titer cold agglutinin. **Acute EBV infection (infectious mononucleosis)** can produce an impressive hemolytic anemia secondary to marked cell-mediated immune response or proliferation/activation of the macrophage system.

B. DRUG-INDUCED HEMOLYSIS:

Drugs induce hemolysis by an immune mechanism or by challenging metabolic machinery of the red blood cell. The latter is a very common scenario in patients with G6PD or GSH deficiency. Drugs associated with acute hemolysis in G6PD deficient patients are listed in Table 11–6. They all share the characteristic of being oxidant compounds that overwhelm the phosphogluconate pathway, which results in denaturation of hemoglobin. Chemicals and drugs such as dapsone, phenylhydrazine, aniline dyes, and potassium or sodium

chlorates can produce hemolysis in normal individuals by the same mechanism.

1. X-linked A-variant G6PD deficiency—The most common form of G6PD deficiency in the United States is the X-linked A-variant. Up to 10% of African American males are at risk. Typically, A-variant G6PD deficient patients, who have normal basal hemoglobin levels, will demonstrate a decrease in the hemoglobin to 9–11 grams per deciliter in association with an acute illness, often while taking one or more oxidant drugs (see Table 11–6).

The mechanism involved is a failure to generate sufficient NADPH to maintain GSH levels and prevent hemoglobin oxidation. Intracellular aggregates of denatured hemoglobin, called **Heinz bodies,** form and result in red cell trapping and destruction within the spleen. Hemolysis is self-limited once the population of older cells that have low G6PD levels are lost from circulation. In the A-variant form of the disease, younger red blood cells have normal or even high G6PD levels (reticulocytes). Therefore, the patient is able to increase red blood cell production and correct the anemia, even when the causative drug is continued.

Table 11–6. Drugs associated with hemolysis.

Oxidant drugs—G6PD deficiency
Antibiotics (nalidixic acid, nitrofurantoin, sulfa drugs, dapsone)
Antimalarials (primaquine)
Pyridium
Doxorubicin
Immune-mediated
Drug-specific antibodies—penicillin (cephalosporins, synthetic penicillins)
Antibody-haptene (drug) combination (quinidine)
Autoantibody to Rh antigens (α-methyldopa)
Antigen-antibody complex (stibophen)
Complement-fixing antibody (streptomycin)

The **ability of the patient to recover from anemia** must be recognized both in diagnosis and management. If there is a delay in detecting the anemia, a hematologic evaluation can show a brisk reticulocytosis and return of the hemoglobin level toward normal. In addition, it is **not essential that all drugs with oxidant potential be withdrawn.** For example, in patients who require malarial prophylaxis, the drug(s) can be continued, recognizing that the patient will compensate by developing a compensated hemolytic anemia. Patients (up to 5% of Ashkenazi Jews, Asian, and Mediterranean populations) with the Mediterranean form of G6PD deficiency or severe GSH deficiency are at risk for more severe hemolysis. Drug therapy or fava bean ingestion can precipitate a severe, fatal hemolytic event with both extravascular and intravascular hemolysis.

2. Drug-induced immune hemolytic anemia—Drug-induced immune hemolytic anemia has been observed with several drugs (see Table 11–6). At least four different mechanisms can be involved, including the formation of antibodies specific to the drug, the induction of antibodies to natural antigens on the red blood cell membrane, the formation of an antigen-antibody complex, and the selective binding of the antibiotic to the cell membrane with formation of a complement-fixing antibody. **Penicillin** is the best example of the first phenomenon, because if given in high doses, it binds to the red blood cell membrane. If the patient then forms an antibody against the penicillin, red blood cells will be removed and destroyed by the monocyte-macrophage system. The hemolytic process is rapidly controlled by simply withdrawing the penicillin. Cephalosporins and semisynthetic penicillins show cross-reactivity with penicillin antibodies. Moreover, **second- and third-generation cephalosporins** have been associated with severe autoimmune hemolytic anemia and should be automatically discontinued in any patient who presents with a positive DAT. **Quinidine** can cause immune hemolysis as well as immune thrombocytopenia. The quinidine acts as the haptene for an incomplete anti-red blood cell antibody. Therefore, withdrawal of the drug stops the hemolysis.

α-**Methyldopa** is an example of a drug that somehow alters T-cell suppressor function to induce an autoantibody to the Rh antigens on the red blood cell membrane. Up to 40% of patients taking α-methyldopa will develop a positive DAT; very few patients (less than 1%) ever develop a hemolytic anemia. **Stibophen** appears to act by the formation of antigen-antibody complexes that bind to red blood cells and induce hemolysis. **Streptomycin** binds specifically to the M or D antigens on the red blood cell membrane. If patients develop a complement-fixing antibody to streptomycin, they can demonstrate hemolysis. A common theme in all patients with drug-induced immune hemolytic anemias is presence of a positive DAT for IgG. Patients receiving streptomycin can show positive DAT with both anti-IgG and anti-C3 sera.

C. AUTOIMMUNE HEMOLYTIC ANEMIA:

Autoimmune hemolytic anemias can be anticipated in such clinical situations as viral/bacterial infections and collagen vascular diseases and in association with lymphopoietic malignancies.

1. Patterns of hemolysis—Each clinical situation tends to have a predictable pattern of hemolysis. For example, patients who are recovering from *Mycoplasma pneumoniae* can develop a high titer, cold agglutinin that results in an acute hemolytic episode over several days. **Patients with acute infectious mononucleosis** can develop an IgM cold agglutinin with i specificity some weeks into the illness, associated with both hemolysis and thrombocytopenia.

If the clinician watches and documents the temporal nature of the hemolytic event, the diagnosis should be relatively easy. In both groups of patients, it should be possible to document a rise in the cold agglutinin titer, a negative anti-IgG DAT, and in some patients, a positive anti-C3 DAT. The demonstration of i specificity in infectious mononucleosis patients is diagnostic. On occasion, **acute EBV infection** will stimulate proliferation and activation of the macrophage system with striking hemophagocytosis. These patients can exhibit pancytopenia and marrow hypoplasia, together with severe liver dysfunction and coagulopathies.

Acute and chronic extravascular hemolysis can accompany **collagen vascular disease** and **malignancies of the lymphatic system. Patients with lupus erythematosus** will often present with a DAT-positive hemolytic anemia or immune thrombocytopenia or both. Autoimmune hemolytic anemia is an anticipated complication in the management of patients with **chronic lymphatic leukemia.** The most common presentation of an immune hemolytic anemia is as an **autoimmune idiopathic hemolytic anemia (AIHA).**

2. Autoimmune idiopathic hemolytic anemia (AIHA)—AIHA patients usually have no clinical manifestations of other disease; their only finding is the extravascular hemolytic anemia. In most cases, the **erythropoietic profile** is typical of a relatively severe hemolytic anemia. The marrow E/G ratio is increased to greater than 1:1 and the reticulocyte index to greater than three times normal. Red blood cell morphology is generally normocytic/normochromic, although a varying number of cells may be spherocytic. Fragmentation is not observed and there is little evidence of poikilocytosis. Measurements of cell destruction (ie, the serum indirect bilirubin and LDH levels) are both increased.

Patients with very severe AIHA can show reticulocytopenia in the face of marrow erythroid hyperplasia. In this situation, autoantibody is responsible for the rapid removal of newly released reticulocytes.

AIHA is classified by laboratory testing as being secondary to either a warm-reacting (IgG) or cold-reacting (IgM) antibody. This designation requires DAT testing using monospecific antibodies to IgG and C3 and a measurement of the cold agglutinin titer. **Patients with warm-reacting (IgG) AIHA** show either IgG alone or a combination of IgG and C3 on the red blood cell surface (Table 11–7). **Patients with a cold-reacting (IgM) AIHA** will have a negative DAT for IgG and a positive test for C3.

The subclassification of AIHA is important in both diagnosis and management. **Warm-reacting (IgG) AIHA** is more frequently associated with lymphopoietic malignancies and collagen vascular disorders and is usually responsive to steroid therapy. **Cold-reacting (IgM) AIHA** is more resistant to therapy, is often a preamble to a lymphopoietic malignancy, and can be associated with severe cold intolerance.

Chronic (Lifelong) Extravascular Hemolysis

Patients with inherited defects in cell membrane function, hemoglobin structure, or intracellular metabolism generally present with a lifelong history of anemia. Racial background and family history provide important clues to the nature of the anemia. The erythropoietic profile reflects a compensated hemolytic anemia with marked expansion of marrow erythroid progenitors (E/G ratio greater than 1:1) and a reticulocyte production index that is three times normal or higher. At the same time, the severity of the anemia can be quite variable. For example, patients with hereditary spherocytosis can have near normal hemoglobin levels despite significantly shortened red blood cell lifespans. For

whatever reason, they are able to maintain a level of red blood cell production sufficient to nearly normalize their hemoglobin level.

The detection and diagnosis of a chronic hemolytic anemia is largely a laboratory exercise. It helps to have a well-organized approach to the workup, one that starts with simple tests available from the routine laboratory. From this viewpoint, the **examination of the peripheral blood film for abnormalities of red blood cell morphology** is the best starting point (Table 11–8). Unique red blood cell shape changes such as sickling, targeting, and spherocytosis are obvious clues to the cause of the hemolytic anemia. In fact, when taken in the context of the clinical picture, red blood cell morphology may be enough to make the diagnosis. If not, it at least guides the selection of additional confirmatory laboratory tests. It also helps to systematically **consider the most likely causes** of chronic hemolysis, grouped according to the broad categories of hemoglobinopathies, defects in membrane structure, abnormalities in intracellular metabolism, and disorders of the environment.

A. HEMOGLOBINOPATHIES:

Inherited abnormalities of hemoglobin structure and stability can result in a significant shortening of red blood cell lifespan. When severe, the erythropoietic profile will fit the picture of a chronic hemolytic anemia. Homozygous sickle cell disease is an excellent example of this presentation (see Chapter 7). Patients with thalassemia major or an unstable hemoglobin can also have a hemolytic component to their disease. The laboratory detection and diagnosis of these conditions are discussed more extensively in Chapters 7 and 8. It involves the selective use of laboratory methods such as hemoglobin electrophoresis, brilliant cresyl blue and crystal violet stains for Heinz bodies, and the isopropanol and heat-stability screening tests.

Table 11–7. Antibody testing in AIHA.

	DAT		
AIHA	**Anti-IgG**	**Anti-C3**	**Cold Agglutinins**
Warm-reacting antibody			
70%	Positive	Negative	< 1/256
20%	Positive	Positive	
10%	Negative[a]	Weakly positive	
Cold-reacting antibody	Negative	Positive	1/512–1/10,000

[a] The routine DAT (Coombs' test) will not detect AIHA patients with small numbers of IgG molecules per red blood cell.

Table 11–8. Red blood cell morphology in the diagnosis of hemolytic anemias.

Red Blood Cell Morphology	Possible Diagnoses	Confirmatory Tests
Sickle cells	Sickle cell anemia, SC disease, and S-thalassemia	Hemoglobin electrophoresis
Target cells	Hemoglobin C or SC disease, thalassemia, and severe liver disease	Hemoglobin electrophoresis
Spherocytes	Hereditary spherocytosis, autoimmune hemolytic anemia	Osmotic fragility, incubated autohemolysis, and DAT
Elliptocytes	Hereditary elliptocytosis	—
Stomatocytosis	Cirrhosis, malignancies, cardiovascular disease, and Rh antigen deficiency	—
Acanthocytosis	Cirrhosis/pancreatitis and a beta-lipoproteinemia	Lipoprotein assay
Fragmentation	Heart valves, DIC, malignancies, thermal burns, TTP, HUS	—

B. MEMBRANE STRUCTURAL DEFECTS:

Abnormalities in membrane protein composition can result in lifelong, well-compensated hemolytic anemia. Hereditary spherocytosis (HS) and hereditary elliptocytosis (HE) are the best clinical examples of this disorder.

1. Hereditary spherocytosis (HS)—HS is inherited as either an autosomal dominant (75%) or recessive (25%) trait. It is the most common inherited hemolytic anemia in Europe and the United States, with a frequency of 1 in 2000 individuals. Involvement of multiple gene loci by point mutations, gene deletions, and defects in RNA processing results in a unique mutation for each kindred.

The **principal defect in HS** is a deficiency in spectrin and ankyrin or, less frequently, band 3 protein or protein 4.2, all of which are key membrane skeletal proteins. Most HS patients demonstrate a silencing of the ankyrin gene (HSAnk+), which interferes with spectrin tethering and causes spectrin-rich vesiculation of the red cell membrane. This "vertical defect" results in a progressive loss of membrane lipid and surface area with the formation of microspherocytes (see Chapter 1). Clinically, the condition in these patients is most often detected because of the **spherocytosis on the peripheral blood film** or **an increase in the MCHC** to greater than 35%.

Patients with HS can be clinically silent or have a hemolytic anemia that ranges from mild to quite severe. In the latter case, the patient complains of easy fatigability and loss of vitality, is at risk for episodes of hemolytic or aplastic crisis, and usually develops pigment gallstones. Severely affected patients invariably have splenomegaly and many microspherocytes (elevated MCHC) on the peripheral blood film. With milder disease, blood film morphology is less dramatic,

splenomegaly may or may not be present, and red blood cell production levels are only slightly increased. The incubated osmotic fragility test will bring out the membrane instability defect and is abnormal in most patients.

2. Hereditary elliptocytosis (HE)—Patients with HE have an abnormality of the interaction of spectrin molecules, spectrin with the 4.1 protein, or with glycophorin in the red cell membrane. This abnormality interferes with "horizontal stability" and pliability, making it difficult for the red blood cell to regain its biconcave shape after distortion in the microcirculation (see Chapter 1).

The **diagnosis of the most common form of HE** is usually not difficult. Most red blood cells on the peripheral blood film (better than 50%) take on a uniform elliptical (oval) shape. Occasional rod-shaped cells may also be present. In contrast to other conditions where a few oval cells may be observed (eg, megaloblastic anemias), there is little or no poikilocytosis and the MCV is normal in HE. Only the occasional patient has a significant hemolytic anemia, requiring splenectomy.

Other **less common forms of elliptocytosis** include spherocytic elliptocytosis (a phenotypic hybrid of HS and HE); "homozygous" HE (a compound heterozygote for two spectrin mutations); Southeast Asian elliptocytosis (a band 3 mutation); and **hereditary pyropoikilocytosis (HPP)**. Each has a somewhat different morphology. This is especially true of HPP, which presents as a severe hemolytic anemia with bizarre poikilocytes, budding red cells, and red cell fragments on smear. The name of the disorder is derived from the observation that the red cells have an unusual thermal instability pattern. The underlying defect, however, as in HE, involves a spectrin mutation. Southeast Asian elliptocytosis may have a protective effect against malaria.

3. Laboratory confirmation of HS/HE diagnosis—Characteristic morphology, coupled with a positive family history and an appropriate clinical presentation, can be enough to diagnose HS or HE. Laboratory confirmation using the **osmotic fragility and autohemolysis tests,** or a direct assay of membrane proteins by **polyacrylamide gel electrophoresis,** is only necessary when the clinical picture is atypical. If fragility of the patient's red blood cells is measured, it is important to order an incubated osmotic fragility test to bring out the underlying defect (see Figure 11–4).

4. Acanthocytosis—Acanthocytosis, another disorder of membrane structure, is seen in patients with abetalipoproteinemia (congenital absence of apolipoprotein-β) and as a complication of severe cirrhosis or pancreatitis. It results from accumulation of nonesterified cholesterol or sphingomyelin on the outer layer of the lipid membrane. This distorts the membrane configuration and produces a characteristic spiculated-spur shape of the acanthocyte.

5. Stomatocytosis—Stomatocytosis is seen in patients with cirrhosis, neoplasms, cardiovascular diseases, and as an inherited defect characterized by marked reduction in the expression of Rh antigen on the cell membrane. Congenital stomatocytosis has been associated with vasoocclusive events, especially pulmonary hypertension. Osmotic fragility is increased reflecting a loss of red cell membrane.

C. Intracellular Metabolic Defects:

The principal metabolic pathways of the red cell are described in detail in Chapter 1. **Major functions of these pathways** include maintenance of protein integrity, membrane structure, and cell shape; the continuous reduction of heme-iron to its ferrous state; and production of appropriate amounts of 2,3-DPG. A deficiency in any one of the more than 20 enzymes involved in these pathways can result in a clinical abnormality. However, pyruvate kinase, hexokinase, glucose phosphate isomerase, and phosphofructokinase are the enzymes most often linked to a clinically significant hemolytic anemia.

Pyruvate kinase (PK) deficiency is the most common of the Embden-Meyerhoff pathway enzymopathies. It presents during childhood with a moderately severe hemolytic anemia, jaundice, splenomegaly, and failure to thrive. Red cell morphology is highly abnormal, with spherocytes, acanthocytes, severely dehydrated red cells (**xerocytes**) and fragmented cells dominating the smear. The reticulocyte count is higher than expected (can exceed 30%) due to a delay in the breakdown of reticulocyte RNA. The incubated autohemoly-

sis test (Figure 11–4) will generally distinguish PK from HS. A simple, sensitive screening test is also available to test for pyruvate kinase deficiency.

The other glycolytic pathway enzyme defects are much less common and are usually associated with mild to moderate nonspherocytic hemolytic anemias. **Glucose-6-phosphate dehydrogenase (G6PD) deficiency** is the most common of the phosphogluconate pathway enzyme defects. **Glutathione reductase** and **phosphogluconate dehydrogenase deficiencies** are rare, but should be considered in circumstances of a well-documented oxidant-induced hemolysis when tests of G6PD are normal (see earlier discussion in this chapter under Drug-Induced Hemolysis).

D. Disorders of the Environment:

Autoimmune hemolysis can also present as a chronic hemolytic anemia, the severity of which can be highly variable depending on the underlying disease process, the level of antibody production, and the activity of the antibody. Although this condition in most patients can be detected using routine polyspecific and monospecific DAT measurements, some patients will have relatively small amounts of antibody on the cell surface. Detection in these patients will require the expertise of a hematology laboratory that uses sophisticated immunoassay and radiolabeled antibody tests.

As discussed in the section on intravascular hemolysis, mechanical heart valves can be associated with chronic fragmentation hemolysis. It is also possible to see a chronic hemolytic anemia following an acute episode of hemolytic uremic syndrome or thrombotic thrombocytopenic purpura. One clue to an environmental disorder is the presence of fragmented cells on the peripheral blood film; another is the appearance of both intravascular and extravascular hemolytic components to the disease.

THERAPY

The management of a patient with a hemolytic anemia will vary according to the individual disease state. As a result, an accurate diagnosis is very important. There are also several therapeutic themes that apply to all hemolytic anemias, especially the chronic, well-compensated hemolytic states.

General Guidelines

Whatever the cause of increased destruction of circulating red blood cells, the **erythroid marrow has the capacity to compensate** by increasing production by more than three- to fivefold. This compensation is equal to a transfusion of a unit of red blood cells every

2–3 days. This fact, coupled with the innate ability of red blood cells to increase the oxygen delivery to tissues, allows patients to survive disease states where the red blood cell lifespan is as little as 10–20 days. The capacity to compensate depends, however, on the ability of the marrow to respond and the patient's cardiovascular status.

As with any anemia, an increase in red blood cell production depends on an adequate supply of essential substrates, a normal marrow structure, and an appropriate erythropoietin response. Patients who develop kidney or marrow damage as a part of their disease will be unable to respond and therefore will need transfusion to survive. **Adequate iron and folic acid supplies** are extremely important. The patient with intravascular hemolysis who loses iron into his or her urine will be unable to increase red blood cell production. All hemolytic anemia patients have an increased requirement for folic acid and need to be chronically supplemented (1 mg of folic acid twice a day by mouth). Otherwise, erythropoiesis will become ineffective and red blood cell production will decrease.

Intravascular Hemolysis

The success of treating intravascular hemolysis depends on the cause. In the case of **ABO incompatible blood,** the severity of the reaction will depend on the nature of the mismatch and the amount of blood transfused. The worst reactions are seen in type O patients who are mistakenly transfused with type A blood. If it is detected early and the transfusion discontinued, little needs to be done other than providing sufficient fluid to induce a diuresis and prevent glomeruli and tubular damage. If there is a delay in detecting the reaction, the kidney is at risk for damage from both disrupted red blood cell membranes damaging the glomeruli and the excess of free hemoglobin that can result in acute tubular necrosis. In this situation, diuresis alone is not enough. The patient should also be treated with mannitol to encourage renal blood flow and decrease hemoglobin reabsorption. If renal shutdown does occur, patients can recover function with time. Transfusion of ABO incompatible blood can result in severe hypotension, DIC, and the death of the patient.

The treatment of acute intravascular hemolysis associated with **bacterial or parasitic infections** must focus on the treatment of the primary infection. The hemolysis is usually not associated with renal failure. Transfusion may be necessary if the hemolysis is severe. **Chronic intravascular hemolysis in patients with PNH or mechanical heart valves** can result in iron deficiency and an iron deficiency anemia (Chapter 9). This condition may respond to routine iron therapy or may require transfusion.

Extravascular Hemolysis

Management of an acute or chronic extravascular hemolytic anemia involves both evaluating the patient's ability to physiologically compensate for the anemia and treating the specific condition. For example, acute self-limited hemolysis in patients with G6PD deficiency rarely needs treatment. The anemia that results is relatively mild, and the normal marrow production response will return the hemoglobin level to normal. The more important management issue is patient education regarding the drugs and chemicals that provoke hemolysis. On the other hand, patients with a more severe enzyme deficiency state or autoimmune disease can present with a life-threatening anemia. In this situation, transfusion, aggressive chemotherapy, or both will be required. As with the diagnostic workup, patient management needs to be organized according to the mechanism causing the hemolysis.

A. Hemoglobinopathies:

The management of the patient with a hemoglobinopathy is discussed in Chapters 7 and 8. These patients require lifelong healthcare support and are at constant risk for both hemolytic and aplastic crises in association with various infections and systemic illness. If they have a severe anemia and require long-term transfusion therapy, they have to be simultaneously treated for iron overload.

B. Membrane Structural Defects:

Patients with relatively mild hereditary spherocytosis or hereditary elliptocytosis maintain near normal hemoglobin levels and are generally in good health. **Patients with severe hereditary spherocytosis** will be symptomatic. They are at risk for recurrent hemolytic and aplastic episodes, often associated with parvovirus infection, and are candidates for splenectomy to improve red blood cell lifespan and decrease the severity of their anemia. If possible, splenectomy should be avoided until after the first decade of life. Splenectomy almost always results in marked improvement. The patient feels better, the red blood cell lifespan returns to near normal, and the risk of gallstones and hemolytic/aplastic crises is reduced.

Partial splenectomy has been used to improve red cell lifespan without total loss of spleen phagocytic and immune functions. A sustained rise in the hemoglobin level and fall in transfusion requirement is observed, although the patients still demonstrate elevated reticulocyte counts. The splenic remnant rapidly regrows, reaching normal splenic size by 1 year and twice normal size by 4–6 years. Because of this, a second total splenectomy is necessary in one-third of patients. Any patient who receives a splenectomy must receive polyvalent pneumococcal vaccine prior to operation. If a total splenectomy is performed before age 10, the child should receive oral penicillin prophylaxis (125–250 mg penicillin per day by mouth).

Because **hereditary spherocytosis patients** are at risk for developing pigment gallstones, a prophylactic, laparoscopic cholecystectomy should be considered early in adult life. Elective cholecystectomy should definitely be performed if a patient has even one attack of cholecystitis because of the risk for recurrent disease.

C. Autoimmune Hemolysis:

Management of patients with autoimmune hemolytic anemia will vary according to the nature of the disease process. For example, autoimmune red blood cell destruction associated with drug ingestion stops after withdrawing the offending agent. When the autoimmune process complicates a lymphopoietic malignancy, control of the hemolysis will depend on effective treatment of the tumor. As for AIHA, the choice of therapy will depend on whether the hemolysis is owing to a warm- or cold-reacting antibody.

1. Warm-antibody AIHA—Several therapeutic options are available to treat warm-antibody AIHA. The first choice is always corticosteroids or, in the case of severe disease, steroids plus an immunosuppressive drug such as cyclophosphamide.

a. Treatment with corticosteroids—Corticosteroids act by blocking the reticuloendothelial cell clearance of red blood cells coated with either IgG or C3 and the production of new IgG antibody. Cyclophosphamide acts as a lympholytic agent to reduce antibody production.

Oral **prednisone** in a daily dose of 60–120 mg (1–1.5 mg/kg) is a typical starting regimen. It should be continued at this level for at least 2 weeks with daily measurements of the CBC and reticulocyte count. The patient's response will vary according to the severity and nature of the disease process. More than half of patients will show an increase in reticulocyte index and hemoglobin level within the first 1–2 weeks. Patients with severe AIHA can show little response or even a worsening of their anemia, however.

The **subsequent management of the patient** will depend on the observed response. If initial therapy is effective, the prednisone dose will need to be gradually tapered while closely monitoring the CBC. Warm-antibody AIHA will frequently relapse as the prednisone is tapered. Therefore, the taper should be gradual, reducing the daily dosage by increments of 10 mg or less at weekly intervals. As the dosage falls below 20 mg, severe hemolysis can recur suddenly, requiring an immediate return to a higher prednisone dose and the institution of other therapies. If the daily dosage can be brought below 15 mg per day, it may be possible to switch to an every-other-day schedule and thereby reduce the chance of significant side effects.

b. Treatment with combined chemotherapy or splenectomy—Patients who do not respond to steroid therapy are candidates for **combined chemotherapy** or splenectomy. Cyclophosphamide given in pulse doses of 1000 mg intravenously on one to three occasions may be effective in some patients. It is very useful in patients who present with a severe hemolytic anemia that does not respond to prednisone therapy during the first 2–3 weeks. **Splenectomy** can help in the long-term control of autoimmune hemolysis in the prednisone-refractory patient. It works both by removing the trapping function of the spleen and by reducing the level of antibody production. It should be performed after the patient is stabilized on chemotherapy. Splenectomy is not a cure by itself and will not eliminate the need for chemotherapy. It can, however, reduce the amount of prednisone, cyclophosphamide, or both needed to control the disease.

c. Other therapies—Warm-antibody AIHA can present as a severe, life-threatening anemia. In this situation, other therapies must be considered. **Transfusion with packed red blood cells** is clearly indicated, regardless of the difficulties encountered in adequately crossmatching the patient. An attempt should be made to find units of red blood cells that have minimum activity on the indirect DAT, although it is unlikely that truly "compatible" blood will be identified. Patients can be transfused with type-specific blood when transfusion is required to save the patient's life. It can be anticipated that the survival of transfused red blood cells will be no better or no worse than the survival of the patient's own cells. There should not be a risk of precipitating an intravascular hemolytic event.

Both intravenous immunoglobulin and plasmapheresis have been used with limited success in the treatment of AIHA. **Immunoglobulin** appears to work by acutely blocking the Fc receptors on reticuloendothelial cells and, perhaps, by downregulating antibody production. If therapy is attempted, at least 5 days of 400 mg per kilogram of one of the commercially available immunoglobulin preparations should be given. If there is a response, it may not be observed for several days and can be short lived. **Plasmapheresis** or extracorporeal absorption of IgG using an anti-staphylococcal protein-A-silica column may also be beneficial in the severely ill patient.

2. Cold-antibody AIHA—The treatment of a patient with a cold-antibody AIHA is significantly different. Little needs to be done for those patients who develop a high titer cold agglutinin following an infection with *Mycoplasma* or EBV virus other than to monitor

the severity of the anemia and, if necessary, transfuse the patient. Patients with cold agglutinin disease or lymphopoietic malignancy with a high titer anti-IgM antibody may respond to treatment with an **alkylating agent.** Usually, corticosteroids are of little benefit. When a patient's anemia is very severe, **plasmapheresis** can be life-saving. Because the major portion of the patient's IgM antibody is intravascular, plasmapheresis can be used to significantly reduce the antibody titer, thereby buying time until cyclophosphamide or chlorambucil therapy reduces antibody production.

As with warm-antibody AIHA, patients with cold-reacting IgM antibodies can receive **transfusions** without risk of precipitating a life-threatening hemolytic episode. Cross-matching is usually not as big a problem as that experienced with warm-antibody AIHA. It is very important, however, to recognize the role of fresh complement in the hemolytic reaction. The severity of hemolysis in a patient with cold-antibody AIHA can be suppressed by the depletion of complement in the patient's plasma. If fresh complement is provided as part of a red blood cell transfusion, the hemolysis can increase dramatically. Therefore, as a precaution, cold-antibody AIHA patients should routinely receive transfusions of washed red blood cells that are free of complement.

Patients with cold agglutinin disease can demonstrate dramatic **cold sensitivity.** Even brief exposure of extremities to cold environments can result in an acute hemolytic episode. These patients need to learn how to avoid cold exposure. In addition, any blood product or intravenous fluid must be warmed prior to transfusion. Cold-antibody AIHA is generally manageable but not curable. With time, patients become refractory to chemotherapy and transfusion-dependent. In addition, the survival of transfused red blood cells becomes progressively shorter. This progression does not respond to splenectomy or other therapeutic options used in warm-antibody AIHA.

BIBLIOGRAPHY

Tabbara IA: Hemolytic anemias: Diagnosis and management. Med Clin North Am 1992;76:649.

Drug-Induced Hemolysis

Beutler E: Glucose-6-phosphate dehydrogenase (G6PD) deficiency. N Engl J Med 1991;324:169.

Membrane Structural Defects

Liu SC et al: Alteration of the erythrocyte membrane skeletal ultrastructure in hereditary spherocytosis, hereditary elliptocytosis and pyropoikilocytosis. Blood 1990;76:198.

Palek J, Sahr KE: Mutations of the red blood cell membrane proteins: From clinical evaluation to detection of the underlying genetic defect. Blood 1992;80:308.

Enzyme Defects

Hirono A, Forman L, Beutler E: Enzymatic diagnosis in nonspherocytic hemolytic anemia. Medicine 1988;67:110.

Autoimmune Hemolysis

Besa EC: Rapid transient reversal of anemia and long-term effects of maintenance intravenous immunoglobulin for AIHA in patients with lymphoproliferative disorders. Am J Med 1988;84:691.

Collins PW, Newland AC: Treatment modalities of autoimmune blood disorders. Semin Hematol 1992;29:64.

Engelfriet CP, Overbeeke MAM, vondem Borne AEGKR: Autoimmune hemolytic anemia. Semin Hematol 1992;29:3.

Polycythemia

Polycythemia and erythrocytosis are clinical terms used to describe an abnormally elevated hemoglobin or hematocrit. Just as in anemia, the probability that a patient has an elevated value will be a function of how far the hemoglobin or hematocrit is above normal for the population. The fact that these measurements are ratios of the number of red blood cells to volume of plasma must be kept in mind. An increase in hemoglobin or hematocrit can result from a reduction in plasma volume (**relative polycythemia**) without a true increase in red blood cell mass.

Detection and accurate diagnosis of polycythemia is important regardless of its cause. Even modest increases in the hemoglobin/hematocrit level can have a major impact on whole blood viscosity. Depending on the patient's clinical condition, this can significantly affect blood flow and oxygen delivery to tissues. Therefore, management involves both treating the primary condition and appropriately adjusting the patient's hemoglobin/hematocrit to normal.

NORMAL ERYTHROPOIESIS & BLOOD VOLUME CONTROL

The total number of red blood cells in circulation will vary according to the patient's age, sex, and clinical condition. Just as the erythroid marrow increases red blood cell production in response to anemia, the number of red blood cells produced each day will increase in response to chronic hypoxia. The normal value for a patient must take these factors into account. The normal distribution of hemoglobin or hematocrit measurements will be different for men and women of different ages and for individuals living at higher altitudes (Figure 12–1). In addition, patients with mild to moderate hypoxia caused by lung disease will compensate by increasing the number of circulating red blood cells. Within limits, this physiologic response to decreased oxygen availability to tissues is an effective compensatory mechanism.

The **regulation of normal erythropoiesis and oxygen transport** are discussed in detail in Chapter 1. Specific derangements in hemoglobin-oxygen dissociation, erythropoietin production, and red cell progenitor growth regulation are associated with abnormal red cell

production and, at times, an increase in red cell mass (volume) beyond physiologic limits.

The control of **plasma volume** follows its own rules. Oncotic protein production, salt and water metabolism, and vasomotor tone are key factors in regulating the amount of plasma in circulation. Clinical conditions such as severe dehydration or allergic reactions with loss of plasma proteins from the vascular compartment are associated with elevations in hemoglobin and hematocrit. Even though the red blood cell mass is not increased, a sustained reduction in plasma volume can significantly affect viscosity, blood flow, and oxygen delivery to tissues.

Major **increases in red blood cell mass,** as seen with polycythemia vera, may not be compensated for by a matched reduction in plasma volume. From a physiologic standpoint, this represents a choice between two bad situations. If any increase in red blood cell mass is accompanied by an equal reduction in plasma volume, the patient will quickly experience an increase in blood viscosity. On the other hand, if plasma volume does not decrease, total blood volume will increase significantly, placing stress on the volume capacity of the vascular compartment.

The relationship of **whole blood viscosity** to blood flow and oxygen delivery to tissues is a complex function (Figure 12–2). In a normal individual, maximum tissue blood flow and oxygen delivery is seen at hemoglobin levels of 11–12 grams per deciliter. Below this level, viscosity decreases but, despite a modest increase in blood flow, tissue oxygen delivery declines. At hemoglobin levels greater than 12 grams per deciliter, increases in viscosity reduce blood flow. With hemoglobin levels between 12 and 16 grams per deciliter, this effect is relatively modest. Once the hemoglobin rises above 18 grams per deciliter, viscosity increases dramatically and both blood flow and tissue oxygen delivery rapidly decline.

Individual organ blood flow is also affected by the blood gas pattern. For example, brain blood flow is very sensitive to CO_2 concentration. When the PCO_2 increases, cerebral vessels dilate. With sudden reductions in PCO_2, vessels constrict and further limit the flow of more viscous blood. The interaction of blood viscosity with vessel reactivity is an important part of

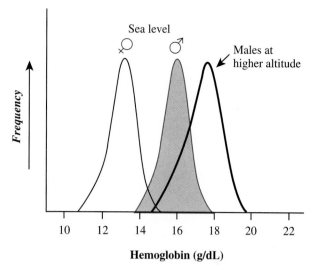

Figure 12–1. **Hemoglobin levels at sea level and higher altitudes.** Population distribution of hemoglobin levels for men and women at sea level will be significantly different from those seen for individuals living at higher altitudes or patients with chronic hypoxia.

the compensation for chronic hypoxia, as seen in patients with chronic obstructive pulmonary disease. Although an increase in the hemoglobin/hematocrit in these patients is associated with increased blood viscosity, the impact on brain blood flow is in part compensated by their CO_2 retention and vasodilation.

CLINICAL FEATURES

The clinical signs and symptoms of an elevated hemoglobin/hematocrit vary depending on disease process and rate of onset. Expansion of the red blood cell mass requires weeks or even months of a sustained increase in

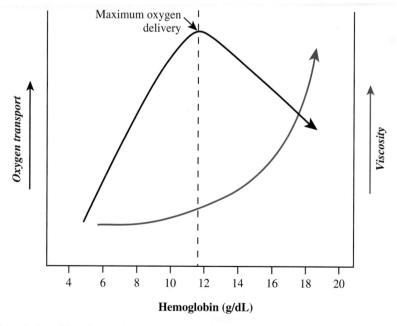

Figure 12–2. **The relationship of oxygen delivery to the hemoglobin level.** Oxygen transport and delivery to tissues is a function of the hemoglobin level and whole blood viscosity. Oxygen transport rapidly decays when the hemoglobin falls to levels below 11–12 grams per deciliter. Whole blood viscosity increases rapidly with hemoglobin levels greater than 12 grams per deciliter. This situation causes a progressive decrease in oxygen transport.

red blood cell production. During this time, the patient's physiology has a chance to adapt. Therefore, patients with modest elevations in hemoglobin/hematocrit secondary to chronic lung disease, a hemoglobinopathy, or polycythemia vera will complain of few symptoms. It is only **when the hemoglobin rises above 18–20 grams per deciliter** that patients report symptoms such as chronic headaches, a general sense of malaise, and easy fatigability.

Hemoglobin levels greater than 20 grams per deciliter can be life-threatening. At this level, viscosity is markedly increased and blood flow to vital organs is compromised. In order to survive, these patients will expand their total blood volume. This situation is a major challenge to the cardiovascular system and can lead to congestive failure. Furthermore, blood volume expansion can lead to thrombotic complications and spontaneous rupture of arterial vessels. Untreated polycythemia vera patients are at risk for excessive bleeding with surgery or trauma.

Patients with a hemoglobin level in excess of 20 grams per deciliter may be recognized from their general appearance. The increase in hemoglobin level and blood volume results in a noticeable facial plethora with prominent, bloodshot eyes and red to purplish mucous membranes. Vessels of the conjunctiva and ocular fundus appear dilated, and venous blood may appear desaturated. In addition, prominent cyanosis is observed in patients who are hypoxic.

Symptoms and signs associated with a primary disease process such as chronic obstructive pulmonary disease or congenital heart disease can help point to the diagnosis. Polycythemia vera patients can complain of **severe itching** almost continuously or especially after a shower. This situation relates to the mast cell proliferation seen with the disease. Most polycythemia vera patients also have palpable splenomegaly.

Laboratory Studies

A routine **complete blood count** (**CBC**) provides all of the information necessary to initially diagnose severe polycythemia. The **upper normal limits** for men and women living at sea level are 18 and 16 grams per deciliter, respectively. Patients who exceed these levels must have an increase in the red blood cell mass or a reduction in plasma volume. If the hemoglobin level is persistently above 20 grams per deciliter in men and 18 grams per deciliter in women, the patient almost certainly has a true increase in the red blood cell mass.

Several other laboratory measurements are important in diagnosing the cause of polycythemia. They may or may not be required, depending on clinical presentation. For example, patients with polycythemia vera can present with a pattern of clinical findings that

Table 12–1. Polycythemia vera diagnostic criteria.

Primary criteria
Increased hemoglobin/(hematocrit)—> 18 g/dL in men; > 16 g/dL in women or red blood cell mass increase (^{51}Cr–red cell volume)—> 36 mL/kg in men; > 32 mL/kg in women
Palpable splenomegaly
No other explanation—renal disease, hypoxia, tumor, etc
And, if present
Abnormal marrow karyotype (10–20% of patients)
Secondary criteria
Thrombocytosis—> 400,000 platelets/μL
Leukocytosis—> 12,000 white blood cells/μL
EPO level less than 9.2 mU/mL
BFU-E hypersensitivity to EPO
Elevated leukoctye alkaline phosphatase[a]
Elevated serum B_{12} level—> 900 pg/mL or elevated transcobalamin level (B_{12} binding capacity)—2200 pg/mL.[b]

[a] Difficult to standardize.

[b] Not specific to polycythemia vera.

is virtually diagnostic for the disease (Table 12–1). The combination of a high hemoglobin level, leukocytosis, thrombocytosis, basophilia, and an increase in the leukocyte alkaline phosphatase in a patient with symptoms and signs such as itching, headaches, malaise, and splenomegaly is virtually diagnostic. The diagnostic finding is the expansion of all three hematopoietic compartments. This situation reflects the fact that polycythemia vera is a clonal malignancy of the stem cell responsible for all hematopoietic cell lines. It separates polycythemia vera from all other conditions where the increase in red blood cell mass results from a pure erythropoietin stimulus. Therefore, additional laboratory studies are most valuable in diagnosing those patients who do not have clear-cut polycythemia vera.

A. RED BLOOD CELL MASS AND PLASMA VOLUME MEASUREMENTS:

The circulating red blood cell mass can be directly measured using ^{51}Cr-labeled red blood cells. By injecting a known amount of labeled cells and measuring their subsequent dilution, it is possible to get an accurate measurement of the total red blood cell mass. In a similar fashion, ^{131}I-labeled albumin can be used to measure the plasma volume. Normal values for adult men and women are summarized in Table 12–2.

These measurements are expensive, involve exposure to radioactivity, and are difficult to complete. Therefore, they should only be used in those situations where the reason for an elevated hemoglobin level is unclear. Most often, this arises when the hemoglobin level is between 18–20 grams per deciliter in men and 16–18

Table 12–2. Red blood cell, plasma, and total blood volumes [(mL +/− 1 SD[a])/kg].

	Red Blood Cell Volume	Plasma Volume	Total Blood Volume
Men	30 ± 5	35 ± 5	65 ± 8
Women	25 ± 5	35 ± 5	60 ± 7

[a] The standard deviation for each volume measurement includes a ± 5% coefficient of variation for the assay technique as well as individual subject variation. Falsely low values are observed in obese patients when results are expressed as milliliters per kilogram of measured body weight.

grams per deciliter in women. Above these levels, the red blood cell mass is invariably increased.

B. BLOOD GAS MEASUREMENTS:

It is essential to measure **arterial blood gas** in patients with lung or heart disease. Sustained hypoxia sufficient to keep arterial oxygen saturation below 80% will, in a normally responsive patient, stimulate a hemoglobin level greater than 18 grams per deciliter. Patients with congenital heart disease and pronounced right to left shunts show the most dramatic desaturation and highest hemoglobin levels (often exceeding 22 grams per deciliter). A single blood gas determination in a chronic lung disease or a sleep apnea patient may not accurately reflect the severity of the hypoxia. In this situation, repeated measurements over 24 hours or as part of a sleep apnea study may be necessary to evaluate the severity of the desaturation.

A direct measurement of **carbon monoxide concentration in blood (carboxyhemoglobin level)** with a spectrophotometer is important in heavy smokers and individuals at risk of environmental exposure to carbon monoxide. Carboxyhemoglobin cannot be detected by pulse oximetry or standard blood gas measurement; even high levels of carboxyhemoglobin will not be reflected by the calculated percent saturation. Carbon monoxide avidly binds to hemoglobin and displaces oxygen, effectively canceling oxygen-carrying capacity of the molecule.

Point mutations in globin structure can interfere with the respiratory motion of the hemoglobin molecule and binding of 2,3-DPG. Some of these hemoglobinopathies produce an increased hemoglobin-oxygen affinity, thereby stimulating a higher than normal hemoglobin level. This functional abnormality can be detected by **measurements of the hemoglobin P$_{50}$ and intracellular 2,3-DPG levels.** A decrease in the P$_{50}$ value to below 15 mm Hg is associated with increases in hemoglobin in excess of 18 grams per deciliter (Figure 12–3). Up to half of these high-affinity hemoglobinopathies can be diagnosed by hemoglobin electrophoresis. Some unstable hemoglobins show decreased oxygen affinity as demonstrated by the P$_{50}$ measurement (see Chapter 7).

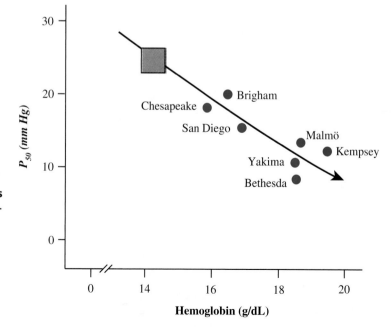

Figure 12–3. Hemoglobinopathies associated with increased hemoglobin levels. Inherited hemoglobin defects with an increased hemoglobin-oxygen affinity will demonstrate high hemoglobin levels. P$_{50}$ values below 15 mm Hg are associated with hemoglobins greater than 18 grams per deciliter.

C. KARYOTYPE ANALYSIS:

Between 10% and 20% of patients presenting with polycythemia vera will exhibit an abnormal marrow karyotype. The most common abnormalities are 20q minus, trisomy 8, trisomy 9, and 13q minus. As for the genetic mechanism underlying the disease, major attention has been given to the role of one or more mutations on the long arm of chromosome 20. Over time with progression of disease, frequency of chromosomal abnormalities increases, especially with evolution to myelodysplasia or acute leukemia. After 10 years, more than 80% of patients will exhibit one or more chromosomal abnormalities.

D. ERYTHROPOIETIN AND STEM CELL ASSAYS:

An accurate measurement of **serum erythropoietin level** is possible by immunoassay. High normal to elevated levels are typically seen with hypoxia, high oxygen-affinity hemoglobins, and erythropoietin-secreting tumors. In untreated polycythemia vera patients, erythropoietin levels are usually depressed, even to the point of being undetectable. Several clinical variables interfere with interpretation of any single erythropoietin level, however. Hypoxic patients will demonstrate a rapid return of the erythropoietin level to normal or even below normal when oxygen delivery to tissues is transiently improved. On the other hand, polycythemia vera patients who are treated with phlebotomy or who become iron deficient can show normal or elevated levels. The pattern of response of the erythropoietin level to phlebotomy can also help identify the cause of the erythrocytosis (Figure 12–4).

Further proof of polycythemia vera is possible using a **stem cell assay.** Expansion of burst-forming unit–erythroid (BFU-E) colonies in marrow culture normally requires the presence of erythropoietin. The malignant cell line of polycythemia vera patients grows in culture with little or no added erythropoietin. Moreover, there may be an increased progenitor sensitivity to insulin growth factor-1 and IL-3. This situation is a direct demonstration of loss of normal regulatory control of erythroid precursor proliferation. Unfortunately, the BFU-E colony assay is difficult to standardize, since BFU-E growth patterns vary considerably among polycythemia vera patients. Also, the assay will not distinguish patients with erythropoietin receptor truncation defects.

E. MISCELLANEOUS STUDIES:

Several other radiologic and laboratory studies can help in differential diagnosis of the polycythemia. **Examination of the marrow by aspirate and biopsy** can provide evidence of myelodysplasia in polycythemia vera patients. **Measurements of the serum vitamin B$_{12}$ level and transcobalamin proteins** provide an indirect measure of granulocytic hyperplasia. Transcobalamins I and III, but predominantly transcobalamin III, tend to be increased.

In the case of secondary polycythemias, studies that help in diagnosing cardiopulmonary disease are integral to the definition of hypoxic erythrocytosis. These studies can include a range of **cardiac imaging studies, heart catheterization, and lung function studies. An intravenous pyelogram and CT scans** of the head and

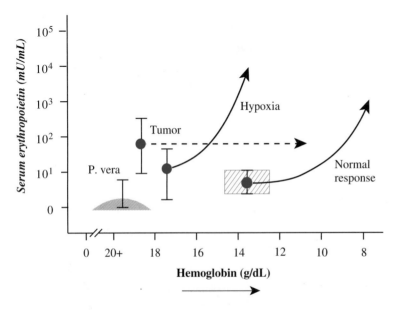

***Figure 12–4.* Erythropoietin measurements in patients with various forms of polycythemia.** When compared with the normal response, polycythemia vera patients present with below normal to absent serum levels. Patients with polycythemia secondary to hypoxia or an erythropoietin-secreting tumor show high normal to elevated levels. The response to phlebotomy is even more distinctive. Polycythemia vera patients essentially follow the normal curve, whereas patients with hypoxia show marked increases in serum erythropoietin levels even while the hemoglobin level is above normal. Patients with erythropoietin-secreting tumors can show a suppressed response.

abdomen will help rule out an erythropoietin-producing tumor or hydronephrosis of the kidney.

Iron studies, including a **serum iron, total iron-binding capacity, and serum ferritin levels,** are essential in the evaluation of any patient with polycythemia. Expansion of the red blood cell mass will deplete iron stores. In women, this is often enough to exhaust stores and result in iron-deficient erythropoiesis. Since a reduction in iron supply suppresses the proliferative capacity of the erythroid marrow, interpretation of any elevation in hemoglobin/hematocrit must take into account iron balance.

DIAGNOSIS

The diagnosis of polycythemia is an excellent test of a clinician's diagnostic skill. Most often, the cause of an increased hemoglobin/hematocrit can be identified from the clinical presentation and routine evaluation of the patient's cardiopulmonary status. Measurements of red blood cell mass and plasma volume, hemoglobin-oxygen affinity, erythropoietin levels, as well as other laboratory and radiologic studies, are only needed in rare cases where the clinical pattern of disease is confusing.

Polycythemia Vera

Patients with polycythemia vera have a stem cell disorder, a clonal malignancy, characterized by the production of an excessive number of mature hematopoietic cells, especially red blood cells. The mutational event appears to involve pluripotent stem cells of the marrow, although some patients demonstrate clonality for all cell lines except T-cells and natural killer lymphocytes. Similar to preleukemic dysplastic anemias, polycythemia vera progresses with time to varying combinations of cell proliferation and cytopenia, myelofibrosis, distorted cell maturation, and even leukemia. Most patients, however, are diagnosed when expansion of the red blood cell mass is the predominant feature.

A. CLINICAL CRITERIA:

Diagnosis of polycythemia vera is usually made based on a handful of clinical criteria (see Table 12–1). These criteria were initially proposed by the polycythemia vera study group for use in clinical trials and continue to evolve.

A direct **measurement of the red blood cell mass** using ^{51}Cr-labeled red blood cells is unnecessary when the hemoglobin exceeds 20 grams per deciliter in males and 18 grams per deciliter in females. At this level, red blood cell mass is almost certainly increased. Red cell mass measurements can be problematic, not only because of the relative inaccuracy of the technique, but

also depending on whether body weight or body surface area is used to express the result. For obese patients, either an ideal body weight or, better yet, the body surface area should be used to avoid a false-negative result. If the red blood cell volume measurement is performed, it should always be accompanied by a direct measurement of the plasma volume using ^{131}I-labeled albumin. This makes it possible to more accurately distinguish true polycythemia from relative polycythemia, where an increase in hemoglobin is caused by a reduction in plasma volume.

Polycythemia vera is almost certainly present whenever a patient demonstrates all of the **primary criteria** (ie, elevated hemoglobin or red blood cell mass, normal arterial oxygen saturation, and splenomegaly, without another explanation) together with some or all of the **secondary criteria** (ie, thrombocytosis, leukocytosis, a lower than normal to absent serum erythropoietin level, an elevated leukocyte alkaline phosphatase, and an elevated serum vitamin B_{12} or transcobalamin-binding capacity level). The secondary criteria are direct demonstrations of the malignant nature of the disease process. Polycythemia vera is a clonal malignancy of the pluripotent stem cell, resulting in abnormalities in all cell lines.

B. MARROW ASPIRATE AND BIOPSY:

Although marrow examination is not necessary to make the diagnosis, marrow aspirate and biopsy will generally show a hypercellular marrow with expansion of all cell compartments. Megakaryocyte proliferation may be striking, with clusters of very large, multinucleate cells. As the disease progresses, cell elements become more dysplastic and the marrow structure can become increasingly fibrotic with an increase in reticulin and collagenous tissue.

C. SERUM VITAMIN B_{12} LEVEL:

An elevation of the serum vitamin B_{12} level provides another indicator of granulocyte proliferation. The elevated B_{12} level is caused by an increase in transcobalamins I and III, predominantly transcobalamin III.

D. IRON STUDIES:

Iron studies are important in diagnosing polycythemia vera. Often, the expansion of the red blood cell mass results in a depletion of iron stores. The Prussian blue stain of the marrow aspirate shows a reduction in reticuloendothelial iron in virtually all cases. A fall in the serum iron and serum ferritin levels to iron-deficient values can occur, as most often seen in women. Significant iron deficiency will restrict expansion of the red blood cell mass and lower the hemoglobin level. From a diagnostic viewpoint, this must be kept in mind. Polycythemia vera patients can present with a relatively normal to slightly elevated hemoglobin/hematocrit but significant microcytosis, a mean cell volume less than 75 fL. The drive to form microcytic red blood cells is another indicator of uncontrolled red blood cell proliferation.

E. Challenges in Diagnosis:

Diagnosis of polycythemia vera can be a greater challenge in patients who present with a **moderate increase in hemoglobin/hematocrit without other clinical criteria.** In this situation, other causes of secondary polycythemia must be excluded using an array of laboratory and radiologic studies. Even with the most careful workup, the condition in some patients will still go undiagnosed. An **assay of stem cell growth patterns** to identify erythropoietin independent/endogenous erythroid colony (BFU-E) growth can be used to distinguish polycythemia vera patients from those with a familial form of polycythemia.

Secondary Erythrocytosis

An increase in the red blood cell mass without evidence of changes in other hematopoietic cell lines is a normal physiologic response to hypoxia, regardless of cause. It can also result from an increased production of erythropoietin by a diseased kidney or an extrarenal tumor.

A. Hypoxic Polycythemia:

Individuals who live at high altitude exhibit an increase in their hemoglobin/hematocrit (see Figure 12–1). Up to altitudes of 7000 feet, the increase in red blood cell mass is physiologically effective and not associated with any clinical abnormalities. At higher altitudes, humans are at risk for both acute and chronic mountain sickness. With rapid ascents, mountain climbers can acutely experience severe headaches, nausea, vomiting, and disorientation secondary to cerebral edema. This is secondary to hyperventilation, producing a respiratory alkalosis, and can be largely prevented by the use of acetazolamide, dexamethasone, or both. Individuals who attempt to live at altitudes of 9000–15,000 feet experience chronic mountain sickness. These individuals demonstrate much higher hemoglobin/hematocrit levels, chronic tissue hypoxia, especially during sleep, and significant problems maintaining nutrition and cardiopulmonary compensation.

Significant cardiopulmonary disease can also result in sufficient tissue hypoxia to induce a hypoxic polycythemia. The most dramatic example of this is in patients with congenital heart disease and cyanosis secondary to a major right to left shunt. These individuals can exhibit hemoglobin levels in excess of 22 grams per deciliter (hematocrit > 75%). Although such patients have very high whole blood viscosities, they appear to have surprisingly few problems with thrombosis or abnormal bleeding. Attempts to therapeutically reduce the hematocrit may be required if patients develop heart failure. Otherwise, patients may feel worse when their hemoglobin/hematocrit is lowered.

Pulmonary disease can also result in a hypoxic polycythemia. The most common clinical scenario is the very obese individual who develops **mechanical hypoventilation (Pickwickian syndrome).** The evaluation of these patients must recognize the intermittent nature of the hypoventilation. A full sleep study may be necessary to document the extent of the patient's arterial desaturation. Most patients with **chronic obstructive pulmonary disease or interstitial lung disease** do not develop a significant erythrocytosis, which reflects not only the severity of their desaturation but also marrow inhibiting effects of their illness.

A rare form of hypoxia-related polycythemia has been described in the Chuvash population of Russia. It presents early in life with a marked increase in the hemoglobin level (20–24 grams per deciliter) and frequent thrombotic and hemorrhagic complications. Chuvash polycythemia appears to represent a congenital defect in the O_2 sensing or angiotensin pathway. Unlike polycythemia vera, erythropoietin levels are generally increased.

B. High-Affinity Hemoglobinopathies:

Patients can develop erythrocytosis secondary to abnormalities in hemoglobin-oxygen binding. Most demonstrate an increase in hemoglobin-oxygen affinity owing to a mutational defect in globin structure or an abnormality in 2,3-DPG production or binding. More than 50 variants have now been described. They are recognized from their **lower than normal P_{50}** (normal P_{50} 526 mm Hg). Once the P_{50} falls much below 20 mm Hg, patients exhibit a significant increase in their red blood cell mass and hemoglobin levels (see Figure 12–3). **Patients with unstable hemoglobins** may also present with a normal hemoglobin level or mild hemolytic anemia, despite an oxygen-binding defect (see Chapter 7). A rare cause of secondary polycythemia is deficiency of 2,3-DPG secondary to an inherited defect in the DPG mutase gene localized to chromosome 7. An assay of DPG mutase will confirm the diagnosis. All patients with increased affinity hemoglobins appear well oxygenated, since their hemoglobin is fully saturated with oxygen. In contrast, **patients with methemoglobinemia, sulfhemoglobinemia, and hemoglobin M disease** (a group of mutant disorders where heme is stabilized in the ferric state) can present with a striking cyanosis owing to reduced hemoglobin-oxygen binding.

C. Methemoglobinemia:

Hemoglobin is at constant risk for oxidation of its heme iron from the reduced ferrous to the ferric state to form methemoglobin. The normal methemoglobin reductase system helps maintain hemoglobin in its reduced state (see Chapter 1). Presence of ferric heme increases the oxygen affinity of ferrous heme, thereby shifting the oxygen dissociation curve to the left, resulting in a compensatory polycythemia.

There are three forms of hereditary methemoglobinemia—hemoglobin M disease, NADH-cytochrome b5 reductase deficiency, and cytochrome b5 deficiency. **Hemoglobin M** is a mutant hemoglobin (usually a His to Tyr substitution in the heme pocket) that is incapable of reversibly binding oxygen. These patients present with asymptomatic cyanosis and, in some cases, a mild hemolytic anemia. Two clinical phenotypes of **NADH-cytochrome b5 reductase deficiency** have been characterized: Type I, where the defect is restricted to erythroid cells; and Type II, where several tissues are involved. The Type I defect is associated with mild cyanosis, whereas Type II disease manifests severe cyanosis, mental retardation, and a progressive encephalopathy.

Symptomatic methemoglobinemia can be seen in otherwise normal individuals who are exposed to strong oxidants in dyes, drugs (Table 12–3), solvents, and fertilizers, as well as in patients with congenital, heterozygous b5 reductase deficiency. Once the methemoglobin level exceeds 10–20%, the patient appears visibly cyanotic and complains of symptoms such as headache, dyspnea, and dizziness. On measurement of the patient's blood gas, arterial blood will appear brownish in color and will not turn red when exposed to oxygen. Oxygen saturation will be reduced while the P_AO_2 **(oxygen tension)** is normal. Exposure to sulfa drugs, acetophenetidin (Phenacetin), and acetylanilid can result in irreversible production of sulfhemoglobin and similar symptoms once levels exceed 30–40%.

Congenital methemoglobinemia can be treated by activating the NADPH-dependent reductase pathway with either ascorbic acid, 300-600 mg/day in 3–4 divided doses or oral methylene blue, 60 mg 3–4 times a day. **Secondary symptomatic methemoglobinemia** is best treated with intravenous methylene blue, 1 mg/kg given over 5 minutes, and then repeated at 1 hour and every 4–6 hours, to a maximum dose of 7 mg/kg.

Table 12–3. Drugs that cause methemoglobinemia.

Analgesics (acetanilid, acetaminophen, phenacetin)
Cardiovascular drugs (nitrates, nitroprusside)
Local anesthetics (benzocaine, lidocaine, etc)
Antibiotics (sulfonamides)

D. Increased Erythropoietin Production:

Renal disease and several erythropoietin-secreting tumors have been associated with secondary polycythemia. Hydronephrosis, polycystic renal disease, renal cysts, and both benign and malignant renal tumors can result in increased production of erythropoietin. Uterine myomas, hepatomas, and cerebellar hemangiomas have also been shown to secrete erythropoietin. Renal patients can develop erythrocytosis post-transplant that is unrelated to erythropoietin production. A role for angiotensin II as a red cell growth promoter has been postulated in this situation, based on the observation that angiotensin-converting enzyme inhibitors will reverse the erythrocytosis.

Surreptitious **use of recombinant erythropoietin by high-performance athletes** can also result in a hematocrit/hemoglobin in the polycythemia range. Measurements of serum erythropoietin levels in any of these patients may show a high normal to elevated value, certainly greater than would be expected if the patient had polycythemia vera. In patients with erythropoietin-secreting tumors, the normal erythropoietin response to anemia may be suppressed (Figure 12–4). This situation is reminiscent of the adrenal suppression observed in patients with steroid-excreting adrenal adenomas. However, definitive diagnosis of a specific tumor or renal disease requires a careful search using appropriate radiologic and laboratory measurements. Any patient who is considered at risk for a non-hypoxic, secondary polycythemia should have an intravenous pyelogram, CT scans of head and abdomen, and both renal and liver function tests.

E. Erythropoietin Receptor Mutations:

An acquired or congenital mutation of the erythropoietin receptor gene can lead to truncation of the cytoplasmic portion of the receptor and a failure to shut off signal transduction following erythropoietin binding. This has the same end result as abnormally high erythropoietin production.

Relative Polycythemia

Moderate elevations of hemoglobin level (16–18 grams per deciliter in men or 14–16 grams per deciliter in women) may be caused by a decrease in plasma volume without a true increase in red blood cell mass. **Acute elevations of hemoglobin/hematocrit** are observed in patients with severe dehydration secondary to salt and water deprivation, diarrhea, excessive vomiting, or all of these. Overly aggressive use of diuretics can also be responsible. A sudden change in vascular permeability secondary to an allergic reaction can dramatically reduce the plasma volume even to the point of increasing hemoglobin to above 20 grams per deciliter, which should be clinically obvious. Patients experiencing **allergic or anaphylactic reactions** exhibit some combination of hives, bronchial spasm, angioneurotic edema, and orthostatic hypotension.

An elevated hemoglobin level may also be seen in **patients with Cushing's disease or pheochromocytoma.** With these conditions, the reduction in plasma volume appears to relate to a hormonally driven increase in vascular tone together with a reduction in the plasma volume. There is no true increase in the red blood cell mass. A similar mechanism has been postulated as the explanation for a condition referred to as "**stress" polycythemia.** This is recognized clinically as an elevation of the hemoglobin level in young to middle-aged males who smoke, are hypertensives, and live a high-pressure lifestyle. Smoking may be the most important factor in causing stress polycythemia. Patients who smoke a pack or more of cigarettes per day will have carboxyhemoglobin levels of 10% or higher. However, increased vascular tone and a reduction in plasma volume can also play a role. Stress polycythemia patients can show symptoms and signs related to increased blood viscosity and decreased brain blood flow. Even without a true increase in red blood cell volume, these patients have been shown to have reduced brain blood flows when their hemoglobins are above 17 grams per deciliter.

THERAPY

Effective management of the patient with polycythemia requires an accurate diagnosis. Although it makes sense to lower the hemoglobin level in patients with polycythemia vera or stress polycythemia, the increase in red blood cell mass in patients with hypoxic polycythemia is usually to the patient's physiologic advantage. In these settings, there has to be a very good reason to go against nature. Several side issues also require attention. Iron balance must be carefully assessed and appropriately managed. In patients with polycythemia vera, problems such as severe itching, erythromelalgia, thrombotic and bleeding complications, and symptomatic splenomegaly must be addressed.

Polycythemia Vera

The mainstay of effective treatment of the polycythemia vera patient is the rapid and sustained reduction of the red blood cell mass. Aggressive phlebotomy is still the best way to achieve this reduction.

A. PHLEBOTOMY THERAPY:

When a polycythemia vera patient is very symptomatic, phlebotomy should be performed daily or every other day, removing 200–500 mL each time, depending on the patient's hemodynamic status. When a patient is unable to tolerate a large-volume phlebotomy but needs a rapid reduction in hemoglobin level, a partial exchange transfusion can be performed by removing whole blood and reinfusing saline or a smaller volume of albumin or plasma. This procedure is most effective if the patient needs to be prepared for emergency surgery.

Although phlebotomy will acutely lower the hemoglobin level, sustained reductions in red blood cell mass require that iron stores be exhausted. Otherwise, new red blood cell production will return the hemoglobin level to its original high level within a short period. Therefore, **phlebotomies must be continued until iron stores are exhausted** and the patient demonstrates a low serum iron and serum ferritin typical of iron-deficient erythropoiesis. A reduction in iron supply will suppress erythroid progenitor proliferation and limit new hemoglobin production. Of course, the drive to make new red blood cells can be so great that the patient's red blood cells will rapidly become microcytic and hypochromic, even while the hemoglobin is above 14–15 grams per deciliter.

Success of long-term phlebotomy therapy will depend on **management of the patient's iron balance.** The amount of iron ingested by the patient will determine the need for periodic phlebotomies. Patients must be educated regarding food and medicinal iron intake. Certainly, any iron supplement must be avoided because it will stimulate a rapid rise in the hemoglobin level. There are also downsides to being chronically iron deficient. Patients may complain of sore mouths, difficulty swallowing, spooning and splitting of the nails, a general loss of energy, and, at times, difficulty sleeping (see Chapter 5). This condition requires very careful treatment. Severely iron-deficient patients should be given one to two tablets of an oral iron preparation daily for 1 or 2 weeks at a time. This regimen can alleviate the symptoms of tissue iron deficiency without stimulating a major increase in the red blood cell mass. The patient must be monitored, however, and phlebotomized if the hemoglobin level rises.

B. CHEMO/RADIOTHERAPY:

Phlebotomy therapy alone may not be appropriate for all patients. Elderly individuals who cannot tolerate phlebotomy because of their cardiopulmonary status, symptoms associated with iron deficiency, or simply the logistics involved in monitoring therapy, are potential candidates for **radiotherapy.** Radioactive phosphorus (^{32}P) can be given as an intravenous bolus in a dose of 2–3 mCi/m^2 to a maximum dose of 5 mCi. Disease control is attained in up to 80% of patients with a single treatment, although some patients may need a retreatment after 3–6 months. The downside of ^{32}P therapy is the **potential for marrow damage.** A few patients will, unfortunately, trade their polycythemia for a transfusion-dependent anemia or pancytopenia.

Chemotherapy is an effective alternative to both phlebotomy and radiotherapy. It is preferred for patients who have very high platelet or granulocyte counts. Platelet counts in excess of 1 million/μL are associated with a higher incidence of both bleeding and thrombotic complications. This condition can be worsened by phlebotomy therapy, since iron deficiency will cause the platelet count to rise further and will increase red blood cell rigidity.

Of the possible **myelosuppressive drugs,** hydroxyurea has performed best in clinical trials. Other drugs including chlorambucil and busulfan, when given over a long period, are associated with an increased incidence of leukemia and pulmonary fibrosis.

1. Hydroxyurea—Most patients treated with hydroxyurea can be effectively controlled with a dose of 500–2000 mg (one to four tablets), given daily. Continuous, uninterrupted therapy is required. Hydroxyurea inhibits the synthesis of DNA and produces megaloblastic, ineffective hematopoiesis. It does not, however, decrease the number of stem cells capable of cell production. Therefore, even a short break in therapy can result in an immediate production of all cell types.

Other **problems associated with hydroxyurea therapy** include gastrointestinal intolerance, stomatitis, hepatitis, rash, fever on occasion, and variable cytopenias. In some patients, anemia or leukopenia can set a limit to therapy despite a continued increase in the production of the other cell lines. The long-term management of hydroxyurea therapy, like phlebotomy therapy, is extremely demanding. Patients must be followed up closely to guarantee compliance with the drug dosage and to monitor the CBC.

2. Interferon-α—Interferon-α has also been shown to be effective in treatment of polycythemia vera. Compared with other therapies, it avoids hematologic complications associated with aggressive phlebotomy or hydroxyurea therapy, and it may delay the development of myelofibrosis if used early in the course of the disease. It also has proved of value in patients with pruritus. This may reflect a better control of megakaryocyte proliferation and platelet production by interferon. Beginning with a dose of 1 million units three times a week, the dose is gradually escalated to 3–5 million units three times a week. In some patients, periodic phlebotomy may still be needed if the dose tolerated by the patient does not give hematocrit control.

C. MANAGEMENT OF OTHER COMPLICATIONS:

Patients with polycythemia vera may report marked **pruritus** that is generalized but not associated with any specific skin lesion. This condition may correlate with a proliferation of mast cells and basophils or a release of prostaglandins and serotonin from platelets. Treatment of this condition can be a challenge. Antihistamines (diphenhydramine or hydroxyzine) may be effective when the condition is mild. When the condition is severe, however, the patient will need combined therapy aimed at both histamine and serotonin blockade with drugs such as doxepin, trifluoperazine, cyproheptadine, and cimetidine. If the pruritus appears to get worse with phlebotomy therapy, a short course of iron therapy may provide some relief. Interferon therapy may offer better control of pruritus in intractable patients.

A few patients with polycythemia vera will complain of **erythromelalgia,** characterized by patchy, localized areas of burning pain and erythema of the skin. This condition is thought to be related to the platelet abnormality. Vascular injury with infarction, gangrene, or skin ulceration may be seen in severe cases. Treatment involves the use of hydroxyurea to lower the platelet count, platelet inhibitors such as aspirin, and vasodilator drugs.

Thrombocytosis and platelet dysfunction can result in both bleeding and thrombotic complications. The higher the platelet count, the more likely there will be a hemostatic defect. The most effective treatment is a sustained reduction in the platelet count using hydroxyurea or anagrelide. If the platelet count cannot be controlled, an antiplatelet agent such as aspirin or ticlopidine may be tried in patients with evidence of thrombotic disease. On the other hand, these agents should not be used in individuals who have a platelet function defect producing a prolonged bleeding time or bleeding tendency.

Gouty arthritis is seen in up to 10% of patients with polycythemia vera. Acute attacks should be managed similarly to primary gout with colchicine and phenylbutazone. Patients with very high uric acid levels who are at risk for recurrent episodes should be maintained on a dose of 300 mg of allopurinol per day.

D. CLINICAL COURSE:

Although polycythemia vera can appear at any age, most patients present during their sixth or seventh decade. Often, the patient presents because of a transient ischemic attack or thrombotic stroke. Median survival for this group of patients is approximately 10 years. **Cause of death** is thrombosis, acute leukemia, myelofibrosis with pancytopenia, or a complication of the illness such as hemorrhage, acute infection, or drug toxicity. When followed over 5–10 years, 30% or more of patients will die of a thrombotic complication, most often a coronary or cerebral artery occlusion. Another 30% will die of cancer, with half of these developing myelofibrosis and acute leukemia. The incidence of acute leukemia is fourfold higher in patients who receive ^{32}P therapy or chemotherapy with the alkylating agent chlorambucil. It is most often an acute myeloid leukemia, which is resistant to antileukemic chemotherapy.

Patients who develop myelofibrosis go through a period where phlebotomy therapy is no longer necessary and then proceed to develop increasing splenomegaly and varying combinations of anemia, leukopenia, and thrombocytopenia. Blood film and marrow findings are similar to those of patients with idiopathic myelofibrosis and include aniso- and poikilocytosis, teardrops, and nucleated red blood cells. The marrow shows progressive fibrosis with increased reticulin and collagen.

Secondary Erythrocytosis

Management of patients with secondary polycythemias will vary according to the specific cause. **Patients with mild hypoxic polycythemia** should be left alone. The rise in the red blood cell mass helps compensate for their hypoxia despite the increase in viscosity. **Patients who present with an erythropoietin-producing tumor** should be treated for the tumor. In the case of the occasional **patient with a hemoglobinopathy associated with a very high hemoglobin level,** phlebotomy may be indicated, but only for patients who have hemoglobins in excess of 22 grams per deciliter.

Stress Polycythemia

Patients with stress polycythemia can show an impressive reduction in brain blood flow that is easily treated by phlebotomy. In most cases, removal of 300–500 mL of blood weekly for 3–6 weeks will be sufficient to lower the hemoglobin level to normal. This treatment will improve brain blood flow and will usually decrease complaints such as headache and generalized fatigue by the patient. Phlebotomy to the point of iron deficiency is unnecessary, whereas smoking cessation is recommended.

BIBLIOGRAPHY

Polycythemia Vera

Asimakopoulos FA et al: Deletions of chromosome 20q and the pathogenesis of myeloproliferative disorders. Br J Haematol 1996;95:219.

Fruchtman SM et al: From efficacy to safety: A Polycythemia Study Group report on hydroxyurea in patients with polycythemia vera. Semin Hematol 1997;34:17.

Landaw SA: Acute leukemia in polycythemia vera. Semin Hematol 1986;23:156.

Marchioli R, for Gruppo Italiano Studio Policitemia: Polycythemia vera: The natural history of 1213 patients followed 20 years. Ann Intern Med 1995;123:656.

Muller EW et al: Long-term treatment with interferon-alpha 2b for severe pruritus in patients with polycythemia vera. Br J Haematol 1995;89:313.

Najean Y, Rain JD: Treatment of polycythemia vera: Use of ^{32}P alone or in combination with maintenance therapy using hydroxyurea in 461 patients greater than 65 years of age. The French Polycythemia Study Group. Blood 1997;89:2319.

Najean Y, Rain JD: The very long-term evolution of polycythemia vera: An analysis of 318 patients initially treated by phlebotomy or ^{32}P between 1969 and 1981. Semin Hematol 1997;34:6.

Silver RT: Interferon alfa: Effects of long-term treatment for polycythemia vera. Semin Hematol 1997;34:40.

Tartarsky I, Sharon R: Management of polycythemia with hydroxyurea. Semin Hematol 1997;34:24.

Wasserman LR, Berk PD, Berlin NA: *Polycythemia Vera and the Myeloproliferative Disorders.* WB Saunders, 1995.

Secondary Erythrocytosis

Brown MM, Wade JPH, Marshall J: Fundamental importance of arterial oxygen content in the regulation of cerebral blood flow in man. Brain 1985;108:81.

Gregg XT, Prchal JT: Erythropoietin receptor mutations and human disease. Semin Hematol 1997;34:70.

Perloff JK et al: Adults with cyanotic congenital heart disease: Hematologic management. Ann Intern Med 1989;109:406.

Porphyrias

The **porphyrias** are caused by inherited defects in the heme biosynthetic pathway that result in excess production of porphyrin precursors. Depending on the type of excess porphyrin produced, patients can experience severe photosensitivity, nerve damage, liver disease, and anemia. Detection requires a high level of suspicion and skill in using the laboratory. Accurate diagnosis is important because there are now effective therapies for several of these defects.

NORMAL PORPHYRIN SYNTHESIS

The normal heme biosynthetic pathway is shown in Figure 13–1. The initial step, condensation of glycine and succinyl-CoA to form δ-**aminolevulinic acid** (δ-**ALA**), is catalyzed by a mitochondrial enzyme, ALA synthase. This is the only enzyme step that requires a cofactor, in this case, pyridoxal-5-phosphate (vitamin B_6).

The next several steps, including formation of porphobilinogen, uroporphyrinogen III, and coproporphyrinogen III, are catalyzed by cytosolic enzymes. The final three steps in the sequence depend on mitochondrial enzymes (coproporphyrinogen oxidase, protoporphyrinogen oxidase, and ferrochelatase). Chelation of iron to protoporphyrin IX depends on an adequate supply of iron; deficient patients accumulate excess protoporphyrin in their red blood cells.

Porphyrin synthesis is regulated by the activity of ALA synthase and the end product, heme. Levels of transcription and translation of ALA synthase in mitochondria are a function of the heme concentration. This is especially true for liver porphyrin synthesis where any reduction in free heme owing to inhibition of heme synthesis or accelerated heme breakdown induces a major increase in hepatic ALA synthase. Defects in any one of the intermediate enzymes in the heme biosynthetic pathway also result in an excess production of porphyrin precursors proximal to the enzyme defect, even while heme synthesis is maintained.

CLINICAL FEATURES

The most prominent clinical findings associated with excess production of porphyrin precursors are cutaneous photosensitivity and nervous system dysfunction. Patients with **porphyria cutanea tarda** (**PCT**) generally present with photosensitivity problems, including appearance of vesiculo/bullous eruptions on the face and hands; white, plaquelike scar formation; hyperpigmentation; and excess hair formation over the face. Symptoms and signs of liver disease and excessive iron loading are also common. **Erythropoietic protoporphyria** (**EPP**) patients experience variable photosensitivity beginning in childhood, characterized by marked itching, burning, erythema, and angioneurotic edemalike swelling of exposed skin areas. Unlike PCT, vesicle formation is uncommon and scarring and hirsutism are not seen. Neuropathic presentations are more typical of patients with **acute intermittent porphyria** (**AIP**), **variegate porphyria** (**VP**), **hereditary coproporphyria** (**HCP**), and **lead poisoning.** Acute intermittent porphyria patients present with recurrent bouts of severe, poorly localized abdominal pain, peripheral and cranial motor neuropathies, seizures, and psychotic episodes. Photosensitivity is not seen with AIP, but does occur in VP and HCP patients.

Laboratory Studies

Measurements of **porphyrin precursors** in urine and stool provide the key to diagnosis. **Other laboratory studies** of importance in the evaluation of a porphyria patient include the routine complete blood count (CBC); serum iron, total iron-binding capacity (TIBC), and ferritin levels; and liver function studies. In patients with neurologic damage, **electroencephalography and electromyography studies** can be important.

Accumulation and excretion of porphyrin precursors in red blood cells, urine, and feces for the various disease states are summarized in Table 13–1. **Screening for excess porphyrin excretion** is best carried out when the patient is symptomatic. This situation is especially true for measurements of δ-ALA and porphobilinogen in patients with AIP, HCP, and VP. Porphyrin excretion is highest when the patient is experiencing a neurologic crisis, especially an attack of abdominal pain. Protoporphyrin measurements in patients with EPP and lead poisoning are easily carried out using a

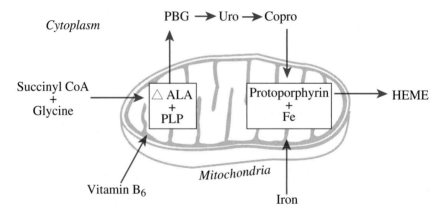

$$PBG \longrightarrow Uro \longrightarrow Copro$$

Cytoplasm

Succinyl CoA
+
Glycine

$\triangle$ ALA
+
PLP

Protoporphyrin
+
Fe

HEME

Mitochondria

Vitamin B_6

Iron

Figure 13–1. **The normal heme biosynthetic pathway.** The first step in the synthesis of heme is the condensation of glycine and succinyl-CoA with pyridoxal 5-phosphate as the coenzyme to form δ-aminolevulinic acid (δ-ALA). This process is carried out in mitochondria catalyzed by the enzyme ALA synthase. The subsequent formation of porphobilinogen, uroporphyrinogen III, and coproporphyrinogen III occurs in the cell cytoplasm. The final steps of protoporphyrin production and the assembly of protoporphyrin IX and iron to form heme depend on mitochondrial enzymes.

standard red blood cell protoporphyrin assay. Detection of elevated porphyrin levels in patients with VP requires a **stool assay.**

The **CBC can be abnormal** in patients with EPP and lead poisoning. Mild hemolysis and a tendency to hypochromia have been observed. Lead poisoning is associated with prominent stippling of red blood cells on the peripheral blood film and the appearance of ringed sideroblasts in the marrow. **Measurements of serum iron, TIBC, and serum ferritin levels** are essential in patients being evaluated for PCT. Excessive liver iron loading leading to cirrhosis is a prominent manifestation of this disease. When iron studies are equivocal, **liver biopsy** may be needed to fully evaluate the sever-

ity of the cirrhosis and the accumulation of iron in hepatocytes.

DIAGNOSIS

Differential diagnosis of porphyria is not difficult once the possibility of its existence is considered. Only five major, inherited forms of porphyria plus lead poisoning need to be differentiated (Figure 13–2). Two of these (PCT and EPP) typically present with **photosensitivity problems,** whereas the others (AIP, HCP, VP, and lead poisoning) present with **neurologic abnormalities.** The specific diagnosis of the individual type of porphyria is usually obvious from the clinical presentation

Table 13–1. Patterns of porphyrin excretion.

	ΔALA/PBG	URO	COPRO	PROTO
Acute intermittent porphyria	↑↑/↑↑	↑	NL	NL
Porphyria cutanea tarda	NL	↑↑	↑	NL
Hereditary coproporphyria	↑/↑	±	↑	NL
Variegate porphyria	↑/↑	↑a	↑a	↑a
Erythropoietic protoporphyria	NL	NL	NL	↑↑b
Lead poisoning	↑/NL	NL	↑↑	↑b

a Excretion predominantly in stool.

b Levels increased in red blood cells.

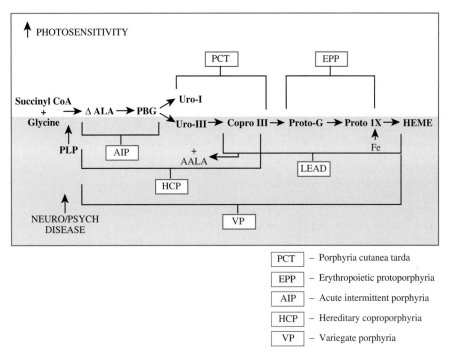

Figure 13–2. Differential diagnosis of the porphyrias and lead poisoning. PCT and EPP present with symptoms and signs of increased photosensitivity. In both situations, excess porphyrins produced include the uro-, copro-, and protoporphyrins. These are highly fluorescent molecules that are found both in red blood cells and in urine and stool. In contrast, AIP, HCP, VP, and lead poisoning present with symptoms and signs of neurologic dysfunction, especially recurrent episodes of abdominal pain and both cranial and motor nerve dysfunction. The common factor in these conditions is the excretion of excess amounts of δ-ALA and porphobilinogen. Those conditions (HCP and VP) where there is also excretion of uro-, copro-, and protoporphyrins show a mixed picture of neurologic dysfunction and photosensitivity.

and routine studies of porphyrin excretion. Actual assay for the enzyme defect is unnecessary.

Porphyria Cutanea Tarda (PCT)

PCT results from a deficiency of hepatic uroporphyrinogen decarboxylase enzyme (URO-D). It is the most common of the porphyrias and can either be inherited as an autosomal dominant trait or occur sporadically in association with hepatitis C virus (HCV) infection or chemical exposure.

The URO-D gene has been located at p34 on chromosome 1. **Familial PCT** results from stable point mutations of the URO-D gene and is transmitted as an autosomal dominant. While URO-D levels are half-normal in all tissues, porphyrins only accumulate in the liver. **Sporadic PCT,** which may or may not have a genetic component and accounts for two-thirds of cases, is associated with HCV infection, excess alcohol intake,

and exposure to estrogens. From 60% to 90% of sporadic PCT cases are anti-HCV positive, and most of these have HCV mRNA in serum by polymerase chain reaction, indicating an active infection. The concentration of URO-D in the liver of sporadic PCT patients is normal despite reductions in enzyme activity, suggesting the presence of a liver-specific inhibitor.

The characteristic clinical feature of PCT is the marked **photosensitivity** with the appearance of vesiculo/bullous eruptions of the face and hands, hyperpigmentation, and excessive hair growth on the face. Some patients develop marked thickening and scarring of the skin reminiscent of scleroderma. Most PCT patients also show **manifestations of liver disease.** In some cases, the appearance of jaundice and mild to moderately advanced cirrhosis can be the event that brings the patient to medical attention. **Excess tissue iron loading** with elevation of the serum iron and serum ferritin levels can also be the first clue to the diagnosis. All patients with PCT should have a full evaluation of liver function including iron studies, and should be considered for a liver biopsy to document both the severity of hepatocellular damage and the level of iron loading of hepatocytes. Excessive iron loading may reflect the simultaneous inheritance of the gene for hemachromatosis; more than 50% of PCT patients are either homozygous or heterozygous for the gene (Cys²⁸²Tyr). The most severe liver dysfunction is seen in patients with a combination of HCV infection, iron loading, and excessive alcohol ingestion, greater than 70 grams per day.

A study of **porphyrin precursor excretion in urine** confirms the diagnosis. PCT patients show an excessive excretion of uroporphyrinogens I and III and to a lesser extent coproporphyrinogen; δ-ALA and porphobilinogen levels are never increased.

Erythropoietic Protoporphyria (EPP)

EPP patients present during childhood with complaints of **itching, burning, and angioneurotic edemalike swelling of skin that occurs almost immediately with sunlight exposure.** Unlike PCT patients, EPP patients tend not to have vesiculo/bullous eruptions or skin scarring. In addition, EPP patients are not at risk for liver disease, iron loading, or neurologic dysfunction.

EPP results from the autosomal dominant inheritance of a deficiency in the ferrochelatase (heme synthetase) enzyme. This inhibits the final step in heme production and results in an accumulation of protoporphyrin in marrow erythroid precursors and adult red blood cells. It does not result, however, in a significant anemia, although red blood cells may be slightly microcytic and hypochromic. A measurement of **red blood cell protoporphyrin levels or demonstration of marked fluorescence of marrow precursors** can be used to confirm the diagnosis of EPP.

Acute Intermittent Porphyria (AIP)

AIP is caused by the autosomal dominant inheritance of a deficiency in porphobilinogen deaminase. It is a relatively common form of porphyria and classically presents with recurrent episodes of poorly defined, **diffuse abdominal pain.** The severity of the presentation can, unfortunately, lead to an unrevealing exploratory laparotomy before the diagnosis is made. Other **neurologic abnormalities** include proximal motor neuropathies with axonal degeneration and loss of reflexes, cranial nerve damage (most often cranial nerves VII and X), bulbar paralysis, and seizures. Acute psychosis during exacerbations of the illness is also seen. **Rarer**

manifestations of AIP include cardiac arrhythmias, inappropriate antidiuretic hormone (ADH) secretion with hyponatremia, and chronic hypertension.

AIP is rarely seen before puberty and tends to be more common in women. This situation may relate to the **tendency for hormones and drugs to induce acute exacerbations of the disease.** Both birth control pills that contain high levels of progesterone and pregnancy are known to induce AIP attacks. Several drugs, including barbiturates, sulfonamide antibiotics, anticonvulsants, and alcohol, also increase the production of δ-ALA and porphobilinogen. Finally, a sudden decrease in caloric intake with dieting or illness can precipitate an attack.

Laboratory diagnosis of AIP is straightforward. A urine sample should be obtained while the patient is symptomatic, especially during an attack of acute abdominal pain, to screen for δ-ALA and porphobilinogen. The excretion of both products should be markedly increased. Screening between attacks is not as reliable, even though most AIP patients do have at least some elevation of both products at all times. Attempts to increase excretion by starvation or drug administration are not advised.

Variegate Porphyria (VP)

VP is caused by an inherited deficiency in protoporphyrinogen oxidase, which is a much less common form of porphyria, being most prevalent in Finnish and South African populations. It can present with **neurologic abnormalities** similar to those of AIP or **skin manifestations** more typical of PCT. In both cases, the disease tends to be milder. An occasional patient can present with **abdominal pain attacks** as severe as those seen in AIP patients, however.

Laboratory diagnosis of VP requires assay of porphyrin precursors in stool. Protoporphyrin and coproporphyrinogen levels are increased at all times; δ-ALA, porphobilinogen, and uroporphyrinogen levels are increased during attacks of abdominal pain. Assays of porphyrin precursors in urine are inadequate to make the diagnosis.

Hereditary Coproporphyria (HCP)

HCP is caused by an inherited defect in coproporphyrinogen oxidase. It is a very uncommon form of porphyria but presents with **symptoms and signs similar to a mild AIP.** Some patients also complain of mild photosensitivity. Diagnosis is confirmed by demonstrating very **high levels of coproporphyrinogen III in urine, as well as δ-ALA and porphobilinogen** during attacks of abdominal pain.

Lead Poisoning

Lead-poisoned patients can present with symptoms and signs that mimic the neurologic abnormalities seen with AIP. Attacks of **severe, diffuse abdominal pain with episodes of paralytic ileus** are the most common manifestation of acute lead intoxication. **Motor neuropathies and central nervous system damage** are also observed. In contrast to AIP, patients with severe lead toxicity usually are anemic. This fact reflects the greater effect of lead on the erythroid precursor heme biosynthetic pathway.

Lead poisoning should always be **suspected in all children or any adult whose occupation puts him or her at risk.** Tests of urinary porphyrins will demonstrate excess excretion of δ-ALA without a comparable increase in porphobilinogen. Coproporphyrin III levels are also increased, not because of a specific toxic effect of lead on the coproporphyrinogen oxidase enzyme but, perhaps, because of induction of an alternate metabolic pathway of coproporphyrin production. With **chronic lead toxicity,** the routine CBC will show mild hemolysis and a tendency to a normocytic, hypochromic anemia. The red blood cell protoporphyrin level is elevated (usually more than 250 μg/dL), and red blood cell stippling should be obvious on blood films prepared from fresh, finger-stick blood. EDTA anticoagulated blood films should not be used, since EDTA makes the stippling disappear. Finally, the **severely lead poisoned patient** can develop a ringed sideroblastic anemia (see Chapter 9). Blood or urine lead levels or both can be used to confirm the diagnosis and provide a measure of the severity of exposure.

THERAPY

There are effective treatments for the major forms of porphyria, including AIP, PCT, and EPP, as well as for lead poisoning. Effective management of infected patients also involves educating the patient regarding risk factors that can increase the severity of the disease process.

PCT

PCT patients with cirrhosis and iron-loading should be **aggressively phlebotomized** to deplete their excess tissue iron. Generally, the magnitude of the iron overload is less than that seen in idiopathic hemachromatosis and removal of 500 mL of blood every 1–2 weeks for 6 months is usually sufficient. Patients should also be advised to **avoid alcohol.** These two precautions can prevent further hepatocellular damage and result in a decrease in the light sensitivity. In some patients, even the cutaneous thickening and scarring will appear to improve.

Treatment with low-dose **chloroquine** (125 mg twice weekly) has also been recommended for treatment of PCT. The mechanism of action is unclear, however. Chloroquine that is concentrated in the liver may complex with the porphyrin or stimulate an increased release from hepatocytes or both. **Interferon therapy** may play a role in patients with active HCV infections. Early case reports have suggested that the level of porphyrin excretion and the progression of the liver disease can be reduced.

AIP

Effective management of patients with AIP requires **close attention to factors that can precipitate attacks or worsen an ongoing attack.** Drugs and hormones that lead to increased production of δ-ALA and porphobilinogen must be avoided. Most narcotics are safe for pain control, and both chlorpromazine and diazepam (Valium) are appropriate to control nausea and vomiting. Since fasting worsens an AIP attack, patients should receive a **high-carbohydrate diet:** at least 300 grams of carbohydrate per day either enterally or parenterally.

Since heme will downregulate δ-ALA and porphobilinogen synthesis, patients can be effectively treated with **intravenous infusions of hematin** given in a dose of 1–4 mg/kg intravenously once or twice daily. Hematin will significantly decrease ALA and porphobilinogen production. The onset of action is somewhat slower than glucose loading, and a full clinical response may not be seen for 48–72 hours. Hematin is primarily indicated for treatment of severe neurologic diseases or major abdominal pain attack. Excessive doses of hematin can cause renal tubular damage.

EPP

Children with relatively mild EPP can be managed by **protecting them from direct sunlight.** β-Carotene given in doses of 120–180 mg per day in adults can help. **Cholestyramine** may be used to interrupt the enterohepatic circulation of protoporphyrin. For patients who have relatively severe hemolysis, **splenectomy** will help decrease the level of red blood cell and protoporphyrin production.

Lead Poisoning

Symptomatic lead poisoning in adults is associated with whole blood lead levels of 80–100 μg/dL or higher. Children are much more sensitive to lead poisoning and can present with more subtle signs of central nervous system damage, including **speech and language deficits and both behavioral and learning problems.** These can be seen when the whole blood level is 50 µg/dL or less. Therefore, aggressiveness of treatment should be based on the patient's age, clinical signs, and symptoms of intoxication.

Obviously, the first and most important step in treating lead poisoning is to **identify and eradicate exposure.** The next step is to use **chelating agents** to mobilize lead from bone and encourage excretion into urine. The principal agents available include edetate calcium disodium, penicillamine, and dimercaprol. Acutely ill patients should receive a 5-day course of 12–24 mg/kg of dimercaprol per day and 0.5–1.5 g/m^2 of edetate calcium disodium per day. After a pause of 2–3 days, this regimen can be repeated until the patient is asymptomatic and demonstrates a blood lead level of less than 40 µg/dL. Penicillamine given in a dose of 20–40 mg/kg but not more than 1 gram per day can be given over several months to further deplete the bone lead pool.

BIBLIOGRAPHY

Beutler E et al: *Hematology,* 6th ed. McGraw-Hill, 2001.

Bulaj ZJ et al: Hemochromatosis genes and other factors contributing to the pathogenesis of porphyria cutanea tarda. Blood 2000;95:1565.

Cribier B et al: Porphyria cutanea tarda and hepatitis C viral infection: A clinical and virologic study. Arch Dermatol 1995; 131:801.

Fauci AS et al: *Harrison's Principles of Internal Medicine,* 14th ed. McGraw-Hill, 1998.

Kushner JP: Laboratory diagnosis of the porphyrias. N Engl J Med 1991;324:1432.

McManus JF et al: Five new mutations in the uroporphyrinogen decarboxylase gene identified in families with cutaneous porphyria. Blood 1996;88:3589.

Mustajoki P: Variegate porphyria. Q J Med 1980;194:191.

Roberts AG et al: Increased frequency of the haemachromatosis Cys[282]Tyr mutation in sporadic porphyria cutanea tarda. Lancet 1997;349:321.

Hemachromatosis

Excessive iron loading of tissues (**hemachromatosis**) can result from a primary genetic defect or as a complication of liver disease and certain anemias. Genetic predisposition to excess iron absorption (**hereditary hemochromatosis**) is transmitted as an autosomal recessive trait in Caucasian populations. Approximately 1 in 10 individuals of Celtic or European stock is a carrier of the trait, whereas 1 of 300 is homozygous. This situation can set the stage for excessive iron uptake in several clinical situations. In addition, patients with liver disease and pancreatic dysfunction can demonstrate significant iron loading, leading to tissue damage. Certain erythropoietic disorders are also characterized by an excessive level of iron uptake even in the absence of a primary genetic defect.

NORMAL IRON BALANCE

The major pathways of iron metabolism are described more extensively in Chapter 5. Most of the body's iron is incorporated in hemoglobin, myoglobin, and iron-containing enzymes (see Table 5–1). The amount of iron bound to transferrin is only 3 mg. Reticuloendothelial iron stores vary according to the patient's sex and diet. Adult males have up to 1000 mg of reticuloendothelial iron stores, whereas children and menstruating females rarely have more than 200 mg.

Iron Storage, Transport and Absorption

Iron is stored intracellularly as ferritin and hemosiderin. **Ferritin synthesis is regulated** according to iron availability by a system of cytoplasmic binding proteins (IRP-1 and -2) and a noncoding iron regulatory element on mRNA (IRE). With iron deficiency, the binding of IRP to the mRNA IRE inhibits the translation of isoferritins. When abundant, iron blocks binding and promotes an increased synthesis of ferritin. In the absence of organ damage, primarily liver damage, serum ferritin is in equilibrium with tissue stores, and can be used, therefore, as an indirect indicator of total body iron stores.

Mucosal cells of the small intestine play a key role in maintaining iron balance. **Iron transport** involves several pathways (Figure 14–1). Heme iron appears to enter mucosal cells directly, where it is metabolized to release ferric iron, while mucin-bound iron binds to β_3-integrin in the membrane, which is then internalized and complexed with mobilferrin to form a ferrous iron compound referred to as **paraferritin.** Another duodenal iron transporter, **DMT1** (also called DCT1 or Nramp2), is responsible for uptake of ferrous iron from the intestinal lumen. Iron can accumulate in the mucosal cell as ferritin or be transported into the plasma. **Hephaestin,** a ceruloplasmin homolog, and plasma ceruloplasmin appear to be involved in transport of iron across the basolateral membrane as well as its oxidation to form ferric iron for binding with transferrin. A second complementary basolateral transporter, **ferroportin 1/Ireg/MTP1,** has recently been identified. Finally, **HFE protein** somehow acts as an overall regulator of mucosal cell iron transport.

The **efficiency of iron transport varies** according to type of iron ingested and body needs. **Mucosal cells regulate iron absorption** according to the level of iron stores. As reticuloendothelial stores expand, iron absorption decreases; as stores shrink, absorption increases. In a normal adult male, where iron losses per day are usually less than 1 mg and stores approach 1000 mg, only a small portion of available dietary iron is absorbed. In contrast, a menstruating female needs to absorb up to 4 mg per day to compensate for menstrual losses. Absorption can increase to levels of 40–60 mg per day in the patient with severe iron deficiency anemia who is receiving maximum oral iron therapy. The level of erythropoiesis also affects absorption. For example, patients with thalassemia who have high levels of ineffective erythropoiesis consistently show increased iron absorption.

Dietary Content of Iron

Dietary content of iron is also an important variable in determining the level of iron absorption and stores in humans. In Western cultures, most available iron comes from meats and meat by-products; much less comes from vegetable sources. Moreover, unlike developing countries, very little iron is incorporated in the diet from cooking in iron utensils or contamination by dirt. Thus, the content of iron in the Western diet is

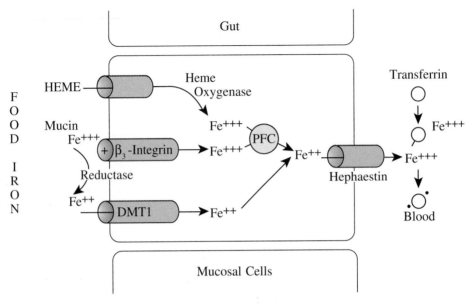

Figure 14–1. **Iron absorption.** Food iron is absorbed by any one of three pathways. Heme iron is transported directly into intestinal mucosal cells, where it is metabolized, releasing ferric iron. Free ferric iron is brought into solution at an acid pH, bound to mucin, and then picked up and transported complexed to β_3-integrin. Membrane ferric reductase also generates ferrous iron, which is then transported by the DMT1 pathway. Intracellular ferric iron is held in a paraferritin complex (PFC) until released for transport as ferrous iron across the basolateral membrane. This is facilitated by Hephaestin (a ceruloplasmin homolog) and plasma ceruloplasmin and appears to be somehow regulated by HFE protein.

relatively low, only 6 mg per 1000 kilocalories, providing the adult male with between 15 and 20 mg of iron per day, but only 8–15 mg per day to the adult female. This situation puts the adult female at a considerable disadvantage and helps explain the absence of significant reticuloendothelial iron stores in menstruating women. Childbearing presents an additional challenge and almost certainly produces iron deficiency unless iron supplements are provided.

HFE Gene & Control of Iron Transport

A single gene (HFE), localized to chromosome 6, is responsible for control of iron transport by mucosal cells and uptake by various tissues. It encodes an atypical major histocompatibility complex class I–like protein (HFE) that binds to β_2-microglobulin and then interacts with transferrin receptors to control iron turnover. The mechanism by which this protein product regulates both iron absorption and iron delivery is still unknown. However, inherited point mutations of the HFE gene (**hereditary hemachromatosis**) are associated with both an increased level of iron absorption and excessive accumulation of iron in vital organs. Mu-

cosal cells of hemochromatosis patients appear to have an increase in ferroportin1, producing a reduction in intracellular ferritin levels and an increase in DMT1 activity.

CLINICAL FEATURES

Symptoms and signs of iron overload reflect the sensitivity of the liver, pancreas, anterior pituitary, joints, and heart to iron toxicity. The original description of hereditary hemachromatosis used the term "bronze diabetes" to highlight the **darkening of the skin** and the appearance of **insulin-dependent diabetes** as two prominent characteristics of iron overload. As listed in Table 14–1, **cirrhosis, gonadal failure, arthritis, and cardiac failure** are also prominent findings. Contrary to past teachings, the clinical expression of the disease is similar for men and women, despite a proposed protective effect of menstrual iron losses. The mean age of presentation (48–50 years) is the same, and the iron load is only slightly less (a mean of 5.5 grams for women versus 8.6 grams for men). Postmenopausal women have the same level of iron loading as men.

The pattern of clinical disease tends to correlate with

Table 14–1. Clinical findings in hemachromatosis.

Arthralgia/small and large joint arthritis	Cardiac failure/arrhythmias
Gonadal failure	Diabetes
Testicular atrophy/impotence	Cirrhosis
	Abdominal pain
Amenorrhea	
Skin pigmentation	

the level of iron accumulation. Patients with hereditary hemachromatosis are usually asymptomatic until 7 grams or more of excess iron has accumulated. The **first symptoms and signs** are **asthenia (unexplained chronic fatigue)**, arthralgia, loss of libido, impotence (or amenorrhea), and a subtle change in skin color secondary to an increase in melanin pigment. **Clinical findings associated with liver, pancreas, and heart damage** tend to occur with iron accumulations of 10–15 grams or more. Women present with complaints of fatigue, arthritis, and increasing pigmentation. Men are more likely to present with signs of diabetes and liver damage.

Arthropathy of Iron Overload

The arthropathy of iron overload is generally not severe when it first appears and is often confused with rheumatoid or osteoarthritis since it involves multiple joints, including small joints of the hands and feet, and several large joints, including the knees, hips, and shoulders. Although joint x-rays are initially normal, with progression, films of the hands show osteopenia, cartilage loss (usually most pronounced in the second and third metacarpal phalangeal joints), cyst formation in metacarpal heads and, on occasion, the development of osteophytes. When large joint arthritis is pronounced, x-rays show chondrocalcinosis with linear and punctate calcification of the lateral meniscus. Large joints can also show cartilage loss, a narrowing of the joint space, and cystic erosions leading to a severe destructive arthritis.

It is important to **consider iron overload in the differential diagnosis of early arthritis.** Studies of large groups of patients presenting with hereditary hemachromatosis have shown a delay of 4–10 years between the patient's first arthritic complaints and the correct diagnosis. Even longer delays to diagnosis have been reported in patients who do not go on to develop other organ damage.

Gonadal Failure & Amenorrhea

Another early manifestation of iron overload is gonadal failure owing primarily to iron loading of the anterior pituitary. Male patients may experience a loss of libido progressing to impotence with testicular atrophy, whereas women will complain of amenorrhea, secondary to iron deposition in the anterior pituitary gland.

Heart Disease

Heart disease, presenting as either congestive heart failure or a cardiac arrhythmia, can be an early manifestation of iron overload. **Congestive failure** is usually biventricular in nature but may resemble constrictive pericarditis with jugular venous distention, hepatomegaly, and ascites. Patients may also present with **atrial fibrillation, a supraventricular tachycardia,** or a **conduction defect.**

Diabetes & Hepatic Cirrhosis

When there is a delay in diagnosis, most patients develop symptoms and signs of both diabetes and hepatic cirrhosis. The **diabetes** is caused by iron deposition in the beta cells of the pancreas and islet cell dysfunction. Insulin resistance is observed and patients usually require insulin therapy. The earliest manifestation of **liver toxicity** is enlargement and tenderness of the liver. Iron tends to concentrate in the parenchymal cells in the periportal areas of the liver. With time, these cells are destroyed and replaced by fibrous tissue, which is accompanied by elevations in the serum levels of alanine aminotransferase and aspartate aminotransferase and later serum bilirubin. One-third or more of patients with iron overload–induced cirrhosis will develop **hepatocellular carcinoma (hepatoma).** This condition occurs late in the disease and is not prevented by iron removal. The clinical appearance of hepatoma is signaled by weight loss, fever, worsening liver function, and right upper quadrant pain.

Hemachromatosis Versus Unusual Presentations

Hemachromatosis often appears in the differential diagnosis of systemic illness not only because the constellation of symptoms and signs involves several organs but also because of several unusual presentations. Excessive iron loading has been associated with **coronary artery disease** and **acute myocardial infarction** in patients at a relatively young age. This does not seem to relate to a concomitant lipidopathy; iron overload may be an independent risk factor. **Right upper quadrant abdominal pain** prior to development of cirrhosis has been reported as a presenting complaint. Although it may mimic acute cholecystitis, it is not associated with an unusual tendency to gallstone formation. **Skin pigmentation secondary to increased melanin forma-**

tion and iron deposition in the skin is another interesting component of the disease. In those patients who develop severe pituitary failure, skin pigmentation may be accompanied by a thinning and wrinkling of the skin that suggests Addison's disease.

Susceptibility to Infections

Hemachromatosis patients also appear to have a greater susceptibility to infections with organisms such as *Listeria, Yersinia,* and *Vibrio vulnificus.* This may reflect an increased growth potential of these organisms in patients with higher than normal serum iron (SI) levels or represent a side effect of iron overload on leukocyte and reticuloendothelial cell phagocytic and lytic activities. Hemochromatotic patients receiving iron chelating therapy have also been reported to be more susceptible to *Escherichia coli* and *Staphylococcus aureus* septicemia. Again, the explanation for this susceptibility is unclear.

Laboratory Studies

The SI, total iron-binding capacity (TIBC), and serum ferritin levels are the mainstays in the laboratory diagnosis of iron overload (Table 14–2). Other important studies in the differential diagnosis and in the evaluation of organ toxicity include bone marrow aspirate, liver biopsy, and the detection of a defective HFE gene.

A. SERUM IRON/FERRITIN STUDIES:

The **normal SI** ranges from 50 to 150 μg/dL with a percent saturation of the TIBC of less than 45%. Patients who are homozygous for hereditary hemochromatosis typically show an increase in the percent saturation to greater than 45% very early in their disease process, which reflects the failure in the regulation of iron transport from the reticuloendothelial cell to transferrin. Children and women may not demonstrate a higher than normal saturation, however, because of the depletion of their iron stores. In addition, any inflammatory disease can still block the delivery of iron from the reticuloendothelial cell and thereby reduce the percent saturation to below 45%.

Although the SI provides information as to the flow of iron to tissues, the **serum ferritin level** is the best indirect measure of total body iron stores. With some exceptions, the serum ferritin correlates well enough that it can be used to estimate total body iron load (Figure 14–2). Each microgram per liter of serum ferritin equates to approximately 10 mg of iron stores. Thus, a normal adult male with a serum ferritin of 100 μg/L generally has 1000 mg of iron stores. **Hereditary homozygous hemachromatosis patients with organ damage** will usually have serum ferritin levels in excess of 1000–2000 μg/L, representing an iron load of greater than 10–20 grams. The correlation of the ferritin level fails once the iron load exceeds 30–40 grams because of an upper limit of inducible isoferritin production. Serum ferritins above 4000 μg/L indicate a release of intracellular hepatic ferritin stores. Very high levels of serum ferritin are seen in patients with **acute hepatic necrosis** where large amounts of intracellular ferritin are released into circulation.

Modest elevations of serum ferritin to 150–300 μg/L are typically seen in patients with **acute and chronic inflammatory states, liver disease, and certain tumors.** Patients with **aplastic anemia or ineffective erythropoiesis** (thalassemia major, megaloblastic and dysplastic anemias) exhibit both high SI levels with elevated percent saturations and high ferritins. In the case of ineffective erythropoiesis, this reflects an increase in iron absorption as well as the increased red cell turnover. Repeated transfusion will also elevate the serum ferritin level; each unit of red blood cells contributes 200 mg of iron to stores.

Table 14–2. Body iron balance.

| | Normal Males | Iron Overload States | |
		Hematopoietic Disease	Hemochromatosis
Erythron iron (mg)	2400	< 2000	2400
Serum iron	Normal	Increased	Increased
Transferrin saturation (%)	< 50	> 50	> 50
Reticuloendothelial stores	3+	> 4+	3+
Serum ferritin (μg/L)	100	> 500	> 1000
Liver iron	Normal	Increased iron in Kupffer cells and hepatocytes	Increased iron in hepatocytes only

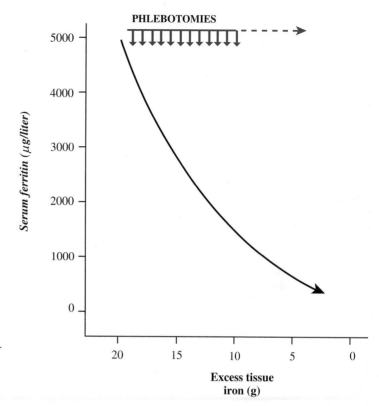

PHLEBOTOMIES

Figure 14–2. Serum ferritin levels and body iron content. The serum ferritin level provides an indirect measure of the total amount of iron in tissues. As a patient with hemachromatosis is phlebotomized, the fall in serum ferritin can be used to estimate the progress in iron unloading.

B. Marrow Iron Studies:

A marrow aspirate or biopsy stained with Prussian blue provides information regarding both the level of reticuloendothelial iron stores and the incorporation of iron into hemoglobin. **Patients with iron overload secondary to a hematopoietic disorder or repeated blood transfusion** typically show a marked increase in marrow iron stores. In fact, the amount of iron in each cell increases to where it obscures normal cell landmarks. In contrast, patients with **hereditary hemachromatosis** show relatively normal amounts of reticuloendothelial cell iron.

A careful **inspection of marrow erythroid precursors** is also important. Patients with defects in globin production (the thalassemias) or mitochondrial function (the sideroblastic anemias) show excessive accumulation of iron in the cytoplasm of basophilic, polychromatophilic, and orthochromatic normoblasts. In thalassemia, excess iron tends to be distributed throughout the cell cytoplasm. Sideroblastic anemias are characterized by precursors with a ring or collar of large iron granules just around the nucleus. These "ringed sideroblasts" are the result of actual iron deposition in the perinuclear mitochondria.

C. Liver Biopsy:

Tissue iron loading and cirrhotic changes can be assessed by liver biopsy. Using the Prussian blue stain, it is possible to characterize the distribution of iron in hepatocytes and Kupffer cells. Patients with **hereditary hemachromatosis** show iron deposits in hepatocytes and bile duct epithelium with lesser amounts in Kupffer cells. Hepatocytes in the periportal area are the most heavily involved. **Fibrosis progressing to cirrhosis** will generally reflect the amount of excess total body iron and the duration of the illness. **Organ damage** can be correlated with a quantitative analysis of iron concentration per gram dry weight liver tissue. Normal individuals have hepatic iron concentrations of 1–2 mg/gram dry weight tissue, whereas hemachromatosis heterozygotes have concentrations of 3–7 mg/gram. Liver damage begins once the iron load exceeds 7 mg/gram and advances rapidly once the concentration exceeds 15 mg/gram. This correlates with total body iron loads of 10–20 grams.

Patients with **iron overload secondary to hematopoietic disorders, excessive transfusion, or alcohol-induced increased absorption** tend to show a greater deposition of iron in Kupffer cells with less involvement of the hepatocytes. Moreover, excessively transfused patients will not develop cirrhosis until iron loads are far greater than 20–30 grams. This situation would appear to reflect the fact that the normal monocyte-macrophage system is able to trap the most of the excess iron and prevent hepatocyte loading.

Patients with **certain hematopoietic disorders** such as thalassemia can show hepatocyte damage at a relatively early age. Because of their high levels of ineffective erythropoiesis, these patients usually demonstrate high SI levels and transferrin saturations of greater than 60% beginning early in childhood. This opens the pathway for parenchymal cell loading despite a normally functioning monocyte-macrophage cell system.

D. OTHER DIAGNOSTIC TESTS:

Patients with marked iron deposition in the liver can be detected by CT scan or MRI. In the latter case, there is a marked attenuation of the T2 signal producing a black image. As a supplement to the SI and serum ferritin levels in screening for iron overload, urinary excretion of iron after an injection of an iron chelator (deferoxamine) is sensitive to both reticuloendothelial cell and tissue iron loading. A dose of 10 mg/kg of deferoxamine is given by subcutaneous injection, and urine is collected for 24 hours to measure total iron content.

E. GENETIC TESTING:

Missense mutations of the HFE gene on chromosome 6 are responsible for 60–100% of the cases of hemochromatosis worldwide (85% of cases in the United States). The HFE gene is closely linked to the HLA-A and -B loci. On average, 73% of patients with the disease will be HLA-A3. HLA-A11, -B7, and -B14 have also been associated with the disease. However, the gold standard test for the diagnosis of hereditary hemochromatosis is the **direct detection of the defective HFE gene.** More than 80% of symptomatic patients are now thought to be homozygous for the single point mutation, $Cys^{282}Tyr$ (C282Y), whereas another 3–5% are compound heterozygotes, $Cys^{282}Tyr/His^{63}Asp$ (C282Y/H63D). Homozygous H63D patients exhibit significant iron overload but usually do not develop the full clinical picture of hemachromatosis. A third mutation, designated S65C, has now been identified. In combination with C282Y (C282Y/S65C compound heterozygotes), it has been associated with mild hemachromatosis. Additional mutations are anticipated, since 10–30% of patients, depending on the population studied, lack any of these mutations.

DIAGNOSIS

Diagnosis and differential diagnosis of an iron overload state is relatively easy (Tables 14–2 and 14–3). Screening tests used to detect the overload state effectively exclude the rare patient with a hereditary absence of transferrin. Hematopoietic disorders are apparent from the patient's past medical history and routine blood count. Severe tissue iron overload is **associated with the more severe anemias,** such as heavily transfused marrow damage, aplastic or dysplastic anemias, and congenital defects in globin production (the thalassemias). Moreover, it is the patients with β-thalassemia major who are at highest risk for tissue iron loading. These individuals are always identified soon after birth, so that the iron-loading manifestation of their disease is anticipated as a part of the treatment of their hematologic disease.

Anemias

Patients with **acquired, dysplastic anemias** present later in life; more than 80% are diagnosed after age 60. Their tendency to iron loading varies and depends on both their transfusion requirement and the nature and duration of their disease. Patients with **ringed sideroblastic anemias** have the highest propensity to tissue iron loading. This correlates primarily with their level of ineffective erythropoiesis and the number of transfusions, although some patients may also be HFE heterozygotes. Whether this increases their tendency to iron loading is unclear. **Sideroblastic anemia** patients are usually recognized from the inspection of the Prussian blue stain of a marrow aspirate. The presence of ringed sideroblasts, ineffective erythropoiesis, and high SI and serum ferritin levels are clear indicators of a propensity for tissue iron loading. A history of **transfusion dependence,** a transfusion requirement of 2–3

Table 14–3. Classification of iron overload states.

Hematopoietic disorders	South African (Bantu) hemochromatosis
Thalassemias	Hereditary atransferrinemia
Sideroblastic anemias	**Secondary iron overload**
Dysplastic/megaloblastic anemias	Transfusion hemosiderosis
Inherited defects in absorption	Porphyria cutanea tarda
Hereditary hemochromatosis	Alcoholic cirrhosis

units of red blood cells each month for a year or more, will predictably result in iron overload. Since each unit contains 200–250 mg of iron, the patient will receive 6–10 grams of iron each year.

HFE Mutations & Routine Screening

In light of the frequency of HFE mutations in Caucasian populations, adult patients should be routinely screened for laboratory evidence of iron loading. A **rise in the percent saturation of transferrin** to a level greater than 45% has been recommended as the most reliable indicator of iron overload, with a sensitivity, specificity, and positive predictive value for the homozygous C282Y mutation of 94%, 94%, and 16%, respectively. The **serum ferritin level** may be more sensitive but is also less specific; several disease states, including liver disease and inflammatory disorders, can result in serum ferritin elevations. **Quantitative analysis of hepatic iron content** is also a sensitive test but, because of the frequency of iron loading with other types of liver disease, has a lower specificity.

Genotypic Analysis

Genotypic analysis is **not recommended for population screening.** While it is highly specific for the diagnosis of hemochromatosis, carriers of the defect do not appear to be at risk. Many homozygotes never develop iron overload, some because of iron loss due to menses or multiple pregnancies and others for reasons that are not clear. In at least one population study of unrelated blood donors, only 50% of individuals homozygous for the C282Y mutation showed clinical features of hemochromatosis. **C282Y heterozygotes who present with clinical disease** should be studied for other diseases that lead to iron loading (iron-loading anemias, excessive alcohol ingestion, porphyria cutanea tarda, etc) and other mutations. The most common double mutation is the C282Y/H63D compound heterozygote. However, other mutations (IVS3+1G-T, I105T, and S65C) may be associated with mild to severe iron loading.

Genetic testing can be used to rapidly confirm the diagnosis of hemachromatosis; results in better than 95% of patients who present with clinical disease will be positive. It replaces liver biopsy unless, because of elevated liver chemistries, there is a need to evaluate the patient for cirrhosis. Genotyping also replaces HLA testing in pedigree studies. It is the most cost-effective approach to detecting family members with clinical disease and can be of value in family planning. Since the prevalence of the HFE gene is so high in the general population, the probability of one heterozygote marrying another heterozygote approaches 10%. However,

genetic testing should only be undertaken with consent of the patient and individual family members after counseling. Moreover, the cost as well as potential implications of a positive finding on insurability are potential reasons to restrict genetic testing to patients and family members with phenotypic disease.

Iron Overload in Blacks

Iron overload in African Americans and sub-Saharan Africans is **not the same as hereditary hemachromatosis in white populations.** It is not associated with C282Y gene mutation. Rather, several factors may play a role, including a high incidence of hepatitis, ingestion of alcoholic beverages containing large amounts of iron, and a second iron-loading gene that is not the same as the hemachromatosis HFE gene defect. Furthermore, the pattern of iron deposition in the liver is different. Both hepatocytes and Kuppfer cells show excess iron accumulations in blacks in contrast to the restriction of iron loading to the hepatocyes in hereditary hemochromatosis.

The **onset of clinical disease can be subtle** in blacks, so the level of clinical suspicion must be especially high. Evaluation of suspected iron overload in black patients should include not only serum ferritin and transferrin saturation measurements, but also a liver biopsy. The range of percent saturations can be lower than that seen in whites, falling below 50%, even with significant iron overload. While testing for the C282Y mutation is appropriate to exclude the HFE mutation, a normal test should not deter a full evaluation, including liver biopsy.

New Phenotypes

Several new phenotypes not linked to the HFE gene have now been described. One of these, called **juvenile hemachromatosis,** appears to be related to a mutation on chromosome 1. Patients present in the second or third decade with cardiac complications, endocrine failure, or both. An inherited "**non–HFE-related hemochromatosis**" has also been described in several Italian families and appears to result from a mutation of the gene that regulates transferrin receptor. Another new genetic disorder, **hereditary hyperferritinemia-cataract syndrome,** has recently been described. Involved family members present with ferritin levels of 500–1000 μg/L or higher and congenital nuclear cataracts. The underlying mechanism is an increased synthesis of serum L-ferritin secondary to a mutation of the L-ferritin IRE on chromosome 19. **Other rare abnormalities of iron metabolism** include hereditary aceruloplasminemia secondary to a mutation of the ceruloplasmin gene on chromosome 3, and "dysmetabolic hepatosiderosis," a syndrome characterized by mild to moderate iron excess in patients with insulin-resistant diabetes. In both cases, serum ferritin levels are elevated but the percent saturations of transferrin are normal. Aceruloplasminemia is also associated with dementia, ataxia, and extrapyramidal signs and is readily diagnosed by demonstration of an undetectable serum ceruloplasmin level.

Other High-Risk Conditions

Patients with **alcoholic liver disease, cirrhosis with portacaval shunt, porphyria cutanea tarda, and aplastic anemia** are also at risk for iron loading and tissue toxicity even without a genetic abnormality. Usually the etiologic relationship of the disease state to the iron loading is clear. However, some patients with end-stage liver disease and a strong alcoholic history may represent a diagnostic dilemma as to whether the iron loading or the alcohol damage came first. Genetic testing can be very valuable in this situation.

THERAPY

Effective treatment of iron overload requires **early detection** and **aggressive iron unloading.** A high SI with greater than 50% saturation of the TIBC or a serum ferritin level greater than 500 μg/L must not be ignored, even when it is discovered in an otherwise healthy patient. Moreover, the fact that the patient is young or female should not be used as an excuse to delay the diagnostic workup. With the definition of the **HLA-H gene,** it is now easy to screen family members of the patient with hereditary hemachromatosis. Homozygous Cys^{282}Tyr family members must be followed up closely with serial SI, TIBC, and ferritin levels, and phlebotomy therapy initiated at the earliest sign of iron loading. Heterozygotes are at very low risk for clinically significant iron overload, unless they also have a condition such as alcoholic cirrhosis, porphyria cutanea tarda, or an iron-loading anemia. Approximately 20% of male and 8% of female heterozygotes will have serum ferritin levels above the 95th percentile for normals.

The first rule of good management is to **aggressively treat any patient with iron overload.** The hereditary hemachromatosis patient with a ferritin level in excess of 1000 μg/L (10 grams or more of excess body iron) deserves maximum therapy. When the iron loading is even greater and organ damage, especially cardiac and liver disease, is present, as much iron as possible should be removed in the shortest possible time. Otherwise, the organ damage will put the patient at risk of death from heart failure, a cardiac arrhythmia, or irreversible liver damage.

Effects of Iron Removal

Rapid removal of iron can **reverse organ damage.** Cardiac arrhythmias and heart failure respond early in the course of treatment. Improvement in liver function can also be seen, even though liver fibrosis and cirrhosis will not significantly reverse and patients will still exhibit complications of their cirrhosis. Moreover, hemachromatosis patients are at increased risk for the development of a primary hepatic malignancy and one-third of patients will go on to die of a hepatoma. This is true even for patients who have been well treated and had their excess iron removed by either phlebotomy or chelation therapy.

Iron removal has **less of an effect on the other manifestations of the disease.** Islet cell function is not restored, even though the patient's insulin-dependent diabetes may be somewhat easier to control. The gonadal failure caused by iron loading of the anterior pituitary is generally irreversible, and patients may require hormonal replacement. The patient's arthropathy may actually worsen during therapy and any joint destruction will be irreversible. Finally, the darkening of skin color will gradually lessen over several years.

Choice of Therapy

The therapeutic approach to hemachromatosis is influenced by the cause of the iron loading, the age of the patient, and the amount of the iron load. The two mainstay treatments are **phlebotomy** and the administration of **deferoxamine.** Whenever possible, phlebotomy therapy is preferred, especially in patients with hereditary hemachromatosis. Obviously, in order to be able to remove iron by repeated bleeding, the patient must have a normal functioning marrow. In patients with thalassemia or a ringed sideroblastic anemia, the primary defect in red blood cell production rules against this approach. In this situation, **chelation therapy** is the only alternative.

Monitoring of Iron Intake

Attention must also be paid to the patient's iron intake. Medicinal iron, including the ingestion of iron as a part of an over-the-counter vitamin preparation or dietary supplement, must be avoided. Patients should be counseled and given a list of approved vitamin preparations. Dietary restriction is less of an issue. Although many vegetables are high in iron content, the bioavailability of this iron is low. Most absorbable iron in Western diets comes from meats and meat by-products. Beer and wines do not contain excess iron. Even the most severe hereditary hemachromatotic patients will only absorb 2–5 mg of iron per day or 500–1500 mg per year on a normal diet. Therefore, once their iron load has been reduced, these patients will require only 2–6 phlebotomies per year to prevent excess iron reaccumulation.

Phlebotomy Therapy

The quickest and least complicated way of removing iron is phlebotomy. In a patient with a hematocrit of between 35% and 45%, the removal of 500 mL of whole blood will remove approximately 200 mg of iron. If the patient is estimated to have 10 grams of excess body iron, 50 or more phlebotomies will need to be performed. To achieve this goal, phlebotomies must be scheduled at least once or twice each week. This rate of blood loss may not be tolerated at the beginning of therapy, especially when the patient is older or of small body size. In this situation, 200–300 mL of blood should be initially removed until the patient develops a tolerance for the procedure. Less-frequent phlebotomies can be scheduled in patients with smaller iron loads: a serum ferritin level less than 1000 µg/L. However, reducing the rate of phlebotomy in hemachromatosis patients with organ damage is poor management.

A. Measurement of the Amount of Iron Removed:

The amount of iron removed can be estimated from the number of phlebotomies. For every five phlebotomies, approximately 1 gram of excess iron will be removed. The serum ferritin level can also be used to monitor the effectiveness of therapy (see Figure 14–2). At the beginning, the serum ferritin level may fluctuate and even appear to increase. However, as stores fall to 10 grams or less, it generally provides a good measure of total body iron. The SI and percent saturation of TIBC can be used as end points to indicate a successful iron unloading. Patients with homozygous hemachromatosis generally show little change in these measurements until their iron load is nearly depleted.

The challenge comes when patients are nearly depleted of their excess iron. At this point, they should be more closely monitored with measurements of CBC, SI, and serum ferritin levels. The **ideal end point** is a serum ferritin less than 50–100 µg/L and a normal SI (less than 50% saturation of the TIBC) in a patient who is not anemic or microcytic. Overly aggressive phlebotomy can easily induce a microcytic, hypochromic anemia secondary to iron deficiency, whereas too little will allow the SI to remain high, with a greater than 50% saturation of the TIBC.

Hemachromatosis patients may show **fluctuating measurements of the serum ferritin level and SI** near the end of unloading therapy. This situation reflects a problem with mobilization of some of the excess iron, so the phlebotomies get ahead of the rate of release. In this circumstance, the frequency of phlebotomy should

be reduced to allow time for iron to mobilize from tissues. The other challenging problem is the propensity of hemachromatosis patients to **increase their SI levels to greater than 50% saturation of their TIBC** even with small accumulations of excess iron. In these patients, serum ferritin levels will need to be reduced to below 40–50 µg/L to keep the SI level within the normal range, even at the risk of a slight anemia. In an occasional patient who does not follow the predicted response, a repeated liver biopsy can help document the effectiveness of therapy.

B. Patient Compliance:

Although there are few complications with phlebotomy therapy, patient compliance can be an issue. Patients will need to be encouraged to **keep up with the phlebotomy schedule.** They should also **maintain a diet with adequate protein** to support albumin production, and should receive a **folic acid supplement.** Once the excess iron load has been removed, it is possible to prevent reaccumulation with a low-iron diet. It is usually more convenient, however, to simply have the patient receive phlebotomy four times a year.

C. Treatment of Porphyria Cutanea Tarda:

Phlebotomy therapy also works very well in treating porphyria cutanea tarda. Usually, the iron load is considerably less and a series of weekly or every-other-week phlebotomies over 4–6 months will result in a significant clinical improvement both in terms of the skin disease and liver chemistries. It is important, however, to be sure that the patient does not have hereditary hemachromatosis, where the iron load is much greater. Therefore, these patients should also be closely monitored with repeated SI, serum ferritin levels, and repeated liver biopsies to document improvement.

Iron Chelation Therapy

Excess body iron can also be removed with chelation therapy. Deferoxamine (DF) is currently the only approved, effective iron chelator for clinical use. The disadvantages of DF are its high cost and the need for parenteral administration. However, oral iron chelators are under development and in the future could offer a much better therapeutic alternative, especially for preventing iron loading.

A. Deferoxamine (DF):

Although DF has a lower binding affinity for iron than transferrin, it can successfully compete for excess iron stored in tissue cells. When injected subcutaneously or intravenously it is rapidly taken up by the hepatocyte, excreted into bile, and reabsorbed by the intestine. At low doses, most of the iron-laden DF is excreted in urine. At higher doses, it also appears in stool.

Since DF is not absorbed orally and has a very short half-life, effective therapy requires that it be **administered either subcutaneously or intravenously by continuous infusion.** To achieve a level of therapy equivalent to two phlebotomies each week, the patient should receive an infusion of 40–50 mg/kg of DF administered over 10–12 hours each night by continuous infusion pump. The DF can be made up in small enough volume that any of the portable pump technologies can be employed. When subcutaneous therapy is used, the drug can be administered with a small-gauge butterfly needle placed just under the skin.

The **response to DF is just as good as the response to phlebotomy therapy.** It is the mainstay for patients with hematopoietic disorders, especially the children with thalassemia (see Chapter 6). The **problems associated with DF therapy** include maintaining patient compliance and a risk of visual and auditory nerve damage. Patients who receive more than 4 grams or 50 mg/kg/day of DF are at risk for an optic neuropathy characterized by increased retinal pigmentation, central scotoma, and night blindness. Less frequently, patients may develop high-tone deafness. These nerve toxicities appear to be dose-dependent and can improve if the dosage is reduced. Serial auditory and visual measurements should be performed whenever high-dose DF therapy is employed. The only other complication of DF therapy is an increased risk of sepsis from organisms such as *Yersinia* and *S aureus.* Treatment with DF is expensive and, if used, should be administered correctly.

B. ORAL CHELATORS:

Several new oral iron chelators are under development but not yet approved for routine clinical use. The most promising of these are the α-**ketohydroxypyridines,** which have a higher binding affinity for iron than DF and are capable of removing iron from tissue cells and transferrin. They are rapidly absorbed, appearing in blood within minutes, where they are then metabolized to the glucuronide. Over the next 24 hours, the iron-drug glucuronide complex is excreted into the urine.

Clinical trials of the α-ketohydroxypyridine L_1 (**deferipone**) have shown that it can be used to remove excess iron from heavily iron-loaded patients. However, it has not been proved effective in preventing iron loading in transfusion-dependent thalassemic patients when given over several years. Adverse effects include muscle and joint pain with effusions, which disappear when therapy is discontinued. There is also a risk of leukopenia, thrombocytopenia, and aplastic anemia. At the same time, this class of drugs has not been associated with neurotoxicity and does not increase the propensity to infections with *Yersinia* and other bacteria. The latter reflects the fact that, unlike DF, deferipone binds iron so tightly that the organisms cannot use it for growth.

CLINICAL COURSE

Survival of patients with iron overload is clearly improved by early diagnosis and effective phlebotomy or chelation therapy. Five-year survivals in patients with **untreated hereditary hemachromatosis** have been reported to be as low as 15–20%. Aggressively treated patients clearly do better, although the extent of organ damage is a major factor. The cumulative survival rate of **patients without cardiac, pancreas, or liver damage** is the same as that for the general population, whereas **patients with cirrhosis or diabetes** follow the survival rates of patients with these same disorders secondary to other causes.

Patients who are not aggressively treated are at risk of an early death from **cardiac complications.** Cardiac disease is also the major manifestation of iron overload in thalassemic patients. Hereditary hemachromatosis patients are at risk for the development of a **liver neoplasm,** either a primary hepatoma or bile duct carcinoma, and up to one-third will die of hepatic malignancy. This condition is usually in patients who have evidence of cirrhosis, but all patients are at risk and the chance of developing malignancy is not diminished by phlebotomy or chelation therapy.

BIBLIOGRAPHY

Clinical Features

Bulaj ZJ et al: Clinical and biochemical abnormalities in people heterozygous for hemachromatosis. N Engl J Med 1996; 335:1799.

Cazzola M et al: Hereditary hyperferritinemia-cataract syndrome: Relationship between phenotypes and specific mutations in the iron-responsive element of ferritin light-chain mRNA. Blood 1997;90:814.

El-Serag HB, Inadomi JM, Kowdley KV: Screening for hereditary hemochromatosis in siblings and children of affected patients. Ann Intern Med 2000;132:261.

Feder JN et al: A novel MHC class 1-like gene mutated in patients with hereditary hemochromatosis. Nat Genet 1996; 13:399.

Gordeuk V et al: Iron overload in Africa. N Engl J Med 1992;326:95.

Mendler MH et al: Insulin resistance–associated hepatic iron overload. Gastroenterology 1999;117:1155.

Milder MS et al: Idiopathic hemochromatosis, an interim report. Medicine 1980;59:34.

Moirand R et al: Clinical features of genetic hemochromatosis in women compared to men. Ann Intern Med 1997;127:105.

Mura C, Raguenes O, Ferec C: HFE mutations analysis in 711 hemochromatosis probands: Evidence S65C implication in mild forms of hemochromatosis. Blood 1999;93:2502.

Olynk JK et al: A population-based study of the clinical expression of the hemochromatosis gene. N Engl J Med 1999;341:719.

Pietrangelo A et al: Hereditary hemochromatosis in adults without pathogenic mutations in the hemochromatosis gene. N Engl J Med 1999;341:725.

Roy CN, Enns CA: Iron hemostasis: New tales from the crypt. Blood 2000;96:4020.

Smith LH Jr: Overview of hemachromatosis. West J Med 1990;152:296.

Therapy

Barton JC et al: Management of hemochromatosis. Ann Intern Med 1998;129:932.

Brittenham GM: Development of iron-chelating agents for clinical use. Blood 1992;80:569.

Nathan DG: Oral iron chelators. Semin Hematol 1990;27:83.

PART II
White Blood Cell Disorders

Normal Myelopoiesis

Normal myelopoiesis is essential to normal host defense. It involves the regulated production of new myeloid cells, including neutrophilic, eosinophilic, and basophilic granulocytes, as well as monocytes and macrophages. The process is driven by several growth factors that control both the rate of cell production and their subsequent function. Thus, an understanding of normal myelopoiesis requires a knowledge of individual cell characteristics and the expected responses of these cells to disease states.

MYELOID STEM CELLS

The myeloid cells share a common progenitor known as the **colony-forming unit granulocyte–monocyte (CFU-GM)**. This cell arises from earlier progenitors, which are capable of giving rise to myeloid, megakaryocytic, and lymphoid lineages, and ultimately from the multipotent stem cell, which is capable of differentiation into all hematopoietic cell lines (Figure 15–1). The progeny of the CFU-GM are capable of differentiating toward granulocytes or monocytes and macrophages. There is a well-recognized pattern of morphology that can be used to evaluate the later stages of differentiation of the myeloid cell lines (Figure 15–2).

MYELOID GROWTH FACTORS

The several growth factors that are known to influence the differentiation of the CFU-GM are shown in Figure 15–1. These growth factors interact with **progenitor cell transcription factor proteins,** which control the expression of the genes involved in cell differentiation. Thus, in order for a progenitor cell to proceed down a unique pathway of differentiation, it must express one or more transcription factors that, when exposed to a growth factor, activate the family of genes required for that pathway.

The **marrow microenvironment (stromal cells)** also plays an important role in cell differentiation and growth factor response. Current methods of studying the marrow structure are still too crude, however, to clearly identify these interrelationships. Still, similar to the response of erythropoiesis to anemia, there are definable limits to the production of myeloid cells in response to infection. Unlike the situation in the erythroid line in which there is a single predominant growth-regulating hormone, erythropoietin, the myeloid growth factors exhibit more complex interactions that do not lend themselves to the simple concept of a feedback regulatory loop.

Most studies of myeloid growth factors have involved use of single or multiple factors given in soluble form so that progenitor cells are exposed to a uniform concentration of growth factor throughout their environment. It is likely that this is not the physiologic mode of action of these substances. Their **principal functions may be more restricted to the local microenvironment,** interacting primarily on surfaces of cells and seldom being present in soluble form. With development of new **immunoassays to detect low levels of humoral growth factors in plasma,** it is possible to show increased levels of granulocyte colony-stimulating factor (G-CSF), granulocyte macrophage colony-stimulating factor (GM-CSF), and monocyte colony-stimulating factor (M-CSF, or CSF-1) in response to infections and inflammation. Thus, myeloid progenitors are probably responding to fluctuating mixtures of growth factors presented in their microenvironment.

Abnormalities in production and regulation of these growth factors may lead to the development of **myeloproliferative diseases.** In particular, there is a cluster of genes on the long arm of chromosome 5 that includes the genes for GM-CSF, interleukin (IL)-3, M-CSF, the

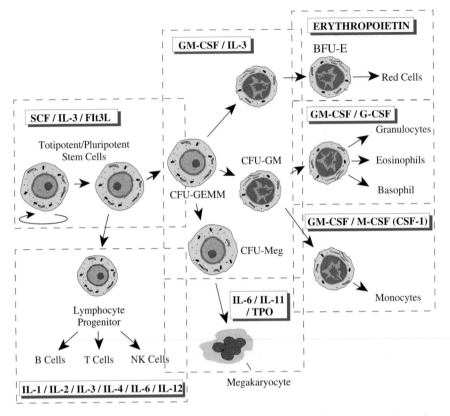

Figure 15–1. **Stem cell differentiation and growth factors.** The central differentiation pathway from totipotent stem cell to committed progenitors is regulated by numerous interleukins and growth factors. With the exception of erythropoietin, none of these factors is entirely specific for a single lineage. They interact with each other and have broad effects at several stages of the differentiation pathways.

receptor for M-CSF (fms), IL-4, IL-5, and others. Deletions in the region (the 5q minus syndrome) are associated with myeloid leukemia (see Chapter 17). Myeloid growth factors also affect the functional activity of mature cells. The **clinical role of growth factors** can be thought of as twofold. In some cases, they stimulate proliferation and increase the numbers of one or more myeloid cells. Alternatively, they can affect the function of the myeloid cells, increasing or decreasing phagocytosis, locomotion, and the ability to kill pathogens.

Granulocyte Macrophage Colony-Stimulating Factor (GM-CSF)

GM-CSF is a 22-kDa molecule that stimulates the production of colonies containing neutrophils, eosinophils, and monocytes. It has a similar effect clinically by causing an increased number of the same cells. It also significantly augments the function of mature neu-

trophils, eosinophils, and monocytes, and appears to be responsible for such systemic effects of inflammation as fever and malaise. It has been shown to be active in mobilizing progenitor cells into the periphery for peripheral blood stem cell harvesting. GM-CSF is produced by several cell types including lymphocytes, myeloid cells themselves, endothelial cells, and fibroblasts. Its production is stimulated by inflammatory cytokines such as IL-1, tumor necrosis factor, and bacterial endotoxin. GM-CSF also may play a role in stimulating megakaryocyte colony formation and, together with erythropoietin, promotes burst forming unit–erythroid growth.

The progenitor receptors for GM-CSF belong to a superfamily of related molecules that includes the receptors for GM-CSF, G-CSF, IL-3, IL-6, and erythropoietin as well as others. In the case of GM-CSF, it is clear that most myeloid cells express the receptor and are capable of binding the molecule, including many

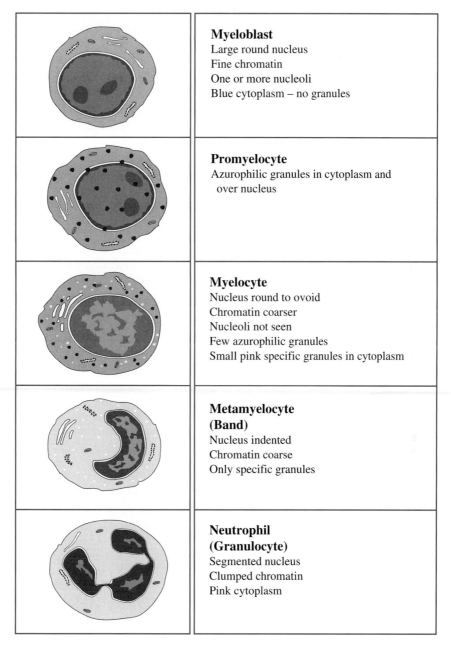

Figure 15–2. The sequence of neutrophil differentiation—morphology. Neutrophils have several stages of differentiation that are easily distinguished by morphology. Changes in staining properties of the granules, the shape of the nucleus, and the chromatin pattern can be used to distinguish each stage, although intermediate stages are commonly seen in normal and abnormal marrow.

myeloid leukemias. A possible autocrine activity of GM-CSF in promoting autonomous growth of leukemic cells has been suggested.

Granulocyte Colony-Stimulating Factor (G-CSF)

G-CSF is a 19- to 20-kDa molecule that, in cell culture systems, stimulates production of granulocyte colonies. It is secreted by a variety of cell types, including endothelial cells and fibroblasts.

Clinically, it promotes the production of granulocytes with fewer systemic effects than GM-CSF. G-CSF also tends to inhibit migration, while strongly activating mature granulocytes. It is widely used in the mobilization of CD34+ stem cells into the circulation for the purposes of transplantation and in promoting more rapid recovery of granulocytes following intensive chemotherapy. When given to normal individuals, G-CSF demonstrates a dose-dependent leukocytosis. A 3- to 4-day course of filgrastim, 6 µg/kg subcutaneously, results in an eightfold increase in the number of circulating granulocytes and monocytes. Long-acting formulations of G-CSF are currently under development; these may prove to simplify dosing and possibly improve efficacy.

Monocyte Colony-Stimulating Factor (M-CSF, or CSF-1)

M-CSF has its primary effect on macrophage colonies. Its clinical activity has not been extensively explored to date. In animal studies it promotes monocytosis and activation of monocytes and macrophages and causes moderate to severe thrombocytopenia. The mechanism of the latter is uncertain. Its receptor is the product of the c-fems oncogene that is expressed on mononuclear phagocytes and shows increased expression in some tumors, particularly ovarian carcinoma. It is heavily glycosylated and, unlike the other colony-stimulating factors (CSFs), is found circulating in blood and in urine from which it may be purified. Because of its effects in activating phagocytes, it is thought that it may eventually have a role in combating infectious diseases as well as tumors.

Interleukin-3 (IL-3)

This molecule was originally called multi-CSF. It stimulates the production of neutrophils, monocytes, eosinophils, basophils, and platelets, and augments the function of mature eosinophils and monocytes. It has systemic side effects similar to those of GM-CSF. IL-3 works together with erythropoietin in the differentiation and proliferation of precursors for erythropoiesis. It is most effective when used in combination with other CSFs, where it shows marked synergy. It is unique among the CSFs because it appears to be produced only by T lymphocytes; hence, its reclassification as an interleukin. Clinical experience with it is limited.

Stem Cell Factor (c-kit Ligand, Steel Factor)

In cell culture systems, this molecule has activities similar to those of IL-3 because it enhances the growth of multiple lineages and appears to have its major activity on very early progenitors. It is being studied for a possible clinical role to improve the mobilization of stem cells for transplantation, perhaps in combination with other cytokines.

Interleukin-5 (IL-5)

IL-5 is the most specific cytokine involved in eosinophil differentiation, marrow release, and survival. Increased levels of IL-5 are associated with helper T-cell and natural killer (NK) cell activity, and both mast cells and eosinophils themselves may secrete IL-5 as a part of the allergic response.

Interleukin-6 (IL-6)

IL-6 is another factor that has multilineage effects and appears to act primarily on early progenitors. One of its most profound effects in animals is to increase platelet production. However, it is unlikely to find clinical utility in this role because both IL-11 and thrombopoietin itself have greater activity in the stimulation of platelet production.

Interleukin-11 (IL-11)

This factor also has multilineage effects in vitro. When given to patients it has two major clinical effects: One is to increase the rate of platelet production; the other is to promote fluid retention by the kidney. IL-11 is approved for use in decreasing the degree of thrombocytopenia induced by chemotherapy. When used in this way, it must be accompanied by diuresis to prevent excessive fluid retention. Although IL-11 is less effective in stimulating platelet production than thrombopoietin, it has come into clinical use because thrombopoietin has not yet been approved by the U.S. Food and Drug Administration.

Flt3 Ligand

This recently discovered factor has been shown to have profound synergism with other growth factors in promoting the growth of very early progenitors. It has been suggested that it may find a role in the support of long-term growth of progenitors in vivo.

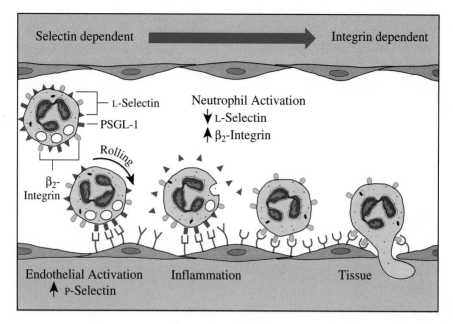

Figure 15–3. **The role of adhesion molecules in margination and migration of neutrophils.** Two major classes of adhesion molecules on neutrophils are the selectins and the integrins. L-Selectin on the neutrophil and P-Selectin on activated endothelial cells are primarily responsible for the loose adhesion of the cell to the endothelium, which leads to rolling and margination. When cells are activated by inflammation, L-Selectin is shed, P-Selectin increases, and β_2-integrin is upregulated, leading to strong adherence of the cell and finally to migration through the endothelium into the tissues.

MYELOID CELL FUNCTION

Myeloid cells may be thought of as having three basic functions. The first is the **ability to migrate out of the circulation into tissues** at sites of infection, damage, or inflammation. The mechanisms by which they do this have recently been shown to involve three classes of adhesion molecules (Figure 15–3). The first, **leukocyte adhesion molecule (LAM-1, or L-Selectin)**, belongs to the selectin class of adhesion molecules and mediates the low-affinity interaction of myeloid cells with endothelium, promoting both margination and a rolling motion along the walls of blood vessels. The second, the **integrin class of adhesion molecules,** mediates a strong interaction of myeloid cells with subendothelial matrix proteins. Third is a mucinlike surface molecule called **P-Selectin glycoprotein ligand (PSGL-1)**. This is expressed on myeloid cells and binds to P-Selectin, which is exposed on activated or damaged endothelial cells. This interaction is essential for the migration of the cells out of the blood vessel and into the tissues. The direction of migration is determined by chemotactic factors, many of which, such as the C5b complement component, are well characterized. New drugs

designed to interfere with these interactions are under development and hold promise of being a new class of powerful anti-inflammatory agents.

The second major function of myeloid cells is **phagocytosis.** Their ability to ingest a particle depends on the nature of the adhesive interactions with the cell surface. Some particles, such as bacteria, seem to have natural surface substances that trigger the phagocytic reaction; others must first be **coated with antibody or complement components (opsonized)** before they can be recognized by phagocytes. Once ingested, particles are isolated in phagocytic vacuoles that fuse with some of the granules within the cell's cytoplasm forming phagosomes. Within these organelles, the particles are subjected to degradation by enzymes and oxidants that kill infectious particles. The ability of myeloid cells to perform phagocytosis and killing of intracellular particles is subject to considerable regulatory control. Thus "activated" cells have markedly enhanced capabilities. Activated status can be achieved by exposure to cytokines, CSFs, and the products of granule release by other myeloid cells.

The third function of myeloid cells is the **release of granule contents,** so-called **exocytosis.** The granules found within myeloid cells are their most clearly defining morphologic feature. Depending on the individual cell type, the granules contain digestive and hydrolytic enzymes and substances capable of mediating the entire range of the inflammatory response. These include chemotactic factors, activators of the complement system, activators of the coagulation system and the fibrinolytic systems, substances that affect vascular permeability and blood flow, and enzymes that are capable of breaking down extracellular matrix proteins. By releasing the content of their granules, myeloid cells trigger and sustain the inflammatory response, recruiting more myeloid cells to the site, and modulating the other components of the organism's reaction to infection, malignancy, and injury.

The **normal myeloid response to a host challenge** hinges on the function of individual myeloid cells. Disease states can be defined according to the capacity and effectiveness of each of these key functions for each of the myeloid cell types. It is important, therefore, to understand the individual characteristics of the myeloid cells.

Neutrophils (Granulocytes)

The mature neutrophil, or granulocyte, is easily recognized by its unique morphology (see Figure 15–2). On the stained film, the cell takes on a nearly round shape with a diameter of 12–16 μm, which is nearly twice that of the red blood cell. The most distinguishing feature is the **segmented nucleus,** where two to three lobes of dense nuclear material are separated by thin, hairlike connections. The other most distinguishing feature is the **large number of granules in the cytoplasm.** Normally this includes a small number of azurophilic, or primary, granules and a greater number of specific, or secondary, granules. **Granule formation is a useful marker** of cell differentiation. Primary granules appear during the promyelocyte stage, whereas specific granules appear during the myelocyte and metamyelocyte stages. By the time the cell reaches maturity, the number and staining properties of the primary granules become less prominent, and the nucleus gradually assumes the lobed configuration.

The granule contents of the neutrophil are a visual demonstration of its functional capabilities (Table 15–1). Primary granules contain abundant myeloperoxidase, in far greater amounts than other myeloid cells. This serves as an excellent histochemical marker for this series; neutrophilic precursors can be differentiated from other myeloid cells by their **strong peroxidase staining** (Table 15–2). Monocytes are also positive but to a far lesser degree. **Leukocyte alkaline phosphatase** is present in mature neutrophils and is markedly increased in most inflammatory states. A reduction of leukocyte alkaline phosphatase is seen in some malignancies, notably **chronic myelogenous leukemia (CML),** and is used as a confirmatory test in making this diagnosis. **Lysozyme (muramidase)** is present in neutrophils (and monocytes) but not eosinophils and basophils. Finally, the pattern of staining for carbohydrate-containing granules using periodic acid–Schiff

Table 15–1. Functions and granule contents of myeloid cells.

Cell Type	Function	Related Granule Contents
Neutrophils	Degradation of pathogens	Lysozyme
		Esterases
		Cathepsin G
		Proteinases
	Generation of oxidants	Peroxidase
	Tissue degradation	Elastase
		Collagenase
Monocytes	Same as neutrophils	
	Clot dissolution	Plasminogen activator
Eosinophils	Same as neutrophils	
	Killing of parasites	Major basic protein
Basophils	Immediate hypersensitivity	Histamine
	? Clot inhibition	Heparin
		Glycosaminoglycans

Table 15–2. Histochemical stains for myeloid cells.

Cell Type	Myeloperoxidase	Specific Esterase	Nonspecific Esterase	Periodic Acid–Schiff
Neutrophil	4+	3+	1+	4+
Monocyte	2+	1+	3+	2+
Lymphocyte	–	–	±	±

stain and two esterase stains (naphthol AS-D chloracetate and α-naphthyl acetate or butyrate) can help **distinguish neutrophils from monocytes** (see Table 15–2). Neutrophils stain positively with **naphthol AS-chloracetate** (specific esterase) but weakly with **α-naphthyl acetate or butyrate** (nonspecific esterase) as a substrate. **Monocytes give the opposite reaction,** that is, a weak or negative reaction with the specific esterase stain but a strong positive reaction to the nonspecific esterase stain.

Myeloid cells can also be categorized according to their **immunologic markers** (Figure 15–4). The marker system is not as extensive as that for the lymphocyte cell line; it is only possible to divide neutrophils into rough stages of immature and mature. The characteristic marker of very immature myeloid cells is **CD34,** and the characteristic markers of mature cells are **CD13 and CD33.** CD34 is lost very early, and the later markers appear simultaneously at a fairly early stage. Thus, these markers are not terribly useful

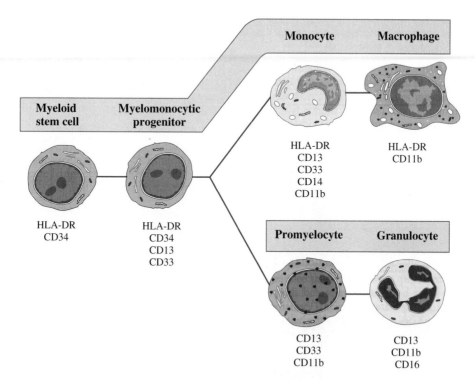

Figure 15–4. **The sequence of neutrophil differentiation—immunologic markers.** Immunologic markers, identified by monoclonal antibodies, can be used to define a maturation sequence for the myeloid cells. Although such markers are most useful in distinguishing very early progenitor cells from mature cells, they do not define the intermediate stages as clearly as does morphology.

in categorizing the maturation sequence of neutrophils. The acquisition of mature markers such as **CD11b and CD16** (an Fc receptor for immunoglobulin) occurs at the metamyelocyte and granulocyte stages.

Monocytes

Mature monocytes also have a distinctive morphology (Figure 15–5). They tend to be somewhat larger than neutrophils on a stained film with a more irregular cell border. The nucleus appears as a horseshoe-shaped structure with chromatin that is less dense than that seen in mature neutrophils. The cytoplasm is a grayish-blue color and contains sparse numbers of pink to purplish granules. When blood is collected in EDTA (purple-topped tube) for laboratory testing, monocytes develop **multiple vacuoles** in the cytoplasm, providing a useful marker of this cell type. Histochemically, monocytes are **best identified by their strong staining with nonspecific esterase.** They stain far less intensely than neutrophils for peroxidase, specific esterase, and acid phosphatase (see Table 15–2). They are rich in lysozyme (muramidase), and very high levels of muramidase can be detected in the urine of patients with monocytosis or monocytic leukemia.

The differentiation of monocytes is less well defined morphologically. It is difficult to distinguish monocyte precursors in the marrow.

A. IMMUNOLOGIC MARKERS:

Immunologic markers of monocytes are similar to those of the neutrophils with the exception of the ac-

quisition of CD14 and the strong expression of class II histocompatibility antigens (HLA-DR) (see Figure 15–4). CD14 is a relatively late marker, and many leukemic cells that appear morphologically and histochemically to be monocytes lack CD14. Of importance is the presence of small amounts of the CD4 molecule on the surface, which serves as a target for HIV. In addition, monocytes have abundant receptors for immunoglobulin (Fc receptors, CD32, and CD64) and are normally coated with considerable plasma immunoglobulin. They also express complement receptors (CD11b, CD18).

B. FUNCTIONS OF CIRCULATING MONOCYTES:

Functions of circulating monocytes parallel those of the granulocytes. Mature monocytes are capable of migration, chemotaxis, phagocytosis, killing, and granule release. They have an important additional role in the immune system. Both circulating monocytes and their progeny, tissue-bound macrophages, are capable of processing and presenting antigens to lymphocytes.

An additional, closely related cell type, **the dendritic cell,** is found in the skin and in germinal centers of lymph nodes. Dendritic cells are specialized in the antigen presentation function. They do this by internalizing antigenic particles, such as bacteria and viruses, partially degrading the molecular components of the antigen and then exposing the degraded and denatured products on their surface noncovalently attached to HLA class II molecules. This molecular complex is recognized by the T cells as antigenic (Figure 15–6). Cul-

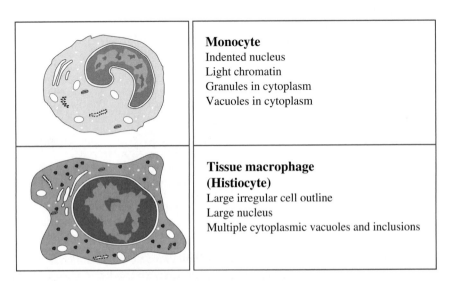

Monocyte
Indented nucleus
Light chromatin
Granules in cytoplasm
Vacuoles in cytoplasm

Tissue macrophage (Histiocyte)
Large irregular cell outline
Large nucleus
Multiple cytoplasmic vacuoles and inclusions

Figure 15–5. **Monocyte and macrophage morphology.** The major functions of monocytes are phagocytosis, killing, granule release, and the processing and presentation of antigen to lymphocytes.

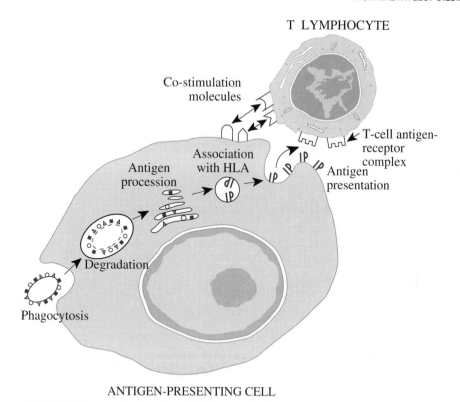

T LYMPHOCYTE

Co-stimulation molecules

Association with HLA

Antigen procession

T-cell antigen-receptor complex

Antigen presentation

Degradation

Phagocytosis

ANTIGEN-PRESENTING CELL

***Figure 15–6.* Antigen presentation by macrophages.** In addition to their role in phagocytosis and killing of pathogens, macrophages play a central role in the immune system by processing antigen and presenting it to the lymphocytes in a manner that facilitates the recognition of foreign material and triggers the immune response. This process involves partial degradation of the antigen, transport to the cell surface, and attachment to the major histocompatibility (HLA) molecules. Lymphocytes recognize foreign antigen as a molecular modification of the normal HLA antigens. Although both macrophages and B cells can perform this antigen-presenting role, the dendritic cells are more highly specialized as "professional" antigen presenters, and are becoming the targets of immunotherapy. The important role of the costimulatory molecules in the induction of immunity and tolerance is also being exploited therapeutically.

tured dendritic cells, and agents that stimulate their function, are being evaluated in the immunotherapy of diseases such as multiple myeloma.

In addition, so-called "**co-stimulatory**" **molecules** have been shown to greatly augment the interaction between antigen presenting cells (APCs) and T lymphocytes. These include CD28 (T cells) and B7 (APCs), CD154 (T cells) and CD40 (APCs), and CD2 (T cells) and CD58 (APCs). Disruption of these interactions using antibodies and recombinant molecules shows considerable promise as a strategy for immunosuppression.

Monocytes also appear to be more capable than the neutrophils in **killing intracellular pathogens** such as *Listeria monocytogenes,* as well as mycobacteria and

yeasts. When activated, they are also able to **kill many tumor cells.** Finally, monocytes **express surface structures that encourage their interaction with platelets** and result in the incorporation of monocytes into thrombi. The purpose of this interaction is unclear; however, monocytes are a source of plasminogen activator and may play a role in limiting clot formation or promoting clot dissolution.

Eosinophils

The eosinophil is easily recognized either in the marrow aspirate or on the stained blood film (Figure 15–7). Their size is similar to a neutrophil and the nu-

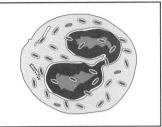

Eosinophil
Bilobed nucleus
Abundant red granules

Figure 15–7. **Eosinophil morphology.** The major function of eosinophils appears to be the defense against multicellular parasites mediated by the release of the highly toxic major basic protein in their granules. In addition, they are capable of scavenging immune complexes and may play a role in the suppression of humoral immune reactions.

cleus is typically bilobed, even though cells with three segmented lobes may be observed. The most distinguishing characteristic, however, is the large number of **bright orange to red specific granules that fill the cell's cytoplasm** to the point of obscuring the margins of the nucleus. When viewed through an electron microscope, the granules contain a crystal composed of an extremely alkaline protein called **major basic protein.**

Although the **principal function of the eosinophil is to kill parasites,** the cell also contains peroxidase and other enzymes similar to those of neutrophils. The production of eosinophils is stimulated by several cytokines, including IL-1, IL-3, and IL-5, as well as by GM-CSF, but IL-5 is the most specific growth factor. Their production and function seems to be more closely tied to the immune system, helper T-cell and NK-cell activity, than the typical antibacterial response of neutrophils.

Eosinophils are **phagocytic** and can kill organisms by phagosome formation. At the same time, when the eosinophil must deal with an organism such as a helminth that is too large to engulf, it will release its granules directly onto the surface of the organism. Eosinophils

also appear to be **involved in immediate-type hypersensitivity reactions.** They are capable of neutralizing histamine and may play a role in down-regulating allergic reactions. When stimulated to excessive levels, eosinophils, perhaps by release of their granules, **can give rise to tissue damage and endomyocardial fibrosis.**

Basophils

Basophils and marrow mast cells are equally distinctive morphologically because of their basophilic granules (Figure 15–8). However, the granules of basophils and mast cells are not identical and it is still unclear just how they are related. Circulating basophils are easily recognized on stained films as cells whose internal structure is largely occluded by a **dense mass of large deep-purple granules.** The cells often appear somewhat smaller than neutrophils. In patients with basophilia, however, the granules may be relatively sparse, revealing a nucleus that resembles that of a monocyte more than a neutrophil. The size of the individual granules is the tip-off; they are much larger than the primary granules of the neutrophils.

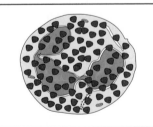

Basophil
Segmented nucleus
Cytoplasm filled by large, dark granules

Figure 15–8. **Basophil morphology.** The major role of basophils and mast cells is the release of vasoactive compounds in response to immunologic stimuli mediated by the crosslinking of IgE.

Circulating basophils appear to play a **major role in immediate-type hypersensitivity reactions.** Their granules contain abundant proteoglycans and histamine. They express high-affinity Fc receptors for IgE and are triggered to release their granule contents by crosslinking of their surface-bound IgE by antigens. Basophils also produce other mediators of acute hypersensitivity such as leukotrienes. Clinically, basophil granule release is **manifested as urticaria, rhinitis, asthma, and anaphylaxis.** Tissue mast cells also play a role in the hypersensitivity response. In addition, **mast cells** contain large amounts of heparin that may serve to maintain blood and extracellular fluid flow, especially in the marrow. Mast cells in the marrow are closely related to the vessels and sinusoids.

Cytokines responsible for basophil production may be similar to those that stimulate eosinophil production. Basophils provide a **useful marker for certain myeloproliferative disorders,** particularly CML. Leukemias restricted to basophils or mast cells are very rare. Many marrow and tissue mast cells are seen in the benign disorder urticaria pigmentosa and the clonal malignancy progressive systemic mastocytosis. Symptoms of these disorders are related to the release of histamine and leukotrienes from the cells, resulting in angioedema, marked pruritus, and hypotension.

MYELOID CELL KINETICS

The kinetics of cell production, egress from the marrow, and survival in circulation is best illustrated for the neutrophils. As with red blood cell production, **marrow biopsy** can be used to evaluate overall cellularity of the pool of leukocyte/monocyte progenitors, whereas a **marrow aspirate** provides information regarding cell differentiation. Overall, there should be approximately three myeloid precursors or mature granulocytes for every recognizable erythroid precursor, the normal ratio of erythroid to granulocytic precursors (E/G ratio) of 1:3. Moreover, in the basal state, about one-third of all of cells observed in a marrow aspirate are mature granulocytes that are being stored and awaiting release in response to an infection-related cytokine.

Figure 15–9 illustrates the relative sizes of the neutrophil precursor compartments, the transit times, and the storage pool for both the normal and infected states. Approximately 1×10^9 neutrophils/kg/day are produced by the **normal adult marrow,** and the total time spent in proliferation, maturation, and marrow storage is estimated to be between 5 and 14 days. **With a severe infection,** however, the maturation time may be shortened to as little as 48–72 hours. This process reflects a shift of the marrow storage pool into circulation, a phenomenon that can be recognized on inspection of the marrow aspi-

rate as a disappearance of mature neutrophils from the specimen even while the E/G ratio shows an increase in the immature granulocyte compartment.

Factors Affecting the Number of Circulating and Stored Neutrophils

Once neutrophils enter circulation, they rapidly equilibrate with the marginated neutrophil pool of approximately equal size. The partition between the marrow storage pool, the circulating neutrophils, and the marginal pool is in constant flux. The number of neutrophils in circulation can increase dramatically in **response to infection** as a result of a shift of neutrophils out of the marrow storage pool that exceeds any increased egress of neutrophils from circulation into the tissues. **Administration of glucocorticoids** will also change the partition by releasing marrow granulocytes into circulation, changing the size of the marginal pool, and slowing the rate of egress into tissues. **Sudden exertion** with release of catecholamines will also change the pool partition and can double or even triple the blood neutrophil count. Finally, **black patients** may have significantly lower neutrophil counts because of variations in the pool sizes, with otherwise normal neutrophil production and delivery into tissues.

Circulating granulocytes leave circulation in a random fashion with a **disappearance time of 6–7 hours.** Once they enter tissue they do not return to circulation, and their survival depends on their reason for homing to that site. At best, it is less than 2–3 days. In response to an infection, they release cytokines, which encourage additional granulocyte migration.

Estimates of Myeloid Cell Production

Even though the kinetics of neutrophil production and survival in circulation are complex, it is possible clinically to estimate myeloid cell production from the count of mature and immature cells in circulation. **Modern automated counters** provide an accurate measurement of the total leukocyte count and a relatively accurate differential count of neutrophils, metamyelocytes (bands), monocytes, eosinophils, basophils, and lymphocytes. A **white blood cell differential** can also be performed by direct counting of a stained blood film. Since a smaller number of cells are counted, the error of this measurement is far larger than the automated differentials. However, automated counters are unable to recognize abnormal cell types, do not accurately distinguish band neutrophils from segmented neutrophils, and may have some built-in methodologic errors that must be taken into account.

Normal values for the leukocyte count and dif-

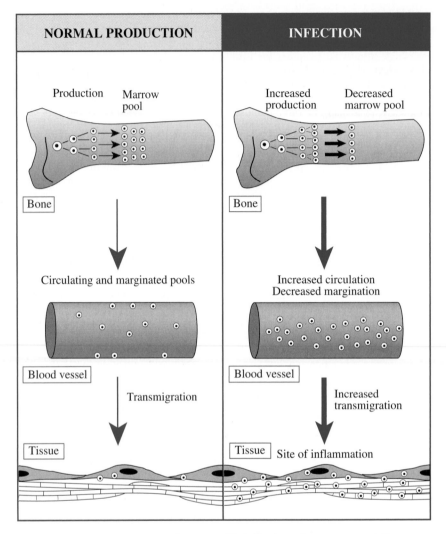

NORMAL PRODUCTION	INFECTION

Figure 15–9. **Neutrophil kinetics in the basal state and in infection.** There are several distinct compartments of neutrophils within the body. These are the proliferating and storage pools in the marrow, the marginated and circulating pools in the blood vessels, and finally those neutrophils in the tissues at the site of inflammation. Infection triggers increased production, depletion of the marrow storage and marginated pools, increase in the circulating pool, and increased transmigration into the tissues.

ferential are summarized in Table 15–3. Clinical laboratories generally report the absolute number of leukocytes and a percent differential of the individual cell types. The **clinician is advised to calculate and use the absolute number** in determining whether the patient has too few or too many cells of a certain type in circulation. This measurement is most important for the accurate identification of a neutropenia or lymphopenia (see Chapters 16 and 20). It is also true in the case of monocytosis, eosinophilia, and basophilia. A **significant monocytosis** is defined as an absolute monocyte count of greater than 1000/µL (1.0 × 10⁹/L), **significant eosinophilia** is greater than 450/µL (0.45 × 10⁹/L), whereas **basophilia** is defined as greater than 50 basophils/µL (0.05 × 10⁹/L).

Table 15–3. The normal leukocyte count.

Cell Type	Percent	Absolute Count
Leukocytes		5–11,000/µL (5–11 × 10⁹/L)
Neutrophils	45–75	4–6000/µL (4–6 × 10⁹/L)
Metamyelocytes (bands)	0–5	
Monocytes	5–10	500–1000/µL (0.5–1 × 10⁹/L)
Eosinophils	0–5	< 450/µL (< 45 × 10⁹/L)
Basophils	0–1	< 50/µL (< 0.05 × 10⁹/L)
Lymphocytes	10–45	2–5000/µL (2–5 × 10⁹/L)

BIBLIOGRAPHY

Anderlini P et al: Biologic and clinical effects of granulocyte colony-stimulating factor in normal individuals. Blood 1996;88:2819.

Babior BM, Golde DW: Production, distribution, and fate of neutrophils. In: Beutler E et al (editors): *Hematology,* 6th ed. McGraw-Hill, 2001.

D'Andrea AD: Cytokine receptors in congenital hematopoietic disease. N Engl J Med 1994;330:839.

Delves PJ, Roitt IM: The immune system, Part I. N Engl J Med 2000;343:37.

Delves PJ, Roitt IM: The immune system, Part II. N Engl J Med 2000;343:108.

Metcalf D: Control of granulocytes and macrophages: Molecular, cellular, and clinical aspects. Science 1991;254:529.

Peters WP: The myeloid colony stimulating factors: Introduction and overview. Semin Hematol 1991;28:1.

Robinson BE, Quesenberry PJ: Hematopoietic growth factors: Overview and clinical applications. Part I. Am J Med Sci 1990;300:163.

Robinson BE, Quesenberry PJ: Hematopoietic growth factors: Overview and clinical applications. Part II. Am J Med Sci 1990;300:237.

Robinson BE, Quesenberry PJ: Hematopoietic growth factors: Overview and clinical applications. Part III. Am J Med Sci 1990;300:311.

Shivdasani RA, Orkin SH: The transcriptional control of hematopoiesis. Blood 1996;87:4025.

Quantitative and Qualitative Disorders of Neutrophils

16

Quantitative disorders of neutrophils are frequently encountered in clinical practice but seldom present a diagnostic problem. For example, **granulocytosis,** which is an acute increase in the number of mature and immature granulocytes in circulation, is an anticipated part of the normal response to any infection. Eosinophilia and monocytosis are seen in association with allergic and inflammatory conditions. On the other hand, granulocytopenia can occur as a side effect of drug administration or as a component of the pancytopenia seen with severe marrow damage. It is an anticipated complication of cancer chemotherapy.

Qualitative disorders of neutrophil function are much less common. Again, they can occur as a complication of drug therapy. Those that result from genetic defects in granulocyte adhesion, migration, or lysozyme function are a greater diagnostic challenge.

NORMAL RESPONSE OF NEUTROPHILS TO INFECTION

The kinetics of normal neutrophil production and destruction are described in Chapter 15. In response to infection or presentation of a foreign antigen, several cytokines (tumor necrosis factor [TNF]-α, interleukin [IL]-1, granulocyte colony-stimulating factor [G-CSF], granulocyte macrophage colony-stimulating factor [GM-CSF], monocyte colony-stimulating factor [M-CSF], and IL-3) are released that affect the kinetics of neutrophil production and the distribution of cells within the circulation and tissues. A single mediator of inflammation cannot be identified; however, the broad effects of TNF-α illustrate how the reaction is coordinated. Administration of TNF-α duplicates essentially all of the signs and symptoms of sepsis, including fever, hypotension, and acute respiratory distress syndrome/pulmonary edema. It is associated with concomitant changes in many other cytokines that mediate the other effects of infection, such as IL-1, which stimulates the immune system, and the colony-stimulating factors (CSFs), which stimulate granulocyte production and function. Interestingly, experimental blockage of

TNF-α can ablate most of the inflammatory effects of sepsis and, in some models, can prevent death from septic shock.

The **earliest response to an infection** is the emigration of granulocytes out of circulation and into the site of bacterial invasion. Granulocytes close to the infected area respond to local chemotactic factors by increasing their rate of margination and migration. They also trigger the full inflammatory response with further release of cytokines capable of stimulating marrow-progenitor proliferation.

The rapidity and magnitude of **the rise in the number of circulating granulocytes in response to infection** is impressive. Within hours of the onset of a severe infection, the granulocyte count can increase by two- to fourfold. Initially, this increase represents a change in the partition between the marginated and circulating pools of granulocytes and the delivery of new granulocytes from the marrow pool (Figure 16–1). In the basal state, mature granulocytes spend 5–6 days in the marrow before entering circulation. With severe infection, this transit time can be shortened to a day or less with release of immature granulocytes (bands or metamyelocytes). With the stimulus of G-CSF, there is a proliferation of committed progenitors and a further shortening of the time delay in precursor maturation. Finally, the response is made more effective by shortening the transit time of granulocytes through the circulation to increase the rate of delivery to a tissue site.

G-CSF, GM-CSF, and M-CSF (CSF-1) can all play a role in the **sustained increase in granulocyte and monocyte production.** The primary effect of **G-CSF** is to stimulate the committed granulocyte precursor pathway. **GM-CSF and M-CSF** promote both granulocyte and monocyte production. As illustrated by measurements of plasma cytokine levels in neutropenic patients, these growth factors appear in sequence, according to the severity of the infection and the rate of use of mature cells. The level of G-CSF rises first. Increases in the levels of GM-CSF and M-CSF occur somewhat later and are most pronounced in patients who become granulocytopenic. They have a wider impact on cell

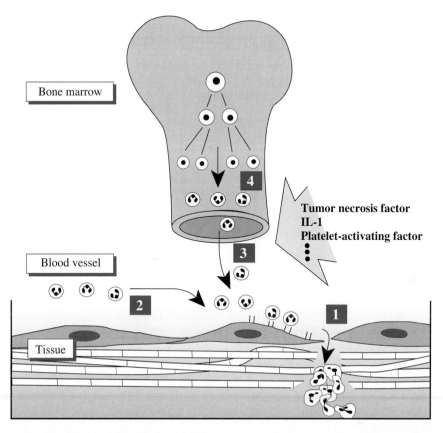

Figure 16–1. Granulocyte response to infection. The response to infection includes (**1**) an increase in cell adherence and migration out of circulation; (**2**) demargination of cells more remote to the site of infection; (**3**) a shift of the marrow granulocyte pool into circulation; and (**4**) a severalfold increase in proliferation of committed progenitors. The response is mediated by several cytokines arising from lymphoid, myeloid, tissue cells, and platelets.

production and are responsible for the increase in the number of circulating monocytes in patients with severe granulocytopenia. In addition to their role as growth factors, they also enhance the phagocytic and cytotoxic functions of granulocytes and monocytes.

■ NEUTROPHILIA

Clinically, **neutrophilia** is defined as an absolute granulocyte count in excess of 7×10^9/L (7000 segmented granulocytes plus bands/μL). The major causes of neutrophilia are listed in Table 16–1. **Tissue damage, inflammation, and infection** follow the normal response pattern of neutrophils to a foreign antigen. This pattern includes changes in cell production, marrow release, and the rate of entry into tissues. **Other causes of neutrophilia** involve changes in only one or two of the steps in the ki-

netic response. For example, the granulocytosis observed with stress is caused by a shift in the pool of marginated granulocytes. The increase in granulocyte count observed in patients with polycythemia vera or chronic myelogenous leukemia (CML) is the product of uncontrolled cell production typical of a clonal malignancy.

CLINICAL FEATURES

An increase in the granulocyte count by itself does not produce specific symptoms or signs, except when the count exceeds 100,000/μL in patients with CML. In this situation, marked leukostasis in the spleen can result in splenic infarction, and sudden activation of granulocytes in circulation can lead to stasis in the lungs with a drop in oxygen diffusion capacity. When present in very large numbers, granulocytes can also accumulate in the skin to produce nontender, purplish

Table 16–1. Neutrophilia.

Cause	Mechanism
Infections/inflammation/tissue damage	Increased production, marrow granulocyte pool release, demargination
Myeloproliferative disease	Increased production
Stress/metabolic disorders (ketoacidosis, eclampsia, etc)	Demargination
Steroid therapy/endotoxin	Marrow granulocyte pool release, demargination, decreased egress
Growth factor therapy (G-CSF, GM-CSF)	Increased production, change in egress
Splenectomy	Decrease in splenic trapping

nodules (**chloromas**). Unlike immature blasts, mature granulocytes do not invade brain tissue.

The clinical features associated with moderate granulocytosis are those of the primary disease. With an acute bacterial infection, the patient is usually febrile and has evidence of a tissue infection (ie, a lung infiltrate, abscess, cellulitis). Similarly, noninfectious inflammatory diseases are accompanied by clinical features particular to the individual condition.

Laboratory Studies

A routine **complete blood count (CBC)** and **white blood cell (WBC)** differential may be all that is needed to diagnose the common causes of granulocytosis. The CBC provides an accurate measurement of the total WBC count, whereas the differential provides a measure of the number of mature granulocytes, metamyelocytes (band forms), monocytes, and eosinophils. **In the basal state,** the absolute number of bands should be less than 500 cells/μL. **Severe infection or inflammation** is associated with an increased release (shift) of marrow metamyelocytes into circulation. **Reactive monocytosis (monocyte counts greater than 1000/μL)** is seen in patients with active tuberculosis, subacute bacterial endocarditis, and severe granulocytopenia. **Parasitic infestations** are typically associated with an elevated eosinophil count, whereas **basophilia (a basophil count greater than 50/μL)** is seen in patients with CML.

A **marrow aspirate** can provide additional supporting information. The shift of marrow granulocytes into circulation and the proliferation of myelocytic precursors are easily detected on inspection of the marrow aspirate film. In the basal state, mature granulocytes make up one-quarter or more of the cells in the marrow. This number is dramatically reduced in patients with acute infection. In addition, the number of early myelocytic precursors increases to shift the ratio of ery-

throid to granulocytic precursors (E/G ratio) to below 1:3 (expansion of the myelocytic portion of the marrow).

Changes in individual cell morphology can also help in the diagnosis. The **appearance of metamyelocytes (bands)** in circulation is one sign of a reactive granulocytosis secondary to cytokine stimulation. Another is the appearance of granulocytes with prominent azurophilic granules, so-called **toxic granulation.** The **leukocyte alkaline phosphatase stain** and **chromosomal analysis** are also of value in distinguishing reactive granulocytosis from a malignant state. Although patients with CML present with varying combinations of granulocytosis, toxic granulation, Döhle bodies, and basophilia, the condition is also accompanied by a decrease in leukocyte alkaline phosphatase activity. In contrast, leukemoid reactions in patients with infection or inflammation demonstrate an elevated leukocyte alkaline phosphatase level. **Cytogenetics** can also separate benign and malignant disorders. For example, most CML patients demonstrate the distinctive translocation of the c-*abl* oncogene from chromosome 9 to chromosome 22 with the reciprocal transposition of the terminal portion of chromosome 22 to chromosome 9 (the **Philadelphia chromosome defect**).

DIAGNOSIS

The diagnosis of granulocytosis associated with an acute infection, inflammation, or major tissue damage is generally straightforward. **Major bacterial infections** are associated with granulocyte counts of 10,000–30,000/μL, together with an increase in the number of band forms. Although a count in excess of 30,000/μL is unusual, very high counts may be observed in patients with **deep-seated infections or peritonitis.** As a rule, granulocyte counts of 50,000/μL or higher indicate a noninfectious, malignant disease process. The appearance of very immature myelocytic cells in circulation and accompanying change in other cell lines (eg, increased or decreased platelets or red blood cells) are also signs of malignancy.

Changes in pool kinetics can result in modest **increases in the granulocyte count** (see Table 16–1). After splenectomy, patients will chronically demonstrate counts of 10,000–15,000/μL. Acute stress in association with trauma, hemorrhage, marked hypoxia, or ketoacidosis will produce a self-limited granulocytosis. This condition involves a catecholamine-induced shift of the marginated granulocyte pool into circulation.

Granulocytosis is an expected **side effect of glucocorticoid therapy** that interferes with the egress of granulocytes from circulation into tissues. There is a clear dose-response relationship since patients who are receiving 60–100 mg of prednisone per day will run WBC counts of 15,000–20,000/μL. Higher doses of **prednisone** can make the WBC count reach levels of 30,000/μL or higher, which is characterized by a marked increase in granulocytes, together with a reduction in lymphocytes and eosinophils. **G-CSF and GM-CSF** are also capable of producing a marked granulocytosis. In this case, the primary cause of the increased count is an increased marrow production. However, G-CSF also influences the rate of egress of granulocytes from circulation and their function in tissues. Daily administration of large doses of either cytokine can raise the granulocyte count to levels in excess of 100,000/μL.

■ EOSINOPHILIA

Clinically significant eosinophilia is defined as a sustained absolute eosinophil count of greater than 1000–1500/μL. Table 16–2 lists the various disease states associated with eosinophilia. **Moderate eosinophilia** is commonly seen with a wide spectrum of disorders, including parasitic infestations, systemic allergic disorders, collagen vascular diseases, various forms of dermatitis, drug reactions, and tumors. Hodgkin's disease and both B-cell and T-cell non-Hodgkin's lymphomas can present with eosinophilia. Even when there is no obvious sign of an underlying lymphoma, up to 25% of patients with apparent idiopathic eosinophilia will have an expanded clone of aberrant T-cells, which produce high levels of IL-5.

Hypereosinophilia (an eosinophil count greater than 5000/μL) is associated with tissue damage secondary to the release of the eosinophil's major basic protein. Irreversible **endomyocardial fibrosis** producing a restrictive myocardiopathy can be anticipated in patients who maintain eosinophil counts greater than 5000/μL. In patients with **eosinophilic leukemia, idio-**

Table 16–2. Eosinophilia.

Allergic disorders
  Asthma
  Allergic vasculitis—polyarteritis nodosa
  Angioneurotic edema
Dermatologic disorders
  Eczema
  Psoriasis
  Dermatitis herpetiformis
  Pemphigus
Parasitic diseases
  Protozoan infections—toxoplasmosis, amebiasis
  Metazoan infections—nematode, trematode, and cestode
    infestations, scabies
Gastrointestinal disease
  Ulcerative colitis/regional enteritis
  Eosinophilic gastroenteritis
Malignancies
  Hodgkin's disease/B- and T-cell lymphomas
  Myeloproliferative disorders
  Carcinomatosis
  Eosinophilic granuloma
Hypereosinophilia
  Eosinophilic leukemia
  Loeffler syndrome

pathic hypereosinophilic syndrome, or Loeffler syndrome, eosinophil counts can reach 20,000–100,000/μL. Widespread **organ dysfunction and rapidly progressive heart disease** can be anticipated with these conditions. These patients need to be treated aggressively with both corticosteroids and hydroxyurea. Leukopheresis can be used acutely to lower the eosinophil count.

■ NEUTROPENIA

Clinically, **neutropenia** is defined as an absolute granulocyte count below 2000/μL in Caucasians or 1500/μL in blacks. It is not until the granulocyte count falls below 500/μL, however, that the patient is at significant risk for **bacterial or fungal infections.** The major causes of neutropenia in the adult involve **abnormalities in cell production and autoimmune destruction.** Changes in pool kinetics play less of a role.

CLINICAL FEATURES

The symptoms and signs of neutropenia depend on the level of the count. When the absolute number of granulocytes is between 500 and 2000/μL, it is unlikely that the patient will develop a serious bacterial infection. The

moderately neutropenic patient may be unable, however, to mount an adequate defense. When challenged by infection, the associated increase in WBC utilization can result in a rapid fall in the granulocyte count. This situation puts the patient at risk for spread of the infection and life-threatening bacteremia.

Once the count falls below 500/μL, the patient is at significant risk for infections of the skin, mouth (teeth and periodontal tissue), pharynx, and lung. As the count falls below 100/μL, the chance of gram-negative or gram-positive sepsis and fungal infections increases dramatically.

Laboratory Studies

The **CBC** and **WBC differential** are the key measurements in diagnosing and managing the neutropenic patient. It is important to **focus on the absolute granulocyte count** and not the total WBC count. Most patients with granulocytopenia will still have normal or near normal numbers of lymphocytes. This level will keep the total WBC count above 2000/μL. Attention should also be given to the number of monocytes. A reactive monocytosis is often observed in patients with drug-induced and cyclic neutropenia. A small increase in the number of monocytes to levels of 500–1000/μL can significantly reduce the risk of fatal bacteremia.

The **marrow aspirate** is the other key test in determining the cause and future course of a neutropenia. Usually, a simple marrow aspirate to look at the marrow E/G ratio and the maturation of myelocyte precursors is adequate. Production defects are associated with a uniform loss of myelocytes at all stages of maturation. The aspirate appears hypocellular with remaining cell elements limited to the red blood cell precursors, lymphocytes, plasma cells, and mast cells. Patients with drug-induced neutropenia often demonstrate "a maturation arrest" where relatively normal-appearing early myelocytic precursors do not progress to more mature myelocyte, metamyelocyte, and granulocyte stages. **Folic acid and vitamin B$_{12}$ deficiency can also produce a maturation abnormality,** characterized by megaloblastic morphology and the appearance of mature granulocytes with an increased number of nuclear lobes (**multilobed polys**).

If an adequate marrow aspirate cannot be obtained, a **marrow biopsy** is required. In patients with severe marrow damage secondary to malignancy, drug damage, or idiopathic aplasia, the marrow biopsy is preferred for the evaluation of total cellularity and structural damage. Patients with myelofibrosis, hairy-cell leukemia, and paroxysmal nocturnal hemoglobinuria will frequently have a dry tap on aspiration and, therefore, can only be diagnosed by biopsy.

Other tests that can help pinpoint the diagnosis include cytogenetics (clonal malignancies of the hematopoietic system), tests for paroxysmal nocturnal hemoglobinuria (Chapter 9), including flow cytometric evaluation of GPI-linked glycoproteins (CD59/55) or a sugar water or acid hemolysin test (or both), serum folic acid and vitamin B$_{12}$ levels (megaloblastic pancytopenia), assays for antineutrophil antibodies (collagen vascular disease), and the Rebuck skin window test to assess the egress of granulocytes into tissues. Turnover measurements are possible using radiolabeled granulocytes. However, this type of measurement is usually limited to the research laboratory. Measurements of circulating cytokine levels (G-CSF, GM-CSF, and M-CSF) by immunoassay are becoming available, but their role in diagnosing clinical conditions is yet to be determined. Marrow culture techniques can be used to study the growth characteristics of colony-forming units as well as the interaction of T-cell subsets with colony growth.

DIAGNOSIS

Neutropenia in Newborns & Children

Several neutropenic syndromes are observed in both newborns and young children (Table 16–3). **Neonatal sepsis** is perhaps the most common cause of severe neutropenia within the first few days of life. A **reversible neutropenia** can be observed in children born to mothers with autoimmune disease or as a result of maternal hypertension, drug ingestion, or both. **Persistent neutropenia** can occur as a result of defects in neutrophil production, maturation, or survival.

Cyclic neutropenia, an autosomal dominant condition, is a particularly well-studied cause of childhood neutropenia. This disorder is characterized by recurrent episodes of neutropenia, which are not always associated with infection and occur in regular cycles of 3–4 weeks. Each episode is characterized by 1 week of reduced granulocyte production, followed by a reactive monocytosis and then a spontaneous recovery of normal granulocyte production. The granulocytopenia can be severe enough to result in recurrent, severe bacterial infections that require aggressive antibiotic therapy. As the child grows older, the cyclical nature of the WBC production can diminish, thereby resulting in a chronic severe granulocytopenia. The postulated mechanism behind cyclic neutropenia is a defect in the feedback mechanism with a decreased capacity of precursors to respond to growth factors such as G-CSF.

Kostmann's syndrome, an autosomal recessive disorder of neutrophil maturation, is another cause of severe congenital neutropenia. These patients appear to have a normal population of early progenitors that are somehow suppressed, inhibiting normal maturation. They are at risk for severe, life-threatening infections.

Table 16–3. Neutropenia in children.

Cause	Mechanism
Newborns	
Isoimmune disease	Immune destruction
Infections	Production defect and increased utilization
Maternal drug ingestion	Production defect
Congenital neutropenias	Production defect
Benign (chronic idiopathic neutropenia)	
Kostmann's syndrome	
Immunodeficiency states	
Chediak-Higashi syndrome	
Autoimmune disease	
Infants and young children	
Infections	Increased utilization
Drug ingestion	Production defect
Vitamin deficiency (vitamin B_{12} folate/copper)	Production/maturation defect
Hematopoietic malignancy	Production defect
Cyclic neutropenia	Intermittent failure of marrow proliferation

Some patients with Kostmann's syndrome have been shown to have a mutation of the G-CSF receptor, although most do respond to therapy with G-CSF. Likewise, **Chediak-Higashi syndrome** is an autosomal recessive disorder with moderate neutropenia, a distinctive appearance of circulating granulocytes (very large azurophilic granules in all myelocytic lineages), and a high susceptibility to bacterial infections.

Neutropenia in Adults

The principal causes of neutropenia in adults are listed in Table 16–4. **Acquired defects in marrow production** are very common and often can be anticipated, as for example, with cancer chemotherapy and in the treatment of AIDS patients with zidovudine (AZT).

This result reflects the impact of specific drugs on stem cell and early myelocytic progenitor proliferation. In most cases, the marrow will recover once the drug or drugs are withdrawn. **Many drugs have been associated with occasional neutropenia.** Among the most prominent of these are the injectable gold salts, chloramphenicol, antithyroid medications (carbimazole and propylthiouracil), analgesics (indomethacin, acetaminophen, and phenacetin), tricyclic antidepressants, and the phenothiazines. Virtually any drug can on occasion produce severe, life-threatening neutropenia, however. Therefore, whenever neutropenia occurs in the course of medical treatment, the possibility that it is drug-induced must be considered.

"**Autoimmune**" neutropenia is observed with a collagen vascular or autoimmune disease. The two most

Table 16–4. Neutropenia in adults.

Cause	Mechanism
Drug-induced	Production, maturation and survival defects
Autoimmune disease	Increased destruction (antineutrophil antibodies)
Hypersplenism	Increased splenic pooling, destruction
Hematopoietic malignancy	Production defects
Leukemias	
Hodgkin's disease	
T-cell malignancies (LGL, etc)	
HIV-1 infection (AIDS)	Production, maturation, and survival defects
Congenital	
Neutropenia in blacks	Maturation defect? increased margination
Chronic idiopathic neutropenia	Production defect

common associations are **lupus erythematosus (SLE)**, where the neutropenia occurs alone or is accompanied by thrombocytopenia, and **rheumatoid arthritis (Felty's syndrome)**, where neutropenia in association with splenomegaly is common. Because the arthritic component of the disease process may be subtle, the appearance of either of these combinations should trigger a careful evaluation for collagen vascular disease as a first step in the differential diagnosis. **Other causes of splenomegaly and neutropenia** include lymphoma, myeloproliferative disease, and severe liver disease with portal hypertension. In all of these situations, it is often difficult to decide whether the granulocytopenia is owing to sequestration alone or an autoimmune component. Splenomegaly may also have an impact on marrow production. Although this connection is not well understood, splenectomy in cases of Felty's syndrome and in patients with myelofibrosis has been reported to significantly improve neutrophil production.

Acute, life-threatening granulocytopenia can occur in patients with overwhelming sepsis. A falling count in a patient with pneumococcal sepsis or peritonitis is a bad prognostic sign. It reflects a rate of granulocyte use that exceeds the ability of the marrow to produce new cells. **Alcoholic patients** are especially susceptible to infection-induced granulocytopenia. In this setting, both folic acid deficiency and the direct toxic effect of alcohol on marrow precursors cripples the patient's ability to produce new cells in response to infection.

Finally, some patients will present with an "**idiopathic**" **neutropenia,** or neutropenia without obvious cause. Usually, the reduction in the number of circulating granulocytes is relatively mild and not associated with life-threatening infections. When the granulocytopenia is accompanied by abnormalities of other blood elements (anemia and thrombocytopenia), it is likely the patient is developing a **myeloproliferative disorder** (see Chapters 17 and 18). **Lymphoproliferative disease,** especially T–suppressor cell malignancies (large granular lymphocyte disease) (see Chapter 21) can also present with granulocytopenia and an increased incidence of skin and mucous membrane infections. **HIV infection** is obviously becoming a common cause of T-cell dysfunction. In these patients, the loss of the T-helper subset and overexpression of the T-suppressor subset is associated with abnormalities of neutrophil production and function.

■ NEUTROPHIL DYSFUNCTION

Patients can present with normal numbers of circulating granulocytes but demonstrate a defect in cell function (Table 16–5). The most common causes of poor granulocyte function fit in the acquired category. Patients with metabolic diseases, especially diabetes mellitus, or those who are alcoholics or have uremia or collagen vascular diseases under treatment with corticosteroids can be shown to have mild to moderate **defects in granulocyte function.** Most often, this defect reflects a decreased responsiveness of the cell to chemotactic signals and a demonstrable reduction in the rate of egress into a site of tissue infection. In diabetic patients, the level of diabetic control may correlate with the functional defect. Patients with myeloproliferative disorders can also demonstrate a

Table 16–5. Neutrophil dysfunction.

Cause	Mechanism
Congenital defects	
Leukocyte adhesion defect	Decreased adherence (CD11/CD18 deficiency)
Lazy leukocyte syndrome	Decreased motility
Chediak-Higashi syndrome	Decreased motility, phagocytosis
Immunoglobulin/complement deficiency states	Decreased phagocytosis
Kartagener's syndrome (immotile cilia syndrome)	Decreased chemotaxis, motility
Specific granule deficiency	Decreased chemotaxis, killing
Chronic granulomatous disease	Decreased killing
Acquired defects	
Drug-induced (prednisone, etc)	Decreased migration
Alcoholism	Decreased motility, phagocytosis
Metabolic disorders (diabetes, uremia, malnutrition, autoimmune disease, glomerulonephritis)	Decreased adhesion, motility, and phagocytosis
HIV infection	Decreased motility, phagocytosis, and killing; poor monocyte function
Myeloproliferative disorders	Decreased phagocytosis and killing

functional defect of their granulocytes with or without granulocytopenia. Patients presenting with recurrent pyogenic infections are frequently suspected of having neutrophil dysfunction. Most cases do not demonstrate any specific defect.

The most defined disorders of neutrophil dysfunction are **genetic** in nature. Some are characterized by structural changes in the cell that can be easily observed on blood films (Chediak-Higashi syndrome), whereas others involve **biochemical abnormalities.** The latter includes **leukocyte adhesion deficiency (LAD),** in which neutrophils lack an important adhesive molecule (the CD11/CD18 integrin) that mediates the binding of the cell to the subendothelium and its subsequent migration out of the vasculature. At least two types of LAD have been described. In LAD type 1 leukocytes roll normally but do not adhere or migrate out of the circulation, while LAD type 2 patients demonstrate defects both in rolling and adhesion. Recently, a child with a **defective cell surface adhesion factor,** E-Selectin, has also been described. Clinically these defects result in an accumulation of granulocytes in circulation and an inability of cells to migrate to the site of infection. Patients have recurrent pyogenic infections but do not form pus.

Chronic granulomatous disease is another genetic disorder in which the granulocytes lack the ability to generate reactive oxygen species. It can result from any one of several distinct genetic abnormalities with different modes of inheritance. The patient's granulocytes are capable of migrating to a site of infection and ingesting organisms, but they are unable to kill them. Therefore, *Staphylococcus aureus* and certain gram-negative bacteria that are normally killed by granulocyte phagocytosis and lysosome digestion are responsible for most of the infections in these patients. The condition is usually diagnosed during childhood or early adult life when patients present with recurrent microabscesses and chronic granulomatous inflammation.

DIAGNOSIS

Patients suspected of neutrophil dysfunction should have an **evaluation of their immune system** (especially the level of serum immunoglobulins) because a lack of antibody production can result in poor opsonization and phagocytosis that give the same symptoms as primary neutrophil dysfunction. In addition, **phenotypic analysis of the neutrophils,** with special attention to the expression of CD11 and CD18, should be performed. Structural abnormalities of neutrophils are best determined by careful examination of the **blood film.** More subtle neutrophil defects such as abnormal phagocytosis or chemotaxis can be evaluated by specialized testing such as the **Rebuck skin window and measurement of phagocytosis of beads or bacteria.**

Chronic granulomatous disease has traditionally been diagnosed by observing the ability of neutrophils to reduce nitroblue tetrazolium to form purple intracellular crystals following a phagocytic stimulus. Recently, fluorescence-based tests for the generation of superoxide and other reactive oxygen species have become available.

THERAPY

Patient management needs to reflect the specific cause of the abnormality in neutrophil number or function. The granulocytosis of patients with infections or inflammatory states will respond to the treatment of the primary condition. Marked increases in the granulocyte count as a result of a clonal malignancy need to be treated aggressively with appropriate chemotherapy and leukopheresis (Chapters 17 and 18). The management of patients with neutropenia or a qualitative disorder of granulocyte function can benefit significantly from antibiotic therapy and the appropriate use of recombinant G-CSF.

Antibiotic Therapy

Most patients with neutropenia or a functional defect of granulocytes present with recurrent infections of skin, mucous membranes, and upper and lower respiratory systems. The organisms responsible for the infections are the common organisms found on the skin and mucous membranes. Patients will develop recurrent staphylococcal skin infections, gingivitis, periodontitis, sinusitis, and pharyngitis with common enteric organisms. Because of this, prophylaxis is not very effective. Rather, patients should be aggressively treated with cidal antibiotics that are specific for the site and type of infection. Careful culture and sensitivity testing of bacterial isolates are extremely important to successful therapy.

Growth Factor Therapy

Whenever possible, the cause of the neutropenia should be addressed with appropriate therapy. Any drugs that may be responsible for a production defect should be withdrawn and drugs that can further suppress neutrophil production (Bactrim, H_2 blockers, tricyclic antidepressants, etc) must not be given. Patients with hematopoietic malignancies or autoimmune disease need to be treated with chemotherapy or marrow transplantation. These therapies provide the most effective long-term management strategy.

Recombinant G-CSF (filgrastim) and **GM-CSF** can help in managing the neutropenic patient. The strategy for the use of these growth factors varies for each condition. It is now routine to **use G-CSF as a part of marrow transplantation and multidrug chemotherapy protocols** to encourage the more rapid return of granulocyte production (5–10 μg/kg/day subcutaneously (SC) until the granulocyte count exceeds 10,000/μL). The duration of absolute neutropenia in patients receiving ablative chemotherapy and autologous marrow transplantation for lymphoma can be significantly reduced, thereby shortening the length of time patients spend on antibiotics, the risk of life-threatening bacteremia, and the incidence of fungal infections. **Children with cyclic neutropenia** clearly benefit from G-CSF therapy (5 μg/kg/day SC or less to keep the granulocyte count above 1500/μL). Although the treatment with the growth factor does not stop the cycling of the granulocyte count, it does decrease the severity of the granulocytopenia. By not allowing the granulocyte count to fall to below 1000/μL, children stop having recurrent infections. G-CSF therapy has also been approved for the **reversal of the neutropenia associated with HIV infection** (1–4 μg/kg/day SC) and the **prevention of worsening neutropenia** with therapy (300 μg/day). The use of growth factors in managing patients with qualitative disorders of granulocyte function still needs to be determined.

BIBLIOGRAPHY

Bone RC: The pathogenesis of sepsis. Ann Intern Med 1991;115:457.

Peterson L, Foucar K: Granulocytosis and granulocytopenia. In: Bick RL (editor): *Hematology: Clinical and Laboratory Practice.* CV Mosby, 1993.

Simon H et al: Abnormal clone of T-cells producing interleukin-5 in idiopathic eosinophilia. N Engl J Med 1999;341:1112.

Watts RG, Howard TH: Functional disorders of granulocytes and monocytes. In: Bick RL (editor): *Hematology: Clinical and Laboratory Practice.* CV Mosby, 1993.

Welte K et al: Filgrastim (r-metHuG-CSF): The first 10 years. Blood 1996;88:1907.

The Acute Myeloid Leukemias

The acute myeloid leukemias (AML) are clonal malignancies that are characterized by the appearance of **increased numbers of immature myeloid cells in the marrow and blood.** Although the fundamental oncogenic event takes place at the level of a very early progenitor cell, the malignant progeny are often capable of considerable differentiation. This has led to classification schemes that emphasize the morphologic characteristics of the cell, patterned after the classification of normal granulocytes.

AML can present as an **acute, catastrophic illness** in a patient who is otherwise healthy. On the other hand, it can be the **final outcome of other myeloproliferative diseases** such as chronic myeloid leukemia, polycythemia vera, myelofibrosis (myeloid metaplasia), or one of the **refractory anemias** (see Chapters 9, 12, and 18). Despite the differences in onset and morphologic appearance, the AMLs generally have a similar clinical presentation, prognosis, and treatment.

LEUKEMIA CLASSIFICATION

The most widely used classification scheme for AML is the "French-American-British" **(FAB) system** (Table 17–1). The FAB system is in reality a morphologic classification. Over the years, however, it has been bolstered by immunohistochemical and immunologic data, using markers for different stages of myeloid differentiation. Each has its strengths and weaknesses. Still, the **overriding principle of leukemia classification** is the placement of the malignant cell in the normal scheme of hematopoietic cell differentiation. Although this is generally satisfactory, lineage infidelity of the malignant cells can result in a mixture of features drawn from different cell lines. Recent modifications of the classification of acute leukemias proposed by a World Health Organization conference emphasize the **use of genetic information to identify subgroups** with considerable prognostic significance. This approach is likely to expand in the future.

Morphologic Classification

The maturation of myeloid cells in the marrow is relatively easily followed based on morphologic criteria (see Figure 15–2). Several characteristics of the maturation sequence are used in classifying the leukemic cell line. The first of these is the **appearance of cytoplasmic granules** in the maturing granulocytes. The most primitive (undifferentiated) myeloblasts have no granules and are difficult to distinguish from lymphoblasts. The earliest cells that can be identified as myelocyte progenitors contain primary (nonspecific) granules that appear as relatively large, purple (azurophilic) granules on the Wright's-Giemsa stain. As the cell line matures to the promyelocyte stage, primary granules become abundant and partially obscure the nucleus. Malignant myeloblasts and promyelocytes can also contain abnormal rod-shaped granules known as **Auer rods.** When present, Auer rods are by far the best criterion for identifying leukemic myeloid cells in the granulocytic lineage. As myelocytes mature further, they acquire **secondary granules** that are smaller and more heterogeneous in their staining properties. When cells follow the monocytic differentiation pathway, cytoplasmic granules are never as prominent as those in granulocytes. They are smaller, scantier, and remain pink to purple. The categorization of leukemias as myelomonocytic reflects the difficulty in distinguishing between immature cells of the granulocyte and monocyte lineages. Finally, **acute eosinophilic and basophilic (mast cell) leukemias** are readily identified from the distinctive granules within the cytoplasm.

Histochemical stains help confirm the granule content of a malignant cell line. The **peroxidase and specific esterase stains** detect the primary granules of myeloid cells. In contrast, the **nonspecific esterase stain** detects esterase activity in monocytes and is only weakly positive in immature myeloid cells. Both the **alkaline phosphatase** and **periodic acid–Schiff (PAS) stains** give a strong reaction with mature granulocytes. These stains are used in conjunction with conventional morphology in the FAB classification system.

The second most important morphologic criterion in the detection of a myeloid leukemia is the **morphology of the nucleus.** The chromatin of immature cells such as myeloblasts is characterized by a very fine, lacy pattern. As the cell matures, the chromatin becomes progressively more coarse or clumped. Moreover, the nature of the clumping is different in granulocytes, lymphocytes, and monocytes. The nucleus in the granulocyte lineage first folds at the metamyelocyte stage and then becomes seg-

Table 17–1. The FAB classification of acute myeloid leukemias.

Cell Type	FAB	Description	Incidence (%)[a]
Undifferentiated	M1	Blasts with bland characteristics	20
Myeloblastic	M2	Blasts with early granulocytic differentiation	30
Promyelocytic	M3	Clear promyelocytic characteristics	10
Myelomonocytic	M4	A mixture of granulocytic and monocytic characteristics	25
Monocytic	M5	Clear monocytic characteristics	10
Erythroleukemic	M6	Blasts with erythroid characteristics	4
Megakaryocytic	M7	Blasts with megakaryocytic properties	1

[a] Percentage of total AML cases.

mented, whereas the nucleus of the developing monocyte remains indented or horseshoe shaped. **Nucleoli** are another sign of immaturity. They are invariably present in immature blasts and are lost during normal maturation. Leukemic cells frequently have a nuclear chromatin pattern that is finer and more immature appearing than that of a corresponding normal cell. They also demonstrate multiple (three to five or more), often large, nucleoli that persist even as the cell cytoplasm matures.

Immunologic Classification

Several normal immunologic markers on myeloid cells can be detected by monoclonal antibodies. There are no markers that are specific for malignant myeloid cells. Therefore, the immunologic classification of a leukemia, like the morphologic classification, is an exercise in matching the malignant cell line to the normal pattern of hematopoietic cell differentiation.

The most commonly used **immunologic markers** for myeloid cells are summarized in Table 17–2. They are most useful in distinguishing myeloid from lymphoid leukemias and in helping determine the lineage of the myeloid leukemias. The immunologic classification of an acute leukemia does not always correlate with the morphologic appearance. For example, cells expressing monocyte markers may or may not have a morphology that suggests monocytic leukemia, and the

Table 17–2. Immunologic markers on myeloid cells and leukemias.

CD	Other Names	Normal Cells	Utility in AML
13	My7	Mono and myeloid	Distinguish AML from ALL
14	My4	Mature monocytes	Monocytic leukemias
15	My1	Mono and myeloid	Distinguish AML from ALL
33	My9	Mono and myeloid	Most consistent marker in AML
34	My10	Progenitor cells only	Most primitive marker, poor prognosis
41	GPIIb/IIIa	Megakaryocytes	Megakaryocytic leukemia
42	GPIb	Megakaryocytes	Megakaryocytic leukemia
45	HLE	All leukocytes	Frequently decreased in leukemias
117	cKit	Progenitor cells	Expressed with CD34 in most AML
—	HLA-DR	Mono and myeloid	Nearly always present on AML and ALL
—	Glycophorin	Erythrocytes	Erythroleukemia

degree of maturation suggested by the surface markers may not match morphologic features such as cytoplasmic granules and nuclear chromatin. Myeloid leukemias can also show **lineage infidelity** in that they express markers that are normally not present on the same cell or because they lack markers that should be present on the cells of a given lineage. Finally, it is common to find a heterogeneous expression of markers within the leukemic population. A patient who has nearly 100% blasts by morphology may show only 50% blasts by marker studies. This condition is usually owing to variations in the intensity of expression of the markers on the cells but could reflect true clonal diversity within the leukemic population.

Cytogenetic Abnormalities

Most cases of AML show some cytogenetic abnormality (Table 17–3). There is a great deal of diversity, however, in the types of abnormalities observed, and as yet, there are only a **few correlations between cytogenetic markers and either prognosis or response to therapy.**

A common abnormality in AML, present in about 10% of cases, and associated with a relatively poor prognosis, is trisomy of chromosome 8. The t(8;21) (q22;q22) translocation, seen in 40% of M2 AMLs, is associated with a somewhat better prognosis. Abnormalities of chromosome 11 are often found in secondary M4 and M5 AMLs after exposure to topoisomerase II inhibitors, whereas abnormalities of chromosome 16 are associated with a variant of M4 that shows pronounced eosinophilia. Several of the **key genes affected by these abnormalities** have been identified (Table 17–3). An important example is the translocation between chromosomes 15 and 17 t(15;17) q(22;11) that can be detected in most cases of promye-

locytic leukemia. It involves a gene that is part of the receptor for retinoic acid. **Retinoic acid** is a factor that induces differentiation in some cells and that has therapeutic activity in promyelocytic leukemia. It has been learned that most chromosomal abnormalities involve DNA transcription factors, oncogenes, and genes coding for myeloid growth factors. It is likely that the significance of these findings will increase in the future.

CLINICAL FEATURES

The AMLs usually present with some combination of **granulocytopenia, anemia, thrombocytopenia,** and the appearance of **immature cells (blasts)** in blood and marrow. The disease can present at any age but is uncommon in children. The classic presentation of AML in an otherwise healthy patient is most often seen in young adults. Older patients can present with atypical aspects such as a pre-existing myelodysplastic syndrome or a slow onset of the disease (**smouldering leukemia**). The incidence of AML increases dramatically after age 50 years; the median age of onset is now 64 years.

AML in younger patients is a catastrophic illness. The entire clinical history is seldom more than a few weeks long and is characterized by the sudden appearance of fatigue, fever, bacterial infections of the upper respiratory tract, bone pain, and various bleeding manifestations. These are signs and symptoms associated with marked anemia, granulocytopenia, and thrombocytopenia.

Less common presentations are seen in patients with various **subtypes of AML or monocytic leukemia.** Rarely, an AML patient will present with a tumor mass of myeloblasts, known as a **chloroma,** involving spinal column or orbit. Monocytic leukemia is more fre-

Table 17–3. Acute myeloid leukemias with recurrent cytogenetic abnormalities.

Abnormality	Approximate Frequency	Genes Involved	Prognostic Significance
t(8;21)(q22;22)	40% of M2 AML	AML1/ETO	Favorable
t(15;17)(q22;q11-22) (Promyelocytic)	10% of AML	PML/RARα	Favorable
inv(16)(p13q22) or t(16;16) (p13;q11)	Most M4 with abnormal marrow eosinophils	AML1/MYH11X	Favorable
11q23 abnormalities	6–8% of primary AML and 85% of secondary AML	MLL (mixed lineage leukemia)	Intermediate or unfavorable
del(5q) or monosomy 5	More common in older patients and secondary AML	Growth factor cluster	Unfavorable
Trisomy of chromosome 8	10% of AML	? AML1	Unfavorable

quently associated with malignant cell infiltrates in skin, gingiva, and central nervous system. Patients with high levels of primitive blasts (greater than 100,000/µL) can present with a leukostasis syndrome characterized by ischemia of multiple organs and both pulmonary and central nervous system dysfunction (**Ball's disease**). This situation is a true hematologic emergency and needs to be treated immediately with combination chemotherapy and leukopheresis to prevent death.

Most patients with AML develop bleeding because of their thrombocytopenia. Therefore, the **most common bleeding manifestations** are petechiae, gum bleeding, nose bleeds, and in women, menorrhagia. **Patients with acute promyelocytic leukemia are an exception** to this rule. They can present with significant prolongations of their prothrombin time (PT) and partial thromboplastin time (PTT) secondary to ongoing disseminated intravascular coagulation (DIC). These patients can have more prominent bruising and much more severe mucous membrane bleeding.

Physical findings in the AML patient include pallor from the anemia, skin and mucous membrane bleeding, aphthous ulcers, gingivitis and pharyngitis, and, on occasion, sternal tenderness. Lymphadenopathy and hepatosplenomegaly are seen in less than 20% of patients, and mediastinal lymphadenopathy is extremely rare, helping distinguish AML from a lymphopoietic malignancy.

Laboratory Studies

The key to the diagnosis of any leukemia is the study of blood and marrow morphology. When AML presents as a precipitous illness in a young or middle-aged adult, the blood film morphology may be enough to make the diagnosis. A **complete workup** should always include a marrow aspirate and biopsy for routine morphology, histochemical staining, and both immunophenotyping and chromosomal analysis. In patients who present with extensive bruising or severe mucous membrane bleeding, a **full coagulation profile** should be obtained to look for DIC.

A. COMPLETE BLOOD COUNT (CBC):

The CBC will demonstrate varying combinations of anemia, granulocytopenia, and thrombocytopenia, together with the appearance of abnormal immature cells (blasts) in circulation. The **total number of blasts will vary** from a small percentage of the circulating cells to an overwhelming, uniform population of primitive blasts, exceeding 50,000/µL. **Loss of other normal cell elements** also helps make the diagnosis. The malignant event responsible for proliferation of the leukemic cell line also blocks normal granulocyte, red blood cell, and platelet production. At the same time, small num-

bers of normal lymphocytes will still be present. **Presence of lymphocytes but absence of normal granulocytes** in circulation suggests involvement of the myeloid cell line in the leukemic process.

Up to 10% of leukemias can present as **aleukemic leukemia,** that is, as pancytopenia with few if any blasts in circulation. In this situation, **marrow aspirate and biopsy** invariably give the diagnosis. In patients who gradually evolve to AML as an endpoint of a myeloproliferative disorder, the pattern of the cytopenia may be quite variable. In addition, some of these patients will demonstrate a macrocytic anemia, marked poikilocytosis with nucleated red blood cells on the peripheral film, or both.

B. MARROW ASPIRATE AND BIOPSY:

A marrow aspirate and biopsy should be obtained in all patients. Sufficient material should be collected for routine morphology and histochemical staining, immunophenotyping, and chromosomal analysis. This process will require several aspirations and may involve several placements of the marrow aspirate needle.

A **marrow biopsy core** should be obtained from a separate site at some distance from the point of marrow aspiration to guarantee an adequate specimen. The biopsy is important to determine overall cellularity, the distribution of the malignant process, and any tendency to fibrosis. Rarely, an AML patient will present with a packed or even necrotic marrow that defies aspiration. In this case, the biopsy is critical.

C. HISTOCHEMICAL STAINS:

Histochemical staining of blood and marrow aspirate films is an integral part of the FAB classification of leukemia (Table 17–4). The most commonly used stains are the following:

1. Peroxidase stain—This stain **detects the myeloperoxidase enzyme** contained in the primary granules of myeloid cells. In the presence of hydrogen peroxide, myeloperoxidase releases free oxygen that can then be detected with benzidine or 3-amino-9-ethyl carbazole. The latter reagent gives a reddish-brown reaction product, whereas the benzidine reagent produces a bluish-black product. Myeloperoxidase is abundant in nearly all mature and immature myeloid cells and is also present in monocytes to a small extent. Recently, it has become possible to detect myeloperoxidase using a **monoclonal antibody and flow cytometry.** The increased sensitivity of this method has proven very useful in identifying even very immature myeloid leukemias that appear to be peroxidase negative by histochemistry.

2. Combined esterase stain—This stain uses two substrates, α-naphthyl acetate and naphthol ASD chloracetate, to distinguish myelocytes from monocytes. The

Table 17–4. Histochemical stains in the FAB classification of AML.

			Combined Esterase		
Cell Type	FAB	Peroxidase	Specific	Nonspecific	+NaF
Undifferentiated	M0	0	0	0	—
Minimal differentiation	M1	> 3%+	0–1+	0	—
Myeloblastic	M2	4+	4+	0	—
Promyelocytic	M3	4+	4+	1–2+	1–2+
Myelomonocytic	M4	3–4+	3+	3+	1–2+
Monocytic	M5	0–1+	0–1+	4+	0
Erythroleukemia	M6	0	0	0	—

chloracetate esterase stain (specific esterase) identifies the primary and secondary granules in myeloid cells. It gives a negative or very weak reaction in monocytes. Furthermore, it is resistant to treatment with sodium fluoride. The α-**naphthyl acetate stain** (nonspecific esterase) produces a strong reaction in monocytes, which is positive to a varying degree in mature and immature myeloid cells. The monocyte reaction is inhibited by sodium fluoride.

3. Periodic acid–Schiff (PAS) stain—This stain **involves the oxidation of carbohydrates by periodic acid to aldehyde products.** Mature myeloid cells stain intensely red; myeloblasts are usually negative. The PAS stain is useful in separating AML from acute lymphocytic leukemia; lymphoblasts can show heavy blocklike staining.

4. Leukocyte alkaline phosphatase stain—This stain is primarily **used in the differential diagnosis of chronic myelogenous leukemia from secondary leukemoid reactions.**

The interpretation of the histochemical stains requires considerable experience and judgment. Although they are a major component in the FAB classification (see Table 17–1), they must always be interpreted in the light of the overall morphology.

D. IMMUNOPHENOTYPING AND CYTOGENETICS:

Both **blood and marrow specimens** should be collected for immunophenotyping and cytogenetic studies. The most important immunologic markers on myeloid cells and their usefulness in the diagnosis and management of AML are listed in Table 17–2. **Chromosomal analysis** should be performed using high resolution banding techniques in order to identify common translocations. The **FAB classification** of leukemia is not based on either the immunologic or cytogenetic

studies. The information gained from these measurements, however, can in many circumstances confirm the diagnosis and in others provide prognostic information. This type of information is particularly useful in the case of very immature leukemias in which it can be difficult to distinguish between myeloid and lymphoid lineage. The **distinctive phenotype of the malignant cell line** can also be used once the patient enters remission to detect relapse at the earliest possible time.

E. OTHER LABORATORY STUDIES:

The growth of the myeloid cell tumor mass is associated with several metabolic abnormalities. The **serum lactic dehydrogenase (LDH)** level is elevated in most patients without significant changes in other liver chemistries. An elevation mirrors the rate of growth and turnover of the leukemic cells. Another indirect measure of myeloid cell proliferation is the level of **vitamin B_{12} binding proteins,** specifically transcobalamin III. In patients with myelomonocytic or monocytic leukemia, a high tumor burden is associated with an increased **excretion of muramidase (lysozyme)** in urine. This process can result in potassium wasting and hypokalemia. Finally, up to 20% of patients may have an elevated **serum uric acid level.**

DIAGNOSIS

An important element in diagnosing AML is the **speed of the workup.** This is especially true when AML presents as a precipitous illness in an otherwise healthy young adult, because successful management depends on the early initiation of appropriate chemotherapy. The time element is less important in patients who gradually evolve from a myeloproliferative disease into AML. In this situation, it can be to the patient's advantage to delay therapy until it is absolutely necessary.

It is also important to **determine whether the AML is secondary to some other factor** such as previous chemotherapy or radiation exposure. AML is the most common form of secondary malignancy following previous tumor therapy. For example, the risk of AML in patients treated for Hodgkin's disease with combination radiation/chemotherapy is 3–10% at 10–15 years. In addition, the incidence of AML as the final outcome in patients with myelodysplastic diseases, such as polycythemia vera and myelofibrosis, may be increased by treatment with specific chemotherapeutic agents. Both aplastic anemia and AML have also been associated with benzene exposure. These relationships are important since secondary AML generally carries a worse prognosis. The patient may be slow to achieve remission, relapse rapidly, or fail to recover normal hematopoiesis following chemotherapy.

Based on cellular morphology and histochemical staining, it should be possible to categorize a patient's leukemia according to the **FAB classification** (Table 17–1). The key decision points are the following:

- Does the patient have acute myelocytic versus acute lymphocytic leukemia?
- To which FAB category does the patient belong?

Therapy is initiated based on this information; it is unnecessary and unwise to wait for the results from chromosomal analysis. Although these results may affect long-term management and prognosis, they are not important in guiding the initial treatment decision.

The patient should also be **evaluated for a coagulopathy.** This process is very important in patients with acute promyelocytic leukemia (M3). Many of these patients present with ongoing DIC and a severe bleeding tendency, which can worsen in the early phases of treatment. A full coagulation profile including a platelet count, PT, PTT, thrombin time, fibrinogen level, split product or D-dimer level (or both), and both antithrombin III and α_2-antiplasmin levels should be measured prior to initiating chemotherapy.

THERAPY

Therapy for AML should **begin promptly after the diagnosis** is made. Because the disease is rapidly progressive, any delay can decrease the chance of therapeutic success. In elderly patients, the possibility of a sustained remission is less and in the case of extreme age or debility, only symptomatic therapy may be indicated. Age by itself is not a contraindication to therapy, and a sustained remission can be achieved even in patients older than 70 years of age. However, while complete remission rates in patients under age 50 years average 70%, older patients show overall rates of less than

40–50% and survivals of less than 12 months. This can be attributed to a higher incidence of unfavorable cytogenetics, multidrug resistance protein (MDR1) expression, and functional drug efflux.

Other **adverse prognostic factors,** besides age, include AML resulting from prior chemotherapy or myelodysplasia, an initial blast count in excess of 20,000/μL, an elevated LDH, and a poor initial performance status. **Patients who fall in a favorable prognostic group,** with a better than 85% chance of remission and low relapse rate, are younger and have either a t(15;17), t(8;21), or inv(16) mutation. **Unfavorable cases** have mutations involving more than two chromosomes, a deletion or abnormality of the long arm of chromosome 3 or 5, a t11q23 translocation, or monosomies of chromosomes 5 or 7. Regardless of age, these patients have a survival rate of less than 20% at 5 years.

Predictable complications such as anemia, thrombocytopenia, a coagulopathy, or infection should never delay therapy since they are unlikely to improve until a remission is obtained. They should be treated with appropriate transfusions and antibiotics at the same time the chemotherapy is begun. The **goal of therapy** is to ablate the leukemic cell line and allow normal progenitor cells to repopulate the marrow. This process will require a period of marrow aplasia and marked granulocytopenia that can extend for 1–4 weeks or even longer. Because of this, leukemia therapy must be carried out in a hospital setting, preferably in a dedicated cancer nursing unit.

General Guidelines

Reliable vascular access is essential and usually requires placement of an in-dwelling catheter (eg, Hickman-Broviac catheter). The patient should be hydrated and receive allopurinol 300–600 mg/day by mouth to prevent hyperuricemia as tumor cells are lysed. Serum electrolytes and CBCs need to be monitored on a daily or every-other-day basis. In those patients who are at risk for DIC, a full coagulation profile should be measured daily for the first several days of chemotherapy. Hypofibrinogenemia (fibrinogen less than 100 mg/dL) should be corrected by infusion of cryoprecipitate, whereas marked prolongations of the PT and PTT may be corrected with fresh frozen plasma. Promyelocytic leukemia patients may benefit from being prophylactically anticoagulated with heparin using a moderate-dose protocol (see Chapters 34 and 36). If bleeding is life-threatening, the patient should be treated with platelet transfusions and infusions of cryoprecipitate to correct hypofibrinogenemia (fibrinogen levels less than 100 mg/dL).

In the absence of severe cardiovascular disease, the **hematocrit** should remain in the vicinity of 25–30%

to decrease the frequency of red blood cell transfusions. **Platelet transfusions** should only be given when the platelet count falls below 10,000/μL in the patient with little or no bleeding, or 20,000/μL if the patient has significant mucous membrane bleeding or tends to bleed from venipuncture sites.

The **treatment of ongoing infection** must be very aggressive, and potential sources of infection should be eliminated. For example, infected teeth should be pulled, abscesses drained, and foreign bodies such as infected intravenous catheters removed and replaced. Good nursing **care of the mouth, skin, and rectum** is very important. Oral prophylaxis to prevent infection using an oral fluoroquinolone such as ciprofloxacin can be used. It is well tolerated and preserves the anaerobic gastrointestinal flora, thereby avoiding the problem of fungal overgrowth in the intestinal tract. It also appears to be effective in reducing the frequency of systemic infections with gram-negative bacteria.

Prophylactic antifungal therapy with nystatin, miconazole, and ketoconazole has been used in the past to prevent yeast colonization of the gastrointestinal tract as a source for systemic candidiasis. Newer antifungals, including fluconazole, may be more effective. Empiric **antiviral therapy** has also been recommended. Acyclovir, 250 mg/m^2 (5 mg/kg) intravenously every 8 hours, or famciclovir, 500 mg given orally every 8 hours during marked granulocytopenia, has been suggested for patients who are known to be at risk for recurrent herpes simplex oral lesions. Patients should also be tested for their **cytomegalovirus** (CMV) status. CMV negative patients should receive only CMV-negative or adequately leukodepleted blood products to avoid an acute CMV infection. Ganciclovir, given in a dose of 5 mg/kg twice daily, may be effective prophylaxis for CMV infection in those who are CMV seropositive or who have received marrow from a seropositive donor.

Empiric Antibiotic Therapy

If patients are not already febrile at the time of diagnosis, they soon become febrile with treatment. They should have thorough cultures to identify specific organisms. But even before a specific site of infection is identified, they need to receive empiric antibiotic therapy (Table 17–5). The choice of antibiotics will depend to some extent on what organisms are seen in each institution. The usual approach is to provide broad-spectrum coverage for both gram-negative and gram-positive organisms. A popular combination of antibiotics for this purpose is an **aminoglycoside** (gentamicin, tobramycin, or amikacin) **together with an antipseudomonal penicillin** (carbenicillin, ticarcillin, mezlocillin, or piperacillin).

Table 17–5. Empiric antibiotic therapy.

Prophylaxis
Gastrointestinal tract
 Nystatin suspension 20 mL swish and swallow or Clotrimazole troche PO qid
 Norfloxacin 400 mg PO q12h
Herpes simplex prevention
 Acyclovir 250 mg/m^2 IV q8h
Initial fever
Culture negative
 Gentamicin or tobramycin 1 mg/kg IV, followed by 1.5 mg/kg q8h
 Piperacillin 4 g IV q6h[a]
Culture positive for staphylococcus (possible catheter infection) or no response after 2 days
 Vancomycin 0.5–1.0 g IV q12h
Uncontrolled or relapsing fever after 4–6 days
Culture negative
 Amphotericin 0.5 mg/kg IV daily after 1-mg test dose
Culture positive for fungus
 Amphotericin 1.0 mg/kg IV daily
 5-Flucytosine 25 mg/kg PO q6h

---

[a] Alternatives: Double β-lactam or Bactrim plus a β-lactam.

If pseudomonas infection is considered unlikely, a **double β-lactam combination or Bactrim plus an antipseudomonal β-lactam** can be used. This offers the one advantage of decreasing the risk of oto- or nephrotoxicity. At the same time, it is not as effective in coverage of *Pseudomonas aeruginosa*. **Single-drug therapy** with ceftazidime, imipenem, or newer cephalosporins is a third alternative. It has the disadvantage of poor coverage for anaerobes and gram-positive bacteria and runs the risk of inducing β-lactam resistance.

Recent studies comparing oral amoxicillin-clavulanate plus ciprofloxacin to conventional intravenous regimens have shown that **oral antibiotics** can be used with equal efficacy in low-risk patients with neutropenia. However, most patients in these studies had a fever that complicated outpatient chemotherapy for a solid tumor; hospitalized patients with hematological malignancies are usually considered to be high-risk because of the severity and duration of their neutropenia.

Once initiated, **antibiotic coverage must be continued throughout the period of granulocytopenia,** until the absolute granulocyte count is greater than 500/μL. This is true even if the patient becomes afebrile during therapy. For most patients, the opposite will be true. Their fever will be poorly controlled, and in fact many patients will, after a brief period of improvement, experience recurrent chills and fever spikes. A careful examination of the patient, repeated chest x-ray, and blood cultures should be obtained with each episode of chills and fever, and the clinician should look for a drug-resistant bacterium or fungus. However, even when an organism cannot be isolated, **other antibiotics should be added** to the regimen. Vancomycin should be started as empiric therapy for *Staphylococcus epidermidis.* If this has little or no effect after 4–6 days, amphotericin B therapy should be initiated for a presumptive fungal infection.

Remission Induction

Chemotherapy protocols are in a constant state of evolution, and the specific regimen to be used may depend on the protocol in a given institution. Chemotherapy for AML can be divided into several phases: remission induction, consolidation, and maintenance. Marrow transplantation must also be considered as an important option for the younger AML patient (Figure 17–1).

A reasonable remission induction protocol is treatment with cytosine arabinoside and an anthracycline. **A typical protocol** would include cytosine arabinoside 100–200 mg/m² daily for 7 days and either daunorubicin 40–60 mg/m² or idarubicin 12–13 mg/m² for the first 3 days. This will ablate the leukemic marrow in most patients. If after 7–10 days a repeated bone marrow biopsy shows residual leukemic blasts, the regimen should be repeated. Ideally, the patient should undergo a 1- to 3-week period of severe pancytopenia followed by a return of normal hematopoiesis (Figure 17–2). Once a complete remission is achieved, the patient's blood and marrow morphology should appear normal. The frequency of complete remission in AML is currently reported as 65–75% overall; patients under the age of 50 years have a better chance of reaching a complete remission.

GM-CSF and G-CSF have been used postinduction chemotherapy to shorten the duration of severe neutropenia with only modest success—length of stay reductions of 3–4 days. At the same time, they significantly increase the cost of therapy. Growth factors can be given, however, without fear of decreasing the complete remission rate or promoting early relapse. To date, attempts to use growth factors to enhance the effect of chemotherapy by increasing the number of cells in S phase have not been successful. Whether growth factors can be used to increase drug dose intensity with consolidation, resulting in a better outcome, is still not clear.

All-*trans* retinoic acid (ATRA) is a relatively benign drug that induces differentiation in myeloid cells and is capable of inducing remission in 70–90% of cases of promyelocytic leukemia. This would appear to correlate with a chromosomal mutation in promyelocytic leukemia involving the receptor for retinoic acid.

However, studies have also shown that initial treatment with ATRA is followed by a high incidence of relapse. Therefore, it should be used in combination with conventional induction chemotherapy. Combined therapy has resulted in a long-term survival in the range of 70–90%. The **preferred maintenance regimen for promyelocytic leukemia** patients is continuous low-dose 6-mercaptopurine and methotrexate with intermittent ATRA. Furthermore, the incidence of severe coagulopathy would appear to be lower in patients treated with ATRA. **Complications of ATRA therapy** include hyperleukocytosis and an acute syndrome of cardiopulmonary and renal failure (RA syndrome). The syndrome will usually resolve rapidly if the patient is treated with dexamethasone 10 mg twice a day for several days. The hyperleukocytosis will also respond to hydroxyurea or induction chemotherapy.

After the patient achieves remission, the goal becomes one of first consolidating and then maintaining the remission. If the patient is under 50–55 years and has a histocompatible sibling who is willing to donate marrow, the best option is **allogeneic marrow transplantation.** The overall probability of disease-free survival after 5 years following allogeneic transplantation is approximately 45%. Patients between 15 and 35 years of age have disease-free survivals of greater than 70%. This rate is a significantly better result than that achieved with conventional chemotherapy. However, only 10–15% of patients meet the requirements for allogeneic transplantation. Even with the advent of the **nonrelated marrow donor** program, fewer than 30% of patients can receive transplants. Moreover, the use of an unrelated donor increases the risk of severe **graft-versus-host disease** (GVHD). Recent data suggest that high-dose **chemotherapy with autologous stem cell transplantation** offers results nearly as good as allogeneic transplantation and better than conventional chemotherapy.

Allogeneic Marrow Transplantation

The procedure of allogeneic marrow transplantation has become routine in recent years. Patients under the age of 50–55 years who present with AML should be **HLA typed** as soon as they enter first remission. All siblings and the patient's parents should also be HLA typed to identify a potential donor. If an identical or close HLA match is found, **further testing by mixed lymphocyte culture** is carried out to determine compatibility. When a family donor is not available, the patient's HLA type can be submitted for computer matching to the multinational **unrelated donor marrow registry.** This increases the chance of finding a compatible donor. Finally, the newest alternative is the **use of cord blood** from matched or one to three

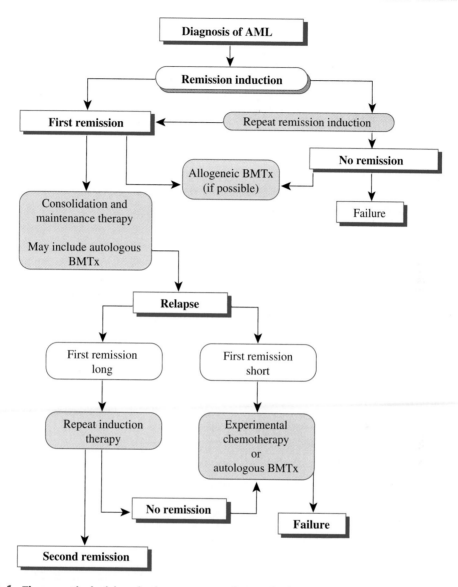

***Figure 17–1.* Therapeutic decisions in the treatment of AML.** The first step in the treatment of AML is to eradicate the malignant cell line and induce a first remission. The younger patients are then considered for allogeneic bone marrow transplantation if a matched sibling is available for marrow harvest. Otherwise, the patient is maintained on varying regimens of chemotherapy with or without autologous bone marrow transplantation.

antigen-mismatched unrelated donors. The greatest number of cord blood transplants have been done in children with acute leukemia or inborn errors of metabolism. The limited number of stem cells in cord blood makes it less useful in the treatment of adults. Even in children, marrow recovery in is slower because of the small number of transplanted stem cells. However, overall results are about the same as with adult un-

related donor transplants. Some evidence suggests that the severity, but not the frequency, of GVHD may be reduced through the use of cord blood stem cells.

The **overall results of transplantation** depend primarily on patient selection (Figure 17–3). In general, 40–70% of younger patients receiving transplants in first remission will experience a long-term disease-free survival, whereas patients who have relapsed and re-

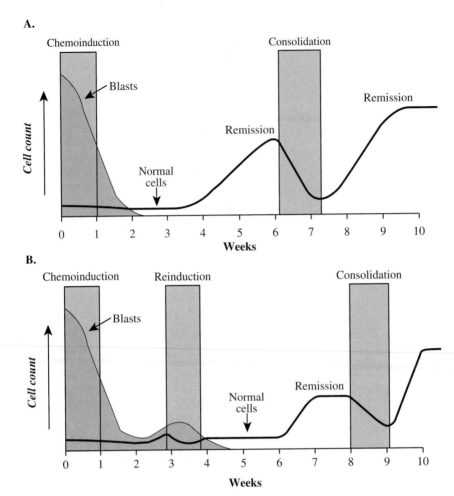

***Figure 17–2.* Remission induction and consolidation.** The patient is initially treated with two or more drugs to eradicate the leukemic cell line. The sequence of drug therapy will depend on the patient's response as follows: **A:** 60% or more of patients will achieve a complete remission with the first chemoinduction course of therapy. They can then be consolidated with a second course of therapy after 6–7 weeks. **B:** Patients who do not achieve a remission with the initial chemoinduction will need a second course of (reinduction) therapy to achieve a complete remission.

ceive transplants in second or subsequent remission have survivals of 20–40%. **Age** is a very important factor. Older patients have more difficulty with GVHD. The **karyotype at the time of diagnosis** is another prognostic indicator. Patients with an abnormal chromosome 5 or 7 (or both) or a hypodiploid karyotype have a far worse outcome.

A. GRAFT-VERSUS-HOST DISEASE (GVHD):

GVHD can be acute (with an onset within weeks or months of transplant) or chronic. Chronic GVHD can occur without a preceding acute phase. GVHD is the result of the engrafted donor immune system reacting

to host histocompatibility antigens. Donor cytotoxic lymphocytes attack normal host tissues, especially the skin, intestinal tract, and liver. Skin involvement can vary widely, from a transient rash to severe exfoliative dermatitis. The most prominent intestinal symptom is usually diarrhea, while liver dysfunction is obstructive in nature with considerable variation in severity.

Treatment of acute GVHD consists of partial immunosuppression with cyclosporin, methotrexate, and prednisone. Any immunosuppressive therapy administered during the first several months following marrow transplant has the unwanted side effect of interfering with reconstitution of normal marrow function and in-

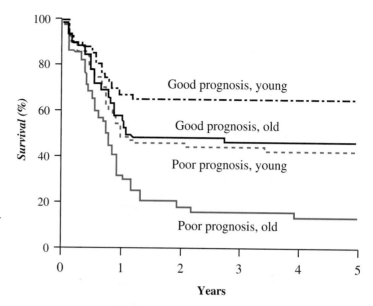

Figure 17–3. **Allogeneic bone marrow transplantation in AML.** Younger patients who respond well to chemotherapy and receive transplants in first remission have an excellent chance of long-term disease-free survival. Older patients, patients with less-responsive tumors, and those who receive transplants later in the disease process have less-successful results. Patients with severe GVHD also have a poor prognosis.

creasing the probability of infection. Still, most cases of acute GVHD can be controlled. The incidence of severe acute GVHD is approximately 25%.

Chronic GVHD most commonly affects the skin with disease that resembles scleroderma, Sjögren's syndrome, or both. Its severity is highly variable and treatment is less satisfactory. Agents such as cyclosporin, steroids, antilymphocyte antibodies, and azathioprine have been used to control it. Patients with chronic GVHD have profound immune dysfunction and remain at risk for opportunistic infections.

A reciprocal **relationship exists between GVHD and relapse,** the two most common complications of transplantation. Measures that are effective in eliminating GVHD, such as removing donor T lymphocytes from the marrow prior to transplantation, invariably lead to a higher incidence of relapse. This result has led to the concept of a "**graft versus leukemia**" **effect,** which is the result of donor cytotoxic T-cells directing their attack against residual leukemic cells. The importance of this effect would appear to be supported by the survival statistics for various donor-recipient pairs. For example, identical twin transplants and HLA-identical sibling transplants without GVHD run a higher incidence of leukemia relapse than those sibling transplants that result in moderate GVHD.

B. OTHER COMPLICATIONS:

The other major clinical complications of allogeneic marrow transplantation are **interstitial pneumonitis** and **venoocclusive disease** (**VOD**) of the liver. The latter condition is a syndrome of mild to very severe liver

dysfunction occurring early after the transplant, in the absence of acute GVHD. Its cause is unclear, but it may be related to the combined effects of high-dose chemotherapy and the radiation therapy used in preparing for the transplant. Treatment has not been very satisfactory, and severe VOD can result in the patient's death. Recent trials of fibrinolytic therapy and the GPIIa/IIIb platelet inhibitors have been encouraging.

Maintenance Chemotherapy/Autologous Marrow Transplantation

In the absence of an HLA-matched donor, or when the patient is above 50 years of age, a chemotherapy protocol consisting of intensive consolidation followed by prolonged maintenance therapy can be offered. Many such **postremission protocols** have been evaluated. They involve the repeated use of cytosine arabinoside plus an anthracycline with the addition of 6-thioguanine, vincristine, prednisone, cyclophosphamide, and other drugs in combinations designed to minimize the development of drug resistance in the leukemic cell line. Unfortunately, no magic combination has been discovered. Most centers report a median duration of complete remission of 12–18 months and a 2- to 3-year survival rate of 20–40%. Long-term survivals are generally thought to be approximately 10–15% or less.

Intensive chemotherapy has recently been **combined with autologous marrow or stem cell transplantation** (see Chapter 22) in an attempt to increase the effectiveness of chemotherapy. The use of the patient's own remission peripheral blood stem cells, which may or may not be treated to remove residual leukemic cells, may offer a viable alternative to the use of allogeneic marrow. Patients treated with autologous transplantation have a higher relapse rate than those undergoing allogeneic transplantation, but have a similar overall survival because of the decrease in procedure-related mortality associated with autologous transplantation. Both forms of transplant appear to be superior to conventional chemotherapy.

Once the patient relapses, the prognosis is poor. It is frequently difficult to achieve a second or third remission. As a rule, if the first remission was a relatively long one (6–12 months), then **standard induction therapy** is used a second time. Newer drugs such as etoposide and mitoxantrone, as well as high-dose cytosine arabinoside, are alternatives. When the patient is younger and in good health, an **autologous marrow transplantation** as a part of the treatment of a first relapse may increase the chances of a second remission. Early results with the use of allogeneic or autologous transplantation to salvage relapsed patients suggest long-term survival rates of 20–25%, which appear to be better than those for conventional chemotherapy. If the patient relapses more than one time, subsequent remissions are usually short and nearly always eventually fatal.

Emerging Therapies

Several innovative therapies are under active investigation, including antibody-based therapy using an unmodified antibody to CD33, antibody-toxin conjugates, radiolabeled antibodies in combination with bone marrow transplantation, antisense nucleotides with sequences complementary to gene-specific mRNA, MDR-1 reversing agents, and tumor vaccines.

BIBLIOGRAPHY

Diagnosis

Baer MR, Bloomfield CD: The clinical significance of biological characteristics of the cells in acute myeloid leukemia. Ann Rev Med 1991;42:381.

Ball ED: Immunophenotyping of acute myeloid leukemia cells. Clin Lab Med 1990;10:721.

Goasquen JE, Bennett JM: Classifications of acute myeloid leukemia. Clin Lab Med 1990;10:661.

Harris NL et al: The World Health Organization classification of hematological malignancies. Report of the Clinical Advisory committee meeting, Arlie House, Virginia, November 1997. Mod Pathol 2000;13:193.

Lowenberg B, Downing JR, Burnett A: Acute myeloid leukemia. N Engl J Med 1999;341:1051.

Stone RM, Mayer RJ: The unique aspects of acute promyelocytic leukemia. J Clin Oncol 1990;8:198.

Therapy

Appelbaum FR: Bone marrow transplantation for acute nonlymphocytic leukemia. Cancer Treat Rev 1990;50:201.

Armitage JO: Bone marrow transplantation. N Engl J Med 1994;330;827.

Casselith PA et al: Autologous bone marrow transplant in acute myeloid leukemia in first remission. J Clin Oncol 1993;11:314.

Clift RA et al: Allogeneic marrow transplantation during untreated first relapse of acute myeloid leukemia. J Clin Oncol 1992;10:1723.

Degos L: All trans retinoic acid as a differentiating agent in the treatment of acute promyelocytic leukemia. Blood 1995;85:2643.

Fenaux P et al: A randomized comparison of all transretinoic acid (ATRA) followed by chemotherapy and ATRA plus chemotherapy and the role of maintenance therapy in newly diagnosed acute promyelocytic leukemia. Blood 1999;94:1192.

Ferrant A et al: Karyotype in acute myeloblastic leukemia: Prognostic significance for bone marrow transplantation in first remission: A European Group for Blood and Marrow Transplantation study. Blood 1997;90:2931.

Freifeld A et al: A double-blind comparison of empirical oral and intravenous antibiotic therapy for low-risk febrile patients with neutropenia during cancer chemotherapy. N Engl J Med 1999;341:305.

Kern WV et al: Oral versus intravenous empirical antimicrobial therapy for fever in patients with granulocytopenia who are receiving cancer chemotherapy. N Engl J Med 1999;341:312.

Leith CP et al: Acute myeloid leukemia in the elderly: Assessment of multidrug resistance (MDR1) and cytogenetics distinguishes biologic subgroups with remarkably distinct responses to standard chemotherapy. A Southwest Oncology Group study. Blood 1997;89:3323.

Schiffer CA: Hematopoietic growth factors as adjuncts to the treatment of acute myeloid leukemia. Blood 1996;88:3675.

Tallman MS et al: All-trans-retinoic acid in acute promyelocytic leukemia. N Engl J Med 1997;337:1021.

Wagner JE et al: Successful transplantation of HLA-matched and HLA-mismatched umbilical cord blood from unrelated donors: Analysis of engraftment and acute graft-versus-host disease. Blood 1996;88:795.

Zittoun RA et al: Autologous or allogeneic bone marrow transplantation compared with intensive chemotherapy in acute myelogenous leukemia. N Engl J Med 1995;332:217.

Myeloproliferative Disorders

Similar to the acute myeloid leukemias, the **myeloproliferative disorders** are clonal malignancies of the hematopoietic stem cell. In contrast to acute leukemia, however, they tend to have a more protracted clinical course and exhibit abnormalities of more than one hematopoietic cell line. It is also clear that many patients can show overlapping aspects of the individual disorders, providing a challenge to the clinician in the classification and management of the disease state.

The diseases that are commonly classified as **myeloproliferative disorders** are displayed in Table 18–1. The list includes chronic myelogenous leukemia (CML), myelofibrosis (myeloid metaplasia), myelodysplasia (preleukemia), polycythemia vera, essential thrombocythemia, and paroxysmal nocturnal hemoglobinuria (PNH). Several of the **dysplastic anemias** also share features with the myeloproliferative disorders. These include the refractory anemias, ringed sideroblastic anemia, refractory anemia with excess blasts, and some instances of aplastic anemia.

CLASSIFICATION

The clinical diagnosis of a myeloproliferative disorder is usually made based on the morphologic pattern of cell involvement (Table 18–2). The names of the several disorders mirror the morphologic abnormalities. Thus, **CML** is characterized by uncontrolled expansion of the myeloid cell lines, whereas **essential thrombocythemia** shows prominent megakaryocyte expansion with excessive platelet production. **Polycythemia vera** (see Chapter 12) is an example of a clonal malignancy resulting in uncontrolled red blood cell production as the predominant feature. These three conditions can share morphologic features, however, which makes the diagnosis more difficult. For example, it is not unusual for polycythemia vera patients to have increased granulocyte and platelet counts. In fact, the platelet count can increase to levels in excess of 1 million/μL, similar to levels in the patient with essential thrombocythemia.

Myelofibrosis (myeloid metaplasia) and **PNH** are disorders that generally present with decreased levels of cell production. They demonstrate varying combinations of anemia, leukopenia, and thrombocytopenia. **Marrow morphology** is very important in their diagnosis, especially myelofibrosis. A dramatic increase in reticulin fibers and collagen together with a loss of normal hematopoietic cells provides the basis for diagnosis. Both myelofibrosis and PNH can appear de novo or develop as part of another myeloproliferative disorder. Therefore, the interpretation of the morphologic findings must be made in light of the patient's clinical course.

Immunophenotyping is generally not helpful in classifying the myeloproliferative diseases. **Genetic analysis** is of particular value in CML. The identification of a morphologically abnormal chromosome, the **Philadelphia (Ph[1]) chromosome,** more than 30 years ago, was a landmark in the use of chromosomal analysis in disease diagnosis. The implications of this chromosome aberration have become clear with time. The Ph[1] chromosome is actually a translocation of the Abelson proto-oncogene from chromosome 22 to the long arm of chromosome 9, t(9;22) (Figure 18–1). The result of this translocation is the approximation of the ABL gene to the **breakpoint cluster region (BCR)** to form a BCR-ABL fusion gene generally with the expression of a p210 fusion protein. This appears to activate the RAS pathway to both increase progenitor cell proliferation and decrease myeloid cell apoptosis. In the early phases of the disease the malignant cells retain the ability to differentiate, giving rise to increased numbers of apparently normal granulocytes. However, over time, there is a progressive failure to differentiate, resulting in increasing numbers of blasts that may appear to be of either myeloid or lymphoid lineage.

Table 18–1. Classification of myeloproliferative diseases.

Chronic myelogenous leukemia
Idiopathic myelofibrosis (myeloid metaplasia)
Myelodysplasia
  Chronic myelomonocytic leukemia (CMML)
  Preleukemia
Primary thrombocythemia
Paroxysmal nocturnal hemoglobinuria
Polycythemia vera (see Chapter 12)
Dysplastic anemias (see Chapter 9)

Table 18–2. Morphologic patterns of the myeloproliferative disorders.

Disease	Morphologic Characteristics
Chronic myelogenous leukemia	Marked increase of myelocytes in marrow and blood Absolute basophilia Normal or increased platelet count Increase in megakaryocytes
Myelofibrosis	Moderate to marked normocytic anemia with nucleated red blood cells and "teardrop" forms Marrow fibrosis (increase in reticulin and collagen) Increase in megakaryocytes
Myelodysplasia (preleukemia, CMML)	Modest increase or decrease in mature granulocytes Increase in "blast" forms in marrow and blood Marrow hyperplasia with increase in myelomonocyte precursors
Primary thrombocythemia	Normal red blood cell, granulocyte counts Marked increase in platelet count, marrow megakaryocytes
Paroxysmal nocturnal hemoglobinuria	Hemolytic episodes leading to an iron deficiency, microcytic anemia Pancytopenia Marrow hypoplasia to aplasia

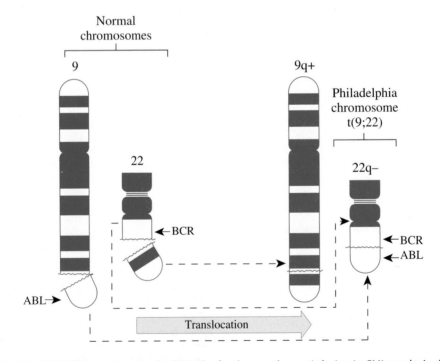

Figure 18–1. **The BCR-ABL translocation in CML.** The fundamental genetic lesion in CML results in the translocation of the ABL oncogene, normally on chromosome 9, to the BCR gene on chromosome 22. The resulting BCR-ABL gene product plays a role in the malignant transformation of the hematopoietic stem cell. The shortened, abnormal chromosome 22 (22q–) is recognized as the Philadelphia chromosome.

More recently, clonal karyotypic abnormalities have been described in several of the other chronic myeloproliferative disorders. Some of the most common of these are shown in Table 18–3.

CLINICAL FEATURES

The clinical presentation of a patient with a myeloproliferative disorder will reflect the pattern of abnormalities in cell production and function. Early in the disease process, **CML patients** demonstrate dramatic **increases in the number of mature and immature myelocytes** in circulation and tissues. The CML patient may complain of **abdominal discomfort secondary to massive splenomegaly.** White blood cells accumulate in the spleen to the point where they jeopardize the normal blood supply. This condition can result in splenic infarction, presenting clinically as moderate to severe left upper quadrant pain made worse with deep inspiration. Patients generally have abdominal tenderness with or without peritoneal signs, and in some cases, a friction rub heard over the spleen with respiration. CML patients may also seek medical attention because of a worsening anemia or, rarely, because of easy bruising and abnormal bleeding.

   Patients with myelodysplasia (preleukemia) or severe **myelofibrosis** (myeloid metaplasia) usually present with symptoms and signs of **severe anemia or pancytopenia.** Myelofibrotic patients can demonstrate impressive **splenomegaly,** especially when there is significant extramedullary hematopoiesis. Unlike CML patients, myelofibrosis patients do not often present with splenic infarction, even when the spleen is so enlarged that it extends below the iliac crest. Preleukemia and myelofibrosis patients can exhibit **thrombocytopenia** or **thrombocytosis** with platelet dysfunction lead-

Table 18–3. Common cytogenetic abnormalities in myeloproliferative disorders.

Syndrome	Abnormality
CML—chronic phase	t(9;22) (Ph[1] chromosome)
CML—blast phase	Extra Ph[1] chromosome
	Monosomy 7, 8, 17, 19
	Trisomy 8
Myelofibrosis	Trisomy 1q
	Deletions 13, 20, and 21
Myelodysplasia	Trisomy 8
	Deletions 5, 7, 9, 20, and 21
	Monosomy 7 or 9
	5q minus syndrome
	Loss of X or Y

ing to an increased bleeding tendency. Generally, this condition manifests as purpura and an increased tendency to mucous membrane and gastrointestinal bleeding. Petechial eruptions are less common.

   PNH patients can present with classic episodes of **nocturnal hemoglobinuria or with a pancytopenia** more reminiscent of a hypoplastic or aplastic anemia. They are at increased risk for thrombosis and can present with a portacaval thrombosis, Budd-Chiari syndrome, mesenteric artery thrombosis, or massive skin infarction (see Chapter 9).

Laboratory Studies

The complete blood count (CBC) and marrow aspirate and biopsy are key studies in the diagnosis of these disorders.

A. COMPLETE BLOOD COUNT (CBC):

The CBC provides an accurate measure of the absolute numbers of the red blood cell, white blood cell, and platelet components. It also will reveal increased numbers of immature myeloid progenitors in circulation. Inspection of the blood film can be very helpful, since automated counters are not as sensitive to the appearance of blasts or the subtle differences between immature myelocytes and monocytes. Furthermore, film inspection will permit a more careful evaluation of red blood cell morphology. This helps in the diagnosis of myelofibrosis where the appearance of teardrop red blood cells, schistocytes, and nucleated red blood cells is characteristic of progressive fibrosis of the marrow and extramedullary hematopoiesis in the liver and spleen.

B. SPECIAL STAINS:

Special stains are not as useful in the diagnosis of myeloproliferative disorders as they are in acute leukemia. An absolute basophil count using a **toluidine blue stain** is of value in diagnosing CML. The normal basophil count should be less than $50/\mu L$; CML patients almost always have basophil counts in excess of $50–100/\mu L$. A **stain for leukocyte alkaline phosphatase** has also been used to diagnosis CML since the chromosomal translocation is somehow associated with a decreased synthesis of the enzyme. At presentation, most CML patients have low to absent levels of leukocyte alkaline phosphatase. This finding is not unique to CML, however. Patients presenting with PNH, myelofibrosis, and other myelodysplastic syndromes can have reduced leukocyte alkaline phosphatase levels. In contrast, patients with secondary leukemoid reactions have normal to elevated levels.

C. MARROW ASPIRATE AND BIOPSY:

The marrow aspirate and biopsy are essential to the diagnosis of the myeloproliferative disorders. The **mar-**

row aspirate provides information as to individual cell morphology and the distribution of cell types. It also provides essential information in diagnosis and management of patients with CML as they become increasingly dysplastic and evolve to acute leukemia. The **marrow biopsy** provides information regarding the overall cellularity and changes in marrow structure. Diagnosis of myelofibrosis depends on the demonstration of increased amounts of reticulin fibers and collagenous tissue. A **silver stain for reticulin fibers** and a **trichrome stain for collagen** can both help in detecting early changes in marrow structure.

D. CHROMOSOMAL STUDIES:

Chromosomal studies of peripheral blood and marrow are important, primarily to distinguish CML from the other myeloproliferative disorders (Table 18–3). The **karyotype of banded metaphase cells** should reveal the presence or absence of the Ph[1] chromosome, as well as other chromosomal abnormalities in patients with CML and other myeloproliferative disorders. The most common abnormalities seen are loss of or deletions within chromosome 5, loss of chromosome 7, trisomy of chromosomes 8 and 9, and deletions within chromosomes 13 and 20. Moreover, the loss of all or part of chromosome 5 (**5q minus syndrome**) appears to be of prognostic importance. This syndrome is associated with a relatively prolonged course, pronounced anemia, and less frequent transformation to acute leukemia.

More sensitive molecular genetics techniques are now available that can detect small numbers of abnormal cells. They have been used to detect residual tumor cells in treated CML patients. For example, the BCR-ABL fusion gene can be identified in small numbers of cells using **polymerase chain reaction (PCR), DNA and RNA blotting techniques, and specific DNA probes.** PCR is capable of detecting translocations in fewer than 1 in 10,000 cells. However, at this level it is also possible to detect mutations that are not clinically important.

E. OTHER LABORATORY TESTS:

Other laboratory signs of increased proliferation of cells typical of myeloproliferative disorders include an increase in the **vitamin B_{12} binding proteins** (transcobalamins I and III) and, because of this, very high vitamin B_{12} levels. **Uric acid** and **lactic dehydrogenase (LDH) levels** may also be increased in patients with large tumor masses. Myelodysplastic patients, especially those presenting with pancytopenia, should be tested for PNH. A simple screening test is the **sugar water test.** This involves adding one part of the patient's blood to nine parts of a sugar water solution made up of 10 grams of sucrose dissolved in 100 mL of distilled water. After a 30-minute incubation at room temperature, the

specimen is centrifuged and the supernatant inspected for hemolysis. The **acid hemolysis test (Ham's test)** can also be used to detect PNH. This test uses a change in pH to detect the sensitivity of the red blood cell membrane to hemolysis (see Chapters 9 and 11). **Flow cytometry measurements of cell-surface antigens** provide a more sensitive and reliable detection method. The underlying molecular defect in PNH is a loss of those surface membrane proteins that are anchored by binding to phosphatidylinositol (the GPI-linked proteins). This leads to the decreased expression of several cell-surface antigens, including CD16, 48, 55, and 59.

DIFFERENTIAL DIAGNOSIS

The diagnosis of the individual myeloproliferative disorders can usually be made from the clinical presentation, the routine CBC and marrow aspirate, and, in the case of CML, the chromosomal analysis.

CHRONIC MYELOGENOUS LEUKEMIA (CML)

CML is a disease of middle age; the peak incidence falls in the fifth decade of life. It is observed, however, in younger and older individuals, and the Ph[1] chromosome marker can be found occasionally in children and adults with acute leukemias. CML is a leukemia that may be induced by environmental factors.

CML patients may first be detected from a **routine CBC** or because of **nonspecific complaints** such as weight loss, fatigue, night sweats, abdominal fullness, or episodes of abdominal pain. They usually do not have abnormal bleeding or an increased tendency to infections. On physical examination, most CML patients have **splenomegaly,** whereas fewer than one-third have hepatomegaly. Patients with very large spleens and acute left upper quadrant abdominal pain may have splenic infarction and may demonstrate a splenic friction rub.

Laboratory Studies

A. COMPLETE BLOOD COUNT (CBC):

The CBC usually points to the diagnosis (Table 18–4). The number of circulating mature and immature granulocytes can be markedly increased. Counts of 50,000–200,000/μL or higher are common. Most of these cells are mature granulocytes, although metamyelocytes, myelocytes, promyelocytes, and even a few blasts may be observed. The spectrum of cells in circulation closely resembles the maturation sequence of the myelocyte lineage in the marrow. There are abnormalities, however, in the white blood cell display that can be used to confirm the diagnosis, including an **increase in the ba-**

Table 18–4. Chronic myelogenous leukemia hematopoietic profile.

Complete blood count (CBC)
  Hemoglobin: Normal or slightly decreased
  White blood cell count: Markedly increased
    (50,000–200,000/μL)
  Increased numbers of metamyelocytes, myelocytes,
    promyelocytes, and blasts in circulation
  Platelet count: Normal or increased
  Basophil count: Greater than 50/μL
Marrow
  Hypercellular (decreased fat)
  E/G ratio: 1:4–1:10 (myelocytic hyperplasia)
  Increased numbers of megakaryocytes
  Variable fibrosis, increase in reticulin
Special studies
  Leukocyte alkaline phosphatase: decreased
  Ph^1 chromosome; present in more than 90% of patients

---

sophil count to levels greater than 50/μL **and the loss of leukocyte alkaline phosphatase activity.** Some CML patients may also show an impressive eosinophilia, although this is not diagnostically specific.

At presentation, CML patients are usually not very anemic. In fact, their hemoglobin level can be normal or even slightly elevated. Similarly, the **platelet count** may be low, normal, or elevated. With higher platelet counts, platelet function can be abnormal and associated with a tendency to increase bruising. Although the malignant event responsible for CML involves the most primitive hematopoietic stem cell, there is usually no early evidence of lymphocyte dysfunction. Late in the course of the disease, some patients may become clinically similar to those with acute lymphocytic leukemia (ALL).

B. OTHER TESTS:

Even when the clinical diagnosis is easy, the patient's **peripheral blood and marrow should be studied** for the presence of the t(9;22)-(q34;q11) translocation to form the BCR-ABL hybrid gene (Ph^1 chromosome) and other **chromosomal abnormalities.** The fusion mRNA that results is translated into a chimeric protein called **p210.** This protein then interacts with **RAS,** a guanosine triphosphate-binding protein responsible for cell proliferation and differentiation. By standard banded karyotype technique, approximately 5–10% of CML patients will appear to be Ph^1-negative. Some of these patients can be shown by DNA probe techniques to still demonstrate BCR-ABL fusion products, whereas others are truly negative and probably represent patients with refractory anemia with excess blasts (see Chapter 9) or an evolving preleukemic state.

Although the **t(9;22) translocation** is the hallmark of CML, it is also detected in 10–20% of adults and 2–5% of children with ALL. Most of these patients have a unique breakpoint **BCR-ABL translocation** resulting in a smaller p190 fusion protein. Expession of p190 can also be associated with a pronounced monocytosis in some patients. Another CML variant, Ph^1-positive chronic neutrophilic leukemia with thrombocytosis, demonstrates a novel breakpoint BCR-ABL translocation with a p230 protein product. In general, the clinical character of the disease reflects the size of the BCR fragment and protein product. Larger BCR fragments are associated with larger protein products and more mature disease phenotypes.

Phases of the Disease Process and Genetic Factors

Initially, CML is a slowly progressive disease. The excessive proliferation of marrow progenitors, the expansion of the mature granulocyte and platelet pools, and the tendency to hepatosplenomegaly are the major manifestations of the clonal defect. Early release of marrow granulocytes and their precursors and reduced apoptosis also play a role in producing the very high peripheral white blood cell counts. **Prognostic features at the time of diagnosis** include age greater than 60 years, massive splenomegaly, a platelet count less than 150,000 or greater than 700,000 μL, increased numbers of blasts or metaphases in the marrow, basophilia (greater than 7% on the CBC or greater than 3% mast cells in the bone marrow), and chromosomal abnormalities other than the Ph^1 chromosome.

A. CHRONIC PHASE:

As long as the granulocyte and platelet counts are kept under control with chemotherapy, the patient is asymptomatic. This is referred to as the **chronic phase** of CML. Depending on the mix of prognostic features, it can last for less than 1 year or, in the occasional patient, more than a decade.

B. ACCELERATED PHASE:

On the average, the chronic phase of CML lasts for 3–5 years before symptoms and signs of more aggressive disease (the **accelerated phase**) appear. At this point, the patient complains of fatigue, weight loss, night sweats, and at times, bone pain. Hepatosplenomegaly worsens with accompanying abdominal discomfort, and control of the proliferation of both granulocytes and platelets becomes much more difficult. Counts rise to high levels, which places the patient at risk for widespread tissue infiltration by white blood cells. Patients can develop lymphadenopathy and nodular tumors of the skin (**chloromas**) that on biopsy have the appearance of marrow tissue. Some patients may also exhibit progressive fibrosis of the marrow that further stimulates the development of extramedullary hematopoiesis and tissue infiltrates.

C. BLAST CRISIS:

As the disease progresses, the number of primitive blasts in the marrow and peripheral blood continues to increase. In less than 1 year in the accelerated phase, most patients will evolve to an acute leukemia–like picture, referred to as a **blast crisis.** The number of blasts needed to declare a blast crisis is unclear. However, once the patient demonstrates other manifestations of leukemia, including worsening anemia, thrombocytopenia, and a sufficient loss of mature granulocytes to put the patient at risk for infections, there is no question that the patient is in the final phase of his or her illness.

D. GENETIC TESTS:

Most terminal leukemias in CML involve the myeloid lineage, although 20–30% appear to be lymphoblastic in nature. Since the latter are more responsive to therapy, it is important to **phenotype the blasts to characterize their lineage,** whether myeloid or lymphoid. **Genotyping** is also important. Cytogenetic changes including monosomies or trisomies of chromosomes 7, 8, 17, and 19, additional translocations, and the appearance of an extra Ph[1] chromosome occur in 50–80% of patients. Trisomy 8 is the most common finding in patients undergoing transformation to blastic stage. The appearance of multiple chromosomal defects is another poor prognostic sign.

Detection of the BCR-ABL translocation by PCR has also been used to assess the patient's response to therapy. A PCR assay of minimal residual disease is the most sensitive measure of the effectiveness of treatment. Up to 80% of bone marrow transplant patients will demonstrate a negative PCR for the BCR-ABL translocation. In contrast, most patients treated with interferon show residual disease even after a year of therapy. Furthermore, a cytogenetic relapse by PCR will usually precede a recognizable clinical relapse, allowing earlier salvage therapy.

MYELOFIBROSIS (MYELOID METAPLASIA)

Myelofibrosis can present as a de novo illness or as a secondary manifestation of CML or polycythemia vera. Like both of the other disorders, it is a disease of the middle-aged and older patient populations. Studies of G6PD isoenzymes and cytogenetic abnormalities have shown that it is a clonal malignancy involving all hematopoietic cell lineages. However, although marrow fibrosis is its most distinguishing feature, the malignant change does not involve the fibroblasts and marrow reticuloendothelial cells. Instead, the **fibrosis** appears to be a reaction to the malignant stem cell line, especially the proliferation of megakaryocytes, and is **associated with the release of several growth factors** (transforming growth factor-β, platelet-derived growth factor, interleukin-1, and fibroblast growth factor). Recently, high levels of thrombopoietin have been demonstrated in patients with myelofibrosis, suggesting perhaps a cause for the megakaryocyte expansion. Even advanced marrow fibrosis has been shown to reverse with bone marrow transplantation or 2-CdA therapy.

Patients with **idiopathic myelofibrosis,** like CML patients, present with **nonspecific symptoms** and signs of easy fatigability, malaise, abdominal distention, and at times, abdominal pain. **Marked splenomegaly** that results from extramedullary hematopoiesis is a hallmark of the disorder. Patients frequently complain of a dragging sensation in the abdomen, left upper quadrant tenderness or pain, and early satiety. At the same time, they appear to be less prone to splenic infarction than CML patients. Patients with rapidly progressive, acute myelofibrosis can complain of **bone pain** and bone tenderness, especially over the sternum.

Laboratory Studies

A. COMPLETE BLOOD COUNT (CBC):

The routine **CBC** helps distinguish the myelofibrotic from the CML patient (Table 18–5). Patients present with a moderate to severe normochromic, normocytic anemia with prominent anisocytosis and poikilocytosis. Presence of nucleated red blood cells and teardrop-shaped red blood cells on the peripheral film is characteristic and suggests extramedullary hematopoiesis in

Table 18–5. Myelofibrosis hematopoietic profile.

Complete blood count (CBC)
  Hemoglobin: moderate to severe normocytic anemia
  Red blood cell morphology: prominent aniso-/poikilocytosis, with nucleated red blood cells and "teardrop" cells
  White blood cell count: near normal
  Platelet count: normal to increased or decreased
Marrow (biopsy)
  Patchy cellularity: islands of hypercellular marrow
  Increased reticulin and collagen
  Marked increase in megakaryocytes
Special studies
  Leukocyte alkaline phosphatase: normal
  Ph[1] chromosome: absent unless fibrosis is a late complication of CML

the spleen. Giant platelets and dysplastic leukocytes (**Pelger-Huët anomaly**) may also be present.

Unlike CML, the myelofibrotic patient will present with a normal or only moderately increased **leukocyte count.** With disease progression, the white blood cell count can fall to subnormal levels as a result of both poor production and increased destruction by the spleen. The **platelet count** may be low, normal, or high when the patient first presents. With treatment and disease progression, it can fall to very low levels or increase dramatically to levels in excess of 1 million/μL. Marked thrombocytosis (platelet counts of several million) is observed in patients who have had a therapeutic splenectomy.

B. MARROW BIOPSY:

Definitive diagnosis of myelofibrosis rests with the marrow biopsy. The marrow is often difficult or impossible to aspirate and a core biopsy is required. Depending on stage of the disease process, a biopsy can show variable distortions of the marrow structure ranging from complete fibrous replacement to patchy losses of hematopoietic and fat cells with islands of residual hyperplastic marrow. Proliferation of immature and abnormal-appearing megakaryocytes can be impressive. Both **trichrome and silver stains** should always be performed to better define the amount of collagen and reticulin fibers in the marrow structure. Increases in reticulin and collagen will depend on the severity and progression of the disease process.

Myelofibrosis can develop as a **secondary manifestation in CML and polycythemia vera patients.** In this setting, appearance of the peripheral blood and marrow is similar to that of idiopathic myelofibrosis. Proliferation of megakaryocytes is a prominent component, suggesting a key role for megakaryocyte and platelet growth factors in stimulating the fibrosis. Patients with widespread malignancies can also develop significant marrow fibrosis. It is essential, therefore, to carefully inspect the marrow biopsy for nests of malignant cells. **Other diseases** that can present with a hematologic picture similar to that of idiopathic myelofibrosis are T- and B-cell lymphomas, especially hairy-cell leukemia, and miliary tuberculosis.

C. OTHER TESTS:

Chromosomal analysis is a less rewarding exercise in the diagnosis of idiopathic myelofibrosis. Although there are often chromosomal abnormalities (Table 18–3), these patients do not show a predominant karyotype. Other laboratory measurements follow the pattern of the other myeloproliferative disorders. For example, these patients can show an increase in **LDH and blood uric acid levels.** In patients with very high platelet counts, it may be possible to demonstrate **defects in platelet aggregation.** A few patients may manifest a hypercoagulable state.

Disease Course

Most patients with idiopathic myelofibrosis follow a protracted course with a median survival between 5 and 8 years. Because it is a disorder of older patients, death may be from such natural causes as myocardial infarctions or stroke; one-third or less of patients will die of complications resulting from their hematopoietic disorder. Unlike CML, 10% or less of patients will progress to acute leukemia.

PRIMARY THROMBOCYTHEMIA

Primary thrombocythemia (essential thrombocythemia or thrombocytosis) is defined by the presence of a markedly elevated platelet count (600,000/μL to more than 1 million/μL) in the absence of any other cause. Because it is a diagnosis of exclusion, any known cause of reactive thrombocytosis must be considered. This includes iron deficiency, chronic inflammatory disorders, chronic infectious diseases, malignancy, and the other stem cell disorders such as polycythemia vera, CML, and idiopathic myelofibrosis. As with the other stem cell disorders, primary thrombocythemia has been shown by G6PD isoenzyme studies to be a clonal disorder involving all of the hematopoietic cell lines in most patients. However, some patients with clinically similar disease have been shown to be polyclonal. Whether the course of their disease is different still needs to be defined.

Most patients with primary thrombocythemia are first detected on routine CBC. They are almost always asymptomatic. When the **platelet count reaches very high levels,** the most common symptoms are those associated with bleeding owing to platelet dysfunction or the appearance of a hypercoagulable state. The latter includes both venous (deep venous thrombosis) and arterial thrombotic events, ranging from distal vessel thromboses, to strokes and coronary artery occlusions, to unusual presentations such as Budd-Chiari syndrome or skin necrosis. Patients with higher platelet counts can complain of vasomotor symptoms such as headaches, dizziness, syncope, visual disturbances, paresthesias, acrocyanosis, and erythromelalgia. These events are related to platelet activation and are usually responsive to treatment with aspirin.

Most patients will have some splenic enlargement, but it is never as prominent as that seen in CML or idiopathic myelofibrosis. The very high platelet counts can result in **splenic infarction and a loss of splenic function.** This will result in the appearance of Howell-Jolly bodies, nucleated red blood cells, and target cells on the peripheral film.

Laboratory Studies

A routine **CBC** and **marrow examination** should distinguish primary thrombocythemia from CML, polycythemia vera, and idiopathic myelofibrosis. The very high peripheral platelet count is not accompanied by major changes in the white blood cell or red blood cell lines, although an absolute basophilia is observed in some patients. The marrow may be normo- or hypercellular, with a normal ratio of erythroid to granulocytic precursors and a normal display of myelocytic precursors. At the same time, the number of megakaryocytes should be dramatically increased. Their morphology is usually normal, but it is common to see large platelet aggregates dispersed throughout the marrow aspirate.

Since diagnosis of primary thrombocythemia is by exclusion of other disease states, laboratory evaluation should include **iron studies** to rule out iron deficiency or an inflammatory state, **chromosomal analysis** to rule out CML and myelodysplasia, and a **bone marrow biopsy** to exclude a diagnosis of myelofibrosis (myeloid metaplasia). Patients with polycythemia vera can present with a normal hemoglobin level and red blood cell mass and marked thrombocythemia secondary to acute and chronic blood loss. These patients may be recognized because of the marked disparity between the severity of their microcytosis and their degree of anemia (see Chapter 12). Rarely, polycythemia vera will not be detected until after iron replacement is initiated and the hemoglobin level rapidly increases.

Spontaneous in vitro formation of megakaryocyte colonies (**CFU-MK**) in the absence of added growth factors has been reported in patients with primary thrombocytosis, perhaps suggesting a hypersensitivity to thrombopoietin in vivo. While it has been suggested as a diagnostic test for the disease, the phenomenon has also been observed in patients with other myeloproliferative disorders.

Disease Course

The overall life expectancy of essential thrombocytosis patients is near normal. However, older adults (over age 60) and patients with a history of thrombosis and a platelet count greater than 1.5 million/μL are at a significant increased risk of thrombohemorrhagic complications and need to be treated. Transformation into polycythemia vera, myelofibrosis, or acute leukemia, even with prolonged chemotherapy, is seen in fewer than 5% of patients. There would appear, therefore, to be little downside to extended chemotherapy.

PRELEUKEMIC STATES

Several hematopoietic stem cell disorders are best classified as preleukemic states. This includes the spectrum of disorders that present as **dysplastic anemias** (see Chapter 9), the **chronic myelomonocytic leukemias,** and some patients who present with **PNH.** Although the clinical presentations appear to be quite different, these disorders tend to be more common in middle-aged and elderly individuals. They tend to follow an indolent course and with time evolve toward a blastic phase characterized by a progressive failure of mature hematopoietic cell production.

The **classification of the preleukemic states** involves integration of distinguishing features from film and marrow morphology, chromosomal analysis, and tests for PNH. The **refractory or dysplastic anemias** are recognized from the distinctive abnormalities of red blood cell morphology (see Chapter 9). Patients are classified as having **chronic myelomonocytic leukemia (CMML)** based on the predominant proliferation of immature myelocytes and monocytes in the marrow, an abnormal chromosomal karyotype without a Ph[1] chromosome, and a tendency over time to evolve into an acute myeloid leukemia (AML)-like picture. Patients with **PNH** demonstrate a highly variable hematologic picture (Chapter 9). Some PNH patients present with pancytopenia or a marrow morphology that suggests dysplasia, aplasia, or myeloproliferative disease. To rule out PNH, red cell surface antigens such as CD48, CD55, CD59, and the FcRIII (CD16) receptor should be measured by flow cytometry.

THERAPY

The most important elements of good management of a patient with a myeloproliferative disorder are the accurate diagnosis of the condition and a sense of when to treat the disease. Since many patients are elderly at the time of presentation, multidrug chemotherapy and marrow transplantation are often not feasible. Therefore, watchful waiting with blood product support and single-drug chemotherapy are often more appropriate. The selection of drugs also varies according to the individual disease process. This is especially true for CML, for which therapy has become increasingly effective.

Chronic Myelogenous Leukemia

Several drugs are effective in treating CML. Prolonged survivals can be attained using combinations of drugs such as interferon-α, cytosine arabinoside, busulfan, and hydroxyurea. Durable disease-free survivals can be attained in patients receiving interferon-α, allogeneic marrow transplantation, or both. Success depends on several factors including the patient's age, the timing of the treatment according to the phase of the disease, and the innate responsiveness of the tumor. In essence, younger patients who are diagnosed and treated early in

COLOR PLATES

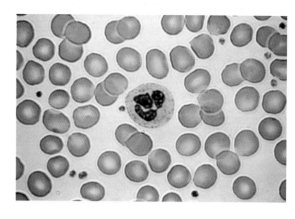

1. NORMAL BLOOD SMEAR.

(Wright's stain). High-power field showing normal red blood cells, a single leucocyte, and several platelets.

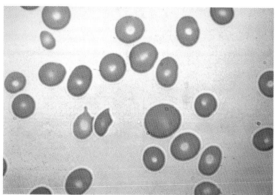

2. POLYCHROMASIA.

A single polychromatic macrocyte (marrow or shift reticulocyte) surrounded by normocytic and microcytic cells.

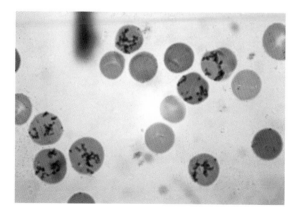

3. RETICULOCYTE COUNT PREPARATION.

A new methylene blue–stained blood smear showing large numbers of heavily stained reticulocytes (cells containing dark blue–staining precipitates of RNA).

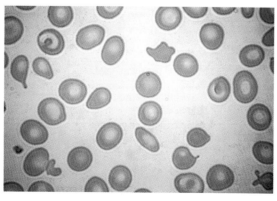

4. MICROCYTOSIS.

Microcytes are smaller than normal (cell diameter less than 7 μm) and may be poorly hemoglobinized (hypochromic). Both anisocytosis and poikilocytosis are present. The target cells suggest thalassemia minor.

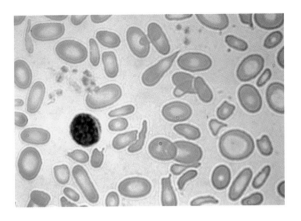

5. SEVERE IRON DEFICIENCY ANEMIA.

Marked microcytosis and hypochromia with pronounced aniso- and poikilocytosis are seen with severe iron deficiency. The presence of cigar-shaped red blood cells and the absence of target cells are also characteristic of iron deficiency and rule against thalassemia.

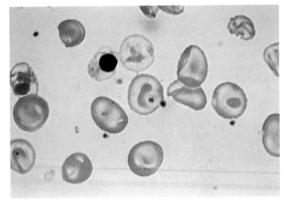

6. THALASSEMIA MAJOR.

Marked microcytosis, with MCVs below 70 fL, together with severe hypochromia and prominent targeting, is typical of thalassemia major. The apparent diameter of the red blood cells on the smear can be deceptive. This effect is caused by the marked deficit of hemoglobin within the cell, producing a flattened cell on the glass surface.

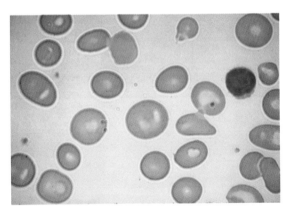

7. MACROCYTOSIS.

Macrocytes are larger than normal red blood cells (cell volume greater than 100 fL and cell diameter greater than 8 μm) and are often oval-shaped (macroovalocytes) and well hemoglobinized.

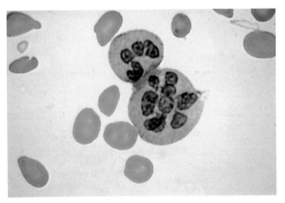

8. HYPERSEGMENTED NEUTROPHILS.

Hypersegmented neutrophils (multilobed polymorphonuclear leukocytes), commonly seen in patients with folic acid or vitamin B_{12} deficiency, are larger than normal neutrophils and contain five or more nuclear lobes.

9. HOWELL-JOLLY BODY.

Howell-Jolly bodies are tiny nuclear remnants that are normally removed by the spleen. They appear on the blood smear after splenectomy and in patients with maturation/dysplastic disorders.

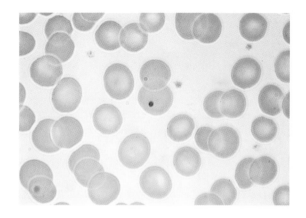

10. MYELOFIBROSIS.

A teardrop-shaped red blood cell *(left panel)* together with a nucleated red blood cell *(right panel)* as typically seen in patients with myelofibrosis and extramedullary hematopoiesis.

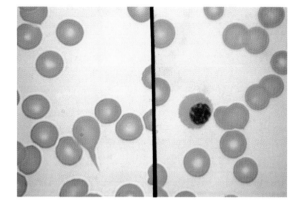

11. SPHEROCYTOSIS.

Spherocytes are small, dense red blood cells that lack the central pallor of a normal biconcave red blood cell. They are smaller than normal and show a higher mean corpuscular hemoglobin concentration (MCHC) because of a loss of cell water.

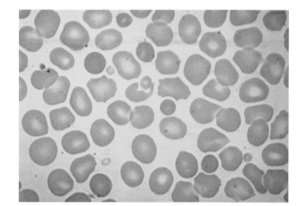

12. ELLIPTOCYTOSIS.

Elliptocytes are recognized by their uniform ellliptical shape but otherwise normal appearance and cell indices.

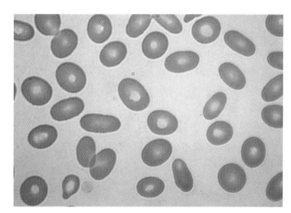

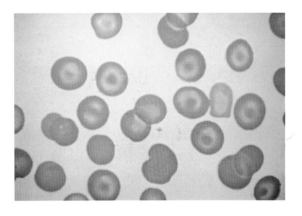

13. TARGETING.

Target cells, commonly seen with hemoglobin C and liver disease, are recognized by the bull's-eye appearance of the cell.

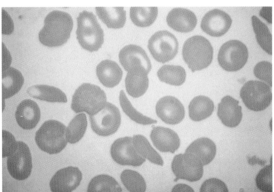

14. SICKLE CELLS.

Sickle cells in a patient with sickle cell anemia.

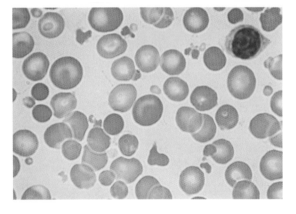

15. FRAGMENTATION.

Marked anisocytosis, poikilocytosis, microspherocyte formation, and polychromasia in a patient with a thermal burn.

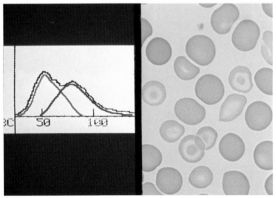

16. MIXED POPULATIONS OF RED BLOOD CELLS.

Red blood cell volume display and smear from a thalassemic patient after transfusion that shows an admixture of normal and microcytic red blood cells. This pattern is also seen with hereditary sideroblastic anemia.

17. MALARIA.

Trophozoite form of *Plasmodium vivax* in an adult red blood cell.

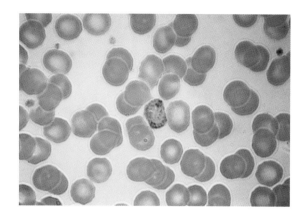

18. ROULEAUX.

Marked rouleaux, red blood cells in a "stack of coins" formation, suggests a proteinopathy.

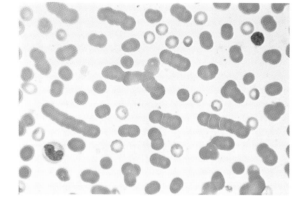

19. AGLUTTINATION.

Clumping of red blood cells in a disorganized mass is typically seen in patients with cold agglutinins.

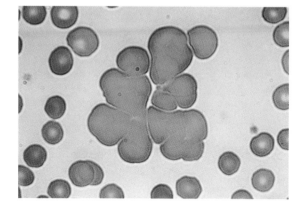

20. GIANT PLATELETS.

Giant platelets, together with an increase in the platelet count, are seen in patients with myeloproliferative disorders, especially primary thrombocythemia.

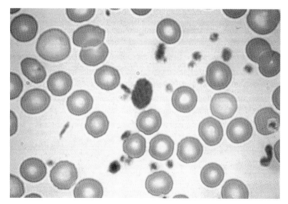

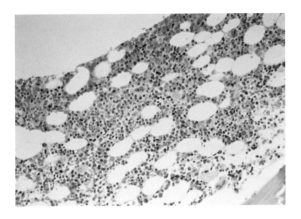

21. NORMAL MARROW BIOPSY AT LOW POWER.

(H & E stain). Low-power view of normal adult marrow, showing a mix of fat cells (clear areas) and hematopoietic precursor cells.

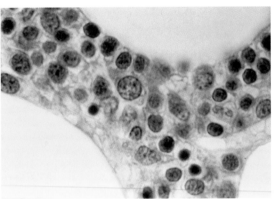

22. NORMAL MARROW BIOPSY AT HIGH POWER.

(H & E stain). High-power view of a marrow biopsy specimen showing the normal admixture of myeloid and erythroid precursors.

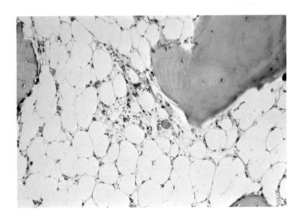

23. APLASTIC ANEMIA.

Normal hematopoietic cells are absent, leaving behind fat cells, reticuloendothelial cells, and the underlying sinusoidal structure.

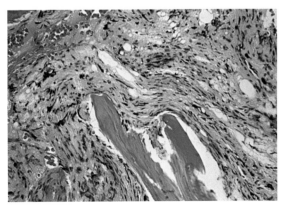

24. MYELOFIBROSIS

(H & E stain). Total replacement of marrow precursors and fat cells by a dense infiltration of reticulin fibers and collagen.

25. MYELOFIBROSIS—RETICULIN STAIN.

Silver stain of a myelofibrotic marrow showing an increased density of reticulin fibers (black staining).

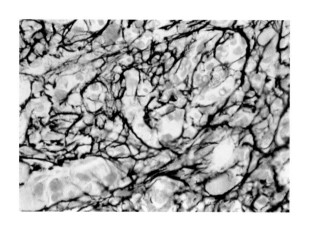

26. METASTATIC CANCER.

Marrow biopsy specimen infiltrated with metastatic breast cancer and reactive myelofibrosis.

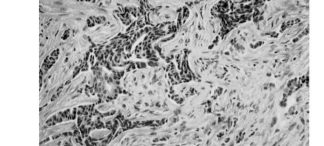

27. LYMPHOMA.

Low-grade, nodular (follicular) lymphoma infiltrate in a marrow biopsy specimen. Note the characteristic paratrabecular distribution of the lymphoma cells.

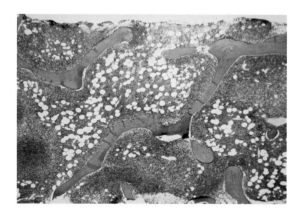

28. TUMOR CELLS.

(Wright's stain). A clump of tumor cells (high-power) in a marrow aspirate specimen.

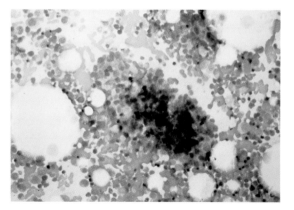

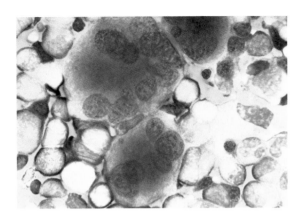

29. MEGACARYOCYTES.
(Wright's/Giemsa stain). Marrow aspirate smear showing an erythroid/granulocytic ratio (E/G ratio) greater than 1:1.

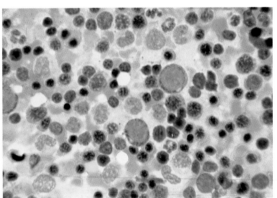

30. ERYTHROID HYPERPLASIA.
(Wright's stain). Marrow aspirate smear showing an erythroid/granulocytic ratio (E/G ratio) greater than 1:1.

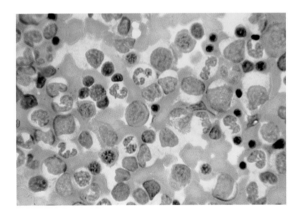

31. GRANULOCYTIC HYPERPLASIA.
E/G ratio less than 1:3.

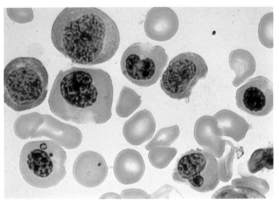

32. MEGALOBLASTIC ERYTHROPOIESIS.
High-power view of megaloblastic red blood cell precursors in a patient with a macrocytic anemia.

33. MARROW IRON STORES.

(Prussian blue stain). Low-power view of marrow specimen stained for iron. Blue-black staining material (iron stores) is concentrated in the reticuloendothelial cells.

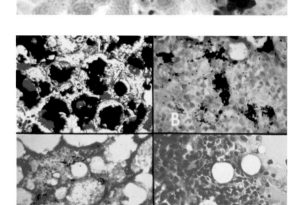

34. GRADING IRON STORES.

Iron stores can be graded on a scale of 0 to 4+. The *upper left panel* shows a marrow with little or no iron stores (grade 0); the *upper right panel* shows 1+ stores; the *lower left panel* shows 2 to 3+ stores; and the *lower right panel* shows greater than 4+ stores.

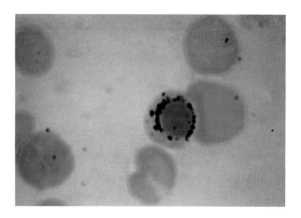

35. RINGED SIDEROBLAST.

Orthrochromatic normoblast with a collar of blue granules (mitochondria encrusted with iron) surrounding the nucleus.

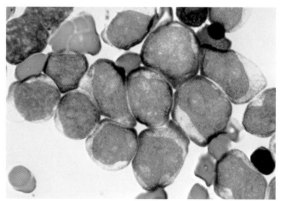

36. ACUTE MYELOCYTIC LEUKEMIA.

Primitive blasts containing multiple, large nucleoli in a patient with acute myelocytic leukemia (AML).

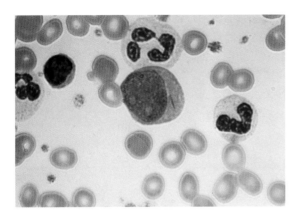

37. AUER ROD

Leukemic myeloblast with a single rod-shaped crystal (Auer rod) in the cytoplasm.

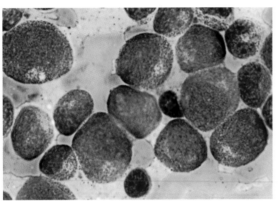

38. PROMYELOCYTIC LEUKEMIA.

Uniform population of malignant promyelocytes with a heavy concentration of primary granules in the cytoplasm.

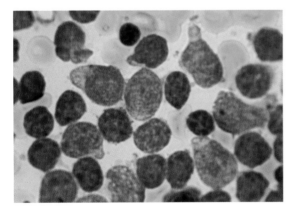

39. ACUTE LYMPHOCYTIC LEUKEMIA.

Lymphoblasts in the marrow of a patient with acute lymphocytic leukemia (ALL).

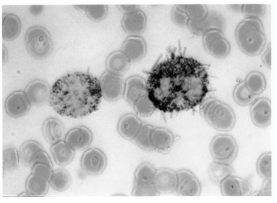

40. MYELOPEROXIDASE STAIN.

Granules in the cytoplasm of myeloblasts from a patient with AML stain positively (blue) for peroxidase.

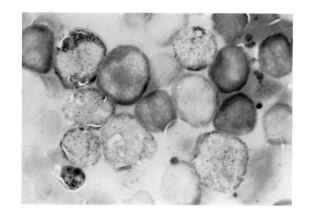

41. COMBINED ESTERASE STAIN.

Blast forms stain positively for esterases with myelomonocytic leukemias.

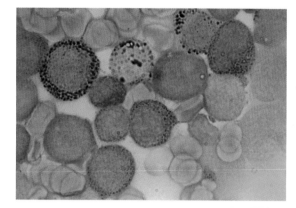

42. PERIODIC ACID—SCHIFF (PAS) STAIN

Lymphoblasts (ALL) and erythroblasts (erythroleukemia) can stain positively (bright red granules) with PAS.

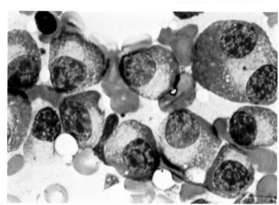

43. MULTIPLE MYELOMA.

High-power view of malignant plasma cells in a patient with multiple myeloma.

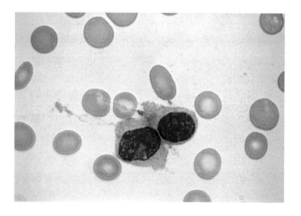

44. HAIRY-CELL LEUKEMIA.

Hairy cells (malignant B cells) with filamentous cytoplasm on a peripheral smear.

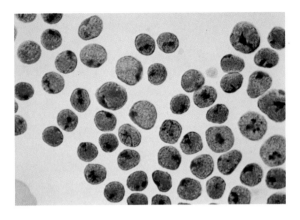

45. ACID PHOSPHATASE STAIN.

Polar staining (red) for acid phosphatase in a patient with T-cell lymphoma. Tartrate resistant acid phosphatase staining is seen with hairy-cell leukemia.

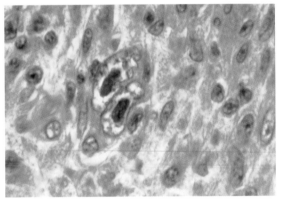

46. REED-STERNBERG CELL.

Binucleate giant cell with prominent staining nucleoli (often bright red) in the lymph node biopsy specimen of a patient with Hodgkin's disease.

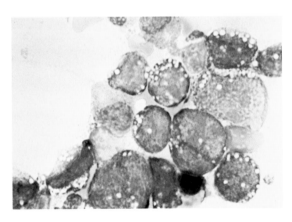

47. BURKITT'S LYMPHOMA.

Heavily vacuolated lymphoblasts in a patient with Burkitt's lymphoma.

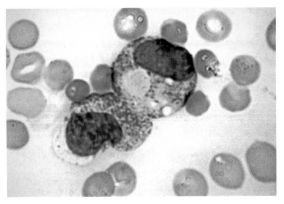

48. ERYTHROPHAGOCYTOSIS.

Red blood cell ingested by a monocyte/histiocyte in a patient with histiocytic medullary reticulosis.

the chronic phase of their illness and who have a very responsive tumor do the best.

A. INTERFERON-α:

Interferon-α has been the preferred drug in the initial treatment of the chronic phase of CML. It improves overall survival by about 20 months when compared with hydroxyurea or busulfan therapy.

1. Assessment of response by CBC and karyotype—Control of the hematologic abnormalities (**normalization of the CBC**) can be achieved in 70–80% of patients. The response can also be assessed by **following the chromosomal karyotype.** By this measure, interferon-α will result in a "complete" loss of the Ph[1] chromosome-positive cell line in up to 30% of patients. The sensitivity of the karyotype measurement must be taken into account, however. Residual malignant cells can be still detected using PCR measurements of the BCR-ABL translocation. Still, although interferon therapy will not eradicate every last Ph[1]-positive cell, the complete cytogenetic response by karyotype studies does predict a durable remission (Figure 18–2). In fact, patients with complete cytogenetic responses may do as well as transplant patients.

2. Effectiveness and dose—The effectiveness of interferon therapy correlates with the maximum dose tolerated by the patient. Lower-dose regimens (2×10^6 U/m² given subcutaneously or intramuscularly three times per week) will improve the blood counts in most patients but will not produce a complete cytogenetic response. A dose of 5×10^6 U/m² given three times a week or, if tolerated, daily is needed to achieve a complete cytogenetic response. The rate of response is slow. If the initial granulocyte count exceeds 100,000/μL, the patient should be first treated with hydroxyurea (see below) to lower the count to below 20,000/μL. The hydroxyurea should then be continued during the first 2–3 months to prevent a count rebound. Interferon therapy is best started at a reduced dose, 3×10^6 U/day for 1–2 weeks, followed by 5×10^6 U/day for another 1–2 weeks, before escalating to full dose. Otherwise, the patient will show poor tolerance for the interferon.

3. Effect on transplantation—Therapy must be given continually for 1 year or more because the maximum response may not occur for 12–18 months. However, when interferon is given for more than 6 months, the success rate of a subsequent marrow transplant may be significantly reduced. Therefore, a **decision regarding transplantation needs to made in the first 6 months** and the transplant completed during the first year. Transplantation should be seriously considered when a significant hematologic remission is not reached by 6 months. If a major cytogenetic remission is achieved, the interferon should continued for 2–3 years. The patient should then be followed off therapy using a sensitive assay (PCR or FISH assay) for the re-emergence of Ph[1]-positive cells. The projected 6- to 8-year survival rate for patients with major cytogenetic responses is better than 85%, and the 10–20% mortality with transplantation is avoided.

4. Side effects—Interferon-α therapy is associated with several side effects. With each injection, patients experience a **flulike syndrome** with fever, chills, and anorexia. **Severe persistent fatigue, depression, weight loss,** and the **appearance of autoimmune-mediated**

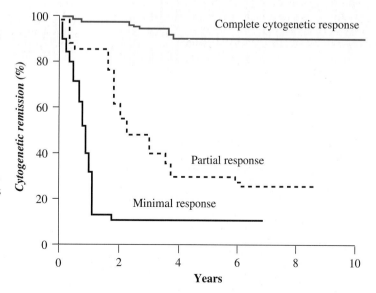

Figure 18–2. **Survival curves in CML.** The quality of remission in CML depends on the degree to which all cells carrying the cytogenetic abnormality can be eliminated. Tests for residual cells carrying the BCR-ABL translocation make it possible to distinguish patients with markedly different outcomes.

organ damage (cardiomyopathy, collagen vascular disorders, hypothyroidism, hemolysis, and thrombocytopenia) will require **dose reductions.** As a rule, the dose administered will need to be cut by 25–50% when there is evidence of organ damage or severe leukopenia or thrombocytopenia (absolute leukocyte count below 2000/μL or platelet count below 60,000/μL). Up to 20% of patients will not be able to tolerate the drug. Rarely, severe organ damage, especially cardiac disease with arrhythmias or congestive failure, will require discontinuation of the drug.

5. Use in combination chemotherapy—In order to reduce the toxicity and at the same time improve the overall effectiveness of interferon-α, studies have looked at combination chemotherapy with drugs such as busulfan, cytarabine, and hydroxyurea. The combination of low-dose cytarabine (20 mg/m² daily or for 10 days each month) with interferon-α (5×10^6 U/m² daily) has now been shown to provide a better and more rapid cytogenetic response and is well tolerated. Busulfan and hydroxyurea combinations are more toxic and add little to the overall outcome.

B. BCR-ABL Tyrosine Kinase Inhibitors:

A specific inhibitor of the Ph¹ chromosome BCR-ABL tyrosine kinase, STI-571 (Gleevec, Novartis), has shown significant activity in both the chronic and blast phases of CML and in the treatment of Ph¹-positive ALL. It has also been shown to be effective in patients who have failed interferon-α therapy. In a dose escalation study of patients with chronic-phase CML, all of whom had failed interferon therapy, 53 of 54 patients who received daily oral doses of 300 mg or more demonstrated a complete hematologic response during the first 4 weeks. One-third of these patients showed a cytogenetic response, with 7 patients achieving a complete cytogenetic remission. Responses have also been reported in more than 50% of patients with myeloblastic crises and 70% of patients with lymphoblastic crises or Ph¹-positive ALL. However, unlike chronic-phase patients, most blastic crisis patients relapsed while receiving therapy. Adverse side effects are described as minimal and include nausea, myalgias, edema, diarrhea, and in some patients, abnormal bleeding.

The role of Gleevec in the management of CML is still being defined. It is the therapy of choice for the patient who cannot tolerate or fails interferon-α therapy. Gleevec may well replace interferon-α as first-line therapy if additional clinical trials confirm its efficacy. No data are yet available on the sustained effect of the drug and its impact on mortality.

C. Hydroxyurea and Busulfan:

Both hydroxyurea and busulfan have been used to treat CML.

1. Hydroxyurea—Hydroxyurea is easier to use than either interferon or busulfan, and it will lower the leukocyte count faster. It also has a wider therapeutic safety range. Evidence shows that patients who become resistant to hydroxyurea may still respond to busulfan, whereas the reverse may not be true. Initially, hydroxyurea is given in a dose of 2–8 grams orally for several days. The CBC is monitored each day, and the dose is tapered as the granulocyte count falls toward normal. Once the granulocyte count is below 10,000–15,000/μL, the patient should be controlled with a maintenance regimen of 500–1500 mg of hydroxyurea by mouth daily for 5 out of every 7 days.

Hydroxyurea is an inhibitor of DNA synthesis and acts by blocking cell division and marrow precursor maturation. It does not affect the malignant stem cells and, therefore, does not produce a cytogenetic remission. Moreover, because hydroxyurea blocks maturation of all hematopoietic cell lines, patients become markedly megaloblastic and develop a macrocytic anemia. The drug also works to reduce the platelet count in most patients secondary to ineffective thrombopoiesis. Although hydroxyurea in doses less than 2 grams per day has few if any other side effects, its long-term use can be limited by its effect on the other hematopoietic cell lines, especially platelet production.

2. Busulfan—For many years, busulfan was considered the drug of choice for the initial treatment of the chronic phase of the disease. When given in a dose of 4–6 mg/day as a single dose by mouth in a treatment course lasting 10–20 days, it can bring the granulocyte count down to below 10,000–15,000/μL. Early in the chronic phase of the disease, the initial course of busulfan therapy is usually followed by a period of hematologic remission that is sustained without maintenance chemotherapy. However, as the disease progresses, more of the drug will be required even to the point where intermittent therapy must be replaced by a daily maintenance dose.

Busulfan therapy is associated with **significant side effects** when given over a prolonged period. The side effects include a high incidence of pulmonary fibrosis and the induction of an addisonian-like syndrome with skin pigmentation, fatigue, anorexia, and weight loss. In addition, the patient must be closely monitored during therapy to avoid the administration of too much drug. Excessive doses of busulfan can result in a loss of stem cells and an irreversible aplastic anemia. The risk for this complication is highest when the drug is given continuously without close monitoring of the peripheral blood counts.

3. Choice of the appropriate chemotherapy agent—The objective of management of CML patients during the chronic phase of their illness is to achieve control of their hematologic abnormalities without significant side effects. The choice of the appropriate chemotherapy agent should take into account the patient's age, the phase of his or her disease, and the presence or absence of other prognostic factors (Figure 18–3). The younger the patient and the more responsive the tumor, the more aggressive the therapy. In this situation, bone marrow transplantation, interferon-α alone, or interferon with low-dose cytarabine has been recommended. Older patients, patients with disease that has progressed and who are less responsive, or patients who have failed interferon-α therapy should be managed with single-agent chemotherapy using drugs like Gleevec, hydroxyurea, and busulfan. Patients in blastic crisis may respond to Gleevec therapy alone or may be managed in the same way as patients presenting with de novo acute myeloblastic or lymphoblastic leukemia. Their prognosis is very poor.

CML patients with very high platelet counts can present a greater therapeutic challenge. This is especially true when chemotherapy successfully controls the granulocyte proliferation but does not lower the platelet count. With some patients, the thrombocytosis can be controlled by changing drugs or by adding short courses of a second drug. Agents that can be used to control very high platelet counts include **alkylating agents** such as melphalan, thiotepa and uracil mustard, or **anagrelide,** a platelet-specific chemotherapy agent, given in a dose of 0.5–1.0 mg four times a day by mouth. A response is seen in most patients within 7–14 days. Although anagrelide is highly effective, it is very expensive and cannot be discontinued without the risk of a dramatic rise in the platelet count.

D. BONE MARROW TRANSPLANTATION:

Allogeneic marrow transplantation using an HLA-matched sibling or nonrelated HLA-matched donor can result in a prolonged disease-free survival in 40–65% (60–70% when under age 50) of patients for whom a donor can be found, which in the case of a matched sibling will be fewer than 50% of patients. As with transplantation in AML, the success rate depends on factors such as the patient's age, the phase of the disease, exposure to previous chemotherapy, and the incidence of graft-versus-host disease (GVHD).

The **best results are seen in younger patients** who, during the chronic phase of their illness, receive a trans-

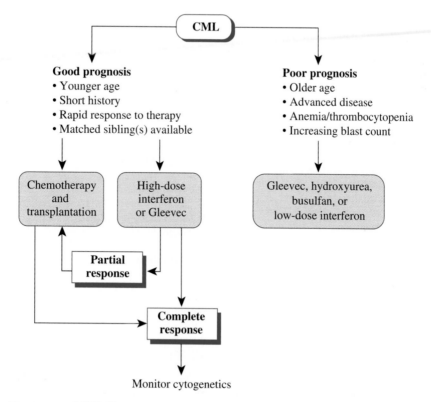

Figure 18–3. **Treatment of CML.** The treatment strategy for CML depends on the age and clinical status of the patient. Interferon therapy and transplantation have improved the outcome in appropriate subsets of patients.

plant from a sibling marrow that produces relatively mild GVHD. It is now recommended that patients under the age of 20 years with a sibling match receive a transplant within the first 6 months of diagnosis, since 70% or more will achieve prolonged, disease-free survivals, if not cures. Most show a full cytogenetic remission; Ph[1]-positive cells will be absent on karyotypic analysis. However, as with interferon therapy, the PCR measurement of the BCR-ABL gene rearrangement marker will still be positive in most of these patients, although this does not necessarily predict relapse.

1. Unrelated HLA-matched donors—Unrelated HLA-matched donors are now being used extensively in the marrow transplantation of CML patients. With a national donor program pool of more than 2 million, a donor can be found for 71% of white patients, 62% of Hispanics, 45% of Asians, but only 24% of blacks. The lower match rate for Asians and blacks is a result of the complexity of their HLA systems, not the racial distribution of the donor pool. In the ideal situation, unrelated donor transplants appear to be as or more effective than an HLA-matched sibling transplant: Disease-free survival is 75% if the transplant is done in the first year. It is self-evident, however, that patients who use the unrelated donor pool for their transplant will often have progressed further in their disease, been exposed to more chemotherapy, and be somewhat older. Because of a higher rate of transplant-associated deaths, overall disease-free survival for patients receiving transplants from unrelated donors is approximately 30–40% at 5 years, and there is a significantly higher incidence of severe GVHD.

2. Relapses—Late relapses are seen in CML patients with transplants, suggesting that transplantation will never result in a guaranteed cure. This situation may reflect a persistence of the rare malignant stem cell or an environmental factor that leads to reappearance of the tumor. The antileukemic effect of acute and chronic GVHD also plays a role. Patients who receive T-cell-depleted marrow transplants have a fivefold increased risk of relapse. This is also true for twin transplants and for patients who receive immunosuppressive therapy for their GVHD. It is perhaps the best example of the **graft versus leukemia** effect (**GVL**) of donor lymphocytes.

In patients who relapse following transplant, **donor lymphocyte transfusions** have been used successfully to reinduce remission. From 70% to 90% of patients with hematologic or cytogenetic relapse will respond, usually after a 2- to 3-month course of multiple transfusions of donor T cells. Patients who develop grade 2 or higher GVHD as a result of the therapy do best, demonstrating a better than 90% remission rate. The mechanism behind this effect is still unclear. Experi-

mental data would suggest, however, that the T-cell GVL effect is distinct from the GVHD effect and that infusions of CD8 (suppressor) T-cell-depleted donor lymphocytes will give the GVL effect with far less GVHD.

3. Autologous marrow transplantation—Attempts to use autologous marrow transplantation have not been effective in CML. In this case, the inability to completely eradicate the malignant cell line with chemotherapy and the absence of a GVL effect may guarantee failure. Recently, it has been observed that during culture in vitro, the Ph[1]-containing stem cells may not survive as well as normal stem cells. This has led to trials of autologous transplantation following in vitro marrow culture. Although promising, this and other new approaches to the use of autologous transplantation in CML require further study.

4. Allogeneic marrow transplantation—Allogeneic marrow transplantation has been recommended as first-line therapy for the younger CML patients with a matched sibling donor. At the same time, transplantation is not without risk. The procedure itself carries a risk of 5–20% acute mortality. In addition, survivors will have to deal with some degree of GVHD in order to achieve the 50–75% chance of a prolonged disease-free survival in patients receiving transplants during the chronic phase. Therefore, a decision to transplant is always a difficult one, and this cannot be avoided by delaying the decision. The best results are achieved when transplantation is carried out early in the chronic phase of the illness. Once the disease progresses, the chance of an effective transplant decreases dramatically. When the patient has had the disease for more than 2 years, a positive result can be expected less than 50% of the time. If the disease enters the accelerated phase, the results fall to 20–50%, and patients in blastic crisis have only a 15–20% chance of achieving a significant remission. The preparative regimen also makes a difference, particularly the blood levels of busulfan. The higher the busulfan blood level, the better the chance of a durable remission.

Myelofibrosis

Patients with myelofibrosis should be managed conservatively. Most often, the disease process follows a chronic, slowly progressive course, and patients can simply be observed. **Symptomatic anemia** will respond adequately to periodic red blood cell transfusion, unless the patient develops hypersplenism with an increased rate of red blood cell destruction.

Patients who develop **hypersplenism** may be candidates for **splenectomy.** Splenectomy may also play a role in decreasing the rate of progression of the marrow fibrosis. It is difficult, however, to predict the outcome of a splenectomy. Often, the patient's condition is worsened both by a spread of the extramedullary hematopoiesis to the liver and other tissues and a postsplenectomy rise in the platelet count to levels in excess of 1 million/μL. Splenectomy is most successful in those patients with symptomatic splenomegaly, with overt portal hypertension, and progressive, transfusion-dependent anemia. Severe thrombocytopenia and a hypocellular marrow are adverse indicators for response to splenectomy. Splenic irradiation has been used effectively to control the splenomegaly and hypersplenism. Ninety percent of patients will respond to repeated treatments. However, splenic irradiation is associated, at times, with severe myelosuppression.

Marrow transplantation has been used successfully in young patients with myelofibrosis. Of interest, the marked fibrosis of the marrow does reverse if the patient's malignant cell lines are eliminated and a successful transplant is achieved. The number of patients who are reasonable candidates for transplantation is relatively small, however. Since myelofibrosis is an illness of middle-aged and older patients, the risk of procedural death and severe GVHD is also very high. **Autologous transplantation** has been shown to result in clinical response, decreased transfusion requirements, and regression of fibrosis in selected patients. It has been reported that **2-CdA therapy** will also result in a decrease in marrow fibrosis. Trials of new drugs that inhibit fibrosis, angiogenesis, or both are currently under way.

Primary Thrombocythemia

Age greater than 60 years, a history of at least one past thrombotic event, or platelet counts greater than $1-1.5 \times 10^9$/μL are adverse prognostic signs that dictate treatment. Patients with primary thrombocythemia can usually be controlled with **chemotherapy.** Several single-agent drug regimens have been used, including hydroxyurea, anagrelide, interferon-α, and in selected cases, alkylating agents. Since the course of the disease can be prolonged, **hydroxyurea** may be considered the drug of choice to initiate therapy. Although it is the least expensive, it is not as effective as some of the other agents, and its use is associated with the development of both anemia and granulocytopenia. Recent reports have raised the issue of hydroxyurea-induced acute leukemia or myelodysplasia in patients receiving long-term therapy. The use of regimens containing alkylating agents is discouraged because of the even higher risk of second malignancies.

Anagrelide is a very effective therapy in resistant patients. If one begins with a daily oral dose of 0.5 mg two to four times per day and then escalating the dose by 0.5 mg/day at 1- to 2-week intervals, the platelet count should fall below 600,000/μL within 1 month.

Continuous maintenance is required, since like hydroxyurea, anagrelide interferes with platelet maturation, not megakaryocyte proliferation. Side effects include headache, fluid retention, diarrhea, nausea, abdominal pain, and, in elderly patients, congestive heart failure. Patients with known heart disease should be given the drug with caution. Interferon can be used in hydroxyurea or anagrelide failures, but at considerable cost and toxicity. Treatment is initiated with 3 million units subcutaneously three times a week.

Use of **antiplatelet agents** in the treatment and prevention of thrombotic events is somewhat controversial. **Aspirin** is probably indicated and effective in patients with recurrent thromboses, especially arterial thrombi, or microvascular ischemia. It is contraindicated in patients with a history of abnormal bleeding.

Preleukemic States

Management of patients with conditions that fall within the category of preleukemic myeloproliferative states will vary depending on the patient's age, the rate of progression of their disease state, and specific, associated complications. The older patient with a **CMML-like picture** who is not severely pancytopenic may simply be observed. **Symptomatic anemia** can be treated with red blood cell transfusions and **thrombocytopenia** with periodic platelet transfusions. This approach is also recommended for those patients with the **5q minus syndrome** because of its prolonged course and slow progression.

A. GROWTH FACTOR THERAPY:

Studies have shown that a significant number of patients with myelodysplastic and myeloproliferative disorders will respond to treatment with growth factors such as granulocyte macrophage colony-stimulating factor, granulocyte colony-stimulating factor (G-CSF), and erythropoietin. The combination of G-CSF and erythropoietin has produced an increase in circulating neutrophils and decreased transfusion requirements in 40–50% of patients. For those patients with anemia, neutropenia, or thrombocytopenia, growth factor therapy may decrease the need for transfusions and may decrease the possibility of infection. Initial concerns that such treatment might hasten the development of acute leukemia have not been borne out. There is no evidence at this time for long-term benefit from such treatment, however.

B. CHEMOTHERAPY:

If chemotherapy is attempted, single-drug regimens such as oral hydroxyurea or low-dose cytosine arabinoside should be used. Ablative, multidrug chemotherapy is not advised because it frequently results in a prolonged period of marrow hypoplasia and pancytopenia that is unresponsive to growth factor therapy. Older patients cannot survive prolonged periods of absolute neutropenia, and the chance of inducing a complete or partial remission of any significant duration is very low.

C. OTHER THERAPIES:

Immunotherapies, using either immunosuppressive agents such as antithymocyte globulin, or monoclonal antibody against the myeloid antigen CD33, are under investigation. Young patients have shown long-term disease-free survival after **allogeneic marrow transplantation.** For those without a matched donor, promising early results have been reported after **autologous transplantation.**

D. MANAGEMENT OF PAROXYSMAL NOCTURNAL HEMOGLOBINURIA (PNH):

The management of the PNH patient should also be tailored to fit the characteristics of the disease. Patients who present with hemolytic anemia with hemoglobinuria, iron loss, and iron deficiency will require appropriate therapy for the anemia and their iron deficiency state (see Chapters 5 and 9). With the initiation of **iron therapy,** the release of increased numbers of red blood cells with the PNH membrane defect can result in an exacerbation of the patient's hemolysis and hemoglobinuria. This should be recognized as a necessary side effect of iron replacement.

PNH patients who present with **thrombotic disease** will require effective anticoagulation to prevent severe tissue or organ damage. The **severely pancytopenic patients** will need blood component support and may be candidates for marrow transplantation. The latter is only successful, however, in younger patients with severe disease who are willing to face the risks of early mortality and lifelong GVHD.

Patience is always a virtue in managing PNH patients. This adage is true with this disease because PNH can spontaneously remit and relapse, so **minimal therapy is advised.** At the same time, the occasional patient can present with a life-threatening illness characterized by widespread thrombosis involving skin and visceral organs or marked pancytopenia. In this situation, **transplantation** may be the patient's only chance for survival.

BIBLIOGRAPHY

Chronic Myelogenous Leukemia

Bhatia R et al: Autologous transplantation therapy for chronic myelogenous leukemia. Blood 1997;89:2623.

Cannistra S: Chronic myelogenous leukemia as a model for the genetic basis for cancer. Hematol Oncol Clin North Am 1990; 4:337.

Druker BJ et al: Activity of a specific inhibitor of the BCR-ABL tyrosine kinase in the blast crisis of chronic myeloid leukemia and acute lymphoblastic leukemia with the Philadelphia chromosome. N Engl J Med 2001;344:1038.

Druker BJ et al: Efficacy and safety of a specific inhibitor of the BCR-ABL tyrosine kinase in chronic myeloid leukemia. N Engl J Med 2001;344:1031.

Enright H et al: Relapse after non T-cell-depleted allogeneic bone marrow transplantation for chronic myelogenous leukemia: Early transplantation, use of an unrelated donor, and chronic graft-versus-host disease are protective. Blood 1996;88:714.

Faderl S et al: The biology of chronic myeloid leukemia. N Engl J Med 1999;341:164.

Faderl S et al: Chronic myelogenous leukemia: Biology and therapy. Ann Intern Med 1999;131:207.

Giralt S et al: CD8-depleted donor lymphocyte infusion as treatment for relapsed chronic myelogenous leukemia after allogeneic bone marrow transplantation. Blood 1995;86:4337.

Goldman JM et al: Choice of pretransplant treatment and timing of transplants for chronic myelogenous leukemia in chronic phase. Blood 1993;82:2235.

Greenberg PL: Treatment of myelodysplastic syndromes with hematopoietic growth factors. Oncology 1992;19:106.

Kantarjian HM et al: Treatment of chronic myelogenous leukemia: Current status and investigational options. Blood 1996; 87:3069.

Kolb H et al: Graft-versus-leukemia effect of donor lymphocyte transfusions in marrow grafted patients. Blood 1995; 86:2041.

McGlave PB: Therapy of chronic myelogenous leukemia with related or unrelated donor bone marrow transplantation. Leukemia 1992;6:115.

Melo JV: The diversity of BCR-ABL fusion proteins and their relationship to leukemia phenotype. Blood 1996;88:2375.

Savage DG, Szydio RM, Goldman JM: Clinical features at diagnosis in 430 patients with chronic myeloid leukemia seen at a referral centre over a 16 year period. Br J Hematol 1997; 96:111.

Silver R: Chronic myeloid leukemia: A perspective of the clinical and biologic issues of the chronic phase. Hematol Oncol Clin North Am 1990;4:319.

Silver RT et al: An evidence-based analysis of the effect of busulfan, hydroxyurea, interferon and allogeneic bone marrow transplantation in treating the chronic phase of chronic myeloid leukemia: Developed by the American Society of Hematology. Blood 1999;94:1517.

Slavin S, Naparastek E, Nagler A: Allogeneic cell therapy with donor peripheral blood cells and recombinant interleukin-2 to treat relapse after allogeneic marrow transplantation. Blood 1996;87:2195.

Szydio R et al: Results of allogeneic bone marrow transplants using donors other than HLA-identical siblings. J Clin Oncol 1997;15:1767.

Myelofibrosis and Myelodysplasia

Heany ML, Golde DW: Myelodysplasia. N Engl J Med 1999; 340:1649.

Negrin RS et al: Treatment of the anemias of MDS using recombinant human granulocyte colony stimulating factor in combination with erythropoietin. Blood 1993;82:737.

Tefferi A: Myelofibrosis with myeloid metaplasia. N Engl J Med 2000;342:1255.

Essential Thrombocythemia

Anagrelide Study Group: Anagrelide, a therapy for thrombocythemic states: Experience in 577 patients. Am J Med 1992;92:69.

Frenkel EP: The clinical spectrum of thrombocytosis and thrombocythemia. Am J Med Sci 1991;301:69.

Tefferi A, Silverstein MN, Hoagland HC: Primary thrombocythemia. Semin Oncol 1995;22:334.

Normal Lymphopoiesis

Normal lymphopoiesis is an essential component in host defense. It involves the proliferation and function of several types of lymphoid cells including **B cells,** which are the antibody-producing cells; **T cells,** which carry out cell-mediated immune functions and are largely responsible for regulatory control of the immune system; and the **natural killer (NK) cells,** which function in a more macrophage-like role in host defense against infection and malignancy. An understanding of normal lymphopoiesis requires a knowledge of individual cell characteristics and expected responses of these cells to disease states.

LYMPHOID STEM CELLS

The earliest lymphoid stem cell is derived from the totipotent stem cell pool of the marrow. However, both B cells and T cells then mature in other lymphoid tissues. The **thymus** plays a major role in developing T cells. Precursors leave the marrow and migrate to the thymus, where they develop into immunocompetent cells. It is in the environment of the thymus that the T cell develops its critical ability to distinguish self from nonself and where errors in development form the basis for most, if not all, autoimmune disease. The stages of T-cell development in the thymus are well defined and form the basis for clinical approach to the classification of T-cell malignancies.

B-cell development takes place in both marrow and peripheral lymphoid tissues, the nodes, and spleen. The stages of B-cell development are not as clearly defined as those of T cells, forming more of a continuum leading to the end stage plasma cell. In addition to their classical role in the production of antibodies, B cells also serve as **antigen-presenting cells.** They have the ability to localize and process antigens from the environment and to present these antigens to other cells of the immune system just like macrophages. Their development and function are largely controlled by regulatory T cells. Therefore, it is sometimes difficult when presented with a disease secondary to immune dysfunction to assign root cause to the B- or T-cell system simply because the two systems are so intimately intertwined.

The Immune Network

An important concept in thinking about disorders of the immune system is that of the "**immune network.**" Cells of the immune system make no basic distinction between internal antigen (ie, a component of self) and external antigen (ie, a pathogen or molecule arising from mutation or transplantation). All chemical structures in the body, including proteins, carbohydrates, and to a lesser extent, lipids, are recognized by immune cells. This includes the components and products of the immune cells themselves. The "immune network" is balanced in such a way, however, that those cells that recognize self antigens are suppressed but not eliminated, and those cells recognizing foreign antigens are stimulated but not allowed to become predominant. Thus, the immune system can be looked on as a balanced network of positive and negative interactions that is controlled by intertwined feedback systems (Figure 19–1).

Although we understand the principles that control the immune network, and have some clear examples of how it functions, it is too complex to describe completely. Autoimmunity is a necessary, even critical, part of the immune system. Disease results from a disruption of the normal balance, that is, emergence of uncontrolled autoimmunity, inappropriate suppression of the ability of cells to recognize a foreign antigen, or uncontrolled proliferation of one or more clones of lymphocytes. However, simple disease explanations, such as "too many suppressor cells" or "too few helper cells," are viewed with great skepticism because they do not present the complete clinical picture of immune dysfunction.

Lymphoid Cell Development

Another important concept in development of the immune system is that it is not a linear process. Development of erythrocytes or neutrophils is characterized by a series of recognizable steps in maturation with no possibility of return to a more immature cell form or independent clonal expansion. This characteristic has served as the foundation for classifying myeloproliferative disorders. This is not true, however, for lymphoid

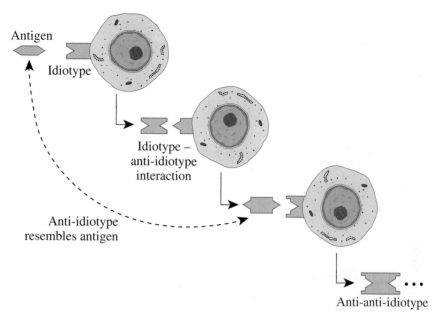

Figure 19–1. The "immune network." The immune network consists of a cascade of interacting cells with specificity for antigen and for each other. The first cell that responds to antigen creates an antibody that is itself antigenic for other cells. The idiotype of this antibody stimulates production of "anti-idiotype" antibodies that resemble, antigenically, the original antigen. This series of interactions continues and results in a balanced network of stimulatory and suppressive interactions that control the immune system.

cells. Both B cells and T cells develop in a three-dimensional manner (Figure 19–2). This complex maturation can be simplified to a linear, recognizable morphologic pathway (Figure 19–3). However, unlike myelocytes, developing lymphoid cells, by the process of gene rearrangement, are able to program themselves to respond to a wide variety of antigens. This results in the appearance of clones of lymphocytes with the ability to recognize and react to a specific antigen. Whenever these cells encounter that antigen, they are stimulated to begin a new round of proliferation and differentiation typical of the mature immune response, both cellular and humoral.

This complex pattern of proliferation and differentiation makes it difficult to determine the history and future of a lymphoid cell simply from its morphology. For example, an activated, proliferating T cell can be a cell that has never encountered antigen but is proliferating in the normal course of expanding the number of antigen-reactive cells. On the other hand, it may be a T cell that has recently encountered antigen and is proliferating to give rise to programmed cytotoxic effector and memory cells. Or it may be a cell that has undergone an oncogenic mutation and is on the way to produce a lymphoma. In each case, we would call such a

cell a blast and the morphologic, immunologic, and cytogenetic tools that we now have could not distinguish between the several possibilities. In order to clinically define the condition, whether benign or malignant, the entire pattern of the disease process must be examined.

LYMPHOID GROWTH FACTORS

Several growth factors (**interleukins**) that regulate the development and function of lymphocytes have now been identified. The precise regulatory roles of each of the interleukins still need to be defined. It is apparent that they function in a complex and overlapping way to control lymphocyte development. In some cases, interleukins affect other cell lineages, as for example, the role of interleukin-3 in myelocyte and erythrocyte production. Thus, the descriptions that follow are not meant to be exhaustive but simply to provide examples of the roles of some of these growth factors in cell development and function.

Interleukin-1 (IL-1)

IL-1 is produced by several different cell types and has a wide range of effects as part of acute and chronic

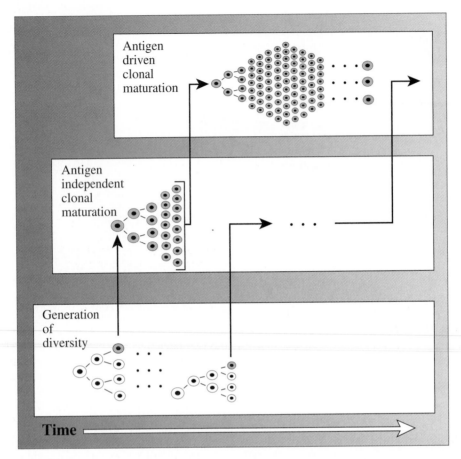

Figure 19–2. **Lymphocyte development.** Both B and T cells develop along a multidimensional pathway. On the first level is the continuous process of gene rearrangement, taking place in lymphoid progenitors, which results in the generation of the diverse repertoire of the immune response. This process begins in the fetus and continues throughout life. As cells with new specificities arise, their development moves to the level of antigen-independent clonal maturation, which results in the production of a clone of cells with the same specificity capable of recognizing a specific antigen. Although all of the cells of a given specificity will have the same antigen-receptor molecules, they may differ in other respects depending on their stage of maturation at this level. Finally, when the cells of a given clone encounter specific antigen, they begin to mature on a new level with the result that they give rise to both the fully differentiated cells of the immune system (plasma cells in the case of B cells and effector T cells) and also to memory cells. As the antigen-driven clonal expansion fades, the memory cells survive and are capable of mounting a secondary response should antigen reappear.

inflammation. For example, IL-1 induces proliferation of thymocytes and fibroblasts, activates osteoclasts to enhance bone reabsorption, increases levels of acute phase reactants, and activates neutrophils. It also stimulates the production of IL-2 by T cells and synergizes with myeloid growth factors to stimulate marrow stem cells.

Interleukin-2 (IL-2)

IL-2 is the interleukin most clearly associated with lymphoid functions. It is produced by activated T cells and in turn stimulates the proliferation and differentiation of both T and B cells. It serves to amplify the immune response and is required for T-cell responses and the

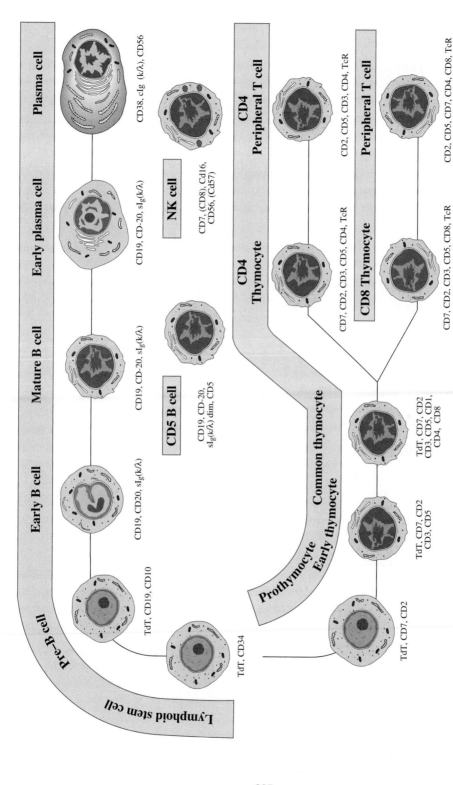

Figure 19–3. Morphologic and phenotypic differentiation of B and T cells. The lymphocytic stem cell can differentiate along a B- or T-cell pathway, characterized by changes in morphology and cell phenotype. Surface markers can be helpful in diagnosing lymphoproliferative disorders, malignancies of the B- and T-cell lines, and immune deficiency states (sIg, surface immunoglobulin; cIg, cytoplasmic immunoglobulin).

stimulation of NK cells. The measurement of IL-2 and its receptors has been used to monitor the activity of the immune system. Drugs and antibodies that inhibit IL-2 or block its receptors may play a role as immunosuppressive agents. On the other hand, IL-2 itself has been used therapeutically as an antitumor agent.

Interleukin-3 (IL-3)

IL-3 is a growth factor for B cells. It induces proliferation of antigen-activated B cells, increases antibody synthesis, and synergizes with IL-2. It also stimulates the proliferation of T cells, predominantly of the CD8 subtype. IL-3 plays a synergistic role in early myeloid and erythroid progenitor proliferation and differentiation (see Chapters 1 and 15).

Other Interleukins

Several other interleukins are now being investigated. **Interleukin-5** appears to induce B-cell maturation with its major effect on IgA production. Its major clinical effect in humans is on eosinophil differentiation. **Interleukin-6** affects B-cell growth and differentiation but also stimulates the growth of hepatocytes and neurons. **Interleukin-7** has stimulatory effects on early B cells and may affect lymphoid progenitors of both B- and T-cell pathways. **Interleukin-11** functions as a generalized hematopoietic growth factor and may have a role in thrombopoiesis. **Interleukin-12** has potent stimulatory effects on lymphoid cells, especially cytotoxic T cells. It is being investigated in the treatment of infectious disease, immunodeficiency, and autoimmunity.

Both lymphocytes and myeloid cells are also capable of producing interferons as a part of host defense. The **interferons** function as stimulators of T- and NK-cell function. At the same time, they have a suppressive effect on hematopoiesis, reducing red blood cell and white blood cell proliferation at the same time they stimulate cell functions such as cytotoxicity and phagocytosis.

LYMPHOCYTE ADHESION MOLECULES

In addition to the growth factors, several adhesion molecules govern the migration, localization, and function

Table 19–1. Major families of adhesion molecules.

Family	CD Numbers	Names	Ligands	Functions
Immunoglobulin-like	CD56	N-CAM		Cell-cell adhesion
	CD54	I-CAM1	LFA-1	Cell-cell adhesion
	CD31	P-CAM		On platelets
	CD58	LFA-3	LFA-2	T-cell signaling
	CD2	LFA-2	LFA-3	T-cell signaling
		V-CAM	VLA-4	Cell-cell adhesion
Integrins β1 Family	CD29/49	VLA1-6	Collagen Fibronectin Laminin	Adhesion to matrix proteins
β2 Family	CD18/11	LFA-1 MAC-1 p150,95	I-CAM1 C3bi	Leukocyte adhesion Complement receptor
β3 Family	CD61/51		Vitronectin	
	CD61/41		Fibrinogen	Platelet–platelet adhesion
Selectins	CD69P	P-Selectin	Carbohydrate	Platelet–leukocyte adhesion
	CD69E	E-Selectin	Carbohydrate	Leukocyte–endothelial cell adhesion
	CD69L	L-Selectin	Carbohydrate	Lymphocyte–endothelial cell adhesion

of lymphocytes and other blood cells. These appear to fall into several families of related molecules (Table 19–1).

Ig Super Family

The **Ig super family** contains molecules that are structurally related to immunoglobulins. In general, these molecules appear to be involved with cell-cell adhesive interactions, although in some cases they also serve as receptors for soluble complement components.

Integrins

The **integrins** are a large family of heterodimers with closely related structures. They derive much of their diversity from different combinations of the two component molecules, the α- and β-chains. They mediate interactions between cells and molecules of the vascular subendothelium and serve as receptors for coagulation proteins such as fibrinogen and factor VIII.

Selectins

The **selectins** are molecules that are structurally related to lectins that bind to carbohydrates. They are involved in interactions between leukocytes, platelets, and endothelial cells, playing a key role in granulocyte adhesion and egress from circulation (see Chapter 15).

Cadherins

The **cadherins** are a family of molecules that bind to themselves. They appear to be involved largely in the interaction of cells within tissues. They play an essential role in the immune network, controlling lymphocyte circulation and their function in immune surveillance. They act as homing receptors to govern migration of lymphocytes into lymph nodes and Peyer's patches.

The **L-Selectin** molecule plays a role in the binding of lymphocytes to the high endothelial venules of lymph nodes. Another molecule, **CD44,** has been implicated in the preferential binding of gut-associated lymphocytes to the endothelium of Peyer's patches. These molecules are expressed on mature migratory lymphocytes but not immature thymocytes or marrow lymphocytes.

B CELLS

Lymphocytes can be characterized according to their functional differentiation, surface phenotype, and gene rearrangement pattern. Each of these needs to be considered when diagnosing an immune deficiency state or clonal malignancy.

Functional Differentiation

A. ANTIBODY PRODUCTION:

The principal role of the B cells in the immune system is to produce antibodies. Early in its development, the B cell acquires, by rearrangement of its immunoglobulin genes, the ability to make a specific antibody. It subsequently displays a small sample of this antibody on its surface (about 100,000 molecules per cell). This antibody serves as an **antigen receptor** for the B cell. Whenever the cell encounters that antigen that binds to the receptor, it is stimulated to begin a process of differentiation leading to the conversion of the B cell into a plasma cell. The **plasma cell** is then a stable factory for manufacturing a constant amount of the same antibody for excretion. This capability of B cells to recognize antigen and respond with a production of antibody is to some extent autonomous, although it is markedly influenced by interactions with T cells, which also recognize the same or closely related antigens. B-cell responses are augmented by the "helper" T cells and are suppressed by interactions with "suppressor" T cells.

B. AUGMENTATION OF THE IMMUNE RESPONSE:

Augmentation of the immune response involves several mechanisms. The antibody receptor of B cells can interact directly with antigen to trigger B-cell differentiation. B cells are also capable of internalizing some of the antigen and processing it in the same way that macrophages process antigen by digestion with proteases. The cell then reexpresses partially degraded and denatured antigen on the surface for recognition by T cells. Thus, **B cells have an antigen-presenting function** that stimulates T-cell activity.

C. MATURATION SEQUENCE:

Finally, once B cells are triggered by antigen, they undergo a **maturation sequence** leading to changes in class, but not specificity, of antibody they produce. Early in the immune response, B cells give rise largely to IgM antibodies. With maturation, there is an increase in the proportion of B cells producing IgG, IgA, and IgE. This occurs by a process called **class switching** that involves further alteration at the DNA level and by RNA splicing. The end result is production of **memory B cells.** These cells are capable of recognizing antigen upon reexposure so as to give rise to an accelerated (secondary) immune response consisting of a magnified production of IgG.

D. TOLERANCE TO ANTIGENS:

There are also defined mechanisms by which B cells fail to respond to a given antigen, that is, demonstrate "**tolerance.**" A first mechanism is an active **suppression of the response mediated by T cells** that recognize the same or similar antigen and actively suppress the response. A second mechanism is **clonal deletion,** in which all of the B-cell clones capable of interacting with antigen are destroyed.

Suppression is the normal mechanism by which an organism prevents its immune system from responding to self antigens. It is an active, continuous process that requires the proper functioning of the immune network. A failure in network control gives rise to autoimmune disease. Immune deficiency or tolerance can also develop because of **clonal deletion.** It can result because of a lymphopoietic malignancy or following chemotherapy. This is not necessarily irreversible. The continuous process of regeneration of diversity by gene rearrangement at the level of the lymphoid progenitor cells will eventually give rise to new clones capable of responding to specific antigens. Thus, no form of tolerance is likely to persist for the life of the patient.

Phenotypic Classification

The normal sequence of maturation and phenotypic expression of B cells is illustrated in Figure 19–3. The listed antigenic markers are those that are most often used clinically in categorizing disease processes. There are many other markers that are not indicated because they are not unique or are of unknown significance.

A. Pre–B Cell:

The earliest recognizable B cell, the **pre–B cell,** is recognized by the presence of cytoplasmic μ heavy chain but no light chain, together with an absence of intact immunoglobulin on its surface. Its surface markers consist of CD19 (but not CD20), HLA-DR, CD34, and CD10 (CALLA). The cell also expresses the nuclear enzyme **terminal deoxynucleotide transferase** (**TdT**), which may be one of the enzymes involved in the gene rearrangement process. This stage of B-cell maturation matches the level of cell development seen in the most common form of acute lymphoblastic leukemia.

B. Mature B Cell Without Antigen:

As the B cell matures, it loses CD34 and TdT and acquires surface immunoglobulin, first IgM and then IgM and IgD. It also acquires CD19 and then CD20. This process takes place in the marrow and in lymph nodes and spleen. It results in a mature B cell that has not yet been exposed to antigen with phenotypic markers of CD19, CD20, HLA-DR, sIgM, and sIgD. This is the most common B cell found in the lymphoid tissues of adults.

C. Mature B Cell With Antigen:

Once a B cell encounters antigen, it continues to express CD19 and CD20, but expression of surface im-

munoglobulin may include IgM, IgG, IgA, or IgE. In addition, these cells can express any number of activation antigens. One that has become of some importance in the classification of lymphomas (see Chapter 22) is **CD23,** which serves as a receptor for the Fc portion of IgE and appears on some activated B cells. This diversity of response is reflected in the diversity of phenotypes seen with B-cell lymphomas. For the purposes of clinical diagnosis, the most consistent and reliable markers for mature B cells at any stage of development are CD19, CD20, and the expression of κ- and λ-immunoglobulin light chains.

D. Plasma Cell:

Once B cells differentiate to become plasma cells, they devote nearly all of their synthetic energy to immunoglobulin production and cease expression of other B-cell markers. Therefore, the best marker for plasma cells is the abundance of **cytoplasmic immunoglobulin** and the intense expression of **CD38,** an activation marker involved in signaling leading to activation and proliferation of lymphoid cells.

E. CD5-Positive B Cell:

A major B-cell subset that does not fit easily into the sequence of B-cell development is characterized by the expression of **CD5.** This antigen is also expressed by T cells. CD5 positive B cells are abundant in the fetus and represent 10–20% of B cells in the adult. They express CD19, CD20, sIgM, and sIgD much like conventional B cells. An expansion of this subset of B cells is associated with a production of autoantibodies in diseases such as rheumatoid arthritis and systemic lupus erythematosus. This is also the phenotype associated with chronic lymphocytic leukemia.

Gene Rearrangement Pattern

The lymphoid stem cell gives rise to the earliest recognizable B cell in the marrow, fetal liver, and spleen. This pre–B cell has already undergone the process of gene rearrangement of both its immunoglobulin heavy- and light-chain–variable regions. The rearrangement normally proceeds in an orderly fashion in which the cell rearranges each of its genes in sequence until it either produces a pair of functional heavy- and light-chain genes or has failed. Because of the uncertainties of splicing the rearranged DNA segments, there is a significant probability that some rearrangements will not give rise to functioning molecules. Even when it is successful, there is a good chance that the gene product will be slightly different from that encoded by the original germline gene sequences. This process of "**generation of diversity**" gives rise to an enormous variety of different antibodies produced by the mature immune system.

From a clinical point of view, studies of the gene rearrangement pattern are important in diagnosing lymphoproliferative diseases. They can be used to answer two important questions:

- Are the malignant cells B, T, or NK cells?
- Do the cells belong to a single clone, which would strongly suggest malignancy?

Although these questions can in part be answered using immunologic markers, they are more directly answered by **analyzing the gene structure of the cells.** Gene rearrangement is independent of the stage of maturation of the lymphocytes since it is the first defining event in a cell's life. In addition, gene rearrangement is unaffected by any of the later events in the life of the lymphocytes such as antigen exposure. Thus, it defines clonality in an irrefutable way.

Recently, information about the genetic structure of malignant B cells has begun to provide prognostic, as well as diagnostic, information. It has been observed that some cases of **chronic lymphocytic leukemia (CLL)** have un-rearranged (germ-line) immunoglobulin heavy-chain genes and thus most likely represent naive B cells that have not previously encountered antigen. This variant of CLL appears to have a significantly worse prognosis than the more common variety in which the heavy-chain genes have undergone somatic mutation as described above.

T CELLS

As with B cells, T cells can be characterized according to their function, surface phenotype, and gene rearrangement pattern. Clinically, classification of the cell type and function is essential for understanding an immune deficiency state or diagnosing a malignancy.

Functional Differentiation

There are two fundamental roles for T cells in the immune system. The first is their **regulatory role.** They modulate the function of all of the cellular components of the immune system, including macrophages, other T cells, and B cells. The second is their role as **effectors of cellular immunity.** They are responsible for carrying out delayed-type hypersensitivity reactions, cytotoxicity, and both graft and tumor rejection, that is, all of the immune functions that are not mediated by antibodies.

A. ANTIGEN RECOGNITION AND "ALTERED SELF":

T cells directly recognize antigen using receptors that are similar to the immunoglobulin antigen receptors of B cells. However, rather than recognizing native, soluble antigen, they respond to antigen processed by macrophages and presented on the surface of the cell in association with the **major histocompatibility complex (MHC) molecules** (HLA-A, HLA-B, and HLA-DR). By way of this close association, the T cell actually senses an alteration of the normal cellular histocompatibility molecules (ie, an "**altered self**"). This concept is integral to the proper functioning of the immune system.

B. CYTOKINE SECRETION AND SUPPRESSION OF IMMUNE RESPONSE:

Once a T cell recognizes a specific antigen, it secretes cytokines that increase the activity of macrophages, recruit more T cells, and augment the function of B cells. Thus, T cells are responsible for initiating the immune and inflammatory response to an antigen. In addition, once the immune response is exhausted, usually by elimination of the antigen, T cells have an important role in signaling the termination of the response. The suppression of the immune response is an active process mediated by T cells.

In the absence of normal balanced T-cell function, an immune response once initiated will not terminate even after the antigen is eliminated. This **failure of suppression** is central to many, if not all, autoimmune diseases. It is important to recognize that the "helper" and "suppressor" functions are not restricted to specific subsets of T cells, as was once thought, but are distributed throughout the T-cell system. A given clone of antigen-reactive T cells will contain both helper and suppressor functions. The dominance of one over the other will depend on the antigenic stimulus, its concentration, and complex interactions within the immune network.

C. ROLE IN INFLAMMATION AND CYTOTOXICITY:

The effector functions of T cells are important in initiating inflammation and for killing other cells (**cytotoxicity**). **Inflammation** is in part mediated by the secretion of cytokines such as IL-1, which recruit and activate other cells of the inflammatory response. T cells also mediate the local delayed hypersensitivity reaction seen when antigen is injected into the skin (eg, the **tuberculin reaction**). The induration and erythema result when T cells recognize the tuberculin protein on the surface of local macrophages and then initiate the recruitment of other T cells, macrophages, neutrophils, and monocytes to the site.

The **cytotoxic function** of T cells is initiated when a programmed T cell recognizes foreign histocompatibility antigens, viral antigens, or tumor-associated antigens on the surface of a target cell. The lymphocyte is then stimulated to secrete cytoplasmic granules that contain enzymes to lyse the target cell. This reaction is at the basis of T-cell elimination of transplanted tissue, tumors, and virus-infected cells. Cytotoxicity is not restricted to a specific subset of T cells. Instead, many if not all T cells are capable of cytotoxicity when appropriately activated by cytokines such as IL-2.

Phenotypic Classification

The differentiation sequence of T cells is illustrated in Figure 19–3. The list of phenotypic markers shows those most often used in the clinical classification of T cells. By the time T-cell markers are first expressed, the cell has already undergone rearrangement of the receptor genes. The presence of TdT as a nuclear marker, and the presence of the common progenitor cell marker CD34, are not unique to the T cell but are shared with the pre–B cell. **CD7** is the earliest marker that characterizes a T-cell lineage.

The CD7 marker is conserved throughout T-cell development; however, it is most strongly expressed on immature T cells and is the best marker for T-cell acute lymphocytic leukemia. **CD2** is the marker originally described as the sheep erythrocyte rosette receptor. It also appears early and is highly conserved. It has a role in signaling activation of the T cell. Early T cells express cytoplasmic but not surface CD3. The **CD3** marker is the best marker for mature T cells and is an integral part of the complex of molecules that constitute the T-cell antigen receptor.

The most abundant cell in the thymus, the **common thymocyte,** expresses a wide array of markers that are common to all T cells, including CD1, CD2, CD3, CD5, and CD7. This panel of markers is useful in differentiating normal from abnormal mature T cells. Malignant T cells are often revealed by the absence (or low expression) of one or more of these markers. The only unique distinguishing characteristic of the common thymocyte is the simultaneous presence of CD4 and CD8.

Later in thymic differentiation, the **maturing T-cell loses either CD4 or CD8,** thereby declaring itself as a member of one of the two major subsets referred to as **helper** (CD4 positive) and **suppressor** (CD8 positive) T cells. The actual role of these two antigenic molecules has to do with the recognition of HLA class II or class I (respectively) histocompatibility molecules and is not directly related to helper or suppressor function.

Mature T cells leave the thymus and circulate in the periphery as **either CD4 or CD8 subsets.** This distinction is very useful clinically. Attempts to further subdivide T cells with finer functional distinctions or markers have not proved to be clinically useful. For example, although most peripheral T cells (80–90%) use a pair of receptor molecules referred to as the α/β-receptor, 10–20% of cells use a different pair known as the γ/δ-

receptor. γ/δ T cells are more often found in skin, but the functional significance of this is not yet clear. The exclusive presence of γ/δ T cells in a tumor mass may suggest clonality, but this is only occasionally useful because of the predominance of the α/β subset.

Mature T cells also express an array of new antigens when activated. The most frequently noted antigens are the reappearance of **HLA-DR** and the new expression of the **IL-2 receptor** (**CD25**). In general, these activation markers are found on cells activated by exposure to antigen. They have also been described on malignant T cells, however. The effector stage of T-cell maturation is not distinguished by any unique markers. Although CD57 is found on cytotoxic T cells, it is not unique.

Gene Rearrangement Pattern

Although the receptors of T cells are different from those of B cells, the principles that govern their genetics are very similar. Thus, T cells undergo a process of sequential rearrangement of their T-cell receptor genes that is analogous to the rearrangement of the B-cell immunoglobulin genes. Identification of rearranged gene sequences by polymerase chain reaction and Southern blot analysis is important clinically in the diagnosis of malignancy. Since studies of T-cell surface markers are poor indicators of malignancy, proof of clonality rests in showing a common gene rearrangement pattern.

NK CELLS

Approximately 10% of circulating lymphocytes do not fall into the T- or B-cell categories, by either surface markers or genetic analysis. These cells **share some properties of T cells and macrophages.** They are very active in cytotoxicity and have been shown to be important in host defense, especially against tumors and virus-infected cells. They appear early in ontogeny and reappear following ablation of the immune system (eg, following marrow transplantation). They may, therefore, be thought of as the more primitive relatives of the true immune system.

NK cells do not have antigen-specific receptors, and they do not show evidence of immune memory. Their ability to kill target cells is not affected by prior exposure to antigen, thus the name *natural killer* cells. NK cells have receptors for MHC class I molecules that are inhibitory, that is, they recognize and kill cells that are deficient in MHC class I expression. Target cells expressing low levels of HLA-A and -B are, therefore, better targets for NK-cell killing. Many tumor cells and virus-infected cells share this property of low level class I expression. The actual act of killing by NK cells is similar or identical to that of activated macrophages and cytotoxic T cells, involving the release of toxic substances from cytoplasmic granules.

NK cells bind to soluble antibody and are thus capable of attaching to and killing any cell expressing antigen recognized by that antibody. This property of being "armed" by antibody (antibody-dependent cytotoxicity) is shared with monocytes and macrophages. NK cells also **respond to and are activated by IL-2.** IL-2-activated NK cells, referred to as **lymphokine-activated killer** cells, have been used effectively in the treatment of certain malignancies.

BIBLIOGRAPHY

Chin YH, Sackstein R, Cai JP: Lymphocyte homing receptors and preferential migration pathways. Proc Soc Exp Biol Med 1991;196:374.

Fackler MJ, Strauss LC: Lymphohematopoiesis: Role of growth factors in leukemogenesis and therapy. Hematol Oncol Clin North Am 1990;4:849.

Gordon J, Cairns JA: Autocrine regulation of normal and malignant B lymphocytes. Adv Cancer Res 1991;56:313.

Hamblin TJ et al: Unmutated Ig VH genes are associated with a more aggressive form of chronic lymphocytic leukemia. Blood 1999;94:1848.

Henney CS: The interleukins as lymphocyte growth factors. Transplant Proc 1989;21:22.

Lymphopenia and Immune Deficiency

20

With the advent of the human immunodeficiency virus epidemic, the diagnosis and treatment of acquired immunodeficiency has become a major preoccupation for many medical subspecialties, including hematology. In addition to HIV-induced AIDS, several congenital and acquired immunodeficiency states may be encountered. In general, the genetic immune defects are well defined, whereas many of the acquired defects are poorly understood.

Lymphopenia is seen in those forms of immune deficiency that are characterized by a failure in the development of a major subset of lymphocytes or by wholesale destruction of lymphocytes. At the same time, patients may manifest profound immune defects with normal numbers of lymphocytes and normal levels of lymphocyte subsets. A failure in cellular interactions, defective production of cytokines, or intrinsic cellular defects probably underlies many of such cases. Tools to diagnose and treat immune deficiency states have been steadily improving. Nevertheless, treatment either is aimed at the underlying disease or is designed to combat infection and replace missing immunoglobulins rather than correct the basic immunologic defect.

NORMAL LYMPHOCYTE KINETICS

The pathways of lymphocyte development are described in detail in Chapter 19. **Lymphocytes** arise from progenitors in the marrow and develop in the lymphoid organs; **T cells,** predominantly in the thymus early in life and then in lymph nodes; **B cells,** in the marrow and lymph nodes. The lymphocytes found circulating in the peripheral blood are not representative of all lymphocytes but rather are particular subsets that circulate for specific reasons (Table 20–1).

They consist predominantly of **T cells** (70–80%) that are in a constant state of circulation from blood through the lymph nodes, tissues, and lymphatics, and back to blood. They exit the blood in specialized postcapillary venules within the lymph nodes, percolate through the nodes, and then return via the lymphatics. T cells are also found in perivascular locations in tissues throughout the body and are found to be markedly increased in sites of inflammation. Most T cells can live for many months to years under normal conditions. Their role in the immune system may be thought of as spreading the immune response against a particular antigen throughout the body.

B cells are much less common in the blood (10–15%) and do not appear to circulate through the tissues as do T cells. There is some evidence that many of the B cells found in blood are a distinct class of B cells, although this is not well established. Since they account for about 50% of the lymphocytes in the nodes, the relatively small numbers that circulate probably serve a special purpose. Blood B cells appear to be enriched for that subset that has been implicated in autoimmunity (**CD5 cells**). B cells, like T cells, are relatively long lived. When they become fully differentiated to plasma cells they no longer circulate, but are confined to lymphoid tissues and the marrow.

Another major class of blood lymphocytes is the natural killer (**NK**) **cells** (10–15%). These share some properties of macrophages and also express antigens and functions that are similar to those of T cells. They appear to mediate a type of immunity that is less antigen-specific than that of T and B cells, and they lack the property of immunologic memory. They may be thought of as more primitive than T or B cells. Nevertheless, they appear to be a major host defense mechanism against many viral infections and some tumors. The fact that very few patients have been described with severe defects of NK-cell function may be testimony to their importance in host defense. Their lifespan and circulation patterns are not well defined.

CLINICAL FEATURES

Significant lymphopenia or lymphocyte dysfunction is usually suspected because of the occurrence of repeated episodes of infection. **Pyogenic, gram-positive bacterial infections** suggest a defect in antibody production, which may or may not be accompanied by a hypogammaglobulinemia. Since an antibody specific for even a

Table 20–1. The normal distribution of lymphocyte subsets in blood.

Subset	Percentage of Lymphocytes	Absolute Count (cells per µL)
Lymphocytes	100	1500–2500
T cells	65–75	1300–1500
B cells	10–15	200–300
NK cells	10–20	200–400
CD4 T cells	35–45	700–900
CD8 T cells	30–40	600–800

complex bacterial antigen usually represents far less than 10% of the total circulating immunoglobulin, it is difficult to detect a failure of specific antibody production by measuring total immunoglobulins. In fact, there would appear to be a feedback mechanism that increases the levels of other immunoglobulins in the face of many forms of immunodeficiency so that an affected patient may well have elevated immunoglobulins.

Repeated episodes of **viral, fungal, or other opportunistic infections** suggest a defect in T-cell function. Again, the number of T cells reacting specifically against any one antigen represents a very small proportion of the total T-cell pool, so profound T-cell defects may not be reflected by lymphopenia or decrease in any T-cell subset. Thus, **clinical evaluation of any patient suspected of immune deficiency** must rely on a detailed past medical history to define the nature and frequency of infections, a family history to identify a possible genetic disorder, and a careful examination for signs or symptoms suggestive of a lymphoproliferative disorder.

Laboratory Studies

The laboratory evaluation of these patients should include a routine complete blood count (CBC) and white blood cell differential, a measurement of the major lymphocyte subsets in the blood, and a quantitative measurement of each of the major immunoglobulin classes. The distribution of lymphocyte subsets in the blood and the absolute number of cells for each subset are listed in Table 20–1. **Absolute lymphopenia** is defined as a count less than 1500/µL. Even when the total lymphocyte count is normal, however, a deficiency of one of the lymphocyte subsets can result in significant immune deficiency.

Measurement of total levels of the major immunoglobulin classes (IgG, IgM, IgA, etc) is relatively insensitive to the detection of immune deficiency. A more sensitive measure of the ability of the immune system to make specific antibodies can be obtained by **quantitating levels of antibody against antigens** that the patient is known to have encountered. This can be done by measuring antibody titers against known infectious agents (*Candida,* mumps, rubella, Epstein-Barr, herpes, or cytomegalovirus) or by measuring antibody levels before and after intentional immunization (Pneumovax, tetanus toxoid, hepatitis B, etc).

Laboratory testing of T-cell function will depend on the level of laboratory services available. **Skin testing with antigens** such as *Candida* and PPD can be used, but their interpretation is highly subjective and a lack of responsiveness may indicate generalized suppression of the inflammatory response rather than a specific immune defect. The ability of T cells to proliferate in vitro in response to mitogens such as phytohemagglutinin, soluble antigens such as tetanus toxoid, or allogeneic T cells (the **mixed lymphocyte response**) provides a more quantitative and reproducible measure of T-cell function. The ability of T cells to kill allogeneic cells after exposure in vitro (so-called **cell-mediated lympholysis**) is a measure of the ability of T cells to both respond to an antigen and to generate fully differentiated effector cells. It is also possible to measure the ability of the T cells to produce cytokines such as interleukin-2 (**IL-2**) in response to soluble antigen or allogeneic cells. **NK-cell function** is usually measured by the ability of lymphocytes to kill certain tumor cell targets or virus-infected cell lines.

CONGENITAL IMMUNODEFICIENCY DISORDERS

Several rare, inherited immunodeficiency disorders may be diagnosed during the first year of life. They present with recurrent bacterial and fungal infections and are often associated with one or more other congenital abnormalities (Table 20–2).

Table 20–2. Congenital immunodeficiency disorders.

Disease	Major Manifestation	Cellular Abnormality	Therapy
X-Linked hypogammaglobulinemia	Pyogenic infections in infancy, absent IgM, IgA, IgD, and IgE, very low IgG	B cells absent	IV gamma globulin Antibiotics
IgA deficiency	Usually asymptomatic, very low IgA	None	None; risk of anaphylaxis when given blood products
Thymic aplasia (DiGeorge syndrome)	Hypoparathyroidism, abnormal facies, opportunistic infections	Decreased T cells	Fetal thymus transplant
Chronic mucocutaneous candidiasis	Chronic *Candida* infection, multiple endocrinopathies	Normal T cells but failure to respond to *Candida* antigens	Antibiotics
Severe combined immunodeficiency	Recurrent viral, bacterial, fungal, and protozoan infections	Absent or very low T and B cells Several mechanisms	Marrow transplantation
Ataxia-telangiectasia	Telangiectasia, neurologic abnormalities, recurrent sinopulmonary infections	Decreased T cells, often low IgA levels	Antibiotics
Wiskott-Aldrich syndrome	Eczema, thrombocytopenia, recurrent pyogenic infections	Abnormal CD43 antigen on lymphocytes and platelets	Marrow transplantation

Defects in Immunoglobulin Production

Children with defects in immunoglobulin production generally present with recurrent, severe pyogenic infections once their maternally acquired antibody is lost at approximately 5–6 months of age. Infants with **congenital hypogammaglobulinemia,** the most common form of which is X-linked, demonstrate a profound decrease in all classes of immunoglobulin and a near total absence of B lymphocytes. Children with **solitary IgA deficiency** are usually asymptomatic. They do not have pyogenic infections but are at lifelong risk for anaphylaxis if they receive repeated transfusion of blood products containing IgA.

Immunodeficiency Syndromes

Children with immunodeficiency syndromes involving the T-cell system present with recurrent infections involving a variety of organisms including viruses, fungi, and protozoans. They frequently show decreased or absent T cells. **Severe combined immunodeficiency disease (SCID),** involving both the T- and B-cell systems, is now known to arise from several distinct mechanisms of dysfunction of the immune system. The most common of these is **adenosine deaminase deficiency (ADA).** The lack of this enzyme results in the accumulation of adenosine metabolites that inhibit the growth and function of T cells, and to a lesser extent B cells. Some of these patients will respond to exogenous adenosine deaminase provided by red blood cell transfusion or the administration of stabilized preparations of the enzyme. The future treatment of choice is "**gene transplantation,**" however, which involves transfecting autologous hematopoietic progenitor cells with the adenine deaminase gene followed by reimplantation. Recently, it has been recognized that some children and adults with mild to moderate lymphopenia and immune deficiency may be partially ADA deficient. Since this is potentially treatable, measurement of erythrocyte ADA should be done in suspected cases.

Other causes of combined immunodeficiency include deficiencies in IL-1 or IL-2, an abnormality in the receptor for IL-2, absence of class II HLA antigens necessary for antigen presentation, and other defects in T-cell development or function. Because of the central role of the T cells in the immune system, any defect in T-cell development will result in profound immunodeficiency involving both T- and B-cell function. The **Wiskott-Aldrich syndrome** includes a defect in the CD43 antigen found on both platelets and lymphocytes. Although the function of CD43 is not known, the defect does shorten the survival of both T cells and platelets. These patients have recurrent pyogenic infections. They are also at risk for developing lymphomas. Marrow transplantation, which is designed to replace both lymphoid and hematopoietic progenitors, will correct both the thrombocytopenia and the immune deficiency state.

Ataxia-Telangiectasia

Ataxia-telangiectasia is an autosomal recessive disorder that has been shown to result from mutation of a gene known as ATM. Current information suggests that the product of this gene plays a role in monitoring the genome for the presence of DNA damage and protecting the cell from abnormal genetic rearrangements resulting during repair. Patients with this disease have an overall incidence of malignancy of 38% despite a reduced lifespan, and 85% of these are lymphoid leukemias and lymphomas. Most lymphomas demonstrate genetic rearrangements involving the immunoglobulin and T-cell-receptor loci that normally undergo rearrangement (Chapter 22). Thus, abnormal regulation of the gene rearrangement process resulting from mutation of ATM may be the root cause of both the immunodeficiency and the high incidence of lymphoma in these patients. There is some evidence that, even in the heterozygous (carrier) state, ATM mutations may result in an increased incidence of malignancy, including breast cancer.

ACQUIRED IMMUNODEFICIENCY DISORDERS

Acquired immunodeficiency must be considered whenever a patient has recurrent bacterial, viral, or fungal infections. It can occur at any age and may or may not be obviously associated with other disease. In addition to the well-defined immunodeficiency disorders listed in Table 20–3, several other common clinical conditions are accompanied by a relative immunodeficiency. These include advanced age, malnutrition, and chronic inflammatory states associated with autoimmunity or infection.

Hypogammaglobulinemia

Acquired hypogammaglobulinemia or common variable hypogammaglobulinemia is frequently diagnosed in young adults and may be characterized by progressive loss of immunoglobulins with normal or nearly normal lymphocyte subsets. Some cases have been attributed to increased levels of suppressor T-cell function, but many cases go unexplained. The hypogammaglobulinemia may be the result of underlying autoimmune disease or the progression of a clonal malignancy of lymphocytes such as chronic lymphocytic leukemia (CLL).

Chronic Graft-Versus-Host Disease (GVHD)

Graft-versus-host disease is a common complication of allogeneic marrow transplantation and is very rarely seen in immunosuppressed patients who receive unirradiated blood transfusions. The syndrome is characterized by skin disease, diarrhea, hepatic dysfunction, and immunosuppression. It results from the reaction of the engrafted immune system against host histocompatibility antigens. Although young patients who receive fully HLA-compatible marrow transplants usually have little or no GVHD, older patients can develop life-threatening disease. It can occur even following transplants that are fully HLA compatible owing to differences at minor histocompatibility loci.

Table 20–3. Acquired immune deficiency disorders.

Disease	Major Manifestation	Cellular Abnormality	Therapy
Common variable hypogamma-globulinemia	Recurrent pyogenic infections at any age, autoimmune disorders	Hypogamma-globulinemia with normal numbers of B and T cells	IV gamma globulin
Chronic graft-versus-host	Desquamation, hepatospleno-megaly, lymphadenopathy, diarrhea, recurrent infections	Activated T cells	Immunosuppression with steroids, methotrexate, cyclosporine
Secondary to lympho-proliferative disease	Opportunistic or recurrent pyogenic infections	Most common in chronic lymphocytic leukemia and Hodgkin's disease; may be seen in any lymphoma	Chemotherapy for underlying disorder
AIDS	Opportunistic infections	Decreased CD4 T cells	Antiviral drugs

Patients who are immune deficient for any reason are also at risk for acute GVHD acquired from viable lymphocytes in transfusion products such as whole blood, packed red cells, and platelets. This form of GVHD is usually fulminant and carries a high mortality. Any patient thought to have significant immune dysfunction should be transfused with irradiated blood products to prevent this complication.

Acquired Immune Deficiency Syndrome (AIDS)

By far the most common immune deficiency syndrome is AIDS, secondary to infection by HIV. This retrovirus is transmitted by sexual contact, blood and blood product transfusion, and potentially by other body fluids.

The **course of infection** is illustrated in Figure 20–1. Most patients experience an **acute mononucleosis-like syndrome** 3–6 weeks following infection. This syndrome is caused by acute viremia followed by the development of an immune response and the formation of circulating antibody-virus complexes. With the appearance of the immune response, the viremia ceases and a **period of latency** begins that may last several years. During the latency period, the patient is asymptomatic, but the infection persists and progresses and the patient is capable of infecting a sexual partner. Virus can be demonstrated in the patient's lymph nodes, as well as in T lymphocytes and macrophages. The mechanism by which the virus is able to continue to exist and proliferate within the patient's lymph nodes during the latency period is under intense investigation. There is no doubt that the process involves the progressive destruction of CD4-positive lymphocytes by HIV infection. As the disease progresses, the ratio of CD4 to CD8 T cells decreases. In guiding management, critical levels of circulating CD4 T cells are thought to be approximately 500/μL. Certainly, once the CD4 T-cell level falls below 200/μL, the patient is at high risk for opportunistic infections.

After a latency period of 5–10 years, the patient gradually becomes symptomatic because of deterioration of the immune system. The **diagnosis of AIDS** depends on two elements. The first is the demonstration of the **antibody to HIV** indicating previous infection and the second is the appearance of one or more **AIDS-defining illnesses** (Table 20–4). A staging classification for the progression of AIDS has been proposed (Table 20–5). It combines the quantitation of the CD4 T-cell level and the presence or absence of complicating illness.

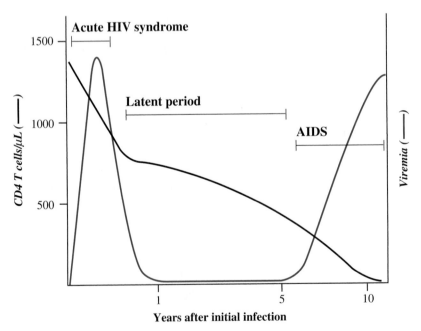

Figure 20–1. **The course of HIV infection.** Initial infection by HIV can be accompanied by an acute viral syndrome, after which the disease enters a prolonged latency phase with no symptoms and no immunologic abnormality. During this time, virus and antivirus antibody can be detected in the tissues. Progression of the disease is characterized by a progressive fall in the CD4 T-cell level and the onset of overt immunodeficiency.

Table 20–4. AIDS-defining illnesses (AIDS indicator conditions).

Candidiasis of bronchi, trachea, lungs, or esophagus
Cervical cancer, invasive
Coccidioidomycosis, disseminated or extrapulmonary
Cryptococcosis, extrapulmonary
Cryptosporidiosis, chronic intestinal for > 1 month
Cytomegalovirus disease other than liver, spleen, or nodes
Cytomegalovirus retinitis with loss of vision
Encephalopathy related to HIV
Herpes simplex, chronic ulcers (> 1 month), bronchitis,
   pneumonitis, or esophagitis
Histoplasmosis, disseminated or extrapulmonary
Isosporiasis, chronic intestinal (> 1 month)
Kaposi's sarcoma
Lymphoma, high-grade or primary in brain
Mycobacterium, any strain, disseminated or extrapulmonary
Mycobacterium tuberculosis, any site
Pneumocystis carinii pneumonia
Pneumonia, recurrent
Progressive multifocal leukoencephalopathy
Salmonella septicemia, recurrent
Toxoplasmosis of brain
Wasting syndrome owing to HIV

A. Hematologic Manifestations:

In addition to the expected lymphopenia, AIDS patients usually show varying combinations of **anemia, granulocytopenia, and thrombocytopenia.** Anemia can be anticipated as the disease progresses. It is usually a hypoproliferative anemia with normocytic, normochromic morphology, low reticulocyte count, and iron studies typical of inflammatory disease. With AZT (zidovudine) treatment, however, the anemia will become more severe and macrocytic. In addition, some patients may be at risk for a true megaloblastic anemia because of vitamin B_{12} malabsorption. The use of erythropoietin in treating the anemia of AIDS is discussed in Chapter 4.

Both **neutropenia and thrombocytopenia** can occur early in the disease process. It is frequently possible to demonstrate increased levels of platelet-associated immunoglobulin. In fact, the presence of IgG, IgM, and complement on the platelet surface, suggesting the presence of immune complexes, is most typical of this disease. A similar mechanism is suspected with neutropenia. Early in the progression of the disease, an examination of the marrow frequently shows normal or increased cellularity. This situation is compatible with a neutropenia and thrombocytopenia owing to peripheral destruction rather than failure of production. However, as complicating illnesses appear, some patients can demonstrate infectious processes such as **mycobacterial or fungal infections** in the marrow, which produce a disordered hematopoiesis. In addition, the marrow may be affected by **lymphoma or Kaposi's sarcoma.**

Another complication of AIDS is the development of a **high-grade lymphoma of the B-cell type.** Indeed, AIDS-related lymphoma is rapidly becoming the major cause of non-Hodgkin's lymphoma. Patients with symptomatic HIV infection have an incidence of lymphoma of 2–6% per year, and a greater than 100-fold increased risk compared with HIV-negative individuals. Despite the advent of highly active anti-retroviral therapy, the incidence of HIV associated non-Hodgkin's lymphoma has not declined.

A large proportion (30–60%) of these lymphomas is associated with the **Epstein-Barr virus (EBV)** genome and may be related to the activation of EBV in the immunodeficient patient. Interestingly, the HIV genome is seldom found in the lymphoma. This apparent role of EBV is similar to that observed in post-transplant patients and some patients with congenital immunodeficiency disorders. However, AIDS-related lymphoma is usually of higher grade, and more often involves a *c-myc* rearrangement than do post-transplant lymphomas. About 20% of AIDS-related lymphomas also show the *c-myc*–associated small noncleaved Burkitt's histology. In general, the prognosis for AIDS patients

Table 20–5. Staging classification for AIDS.

CD4 T-Cell Levels	Asymptomatic	Symptomatic, No AIDS Indicator Conditions	AIDS Indicator Conditions Present
	A	B	C
> 500/μL	A1	B1	C1
200–499/μL	A2	B2	C2
< 200/μL	A3	B3	C3

Note: Categories A3, B3, C1, C2, and C3 meet the criteria for AIDS case surveillance. The other categories are pre-AIDS syndromes.

who develop a lymphoma is poor, although some do respond to conventional multiagent therapy and experience lymphoma-free remissions lasting several years. The central nervous system component of their disease must be recognized and treated early. In addition, the patient's course is very often complicated by opportunistic infections.

Immunodeficiency Secondary to Lymphoproliferative Disease

Most of the lymphomas are associated with relative immunodeficiency due to disruption of the normal lymph node architecture and aberrant secretion of cytokines that regulate the normal immune response, such as IL-1, IL-2, and IL-6. Chronic lymphocytic leukemia (Chapter 21) and Hodgkin's disease (Chapter 23) are often accompanied by a profound immunodeficiency. In **CLL,** the primary defect is in the production of normal antibody responses, leading to recurrent pyogenic infections. In **Hodgkin's disease,** the defect is primarily in T cell responses, leading to anergy and increased susceptibility to viral infections such as herpes zoster, to transfusion-associated GVHD, and to secondary malignancies. Patients with Hodgkin's disease can have a profound immune defect even when only small amounts of tumor are present, and even after successful therapy. The defect can continue for years even in patients who have been cured of their Hodgkin's disease.

Post-Transplant Immunodeficiency

Patients who receive immunosuppressive therapy for repeated episodes of organ rejection following transplantation are at increased risk for lymphoproliferative disease. The intensity of the immunosuppressive therapy is an important factor; patients who receive cyclosporine and the monoclonal antithymocyte antibody OKT3 are at special risk. In virtually all cases, the lymphoproliferative disease is associated with EBV infection.

Three types of post-transplant lymphoproliferative disorders have now been described. The first is a **polyclonal proliferation of plasmacytoid lymphocytes in the oropharynx or lymph nodes.** EBV infection can be demonstrated in multiple genomic sites without immunoglobulin-gene rearrangements or oncogene activation. This type of disease is more responsive to chemotherapy and may spontaneously regress if immunosuppressive therapy is discontinued. Another form is a **polymorphic lymphoproliferative disorder,** presenting in nodal or extranodal sites, secondary to a monoclonal EBV infection. The third type presents as a **widely disseminated monoclonal lymphoma, immunoblastic lymphoma, or multiple myeloma** with alterations in tumor-suppressor and oncogenes.

THERAPY

Treatment of **congenital immunodeficiencies** is directed at replacing the missing or dysfunctional component of the immune system if possible. Although it is possible to supply adequate amounts of antibody to replace B-cell function, it is not possible to replace defective T-cell function except by transplanting a new T-cell system. For **acquired immunodeficiencies,** treatment is directed at the underlying disorder. With the rapid development of cytokine and growth factor therapy, it may be possible in the future to direct therapy toward improving or augmenting the function of the immune cells themselves.

Gamma Globulin

Defective B-cell function and hypogammaglobulinemia can be effectively treated by replacing the antibody with intravenous gamma globulin. These preparations are obtained from very large numbers of donors and thus contain antibodies representative of the normal immune response. They have few side effects and can be given in large amounts. There is some evidence that intravenous gamma globulin, because it arises from a large pool of donors, may contain enough anti-idiotypic antibody and antibody to histocompatibility antigens to be somewhat immunosuppressive. However, its advantages of replacing missing antibodies for patients with B-cell dysfunction far outweigh this drawback.

The **recommended dose** is 100–200 mg/kg every 3–4 weeks. The dose and frequency of administration should be adjusted to achieve near normal levels of serum IgG. It should not be given to patients with isolated IgA deficiency due to the risk of anaphylaxis. In addition to gamma globulins, some patients may require chronic or intermittent **prophylactic antibiotics** to prevent recurrent infections. Bactrim is most commonly used in this setting.

Marrow Transplantation

Children with congenital defective T-cell function can only be treated with marrow transplantation. In **SCID,** the lack of a normal immune system means that there is no need to condition the patient with immunosuppressive therapy prior to the transplant. If a matched donor is available the donor's immune system will replace the defective system, resulting in a stable chimeric state in which the lymphoid cells arise from the donor and the remainder of the hematopoietic cells are of recipient origin.

Drugs for Patients With AIDS

The treatment of AIDS is directed at suppressing the growth of the virus. The drugs that are currently available inhibit viral replication and slow the progression of the disease, but they do not result in cure. They have a limited duration of action owing to the emergence of drug resistance. Thus, the overall strategy for treating AIDS is to have the patient begin receiving therapy at a time that will result in maximal benefit. Treating too early may result in drug resistance prior to the onset of symptoms, whereas treating too late may not prevent the onset of debilitating opportunistic infections. The optimal timing of therapy is still the subject of study.

With the availability of a new class of antiviral drugs known as **protease inhibitors,** it is now possible to give patients therapy with two or three drugs with different mechanisms of action. Such combinations appear to be highly successful at suppressing viral growth and are thus being used at a much earlier stage of the disease. The decision as to when to begin therapy used to depend on the level of CD4 cells, as an indicator of how far the immunodeficiency state has progressed. Now, a direct measurement of the level of viral genome in the blood, a surrogate indicator of total viral load, is taking on greater importance in the therapeutic decision. Many patients with high viral loads now receive therapy long before their CD4 count has fallen into the immunosuppressed range. Such early combination therapy can lead not only to a dramatic fall in viral load but also to a recovery of CD4 T cells with improve-ment in immunologic function. However, it is not yet clear to what extent the immune system can reconstitute itself with control of the HIV viral load. Longer survival and delayed onset of viral drug resistance will almost certainly increase the number of patients surviving with partial immunologic defects.

Bibliography

Drugs for HIV infection. Med Lett 1997;39:111.

Levine AM: Acquired immunodeficiency syndrome related lymphoma: Clinical aspects. Semin Oncol 2000;27:442.

Ozsahin H et al: Adenosine deaminase deficiency in adults. Blood 1997;89:2849.

Pantaleo G, Graziosi C, Fauci AS: The immunopathogenesis of human virus infection. N Engl J Med 1993;328:327.

Sandler AS, Kaplan LD: Diagnosis and management of systemic non-Hodgkin's lymphoma in HIV disease. Hematol Oncol Clin North Am 1996;10:1111.

Scadden DT: Hematologic disorders and growth factor support in HIV infection. Hematol Oncol Clin North Am 1996; 10:1149.

Shibata D et al: Epstein-Barr virus associated non-Hodgkin's lymphoma in patients infected with the human immunodeficiency virus. Blood 1993;81:2102.

Vanasse GJ, Concannon P, Wilerford DM: Regulated genomic instability and neoplasia in the lymphoid lineage. Blood 1999;94:3997.

Chronic Lymphocytic Leukemias

The chronic lymphocytic leukemias (CLL) are relatively common lymphoproliferative diseases with several unique clinical manifestations. They are different from the acute leukemias in terms of both prognosis and therapy. Understanding the various forms of CLL requires familiarity with the major lymphocyte subsets.

LYMPHOCYTE SUBSETS

Three major lymphocyte subsets are found in blood: T cells (approximately 70–80% of lymphocytes), B cells (10–15%), and natural killer (NK) cells (10–15%). **T cells** are responsible for cell-mediated immune reactions and regulation of the immune system; **B cells** are responsible for antibody production; **NK cells** seem to function in a relatively nonspecific way to defend against some viral infections and perhaps against malignantly transformed cells (see Chapter 19).

T cells are subdivided into two major additional subsets identified by the markers CD4 (40–50%) and CD8 (20–30%) and referred to as "helper" and "suppressor" T cells, respectively. Additional markers, each identified by a corresponding set of monoclonal antibodies, can be used to distinguish all of these major subsets. These markers are summarized in Table 21–1. In addition to the lineage-specific markers, there are several nonlineage-specific markers whose presence or absence is particularly useful in classifying lymphoproliferative disorders. These are summarized in Table 21–2. For the purposes of describing the CLLs, the following phenotypes are particularly important.

B CELLS

Mature B cells are identified by their expression of CD19 and CD20 as well as surface immunoglobulin (sIg) heavy chain (predominantly IgM and IgD) and immunoglobulin light chain (κ or λ). Normal B cells express either κ or λ light chains but never both, and the normal ratio of κ- to λ-expressing cells is about 3:2. Therefore, when a population of B cells expresses only one light chain, it can be presumed to be clonal and likely malignant. Even minor distortions of the normal relationship between κ and λ light chain expression (**clonal excess**) can be used to indicate the presence of an abnormal B-cell clone.

CD5 B Cells

CD5 B cells are a subset of B cells that comprise 20–30% of the normal B-cell population in blood. CD5 is a marker usually associated with T cells. This CD5 B-cell subset has been shown to have a propensity to produce autoantibodies such as rheumatoid factor, antiDNA, antiphospholipids, and so on. They are present in large numbers during fetal development of the immune system and when the immune system is reconstituted following marrow transplantation or intensive chemotherapy. They are of importance because most B-cell CLLs have this phenotype.

T CELLS

Mature T cells are identified by their expression of several different markers. The most important is CD3, which is part of the **T-cell antigen receptor** (**TCR**), analogous to B-cell sIg. In addition to CD3 the TCR contains other proteins known as α-, β-, γ-, and δ-chains. The expression of these chains is not nearly as good a clonal indicator as is B-cell sIg light chain because the vast majority of normal T cells express α- and β-chains only. The presence of γ- and δ-chains on a population of T cells is rare but, if found, can be an indicator of clonality. The other major T-cell markers include CD2, CD5, and CD7. Normal mature T cells express all of these, whereas abnormal T cells frequently lack one marker or express it in abnormal amounts. This condition usually indicates a malignancy. The other two major T-cell markers, CD4 and CD8, are found together in normal thymocytes (and some T-cell malignancies) but are mutually exclusive on mature T cells.

CD4 T Cells

CD4 T cells represent 60% of T cells in blood (40–50% of lymphocytes) and are usually referred to as "helper" T cells. This terminology is outdated and somewhat misleading but is useful conceptually. The true role of CD4 on T cells is in recognizing HLA-DR on macrophages and B cells. T-cell-specific retroviruses such as human T-cell leukemia virus (HTLV) and HIV

Table 21–1. Clinically useful lineage-specific lymphocyte markers.

Markers	Lymphocyte Subset	Clinical Utility
CD3	All mature T cells	T-cell CLL
CD4	"Helper" T cells	T-cell CLL, AIDS
CD8	"Suppressor" T cells	T-cell CLL, AIDS
CD19	Mature and immature B cells	B-cell CLL
CD20	Mature B cells	B-cell CLL
sIg	B cells	B-cell CLL

use CD4 as a receptor. Thus, this subset is involved in both the lymphoproliferative and the immunodestructive processes mediated by these viruses.

CD8 T Cells

CD8 T cells represent about 30–40% of T cells (20–40% of lymphocytes) and are referred to as "**suppressor**" **T cells,** again a misleading term. The role of CD8 is in recognizing HLA-A and -B antigens on macrophages and B cells. It is the CD8 subset that is mostly involved in graft rejection, killing of tumor cells, and virus-infected cells. Most of the "atypical" lymphocytes seen in response to viral infections are the CD8 subset. Their numbers are more highly variable in normal individuals in response to even mild viral infections and stress. They are much less commonly involved in malignant processes.

Cytotoxic T Cells

Cytotoxic T cells are a subset of CD8 T cells that specialize in killing tumor cells and virus-infected cells. They are usually activated (ie, they express activation antigens such as HLA-DR and CD38) and frequently express CD57. They can be markedly increased in patients with acute viral infections and are the malignant cell type in large granular lymphocytic (LGL) leukemia or T γ lymphocytosis.

NK CELLS

NK cells represent only 10–20% of blood lymphocytes. They are best characterized by their expression of markers such as CD16, CD56, CD57, and, more importantly, their lack of CD3. True NK cells are not T cells and have not rearranged their TCR genes. They are ca-

Table 21–2. Clinically useful nonlineage-specific lymphocyte markers.

Marker	Lymphocyte Subsets	Clinical Utility
CD1	Thymocytes (immature T cells)	T-ALL
CD2	T cells and NK cells	T-ALL and CLL
CD5	T cells and some B cells	T-ALL, T-CLL, and B-CLL
CD7	T cells and NK cells	T-ALL, T-CLL
CD10	Pre–B cells and immature granulocytes	Common-ALL
CD16	NK cells and granulocytes	NK cells
CD23	Activated B cells	B-CLL
CD38	Activated lymphocytes and plasma cells	Present in many leukemias but not on normal resting lymphocytes
CD56	NK cells and some T cells	Best marker for NK cells
CD57	Some cytotoxic T cells	T γ-CLL
HLA-DR	B cells and activated T cells	Present in most leukemias but not on resting T cells

pable of killing tumor cells and some virus-infected cells by a mechanism similar to that of cytotoxic T cells. They do not, however, use the immune recognition mechanisms of T cells and do not display immunologic memory. They identify abnormal cells by their characteristic deficiency of HLA class I histocompatability antigens. They can be thought of as transitional between the nonspecific role of macrophages and the specific recognition found in T cells and B cells. They represent an important host defense mechanism and can be markedly expanded in response to malignancy and infection. True clonal malignancies involving NK cells are rare.

There are examples of CLL that correspond to each of the major lymphocyte subsets. Each of these has distinct clinical and pathophysiologic manifestations.

■ CHRONIC LYMPHOCYTIC LEUKEMIA (CLL)

In general, CLL is a disease of older adults (90% over 40 years), and its major clinical manifestation is an increase in the number of circulating lymphocytes. The patient with CLL may have varying degrees of lymphadenopathy, ranging from very little to massive.

The **distinction between CLL and lymphoma** is largely semantic. Patients presenting with a marked increase in circulating lymphocytes and less adenopathy are diagnosed as having CLL, whereas patients presenting with prominent adenopathy or a tumor mass and near normal white blood counts may be diagnosed as having lymphoma. If a lymph node biopsy is done, it will be read as typical of a "small cell" or "diffuse well-differentiated" lymphocytic lymphoma. Even when the lymphocyte count is normal, such patients will have some detectable circulating lymphoma cells and thus can be said also to have CLL. Also from a clinical standpoint, there is little difference between patients presenting with lymphoma and those presenting with leukemia. They are, therefore, almost certainly the same disease.

CLL may also present with minimal leukemia or adenopathy but a major immunologic or hematologic abnormality. The most common is a **B- or T-cell immunodeficiency state** resulting in recurrent infections, autoimmune thrombocytopenia or hemolytic anemia, and, less often, granulocytopenia or aplastic anemia. Thus, CLL must be considered in the differential diagnosis of patients with any of these disorders and must be ruled in or out by analysis of lymphocyte markers. It is not uncommon to find patients with a normal level of circulating lymphocytes that are nevertheless largely CLL cells.

There are major **genetic and environmental influences** on the type of CLL that occurs in different populations. In parts of Japan, T-cell CLL (specifically of the CD4 type) is by far the most prevalent. This situation has been associated with the prevalence of HTLV-1 virus as well as a genetic predisposition in some peoples. Conversely, in the Americas and in Europe, the most common form of CLL is of B-cell origin. The awareness, and perhaps the incidence, of T-cell CLL seems to be increasing throughout the world, however. Although specific viruses have not yet been implicated in most forms of the disease, it is likely that more will be identified.

B-CELL CLL

B-cell CLL is the most common form of CLL in the West. It is almost entirely a disease of older adults. With the increasing frequency of lymphocyte marker studies, however, it is being diagnosed earlier and in younger patients. It has a long natural history and is the least "malignant" of the lymphoproliferative disorders.

CLINICAL FEATURES

B-cell CLL patients may present with **nonspecific symptoms** of malaise, easy fatigability, weight loss, and night sweats. More often, they seek medical attention because of **lymphadenopathy** or the condition is picked up on a routine complete blood count (CBC). Symptoms and signs associated with CLL are dependent on the tumor burden both in terms of its metabolic demands and mechanical effects of collections of lymphocytes in the nodes, liver, spleen, and marrow. Very large lymph nodes can occasionally result in airway obstruction. With extensive marrow involvement, patients develop anemia, thrombocytopenia, or pancytopenia. At the same time, most patients with CLL are asymptomatic despite the presence of extraordinarily high numbers of circulating lymphocytes. The absolute lymphocyte count can easily reach levels of 100,000–300,000/μL without impinging on the production of other hematopoietic cell lines.

B-cell CLL patients can also present because of a **functional abnormality of their immune system.** They are usually hypogammaglobulinemic secondary to a suppression of normal B-cell proliferation and are subject to recurrent bacterial infections with encapsulated organisms (eg, *Streptococcus pneumoniae*). More often, however, they present with an autoimmune manifestation such as autoimmune thrombocytopenia or a Coombs' positive hemolytic anemia.

Laboratory Studies

A routine **CBC** *may* be all that is needed to diagnose B-cell CLL. The typical pattern is a marked increase in the number of mature-appearing lymphocytes in circulation with little or no impact on the red blood cell, granulocyte, or platelet counts. Still, the **definitive diagnosis** requires immunophenotyping and gene rearrangement studies.

In patients with very high absolute lymphocyte counts, most cells in circulation will be found to be mature B cells that mark for CD19, CD20, and CD23. In addition, the most striking and nearly diagnostic finding is the presence of CD5, together with abnor-

mally low amounts of sIg. The sIg is usually IgM or IgD or both, less frequently IgG; and always only a single immunoglobulin light chain, either κ or λ, is present. Thus, the finding of an increased number of B cells expressing CD5, with low levels of sIg and a single immunoglobulin light chain, is diagnostic of B-cell CLL (Figure 21–1).

A. IMMUNOGLOBULIN GENE REARRANGEMENT:

The diagnosis of a clonal B-cell CLL can also be made by testing DNA for immunoglobulin gene rearrangement. All B-cell CLLs show rearrangements of one or both immunoglobulin heavy chain genes and either the

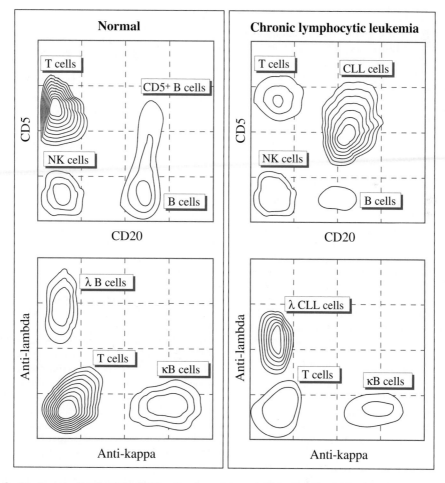

Figure 21–1. **Marker studies in CLL.** CD20, a B-cell marker, and CD5, a T-cell marker, distinguish between normal T cells (CD5+ CD20−) and normal B cells (CD5− CD20+). A subset of normal B cells also expresses lower levels of CD5 (CD5+ B cells). B-cell CLL is characterized by a predominance of CD5+ B cells. Normal B cells express either κ or λ immunoglobulin light chains, never both. CLL is characterized by a population of B cells expressing one light-chain class, usually in decreased amounts.

κ or λ or both immunoglobulin light chain genes. In addition, about 10% of B-cell clones show rearrangement of TCR β-chain gene but rarely the TCR γ-chain gene. Although this technique is both extremely sensitive and specific, it is usually unnecessary in the patient who presents with a large tumor burden. It is of value in situations where there are very few leukemic cells, whether at presentation or following chemotherapy or transplantation. Although the measurement of phenotypic markers and immunoglobulin light chain expression can accurately detect a clone of B cells that makes up only 1% of the circulating population, gene rearrangement studies are more sensitive.

B. Cytogenetic Analysis:

Obtaining cytogenetic analysis of CLL cells has been difficult owing to their very low proliferation in response to mitogens. In the studies that have been done, a variety of chromosomal abnormalities have been described, the most common being deletions of the short arm of chromosome 13 and trisomy 12. Multiple cytogenetic abnormalities indicate a worse prognosis. The clinical significance of the genetic changes may involve the overexpression of the anti-apoptotic protein bcl-2, together with lower levels of the pro-apoptotic protein bax. Drugs that are active in treating CLL would appear to reverse the bcl-2/bax ratio.

An additional genetic prognostic factor has recently been recognized. About half of CLL patients have tumor cells expressing **immunoglobulin molecules that closely resemble the germline DNA sequence** and thus have not undergone somatic mutation. These cells are presumably naive, not having undergone antigen recognition and expansion in germinal centers. This finding has also been associated with high-level expression of CD38 on the cell surface, the presence of trisomy 12, and a significantly worse prognosis. In one study patients with unmutated immunoglobulin genes had a median survival of 8 years, whereas those with mutated sequences had a median survival of 24 years.

C. Other Important Laboratory Studies:

Other important laboratory studies for diagnosing CLL include **serum protein electrophoresis** to detect an M protein and provide an overall assessment of immunoglobulin production. CLL patients can present with diffuse hypogammaglobulinemia or will develop hypogammaglobulinemia during the course of their disease. **Tests for autoantibodies,** including both a Coombs' test and a measurement of platelet-associated immunoglobulin, should be obtained in any patient who presents with anemia or thrombocytopenia. In patients with very large tumor burdens, the **serum lactic dehydrogenase (LDH) level, β$_2$-microglobulin, and uric acid levels** can be elevated.

DIFFERENTIAL DIAGNOSIS

Many of the B-cell lymphomas may have a leukemic component with increased numbers of circulating cells. If adenopathy is a prominent aspect of the clinical presentation, a **node biopsy** is indicated to rule out a more aggressive form of lymphoma. The presence of relatively large amounts of sIg also indicates that the physician is not dealing with typical B-cell CLL. Disorders such as hairy-cell leukemia, prolymphocytic leukemia, and leukemias involving large, less-well differentiated cells are usually easily distinguished on the basis of morphology (Figure 21–2). **Mantle cell lymphoma** is another B-cell malignancy that expresses CD5 but is distinguished from CLL by the absence of CD23, the presence of larger cells, and by a much more aggressive course. Seventy percent of these cases show a t(11;14) translocation involving the bcl-1 locus, which results in the overexpression of cyclin D1—a critical regulator of the cell division cycle.

THERAPY

Staging systems for CLL have been proposed and are useful in protocol studies and in predicting the prognosis of individual patients. **Adverse prognostic factors** include a lymphocyte count greater than 300,000/μL, atypical lymphocyte morphology, lymphadenopathy, a short lymphocyte doubling time, trisomy 12 or more than one cytogenetic abnormality, and a large tumor burden as indicated by an elevated LDH, β$_2$-microglobulin, or both. Autoimmune anemia or thrombocytopenia and frequency of infections also have a major impact on prognosis.

Most patients will have a relatively chronic **clinical course,** some progressing very slowly and succumbing to unrelated disorders, others progressing more rapidly, succumbing to complications of infection, anemia, thrombocytopenia, or chemotherapy. The disease can also undergo transformation to a much more aggressive form of lymphoma such as **diffuse histiocytic lymphoma with massive splenomegaly (Richter's syndrome),** prolymphocytic leukemia, or, very rarely, acute lymphocytic leukemia or multiple myeloma. One of these should be suspected if the patient's course appears to change abruptly.

There is **no curative therapy,** thus all treatment is directed toward palliation of symptoms and prolonging life with minimal morbidity. Patients without symptoms (fever, weight loss, night sweats, fatigue, bulky adenopathy) and without complications such as thrombocytopenia, anemia, or infections should not be treated immediately. Chemotherapy directed entirely at lowering the lymphocyte count will be effective but there is no evidence that it prolongs life or slows pro-

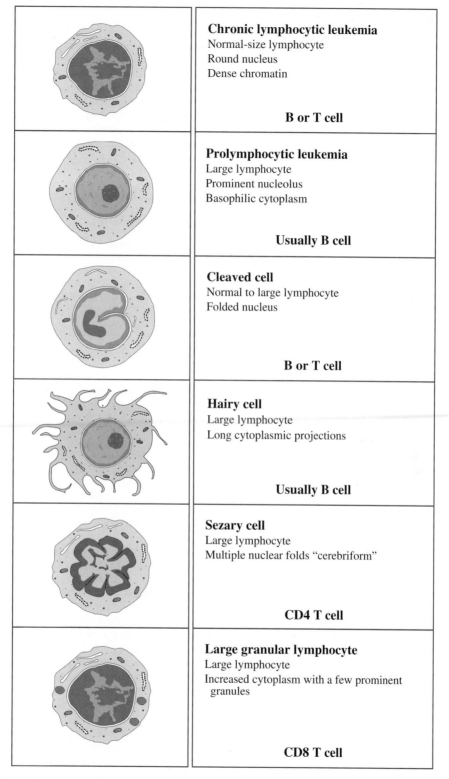

Chronic lymphocytic leukemia
Normal-size lymphocyte
Round nucleus
Dense chromatin

B or T cell

Prolymphocytic leukemia
Large lymphocyte
Prominent nucleolus
Basophilic cytoplasm

Usually B cell

Cleaved cell
Normal to large lymphocyte
Folded nucleus

B or T cell

Hairy cell
Large lymphocyte
Long cytoplasmic projections

Usually B cell

Sezary cell
Large lymphocyte
Multiple nuclear folds "cerebriform"

CD4 T cell

Large granular lymphocyte
Large lymphocyte
Increased cytoplasm with a few prominent
    granules

CD8 T cell

Figure 21–2. **Morphology in CLL.** The morphologic appearance of typical CLL cells is not distinguishable from that of normal lymphocytes. Several morphologically distinctive forms of lymphocytic leukemia, however, correlate to some extent with the immunophenotype.

gression, and it certainly increases morbidity owing to infection and exposes the patient to the risk of second malignancies.

Drug Therapy

When treatment is initiated, it should be designed to reduce and control whatever symptoms gave rise to the necessity for treatment. If symptoms are abolished, there is no need to continue treatment. Traditionally, **first-line therapy has been chlorambucil,** 4–6 mg orally each day for 4–7 days every 3–4 weeks. Higher doses, up to 15 mg/m²/day for 5 days per month, have been used in patients with disseminated disease. This will usually reduce the tumor burden (blood lymphocytosis, node enlargement, and splenomegaly) for many months to years. However, chlorambucil therapy does not extend lifespan; the natural history of CLL is unaffected.

Recent studies have shown that **fludarabine,** a nucleoside analogue, as a single agent is more effective than chlorambucil for initial therapy. It produces a higher rate of complete and partial remissions, and the duration of response is nearly twice that of chlorambucil. Nevertheless, to date there is no evidence for prolonged survival or cure, and fludarabine has the disadvantages of increased expense, intravenous administration, and a higher incidence of both myelo- and immunosuppression. The currently recommended dose of fludarabine is a bolus of 25 mg/m² intravenously for 5 days each month, continuing to best response plus 2 additional months. When used for more than 4–6 months, T-cell subsets should be monitored to prevent a major reduction in CD4 lymphocytes. In addition, prophylaxis with Bactrim and fluconazole is recommended to prevent opportunistic infections. Autoimmune hemolytic anemia and prolonged thrombocytopenia have both been reported as complications of fludarabine therapy. Combinations of fludarabine (30 mg/m² daily for 3 days) with Cytoxan (300 mg/m² daily for 3 days) may give a better response in heavily treated patients.

Other second-line drugs for patients who fail chlorambucil are **2'-chlorodeoxyadenosine (2-CdA)** and **pentostatin (deoxycoformycin).** Like fludarabine, these agents can cause severe immunosuppression. When a patient's disease transforms into a more aggressive lymphoma, combination chemotherapy is indicated. Symptomatic bulky adenopathy will respond promptly to local radiotherapy.

Complications

Complications such as hemolytic anemia and immune thrombocytopenia are treated with corticosteroids in the usual fashion, starting with a high dose of pred-nisone, 60–90 mg orally daily, and then tapering to a minimal daily or every-other-day maintenance dose. Recurrent infections can be decreased by administering intravenous gamma globulin (400 mg/kg every 3 weeks). Owing to its expense, intravenous gamma globulin should be reserved for patients with severe hypogammaglobulinemia and documented recurrent bacterial (encapsulated organism) infections.

T-CELL CLL (CD4 type)

CLINICAL FEATURES

T-cell CLL associated with HTLV-1 is the most common form of CLL in parts of Japan but is rare in Western countries. Although the retrovirus that causes it is closely related to the HIV virus of AIDS, T-cell CLL causes only uncontrolled proliferation of the CD4 T cell rather than its destruction. These viruses use the CD4 molecule as their binding site on the cell, and thus the infection is specific for the CD4 T cell.

Outside of Japan, cases of T-cell CLL are not always associated with the same virus. Their incidence appears, however, to be increasing, and it is likely that there are other related retroviruses involved with these disorders. Reports of involvement by defective retroviruses, herpes virus, and Epstein-Barr virus have appeared, but as yet no common element has been identified. T-cell CLL is a less homogeneous disorder than B-cell CLL and has been classified in several different ways. The typical disease seen in Japan has been called **adult T-cell leukemia.** In the West, it has been called various names depending on the presentation, morphology, and the rate of progression.

The CD4 T-cell leukemias share several clinical characteristics. Most striking is a propensity to involve the skin. The skin disease known as **mycosis fungoides** is an infiltration of CD4 T cells often associated with a leukemic population of CD4 T cells. When the leukemia is prominent and the cells have a characteristic nuclear morphology (ie, a folded or "cerebriform" nucleus), the disease is known as **Sezary syndrome.** Many patients with CD4 T-cell leukemia will have skin involvement ranging from a diffuse erythroderma with exfoliation to patchy plaquelike or nodular infiltration. Infection of the skin lesions is common and is the most common cause of death.

T-cell CLLs in general have a more aggressive course, with more adenopathy, more susceptibility to viral infection and opportunistic infection, and a worse overall prognosis. It is difficult to generalize, however, because of the heterogeneity of the disorders. Some cases are as benign as B-cell CLL but others are rapidly progressive.

Laboratory Studies

CD4 T-cell disease is frequently associated with hypergammaglobulinemia, sometimes to a striking degree and often predominantly IgA. It is tempting to associate this with the "helper" nature of the CD4 T cells, but this is probably an oversimplification. Despite the hypergammaglobulinemia, these patients have poor antibody responses to specific pathogens and have defects in both humoral and cellular immunity. The propensity to autoimmune phenomena seen in B-cell CLL is not observed.

Unlike the situation with B-cell CLL, there is **no immunologic marker for T cells that indicates clonality.** Thus the presence of many CD4 T cells in skin, blood, or nodes cannot be taken as definitive evidence that they are malignant. Since CD4 is the predominant T-cell subtype normally, it is sometimes difficult to be certain whether they are malignant. One useful clue comes from examining several different T-cell-associated markers. Normal mature CD4 T cells also express CD2, CD3, CD5, and CD7. Often, a malignant population will lack one or more of these markers or express them in abnormal amounts, and this may indicate that they are not normal. In addition, normal resting CD4 T cells do not express HLA-DR or CD38. Thus intense expression of these activation markers may indicate that the cells are proliferating abnormally.

At present, the only definitive test for clonality among the T cells is to study the **rearrangement of the T-cell receptor genes.** Most malignant T cells will have a clonal rearrangement of the TCR β and -γ genes that can be detected either by restriction mapping and Southern blotting or more recently by polymerase chain reaction (PCR).

THERAPY

Because of the more aggressive nature of the T-cell CLLs, the relatively passive approach used with B-cell CLL is inappropriate. Treatment aimed at **decreasing the cell count, controlling skin involvement, and reducing adenopathy** should be undertaken. Cures cannot be achieved with combination chemotherapy, however; thus single-agent treatment is usually employed to achieve specific therapeutic goals.

In the early stages of cutaneous T-cell lymphomas, the malignant T cells appear to be dependent on stimulation by epidermal Langerhans cells, and therapy directed entirely to the skin can be highly effective, even though it may be possible to demonstrate malignant T cells in other sites as well. Topical **chemotherapeutic agents** such as corticosteroids, mechlorethamine, or carmustine can be used on localized lesions. More extensive involvement responds to **electron beam irradia-**tion if available. **Phototherapy,** with oral psoralen with UVA irradiation or ultraviolet (UV) B, is often used as first-line therapy and has the advantage of also treating unrecognized subclinical lesions. Because T cells circulate relatively more than B cells, they sometimes respond to repeated **leukapheresis** with decreased skin infiltration and adenopathy as well as decreased cell count. **Photopheresis,** in which the circulating T cells are exposed to UV radiation in an extracorporeal circuit, can achieve compete remissions, even though only a small fraction of the total T-cell pool is being treated. **Systemic chemotherapy** with single alkylating agents such as chlorambucil, cyclophosphamide, or BCNU can be beneficial with or without the addition of glucocorticoids. In more aggressive situations, **combination chemotherapy** including such drugs as methotrexate, bleomycin, and Adriamycin is used. With most treatments, the initial response rate is high (50–70%), but long-term responses are difficult to achieve.

T-cell CLL is uniquely susceptible to several **newer immunologically oriented therapies** that are still being investigated. These include inhibitors of adenosine deaminase such as pentostatin and 2-CdA. In addition, therapy with monoclonal antibodies directed against CD4 or CD52 (Campath-1) has been effective in rapidly lowering the cell count and sometimes inducing remission. A conjugate of diphtheria toxin with interleukin (IL)-2 ($DAB_{389}IL$-2) has been recently approved for treatment of patients who have failed other therapies. It is likely that these approaches will become more attractive with further investigation. Attempts at therapies with stem-cell transplantation, interleukin inhibitors, and antibodies conjugated to toxins are being evaluated.

T-CELL CLL (CD8 type)

Occasionally, patients with what appears to be a typical T-cell CLL will prove to have not CD4, but CD8-bearing T cells. These cases can be distinguished only by immunologic study and not on any reliable clinical grounds. Sometimes such cases will express both CD4 and CD8, thus reflecting an early stage of T-cell maturation normally found only in the thymus. A unique presentation of CD8 T-cell leukemia, however, appears to be increasing in frequency and is clinically distinct. This type has been given various names, the most common of which are **large granular lymphocytic (LGL) leukemia** and **T γ-lymphocytosis.**

CLINICAL FEATURES

LGL leukemia patients may present with lymphocytosis in the same way as other CLLs. However, they usually show only modest lymphocytosis or none at all together with granulocytopenia, aplastic anemia, or pancytopenia. There is evidence that CD8 T cells are capable of directly inhibiting one or more aspects of hematopoiesis and that this gives rise to this unique clinical presentation. In the more common CLLs, hematopoietic failure is not seen until there is extensive marrow infiltration with CLL cells. With LGL leukemia, the offending CD8 T cells may not be present in large numbers. Approximately 25% of these patients will also have pre-existing rheumatoid arthritis or other autoimmune disorder.

The course of LGL leukemia is highly variable. Some patients appear to have little or no progression of the lymphoproliferative process and may only need to be treated for their anemia or granulocytopenia, whereas others have a more aggressive course resulting in progression to florid lymphoma or lymphocytic leukemia or both.

Laboratory Studies

The malignant cells ("large granular lymphocytes") resemble "atypical lymphocytes" of the type sometimes seen in infectious mononucleosis. They are larger than normal lymphocytes, with a more open chromatin pattern and with a few prominent azurophilic granules in their cytoplasm. **Marker studies** show expression of the normal T-cell lineage markers CD3 and CD8. In addition they typically express CD57 and activation markers such as HLA-DR and CD38. In some cases they have low or absent expression of the CD5 that should be present on normal T cells.

This morphology and phenotype are associated with activated cytotoxic T cells. These cells resemble and are sometimes confused with NK cells because they share some of the morphologic characteristics and markers such as CD57. Gene rearrangement studies have shown definitively, however, that they are conventional T cells. The entity of true NK-cell leukemia is rare. Although morphologically very similar, in these cases the cells do not show rearrangement of T-cell receptor genes and do not express CD3. The presentation is much more acute and the course much more aggressive.

THERAPY

Up to one-third of patients may require no chemotherapy directed at the lymphoproliferative disease but only supportive therapy for anemia or recurrent infections owing to granulocytopenia. Others respond to single-agent treatment with chlorambucil or cyclophosphamide, with or without prednisone. With transition to more aggressive disease, combination chemotherapy is indicated; however, the response rate is not high in this situation.

HAIRY-CELL LEUKEMIA (HCL)

HCL was named for its unusual morphology. The malignant lymphocytes have very long filamentous cytoplasmic projections that are sometimes difficult to see in dried stained films but are prominent in wet mounts observed by phase microscopy. HCL has also been called "leukemic reticuloendotheliosis," perhaps because of the tendency for the malignant cells to infiltrate the marrow, liver, and spleen.

CLINICAL FEATURES

Like many of the CLLs, this disorder occurs most commonly in older adults and frequently has a unique clinical presentation characterized by extensive marrow involvement with pancytopenia and relatively prominent splenomegaly. It is more often seen in males than females (4 to 5:1).

Laboratory Studies

The cell that originates HCL has been the subject of considerable investigation. Some HCL cases have cells with properties of both lymphocytes and macrophages in that the cells can be mildly phagocytic and sometimes have markers associated with macrophages. Careful marker studies and gene rearrangement studies have shown, however, that they are always either B or T cells, more commonly B cells. It appears that the disease is not derived from some normal "hairy cell" but rather arises in normal B and T cells just as other CLLs. The **most useful markers** for these cells, in addition to the usual lineage-specific B-cell markers (CD19, CD20, and sIg), are the absence of CD5, CD10, and CD23 and the strong presence of CD11 and CD103.

The initial CBC in the patient with HCL usually shows mild to moderate pancytopenia. The number of abnormal lymphocytes in circulation is not dramatically increased. A careful inspection of the blood film may reveal the classic **hairy cell** (a small lymphocyte with filamentous projections of cytoplasm). A special stain, the **tartrate-resistant acid phosphatase stain,** can be used to confirm the presence of hairy cells in circulation. The characteristic staining pattern is one of a polar deposit of brownish-red material surrounded by unstained cytoplasm.

The diagnosis of HCL can also be made on the **histology of the marrow or spleen.** When the marrow is infiltrated by hairy cells, it usually cannot be aspirated. A marrow biopsy specimen will reveal, however, the typical morphologic pattern of the malignant hairy cell. Once again, the tartrate-resistant acid phosphatase stain can be used to confirm the diagnosis. Occasionally, the diagnosis of HCL is made from liver or spleen tissue obtained by a biopsy or at the time of surgery.

THERAPY

The prognosis of HCL is similar to that of most other CLLs. Some cases are quite indolent and require therapy primarily for complications such as infection, anemia, thrombocytopenia, or symptomatic splenomegaly. Other cases are more aggressive with transitions to aggressive lymphomas. In general, therapy should be begun if the patient is symptomatic or if there is clear progression of the disease.

HCL appears to be unique among the CLLs because it responds very well to therapy with **interferon,** with complete or partial response rates of about 80% but no evidence for cure. Even higher complete remission rates and prolonged relapse-free survival are obtained with **pentostatin** (deoxycoformycin) and with **2-CdA. Fludaribine** has shown similar results and has been effective in patients previously treated with other agents.

Prior to the use of these drugs, splenectomy was considered the initial therapeutic step owing to a high frequency of apparent remissions after splenectomy. In patients with massive splenomegaly or severe hypersplenism, **splenectomy** is still the best first-treatment option. If the patient is not a candidate for surgical splenectomy, **splenic irradiation** is an alternative. When splenomegaly is not pronounced, chemotherapeutic options are available, each of which appears to offer good results. The purine analogues are now preferred to interferon as initial therapy. Overall survival is 80–90% over 5 years for each of the drugs; longer follow-up data are needed to determine if one of the agents can provide substantially longer survival. Patients who relapse may respond to interferon or to another of the purine analogues.

BIBLIOGRAPHY

Bartlett NL, Longo DL: T-small lymphocyte disorders. Semin Hematol 1999;36:164.

Cheson B et al: National Cancer Institute–sponsored working group guidelines for chronic lymphocytic leukemia: Revised guidelines for diagnosis and treatment. Blood 1996;87:4990.

Dhodapkar MV et al: Clinical spectrum of clonal proliferation of T-large granular lymphocytes: A T-cell clonopathy of undetermined significance? Blood 1994;84:1620.

Diamandidou E, Cohe PR, Kurzock R: Mycosis fungoides and Sezary syndrome. Blood 1996;88:2385.

Flinn IW, Grever MR: Chronic lymphocytic leukemia. Cancer Treat Rev 1996;22:1.

Goodman MG et al: New perspectives on the approach to chronic lymphocytic leukemia. Leuk Lymphoma 1996;22:1.

Hamblin TJ et al: Unmutated Ig V_H genes are associated with a more aggressive form of chronic lymphocytic leukemia. Blood 1999;94:1848.

O'Brien S, del Giglio A, Keating M: Advances in the biology and treatment of B-cell chronic lymphocytic leukemia. Blood 1995;85:307.

Rozman C, Montserrat E: Chronic lymphocytic leukemia. N Engl J Med 1995;333:1052.

Tallman MS et al: Treatment of hairy cell leukemia: Current views. Semin Hematol 1999;36:155.

Non-Hodgkin's Lymphomas

The **non-Hodgkin's lymphomas** (**NHLs**) are a heterogeneous group of disorders characterized by malignant proliferation of B or T lymphocytes. From a clinical standpoint, lymphomas generally present as solid tumors of the lymphoid system—the lymph nodes, Waldeyer's ring, spleen, blood, and marrow. Because of the functional heterogeneity of lymphocytes and because lymphocytes by their nature have access to nearly every anatomic site, these diseases may involve any organ and are very heterogeneous. Despite multiple attempts to improve the classification of NHL, it remains **difficult to predict the course of the disease** in an individual patient based on prognostic factors. Perhaps more than any other malignant disease, the treatment of the patient must be individualized based on the behavior of the patient's own disease.

The importance of accurate diagnosis and effective management of lymphomas has been heightened by their increasing incidence, the association of lymphomas with immune deficiency states, and improvements in therapy. The incidence in Western countries has more than doubled in the last 20 years and should increase even further because of the association of B-cell lymphomas with AIDS. The rising incidence may also reflect greater exposure to chemical agents in the environment.

NHL in general is very **responsive to therapy,** and in most cases the physician can offer the patient with NHL both improved survival and improved quality of life. It is an unusual fact that the NHL patient with the most aggressive form of the disease can be offered the possibility of a cure, whereas the patient with indolent lymphoma may never be cured despite a relatively long survival.

Because lymphoma cells tend to be very mobile, silently involving not only lymphoid organs but nearly every part of the body, concepts of staging, remission, and relapse are less useful and less important than in other malignancies. With increasingly sensitive **means of detecting lymphoma cells,** it is frequently possible to demonstrate their presence throughout the body in patients previously thought to have localized disease. Similarly, it is frequently possible to detect lymphoma cells in patients who appear by usual criteria to be in complete remission. Patients with lymphoma will sometimes undergo prolonged periods of quiescent disease punctuated by periods of increased disease activity. In general these patients must be followed up carefully, with a constant suspicion that minor symptoms may indicate progression or relapse.

DIAGNOSIS

Ultimately, a diagnosis of lymphoma depends on finding abnormal numbers of lymphocytes that are destroying the normal architecture of the lymphoid tissues or invading nonlymphoid tissues or both. Detection of lymphoma in its early stages can be more of a challenge. It is difficult, probably impossible, to recognize a single malignant lymphocyte based on morphology alone, because lymphocytes are capable of de-differentiation, proliferation, and differentiation in the course of a normal immune response. A reactive lymph node contains activated lymphocytes that look as malignant as any lymphoma cell.

Thus, in order for one to accurately diagnose lymphoma, an adequate **tissue biopsy** is absolutely required. Lymphoma can be suspected on the basis of cytologic examination of blood, marrow, effusions, and aspirates, but the physician should always make every attempt to obtain a good surgical biopsy of involved lymphoid or nonlymphoid tissue in order to be certain of the diagnosis. When multiple sites are available for biopsy, one should avoid those sites where normal reactive nodes are frequently found, such as the groin and the axilla.

With the availability of **immunologic and genetic tests for clonality,** one can make a strong presumptive diagnosis of lymphoma on the basis of the finding of clonal lymphocytes involving multiple sites, such as marrow and blood, but the finding of clonality does not absolutely prove malignancy, and clonality tells us nothing about prognosis. Therefore, a diagnosis based solely on these criteria should be viewed with caution.

CLASSIFICATION

Over the years, several different classifications of lymphomas have been popularized: the Rappaport classification, the Lukes-Collins classification, the International Working Formulation, the **Revised European American Classification** (**REAL**), and most recently a consensus classification sponsored by the **World Health Organization** (**WHO**), which closely follows the REAL system. The Working Formulation and WHO/REAL classifications are compared in Table 22–1. The Working Formulation and previous systems were based almost entirely on morphologic criteria. The Working Formulation was an advance because it emphasized the clinical behavior of the various lymphomas, grouping them into low-, intermediate-, and high-grade based on their aggressiveness. The REAL

system, for the first time, incorporated immunologic and genetic criteria in classifying the lymphomas, and this has been extended in the WHO system.

The WHO/REAL classification should hold promise in the design of future therapies. However, as can be seen in Table 22–1, it is difficult to correlate the WHO/REAL system with the Working Formulation. As long as the concept of tumor aggressiveness is preserved in the classification, there is extensive overlap and duplication. For example, the B-cell, marginal zone (MALT) lymphomas can present as follicular or diffuse, small- or mixed-cell tumors with low to intermediate

Table 22–1. Lymphoma classification.

Working Formulation	Revised European American (REAL) and WHO Consensus Classification	
	B-Cell Neoplasms	**T-Cell Neoplasms**
Low-Grade		
Small lymphocytic	B-cell CLL/SLL	T-cell CLL
	Marginal zone, mucosa associated (MALT)	Large granular lymphocytic
	Mantle cell	Adult T-cell lymphoma/leukemia
Plasmacytoid	Lymphoplasmacytic	
	Marginal zone (MALT)	
Follicular, small-cell, and mixed-cell	Follicular, grades I and II	
	Mantle cell	
	Marginal zone (MALT)	
Intermediate-Grade		
Follicular, large-cell	Follicular, grade III	
Diffuse, small-cell	Mantle cell	T-cell CLL
	Follicular center, diffuse small-cell	Large granular lymphocytic
	Marginal zone (MALT)	Adult T-cell lymphoma/leukemia
		Angioimmunoblastic
		Angiocentric
Diffuse, mixed-cell	Large B-cell lymphoma	Peripheral T-cell lymphoma
	Follicular center, diffuse small-cell	Adult T-cell lymphoma/leukemia
	Lymphoplasmacytoid	Angioimmunoblastic
	Marginal zone (MALT)	Angiocentric
	Mantle cell	Intestinal T-cell lymphoma
Diffuse, large-cell	Diffuse large B-cell lymphoma	Peripheral T-cell lymphoma
		Adult T-cell lymphoma/leukemia
		Angioimmunoblastic
		Angiocentric
		Intestinal T-cell lymphoma
High-Grade		
Large-cell immunoblastic	Diffuse large B-cell lymphoma	Peripheral T-cell lymphoma
		Adult T-cell lymphoma/leukemia
		Angioimmunoblastic
		Angiocentric
		Intestinal T-cell lymphoma
		Anaplastic large cell
Lymphoblastic	Precursor B-cell lymphoblastic	Precursor T-cell lymphoblastic
Burkitt's lymphoma	Burkitt's lymphoma	Peripheral T-cell lymphoma

growth potential. It is likely that with more experience, the clinical classification and the immunogenetic classification will converge, and the situation will become clearer.

The frequencies with which the more common forms of lymphoma will be encountered in practice are indicated in Table 22–2. When a patient presents with lymphoma it is important to obtain as much prognostic information as possible on the basis of whatever can be measured. This can be divided into histologic features, cytologic features, immunologic features, cytogenetics, and stage or extent of disease.

Histologic Features

The normal architecture of a lymph node and the phenotypic and cytologic features of the lymphocytes found in various regions are illustrated in Figure 22–1. The histologic description of lymphoma focuses on the overall architecture of a lymphoid or nonlymphoid tissue. Perhaps the most useful histologic finding is whether there is nodular (or follicular) versus diffuse morphology. Those lymphomas showing the formation of nodules, reminiscent of normal lymphoid follicles, tend to be more indolent and have a better prognosis than those showing diffuse infiltration. This distinction is true regardless of the details of the individual cells and regardless of the immunologic type of the lymphoma. Therefore, the first question the clinician

should ask of NHL is whether it is nodular (follicular) or diffuse in histology. This distinction can only be made on the basis of an adequate biopsy.

Cytologic Features

The cytologic classification of a lymphoma depends on the appearance of the individual cells. Cells may be described as well versus poorly differentiated (Rappaport classification) or as large versus small, with folded or "cleaved" nuclei (Luke-Collins classification and International Formulation). In general, small, well-differentiated cells are seen with more indolent lymphomas, whereas large, poorly differentiated cells are typical of high-grade, aggressive lymphomas. However, this classification is weakened by the frequent presence of cells of many descriptions scattered throughout the lesion. Overall, the cytologic description of the cells is not as strongly associated with prognosis as is the histologic description (nodular versus diffuse).

Immunologic Features

The immunologic classification of the lymphomas requires use of immunologic markers, genetic analysis, or both (see Chapters 19 and 21) to determine whether the cells are of B- or T-cell origin and to indicate clonality. Most (approximately 80%) NHLs are of B-cell origin. **Clonality in a B-cell lymphoma** can be indicated by uniform expression of a single light chain class

Table 22–2. Frequencies of non-Hodgkin's lymphomas.

Diagnosis	Frequency (%)
Diffuse large B-cell lymphoma	31
Follicular lymphoma	22
Small lymphocytic lymphoma	6
Mantle cell lymphoma	6
Peripheral T-cell lymphoma	6
Marginal zone B-cell lymphoma, MALT type	5
Mediastinal large B-cell lymphoma	2
Anaplastic T-cell lymphoma	2
Lymphoblastic lymphoma	2
Burkitt-like lymphoma	2
Marginal zone B-cell lymphoma	1
Lymphoplasmacytic lymphoma	1
Burkitt's lymphoma	< 1

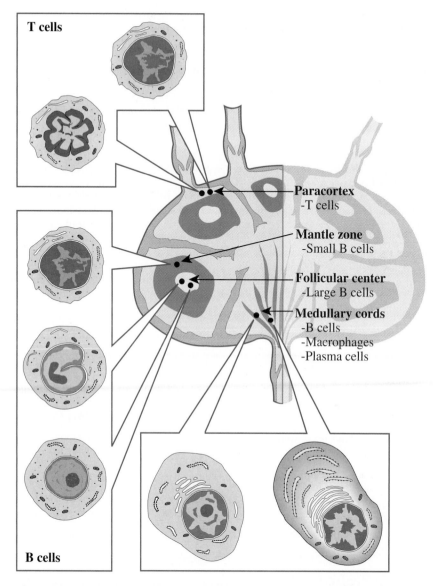

T cells

B cells

Paracortex
-T cells

Mantle zone
-Small B cells

Follicular center
-Large B cells

Medullary cords
-B cells
-Macrophages
-Plasma cells

Figure 22–1. **The normal architecture, histology, and phenotype of a lymph node.** The major lymphocyte subsets are distributed through the lymph node in characteristic regions. Follicular centers contain predominantly large proliferating B cells, whereas the mantle zones of the follicles contain smaller B cells in the resting state. Interfollicular regions and the paracortex contain predominantly T cells. Macrophages are located in the follicular centers and in the medulla of the node. Antigen, and circulating T cells, enter via the cortical afferent lymphatics. Antigen-stimulated T cells reenter the circulation via the efferent lymphatics. Disruption of the normal lymph node architecture is one of the major causes of immunodeficiency in lymphoma.

of surface immunoglobulin (κ or λ) or by the presence of a single immunoglobulin gene rearrangement pattern. **Clonality of the T-cell lymphomas** is suggested by the expression of a single functional class marker (CD4 or CD8) or by a characteristic pattern of expres-

sion and deletion of other T-cell markers, but it is best demonstrated by genetic analysis for T-cell–receptor gene rearrangement.

Immunologic analysis of lymphomas is particularly useful in distinguishing between a reactive process and a lymphoma. It is not uncommon for a lymph node biopsy to show a lymphocyte proliferation that could be a normal reactive process rather than a lymphoma. Since the reactive process is characterized by a heterogeneous collection of T and B cells arising from multiple clones of different progenitor cells, it is easy to distinguish immunologically from a lymphoma, where most cells are of one phenotype and belong to one clone.

Cytogenetic Features

Specific NHL subtypes can also be classified based on **nonrandom chromosomal translocations** (Tables 22–3 and 22–4). Most share one common feature in that they involve the genes responsible for the coding of the immunologic receptors for antigen on the lymphocytes. For the B cells these are located on chromosome 14 (the immunoglobulin heavy chains) and on chromosomes 2 (κ immunoglobulin light chain) and 22 (λ immunoglobulin light chain). For the T cells, the T-cell–receptor genes

are usually involved. Most of these mutations result in the juxtaposition of an immunologic receptor gene and its controlling elements next to a proto-oncogene, resulting in overexpression of the oncogene product. The best examples are the t(14;18) (q32;q21) translocation, which brings the immunoglobulin heavy chain locus next to the BCL-2 proto-oncogene, and the translocations that bring the c-*myc* oncogene next to immunoglobulin genes on chromosomes 14, 2, or 22.

The BCL-2 abnormality occurs in at least 80% of nodular lymphomas, and the c-*myc* translocation is characteristic of Burkitt's lymphoma. **BCL-2** is a gene associated with the inhibition of programmed cell death (apoptosis). Thus, its overexpression in lymphomas leads to prolongation of the life span of the cells and their accumulation to the detriment of the patient. On the other hand, **c-*myc*** is a transcription factor whose overproduction leads to uncontrolled cell proliferation.

Since immunoglobulin and T-cell–receptor genes are always rearranged as a part of the normal differenti-

Table 22–3. Immunologic and cytogenetic features in the REAL classification of B-cell neoplasms.

Disease	Morphology	Immunophenotype	Genotype
Small lymphocytic, CLL	Small, round lymphocytes	Dim sIgM, sIgD CD19, 20, 5, 23+ CD10−	Ig rearrangements Trisomy 12 (30–40%) Deletion 13q14 (50%)
Lymphoplasmacytoid	Small lymphocytes with plasmacytoid features	cIg+, CD19, 20+ CD5, 10−	Ig rearrangements t(9;14) (50%)
Mantle cell	Small to medium irregular lymphocytes	sIgM, sIgD+ CD19, 20, 5+ CD10±, CD23−	Ig rearrangements t(11;14) (70%) involves BCL-1
Follicular center cell	Small, medium, or large, irregular, cleaved cells	sIgM, sIgD+ CD19, 20+ CD10, 23± CD5−	Ig rearrangements t(14;18) (70–95%) involves BCL-2
Marginal zone (MALT)	Small or large, monocytoid lymphocytes	sIgM, sIgD+ CD19, 20+ CD5, 10, 23−	Ig rearrangements Trisomy 3 t(11;18)
Hairy-cell	Small lymphocytes with cytoplasmic projections	sIgM, sIgD+ CD19, 20, 11b, 103+ FMC7+, CD5, 10, 23−	Ig rearrangements
Diffuse large B-cell	Large, irregular lymphocytes	sIgM, sIgD± CD19, 20+ CD5, 10±	Ig rearrangements Rearrangements of 3q27 (BCL-6) (30%)
Burkitt's lymphoma	Medium round cells with abundant cytoplasm	sIgM+ CD19, 20, 10+ CD5, 23−	t(8;14), t(2;8), or t(8;22) involves c-*myc*

Table 22–4. Significance of some chromosomal translocations associated with B-cell neoplasms.

Disease	Translocations	Frequency	Immunoglobulin gene(s)	Proto-oncogene	Mechanism
Lymphoplasma-cytoid	t(9;14)	50%	Ig$_H$	PAX-5 (9q13)	A transcription factor controlling B-cell proliferation and differentiation
Mantle cell	t(11;14)	95%	Ig$_H$	BCL-1 (11q13)	The gene for cyclin D1 that regulates the cell cycle
Follicular cell	t(14;18) t(2;18) t(18;22)	80%	Ig$_H$ or Ig$_L$	BCL-2 (18q21)	A gene that inhibits apoptosis
Diffuse large-cell	t(3;14)	5–10%	Ig$_H$ or Ig$_L$	BCL-6 (3q27)	A gene that appears to control some aspect of germinal center formation
Burkitt's lymphoma	t(8;10) t(2;8) t(8;22)	100%	Ig$_H$ or Ig$_L$	c-*myc* (8q24)	A transcription factor controlling proliferation, differentiation, and apoptosis
MALT lymphoma	t(11;18)	30%	Ig$_H$	API2, MLT	Genes involved in inhibition of apoptosis

ation process of B and T lymphocytes (see Chapter 19), it is reasonable to conclude that the defect in lymphoma is often owing to abnormal rearrangement. This is confirmed by the observation that most of the translocations in B-cell lymphomas involve the J and S sequences of the immunoglobulin genes that are the sites of normal rearrangements. Most of the common genetic alterations seen in lymphomas can be detected by polymerase chain reaction (PCR) techniques or by fluorescence in-situ hybridization.

CLINICAL FEATURES

The clinical manifestations of lymphoma can be considered under several general categories, which are discussed further under Laboratory Studies. The first category is those effects caused by enlargement of lymphoid tissues; second is the immunologic sequelae of the lymphoma; third is those effects caused by invasion of non-lymphoid tissues, particularly marrow; and last, the metabolic and humoral effects of the lymphoma.

Enlargement of Lymphoid Tissues

Most patients with lymphoma present with **painless enlargement of lymph nodes or spleen** or both. The effects of node enlargement vary from the cosmetic to such complications as obstruction of airway or major vessels, compression of the stomach, or obstruction of the intestines. In general the node enlargement is gradual and painless. Lymphomatous infiltration seldom results in an inflammatory response, and thus symptoms such as fever, weight loss, and night sweats are less common than in Hodgkin's disease.

A common clinical situation is the patient who presents with one or more **enlarged nodes** and a history compatible with a recent **viral infection.** Although the only way to confidently rule out lymphoma is to take a biopsy of the node, one is usually reluctant to do this immediately. If the node enlargement has been sudden or painful (tender), a reactive process is more likely than a lymphoma. If the node is very hard to palpate or fixed to underlying tissues, suspect carcinoma rather than lymphoma. In general a reactive process will subside over a few weeks. A node that persists longer than this, and is painless, firm, or grows in size, must undergo biopsy. Lymphomatous nodes can undergo fluctuating enlargement. A history of recurrent enlargement of a node is as compatible with lymphoma as is persistent enlargement. It is also possible to obtain a history of previous node biopsies that were read as reactive followed by a biopsy read as lymphoma. Thus a previous benign biopsy should not weigh against taking a biopsy of a suspicious node.

Multifocal Versus Localized Disease

Nodal involvement in NHL is usually **multifocal,** with involved nodes separated by groups of normal nodes, and early dissemination throughout the body. Thus the concept of metastasis with orderly progression of disease from one node group to another, although useful in Hodgkin's disease, has little use in NHL.

However, a few patients do present with **localized disease,** often in unusual locations. **High-grade B-cell lymphomas** can present in one node area or present as solitary brain tumors or osteolytic bone tumors. **Gastrointestinal lymphomas** can be localized and, if disseminated, tend to preferentially involve gut-associated lymphoid tissue.

Interestingly, low- and intermediate-grade lymphomas are almost always disseminated at the time of presentation. Although the tumor masses associated with **B-cell lymphomas** tend to follow the anatomic distribution of the lymph nodes and lymphatics, **T-cell malignancies** are more likely to show a wider tissue distribution. T-cell malignancies resulting from clonal expansion of CD4-positive T cells generally involve the skin, sometimes with their major manifestation being skin infiltrations (mycosis fungoides). This situation reflects the natural propensity of T cells to migrate through the subepidermal layers of the skin. Both T- and B-cell lymphomas can have a blood (leukemic) component. The **T-cell lymphomas and B-cell chronic lymphocytic leukemia (CLL)** (see Chapter 21) are the most likely to result in high circulating lymphocyte counts, whereas other lymphomas usually have a minor circulating component that may not be reflected in the absolute lymphocyte count.

Other Clinical Features

A detailed history and a physical examination are very important in evaluating the NHL patient. **Exposure to toxic chemicals, chemotherapeutic or immunosuppressive agents,** or **ionizing radiation** can have epidemiologic importance, especially in the younger patient. **HIV infection** is a clear risk factor. A careful physical examination to look for **other enlarged lymph nodes** is essential for any patient presenting with a suspicious node. In addition to the common sites, involvement of retroclavicular nodes, Waldeyer's ring, and thoracic and retroperitoneal nodes should be sought by physical examination, x-ray, and CT scan. Renal and hepatic function tests should be done; however, in the absence of obstruction, involvement of these organs with lymphoma is frequently not reflected by chemistries.

Laboratory Studies

As mentioned in the preceding section, Other Clinical Features, a detailed history and physical examination are important in identifying many manifestations of NHL. **Renal and hepatic function tests** should also be done. The evaluation of patients suspected of having lymphoma should include **examination of blood and marrow** for the presence of lymphoma cells as judged by morphology, **cell surface markers,** and **genetic analysis.** Sixty percent to 80 percent of lymphoma patients have involvement of blood, marrow, or both when sensitive techniques are used. This is true even when the complete blood count is perfectly normal

A. BLOOD AND MARROW TESTS FOR IMMUNOLOGIC EFFECTS:

Most patients with NHL do not develop profound marrow dysfunction even when the marrow is partially infiltrated with malignant cells. **Immunologic testing** of blood and marrow is best performed after the disease has been diagnosed by biopsy so that specific immunologic characteristics of the lymphoma are known. For example, if the lymphoma is of B-cell origin and is expressing λ immunoglobulin light chains, this information can be used to increase the sensitivity of the tests in blood and marrow.

Most patients with lymphoma have or soon develop an **immune deficiency** that is characterized by diffuse hypogammaglobulinemia or by a poor response to new antigens and to infections (or both). However, a significant number of these patients, particularly those with T-cell lymphomas, may have diffuse or specific hypergammaglobulinemia, and a minority (about 5%) have a monoclonal serum immunoglobulin (M protein). Increased susceptibility to viral infection, and reactivation of viruses such as herpes zoster, may occur even prior to the onset of overt symptoms of lymphoma. This situation is owing to depression of cell-mediated immunity. Some lymphomas, particularly low-grade B-cell and CLL, may demonstrate autoantibodies directed against red blood cells or platelets, resulting in hemolytic anemia or immune thrombocytopenia.

B. TESTS FOR LYMPHOMATOUS INFILTRATION OF NONLYMPHOID ORGANS:

The possibility of lymphomatous infiltration of nonlymphoid organs should always be suspected. Because lymphoma seldom elicits an inflammatory response as it invades, the involvement can be extensive before the patient becomes symptomatic. The most common involvement is seen in skin (especially T-cell lymphomas), lung, the gastrointestinal (GI) tract, the liver, bone and marrow, the kidney, and the central nervous system (CNS). Attention should be paid to all of these sites in evaluating a patient with lymphoma, and any otherwise unexplained findings should be fully evaluated by chemical and radiologic techniques. Liver involvement, for example, may be revealed by **CT scan** despite normal **liver chemistries.** Because the patient with lymphoma is subject to unusual and opportunistic infections, one is often faced with a difficult clinical distinction between infection and lymphomatous infiltration, for example, in the lung. These distinctions may require **biopsy** to resolve.

C. SERUM ASSAY TESTS FOR METABOLIC AND HUMORAL EFFECTS:

Some patients with lymphoma develop profound marrow dysfunction even when the marrow cannot be shown to be heavily involved with lymphoma. However, more common is the presence of significant numbers of lymphoma cells in the marrow with relatively normal blood counts. Anemia and thrombocytopenia are more often seen as side effects of therapy than as presenting features. Because lymphocytes produce a variety of cytokines with diverse effects on other cells, patients with lymphoma can display generalized **metabolic and systemic symptoms.**

Most common are unexplained fever, weight loss, night sweats, and chills; less common are hypercalcemia and hypoglycemia. The availability of **serum assays** for lymphocyte-produced cytokines and their receptors may be useful in evaluating patients for these effects.

CHARACTERISTICS OF INDIVIDUAL LYMPHOMAS

Some types of lymphoma have relatively specific profiles of clinical presentation, histology, cell phenotype, and cytogenetic abnormalities. The following descriptions highlight the more important disease states as classified in the Working Formulation or REAL classification. Tables 22–3 and 22–5 summarize the features of many of these lymphoma types.

Low-Grade Lymphomas

The nodular, or follicular, lymphomas dominate this class. In fact, they make up one-third or more of all cases of NHL. **Follicular lymphomas** typically occur in middle-

Table 22–5. Immunologic and cytogenetic features in the REAL classification of T-cell neoplasms.

Disease	Morphology	Immunophenotype	Genotype
T-cell CLL	Small lymphocytes or prolymphocytes	TdT⁻ CD2, 3, 5, 7⁺ CD4⁺8⁻ > CD8⁺4⁻ > CD4⁻8⁻ CD25⁻	TCR rearrangements Inv14 (q11;q32) (75%)
Cutaneous T-cell	Small and large cells with cerebriform nuclei	TdT⁻ CD2, 3, 5⁺, 7± CD4⁺8⁻, CD25±	TCR rearrangement
Large granular lymphocyte	Lymphocytes with abundant cytoplasm and azurophilic granules	TdT⁻ CD2, 3⁺, 5± CD8, 16, 57⁺ CD4, 56, 25⁻	TCR rearrangement
Peripheral T-cell	Small to medium-sized irregular lymphocytes	TdT⁻ CD2, 3, 5, 7± CD4 and/or 8⁺	TCR rearrangement
Adult T-cell	Highly variable	TdT⁻ CD2, 3, 5, 25⁺ CD7⁻, CD4⁺8⁻	TCR rearrangement Integrated HTLV-1
Anaplastic large-cell	Large blastic pleomorphic cells	TdT⁻ CD2, 3, 5, 7± CD25±, CD30⁺	TCR rearrangement t(2;5) (ALK)
Precursor T lymphoblastic	Medium-sized blastic cells	TdT⁺ CD7⁺ CD2, 3, 5± CD4, 8⁺ or CD4, 8⁻	Variable TCR and IgG rearrangement

aged or elderly adults. They usually present as a slow-growing, nontender enlargement of lymph nodes, taking months to years to appear and evolve. More than 75% of patients have disseminated disease at presentation, and 50% or more have marrow involvement. They tend to be resistant to curative chemotherapy, but even so, have a median survival of 7 years as compared with survival of 1–2 years for the intermediate- and high-grade lymphomas that fail to respond to curative chemotherapy or transplantation. With time, the follicular lymphomas can exhibit a change in histology and behavior to a more high-grade tumor class with a concomitant reduction in survival.

Once a diagnosis is made from a node or tumor mass biopsy, a **search for evidence of disseminated disease** should be undertaken, using studies of blood and marrow for cell morphology, immunologic markers, and gene rearrangements. These studies will usually be positive. More complex staging (staging laparotomy or organ biopsy) is unnecessary unless it appears that the disease may in fact be localized.

These tumors are usually of B-cell origin, and their nodular pattern of growth is reminiscent of their origin in the germinal center. The presence of larger cells and mixtures of diffuse as well as nodular architecture suggests a more aggressive variant of the disease. The characteristic **cell phenotypes** are summarized in Figure 22–2. These cells correspond to the phenotype of maturing lymphocytes of both T- and B-cell type (see Chapter 19). The presence or absence of CD5 is important because it is characteristic of B-cell CLL and its presence suggests a less aggressive variant. In addition, there is a rough positive correlation between the intensity of expression of surface immunoglobulin and the aggressiveness of the disease.

The cells display the characteristic **immunoglobulin gene rearrangements** seen in B cells. In addition, most will display a t(14:18) **chromosomal translocation,** which places the BCL-2 proto-oncogene under the influence of the immunoglobulin heavy chain gene locus. The use of PCR technology to detect immunoglobulin gene rearrangements and the BCL-2 translocation permits the detection of very small numbers of malignant cells in clinical specimens.

A. Tissue-Based Variant of B-Cell CLL:

Another low-grade lymphoma is characterized by a diffuse infiltration of small, noncleaved lymphocytes. The tissue-based variant of B-cell CLL is almost always associated with a leukemic phase of varying degree. The presence of the CD5 marker and low levels of surface immunoglobulin are characteristic. Its presentation and response to therapy are identical to that of CLL. In many cases it evolves over time to a more aggressive variant of lymphoma.

B. Lymphoplasmacytoid Variant:

The lymphoplasmacytoid variant is frequently associated with an IgM component that leads to its being considered along with multiple myeloma as a plasma cell neoplasm (see Chapter 25). However, the biology and clinical behavior of this disease more closely resemble that of the low-grade lymphomas.

C. Marginal Zone Lymphomas:

An additional variant of low- to intermediate-grade lymphomas has been brought to the forefront by the REAL classification—the marginal zone lymphomas. Three clinical presentations have now been described, including nodal marginal zone, splenic marginal zone, and extranodal with masses in the respiratory or GI system, involving subepithelial, **mucosa-associated, lymphoid tissue (MALT tumors)**. Patients with MALT tumors generally have a history of autoimmune disease or chronic antigenic stimulation. Sites of presentation include the GI tract, especially the stomach, salivary glands, skin, lung, thyroid, and orbit. Gastric MALT lymphomas commonly present with symptoms of dyspepsia, anorexia, epigastric pain, and GI bleeding. Their pathogenesis is thought to be related to *Helicobacter pylori* infection, and some cases will respond to antibiotic therapy alone. This has raised the issue of whether a protracted course of antibiotics is indicated as initial therapy. When the bacteria are eliminated through the use of combinations of antibiotics and blockade of acid production, a large proportion of these lymphomas will show regression. Unfortunately, less than one-third of patients, usually those with stage I (T1) disease (endoscopic appearance of gastritis), appear to have sustained responses.

Splenic marginal zone lymphoma appears to be another distinct entity, although much less common. It is distinguished by variable lymphocytosis (10,000–40,000/µL) with the appearance of villous lymphocytes in both blood and marrow, moderate to marked splenomegaly, and the presence of a small M component (either IgG or IgM) of less than 30 grams per liter. B symptoms are rare and the lactic dehydrogenase (LDH) level tends to be normal at presentation. Spleen histology shows giant follicles with some red pulp infiltration but not to the degree seen in hairy-cell leukemia. By immunophenotype, the tumor cells are usually positive for sIg and CD22, 24, and 25 (unlike hairy cells, which are CD24 and 25 negative), and negative for CD5, 23, and 76b. No consistent or unique chromosomal abnormalities have been reported.

Intermediate-Grade Lymphomas

The intermediate-grade lymphomas share characteristics of the low- and high-grade tumors. Patterns of dis-

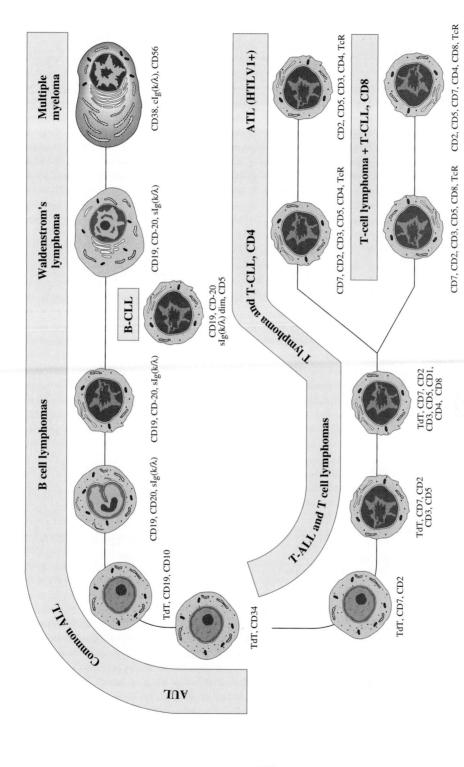

Figure 22-2. Characteristic phenotypes of B- and T-cell lymphomas. Patterns of normal lymphocyte differentiation (see Figure 19-3) can be used as a structure to visualize the relationships between the various lymphoid malignancies. Although the phenotypes of the lymphomas bear some resemblance to their normal developmental counterparts, there are numerous differences that make the comparison only approximate.

Labels within the figure:

B cell lymphomas

Multiple myeloma — CD38, cIg(κ/λ), CD56

Waldenstrom's lymphoma — CD19, CD-20, sIg(κ/λ)

B-CLL — CD19, CD-20, sIg(κ/λ) dim, CD5

CD19, CD20, sIg(κ/λ)

CD19, CD-20, sIg(κ/λ)

TdT, CD19, CD10

Common ALL

AUL — TdT, CD34

T lymphoma and T-CLL, CD4

ATL (HTLV1+) — CD2, CD5, CD3, CD4, TcR

CD7, CD2, CD3, CD5, CD4, TcR

T-ALL and T cell lymphomas

TdT, CD7, CD2, CD3, CD5, CD1, CD4, CD8

TdT, CD7, CD2, CD3, CD5

TdT, CD7, CD2

T-cell lymphoma + T-CLL, CD8

CD2, CD5, CD7, CD4, CD8, TcR

CD7, CD2, CD3, CD5, CD8, TcR

259

ease histology include nodular large-cell lymphoma; a small cell or mixed small and large-cell tumor with diffuse histology; and a diffuse large-cell lymphoma. The latter may be classified as high-grade if the cells are poorly differentiated. The classification of lymphomas as intermediate-grade is done more on the basis of what the tumor is not, rather than on specific characteristics. Thus, when a lymphoma does not fit the profile of either a low- or high-grade lymphoma it is assigned to the intermediate-grade class.

Most of the intermediate-grade lymphomas are of B-cell origin. There are no unique characteristics to the clinical presentation or course other than an intermediate level of aggressiveness of the tumor growth. The physician must observe the patient to determine the pattern and course of the disease over time in order to derive the prognosis for the individual patient. For treatment purposes, intermediate-grade lymphomas are generally considered in the same category as high-grade lymphomas.

Another class of B-cell lymphomas, which has been emphasized by the REAL classification, is **mantle cell lymphoma.** This lymphoma variant is characterized immunophenotypically by the presence of CD5 (like CLL), but, unlike CLL, it does not express CD23. Most mantle cell lymphomas have a t(11;14) translocation that involves the BCL-1 proto-oncogene (see Table 22–3). Patients with this lymphoma respond poorly to therapy and relapse early. Therefore, these lymphomas are clinically very distinct from the low-grade lymphomas, which they otherwise resemble.

High-Grade Lymphomas

Several diseases with unique profiles fall into the high-grade lymphoma category. It is also common to see tumors of both B- and T-cell origin within this grouping. Four of the more important node-based high-grade lymphomas are diffuse large-cell lymphoma, formerly referred to as diffuse histiocytic lymphoma; large-cell immunoblastic lymphoma; lymphoblastic lymphoma; and a very aggressive small-cell tumor called Burkitt's lymphoma. In general, these are all very rapidly growing tumors with a poor prognosis when left untreated.

A. DIFFUSE LARGE-CELL LYMPHOMA:

The large-cell lymphoma patient frequently presents with one or more rapidly developing tumor masses involving nodal or extranodal sites. As is typical of most lymphomas, the mass is not tender and does not cause inflammation or interfere with organ function except by compression. Retroperitoneal disease can obstruct venous drainage of the legs, resulting in edema and thrombophlebitis.

Staging studies should involve a large-volume biopsy of the tumor for histology and cell phenotype studies. Marrow and blood studies for morphology, immunophenotype, chromosomal analysis, and T- and B-cell gene rearrangements should be obtained to prove disseminated disease. Cerebrospinal fluid examination and imaging of the CNS are indicated in patients with neurologic findings. Patients can present with localized involvement of the brain or widely disseminated lymphoma involving the CNS. Ten percent to 20 percent of the large cell lymphomas may be limited to a single node or extranodal site such as bone, Waldeyer's ring, thyroid, lachrymal glands, or the gastrointestinal tract.

The **typical large-cell tumor mass** shows complete effacement of normal lymphoid architecture with a monotonous infiltrate of large lymphocytes. These cells are usually of B-cell origin with a phenotype not distinctly different from that of other lymphomas except for an increased expression of surface immunoglobulin in many cases. Many of these lymphomas have chromosomal rearrangements that involve BCL-6, either alone or in combination with involvement of BCL-2 and, in some cases, c-*myc* (see Tables 22–3 and 22–4). In addition, mutations of the p53 tumor-suppressor gene are seen. This complex genetic background may explain the clinical heterogeneity that characterizes this disease.

B. LARGE-CELL IMMUNOBLASTIC LYMPHOMA:

Some of the diffuse large-cell lymphomas are composed of so-called **immunoblasts,** that is, cells with abundant basophilic cytoplasm and nuclei with a large central nucleolus. Some of these cells resemble plasma cells or plasma blasts. This form is referred to as **immunoblastic lymphoma** and may be of either T- or B-cell origin. It is most commonly seen in older patients, often with pre-existing immunologic disease such as Sjögren syndrome, thyroiditis, or celiac sprue or a previous lymphoproliferative disease such as CLL, myeloma, or angioimmunoblastic lymphadenopathy. In those patients with a T-cell angioimmunoblastic lymphoma, leukopenia and polyclonal hypergammaglobulinemia are often seen. Angioimmunoblastic lymphoma has an extremely poor prognosis, especially in older patients.

C. LYMPHOBLASTIC LYMPHOMA:

Precursor lymphoblastic lymphoma represents another high-grade malignancy with diffuse histology. This condition is a disease of younger individuals and children. It often presents with a bulky, rapidly growing mediastinal mass. The marrow and CNS are frequently involved. On biopsy, the mass consists of a diffuse infiltrate of cells with convoluted nuclei and little cytoplasm. The phenotype of the cells is most often that of a pre–B or T cell. This tumor shares characteristics with acute lymphocytic leukemia (ALL) and is treated with a similar regimen. Patients presenting with lymphoblastic lymphoma frequently have a leukemic component to their disease and may rapidly progress to overt ALL.

D. BURKITT'S LYMPHOMA:

Burkitt's lymphoma, another disease in the high-grade category, is a very aggressive tumor of immature B-cell origin. The characteristic histology is that of a diffuse infiltrate of small noncleaved lymphocytes interspersed with large cells imparting a "starry sky" appearance under low-power magnification. The tumor is associated with a unique chromosomal rearrangement involving the c-*myc* proto-oncogene on chromosome 8 moving to one of the immunoglobulin gene loci, the most common being t(8;14) (see Tables 22–3 and 22–4).

A form of Burkitt's lymphoma occurs endemically in children in Africa. It usually presents as a tumor mass localized to the jaw or retroperitoneum with involvement of bone, kidney, ovaries, and CNS. This endemic form is strongly associated with Epstein-Barr virus infection. In Western countries, Burkitt's lymphoma is a nonendemic disease of children and young adults with no clear connection to the Epstein-Barr virus. It most often presents as a rapidly growing tumor of abdominal lymph nodes, although marrow involvement is generally present at the time of diagnosis.

E. B-CELL LYMPHOMA IN AIDS PATIENTS:

An increasing incidence of B-cell lymphomas is being seen in AIDS patients. They are strongly associated with Epstein-Barr virus and may also show rearrangements involving c-*myc* and mutation of p53. Many of these involve the brain. Clinical staging is important in planning treatment and should be carried out without delay. Patients with a single tumor mass and low LDH indicating a small tumor mass have the best prognosis. Bulky tumor in the abdomen imparts a worse prognosis, and involvement of either marrow or the CNS together with a high LDH predict a high failure rate even with multidrug chemotherapy.

T-CELL LYMPHOMA CLASSIFICATION

As techniques for diagnosing clonal lymphoid malignancies have improved, especially the ability to detect rearrangements of the B- and T-cell antigen receptor genes, an increasing number of tumors of T-cell origin have been identified. **Clinical clues** to the presence of a T-cell malignancy include the presence of B symptoms, leukopenia or aplastic anemia (or both), disseminated disease with marrow involvement, hepatosplenomegaly, and lung and skin involvement.

Several subtypes of T-cell disease have been identified. These are defined largely by their clinical profiles;

however, the ultimate diagnosis of a T-cell lymphoma requires study of **cell surface markers and an analysis for T-cell–receptor gene rearrangement.** The latter is the only certain way of proving a clonal origin for T cells. The array of surface markers can be helpful in that frequently T-cell lymphomas will express some, but not all, of the characteristic T-cell markers. The unexpected absence of a T-cell marker on a population of T cells can be a clue to their malignant nature. In addition, the presence of CD4, CD8, or both provides some help in predicting the signs and symptoms related to lymphomas of T-"helper" (CD4+) or T-"cytotoxic/suppressor" (CD8+) subtypes.

Histologic subclassifications of T-cell lymphoma distinguish between peripheral T-cell lymphoma, several angiocentric forms, and a Hodgkin's disease–like form (Table 22–5). Many T-cell lymphomas are characterized by a pleomorphic cell population, often including large numbers of macrophages. This diverse cell population is probably recruited to the site of the tumor by production of cytokines by the malignant T cells. In addition, production of these cytokines explains the common occurrence of inflammatory signs and symptoms.

Peripheral T-Cell Lymphoma

Most patients present with **peripheral T-cell lymphoma,** which is a diffuse small- or large-cell lymphoma with the phenotype of mature T cells. More than one-half of these patients have B symptoms (fever, chills, weight loss) suggesting active cytokine production by the malignant cells. Widespread lymphadenopathy is the rule, and many patients have involvement of extranodal sites, marrow, blood, liver, spleen, lung, and skin.

Large Granular Lymphocyte (LGL) Disease

Large granular lymphocyte (LGL) disease is a distinct disorder arising from a clonal proliferation of a granular lymphocyte, derived from a CD3+, CD8+ T cell. Although sometimes confused with an NK cell, these are true T cells. The disease presents clinically as a low-grade lymphoproliferative disorder with splenomegaly but little or no lymphadenopathy, pancytopenia complicated by recurrent bacterial infections, and, in a quarter of cases, an autoimmune disorder such as rheumatoid arthritis. LGL disease in patients with rheumatoid arthritis can be indistinguishable from Felty's syndrome. Proliferation of LGL cells has also been reported in association with other hematologic malignancies (monoclonal gammopathy of undetermined significance, multiple myeloma, and myelodysplasia) and with both marrow and organ transplantation.

The **diagnosis** of LGL leukemia can usually be made from the appearance of large numbers of **granular lymphocytes (GL)** in the peripheral blood and bone marrow. Most patients demonstrate GL levels greater than 2000/μL, although when the other clinical features are present, a GL count greater than 500/μL is acceptable (normal GL count 223–699/μL). True NK-cell disease is very uncommon and often presents as a leukemia with a very aggressive course.

Lymphomatoid Granulomatosis & Polymorphic Reticulosis

Less common, angiocentric types of T cell lymphoma include two entities: lymphomatoid granulomatosis and **polymorphic reticulosis (lethal midline granuloma)** of the upper respiratory tract. The latter is characterized by destructive lesions of the nose, sinuses, and nasopharynx. Patients with **lymphomatoid granulomatosis** complain of fever, weight loss, shortness of breath, cough, and hemoptysis. They have single or multiple lung nodules or masses on chest x-ray.

Angioimmunoblastic Lymphadenopathy

Angioimmunoblastic lymphadenopathy is a disease of the elderly that presents with generalized lymphadenopathy, hepatosplenomegaly, B symptoms, polyclonal expansion of B cells with hypergammaglobulinemia, and, in some cases, autoantibodies resulting in hemolytic anemia or thrombocytopenia. It is an aggressive disease that progresses to either overt T- or B-cell lymphoma.

Histiocytic Medullary Reticulosis (HMR) & Lennert's Lymphoma

HMR is primarily a disease of the marrow that results in profound pancytopenia with infiltration of phagocytic cells that characteristically ingest erythrocytes. As with other T-cell lymphomas, it is usually accompanied by fever, weight loss, lymphadenopathy, and hepatosplenomegaly. **Lennert's lymphoma** is characterized by the appearance of large numbers of epithelioid cells mixed with lymphoid cells, often forming granulomas.

Hodgkin's Disease–like T-Cell Lymphoma

Hodgkin's disease–like T-cell lymphoma, as implied by its name, mimics the presentation and histology of Hodgkin's disease. However, the T-cell infiltrate of the involved nodes is clonal. It is important to distinguish this variant since its prognosis is significantly poorer than that of Hodgkin's disease.

Other Presentations

T-cell malignancies can also present as **CLL** (see Chapter 21), **ALL** (see Chapter 24), or as skin disease (**cutaneous T-cell lymphoma/mycosis fungoides/Sezary syndrome**). The presenting skin lesions of mycosis fungoides vary from an eczematous or psoriatic-appearing lesion to plaques with sharply demarcated margins. With time these cutaneous lesions develop into painless nodules that can ulcerate and become infected. Severe itching is the rule, and many patients will develop generalized erythroderma progressing to exfoliation. Survival can range from a few months to several decades, depending on extent of blood, nodal, and visceral disease. When disease is limited to the skin, median survival is in excess of 10 years. However, most patients will in time progress to stage IV with involvement of lymph nodes and visceral organs. Blood and marrow involvement is characterized by the appearance in the circulation of small or large lymphocytes with highly convoluted (cerebriform) nuclei. These cells are acid phosphatase positive and CD4 positive. Their presence signifies progression from mycosis fungoides to Sezary cell leukemia.

On skin biopsy the CD4 T-helper cell lymphomas typically show a lymphocytic or mixed cell infiltrate immediately under the epidermis. In some patients the epidermis is actually invaded by clusters of lymphocytes producing unique lesions called **Pautrier microabscesses.** This pattern is quite different from that seen with B-cell lymphomas, where the cells tend to congregate in the lower dermis, leaving a clear subepidermal zone. T-cell–receptor gene rearrangement analysis can be used to identify the clonal T-cell nature of the infiltrate in unclear cases.

THERAPY & CLINICAL COURSE

The success rate in treating lymphoma is of course related to grade of disease as well as many other prognostic factors. For both high-grade and low-grade lymphomas the most important **prognostic indicators** are summarized in Table 22–6, and the **outcomes** associated with combinations of these factors are shown in Table 22–7. Patients with low-grade lymphomas often have a good prognosis in terms of their long-term survival but are very rarely cured, ultimately dying of their disease. Conversely, patients with high-grade lymphomas, who have a very poor prognosis when untreated, and a much shorter average survival, can often be cured by aggressive therapy (Figure 22–3). Thus, NHL therapy must be tailored to the disease and to the patient. In many institutions these patients will be treated according to research protocols. This permits continuous improvement in therapy as new regimens

Table 22–6. Prognostic indices in high- and low-grade lymphomas.

Adverse Factors for High-Grade Lymphoma	Adverse Factors for Low-Grade Lymphoma
Age > 60 yrs.	Age > 60 yrs.
Serum LDH elevated	Serum LDH elevated
Performance status 2–4	B symptoms or ESR > 30
Stage III or IV	Male sex
Extranodal involvement	Extranodal involvement

for radiotherapy, multidrug chemotherapy, and marrow transplantation are introduced. Successful treatment of the lymphoma also requires a high-quality blood transfusion service to provide red blood cell and platelet support and an aggressive approach to the control of infection in these immunocompromised patients.

Radiation Therapy

Radiation therapy is very effective in destroying sites of bulky disease. Relatively low doses (2000 cGy) will result in spectacular regression of a tumor mass. However, since most patients have widely disseminated disease at presentation, the role of radiotherapy is only palliative, and limited to the treatment of a restricted site of symptomatic disease. The only situation in which radiotherapy may be undertaken with curative intent is in localized (stage I or II) disease, where cures have been reported in high-, low-, and intermediate-grade lymphomas. However, radiotherapy alone can only be recommended after an exhaustive search using radiologic, immunologic, and molecular techniques has failed to find any evidence of dissemination of the lymphoma. Even when there is no evidence for blood, marrow, or other organ involvement, up to 50% of apparent stage I lymphomas will relapse at a distant site and need multidrug chemotherapy with or without transplantation.

Treatment of Low-Grade Lymphomas

Low-grade lymphomas are frequently extremely indolent, with long periods of regression or stable disease interrupted by periods of increased disease activity. No evidence exists that aggressive chemotherapy can cure these patients. Thus a conservative therapeutic approach is indicated, ranging from no therapy at all during quiescent periods to the use of minimal chemotherapy or radiotherapy designed to control flare-ups and eliminate symptoms. Some of these patients will survive for 5–10 years, requiring only brief periods of treatment or none at all. The usual treatment for these patients is local radiotherapy to bulky symptomatic disease and a mild regimen of chemotherapy such as oral chlorambucil or cyclophosphamide or a cyclophosphamide-vincristine-prednisone regimen (see Table 22–5). Chemotherapy should be continued until the disease has regressed and appears quiescent, and then should be stopped and the patient closely observed. Such patients may gradually become more resistant to treatment with shorter periods of remission, or they may convert to a higher grade of lymphoma with a more rapid growth pattern.

Recently there have been reports of a high level of responsiveness in patients with low-grade lymphoma to the newer agents such as **fludarabine** and **2′-chlordeoxyadenosine (2-CdA)**. These agents, which are proving very effective in the treatment of the CLLs (see

Table 22–7. Survival according to prognostic indices.

	High-Grade Lymphoma		Low-Grade Lymphoma	
	2-yr Survival	5-yr Survival	5-yr Survival	10-yr Survival
Low risk: 0–1 factor	84%	73%	89%	70%
Intermediate risk: 2–3 factors	60%	47%	71%	49%
High risk: > 3 factors	34%	26%	47%	8%

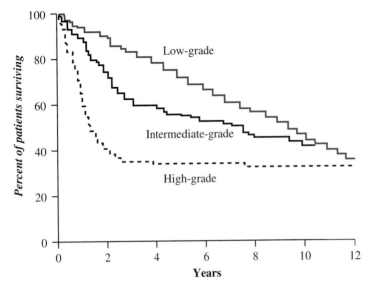

Figure 22–3. **Survival curves in lymphomas.** The success rate in treating high-grade lymphomas depends on the age of the patient, the tumor burden, and the histologic characteristics of the lymphoma.

Chapter 21), now have roles in the therapy of other low-grade lymphomas. These agents are highly immunosuppressive, especially in combination with corticosteroids, and their use increases the risk of opportunistic infections.

Some patients with low- or intermediate-grade lymphoma will show a pattern of continual slow growth of the disease despite therapy (**unresponsive disease**) or will have **brief responses followed by rapid resumption of growth.** These patients have a markedly poorer prognosis. In this case more aggressive chemotherapy protocols are justified in an attempt to achieve longer remissions. Such protocols include chemotherapy capable of crossing into the CNS, such as high-dose methotrexate with leucovorin rescue, cytosine arabinoside, or both. Such multidrug protocols involve a high level of treatment-related morbidity and mortality (up to 5–10%) but do result in prolonged disease-free survival in up to 50% of patients. Because of a tendency to see late relapses it is unclear what proportion of these may be considered cures.

Therapy of the low-grade lymphomas with **monoclonal antibodies** has been attempted in several different ways. It is possible to custom-produce anti-idiotypic antibodies that are specific for an individual's tumor cells. However, this approach has been limited by the necessity to produce a new reagent for each patient and by the ability of the tumor cells to mutate and thus change the idiotypic epitopes. Clinical testing has also been done with more general approaches using monoclonal antibodies against B cells—for example, CD19 or CD20 together or alone, coupled to toxins, or coupled with radioisotopes. **Rituximab,** a chimeric anti-CD20 monoclonal antibody with specificity for the late pre–B stage to plasma cell differentiation, has shown effectiveness in up to 50% of patients with relapsed low grade B-cell lymphomas. Patients with follicular histology showed the best response; 80% of patients who had failed chemotherapy and autologous transplantation responded with minimal toxicity. Although the best use of this agent is still a matter of study, it is typically given in doses of 375 mg/m^2 as a weekly infusion for up to 8 weeks. Its use as a part of combination chemotherapeutic regimens is also being studied. Another approach to immunotherapy involves coupling a radionuclide, such as ^{131}I, to an anti-CD20 antibody. When given in myeloablative doses followed by stem cell rescue, this approach is well tolerated and can produce prolonged remissions in better than 50% of relapsed patients.

Treatment of High-Grade Lymphomas

Patients with high-grade lymphomas have a poor prognosis when left untreated and should be treated with aggressive chemotherapy without waiting to see how the disease responds to milder therapy. A high-dose, multidrug protocol should always be used in these patients. The potential for long-term disease-free survival is now greater than 50%, and many appear to be true cures. An international index of prognostic factors has been applied to these patients and has demonstrated that age (greater than 60 years), elevated LDH, poor performance status, the presence of stage III or IV disease, and the presence of more than one site of extranodal involvement are the most significant factors. Patients with 0 to 1 risk factor show 5-year survivals of greater than 70%, whereas patients with four or more risk factors have survivals of 20–30%. The recent addition of even more aggressive chemotherapy and autologous marrow or peripheral stem cell transplantation offer even high-risk patients a probability of long-term survival approaching 50%.

Extensive research has been done to try to improve the outcome in the high-grade lymphomas by the addition of more aggressive multiagent chemotherapy. Unfortunately at this time, there is no evidence that the use of more than four drugs found in the standard treatment regimens, such as cyclophosphamide-Adriamycin-vincristine-prednisone (CHOP), can improve survival.

Patients with high-grade lymphomas who relapse after chemotherapy are now being treated with very high-dose chemotherapy regimens, sometimes including total body irradiation, followed by peripheral stem cell or autologous marrow transplantation. The success of this **salvage therapy** has been reported by several centers to range from 30% to 50% long-term disease-free survival. Radioimmunotherapy is another promising approach for relapsed high-grade lymphomas.

Autologous Marrow Transplantation/Peripheral Blood Stem Cell Support

Autologous marrow transplantation (ABMTx) has become a major treatment option for patients with high-grade lymphomas and relapsed Hodgkin's disease. The procedure has undergone a gradual transition so that it is now more correctly referred to as high-dose chemotherapy with **peripheral blood stem cell (PBSC)** support. Most transplant protocols now make use of autologous peripheral blood stem cells collected by apheresis, rather than bone marrow. The rate of recovery of the patient's blood counts, especially the platelet count, is more rapid with the peripheral stem cell method.

In essence ABMTx/PBSC support is not a transplant in the usual sense of the word, but is really a strategy for overcoming the major dose-limiting toxicity of chemotherapy, marrow failure, by supporting the patients with infusions of marrow cells, blood progenitor cells, or both. The fundamental rationale is that it may be possible to achieve cures of some diseases by increasing the dose of chemotherapy to 5–10 times that which could be given without replacement of hematopoietic progenitor cells. This has proved to be the case for some diseases. It must be remembered, however, that the procedure cannot be successful if the disease is not responsive to very high-dose chemotherapy.

ABMTx/PBSC support has the **advantage** that it can be used in patients who do not have an HLA-compatible family or unrelated donor, it can be applied to older patients with much greater safety than allogeneic transplantation, and it does not have the complication of graft-versus-host disease. Its major **disadvantage** is the risk of relapse due to small numbers of tumor cells in the autologous marrow or PBSC collection. There is increasing evidence that this is indeed a serious consideration that limits the success of this strategy.

A. PROCEDURE:

ABMTx/PBSC protocols now involve the **collection of PBSCs** in addition to, or instead of, marrow (Figure 22–4). PBSCs are collected from the patient by repeated leukapheresis, usually two to five times over as many days. The timing of these collections is critical since for them to be successful it is necessary to increase the proportion of circulating progenitor cells in the blood. This may be done either by collecting the cells during the period that the patient is recovering from conventional chemotherapy or when the granulocyte count is rising in response to either granulocyte colony-stimulating factor (G-CSF) or granulocyte macrophage colony-stimulating factor (GM-CSF). In either case it is preferable to begin collections when the count is rising sharply, either at the level of 1000–2000/µL following chemotherapy or after 4–5 days of daily colony-stimulating factor injections. The leukocytes from these collections are frozen until needed by the patient. Usually between 1 and 10×10^{10} cells are collected. Enumeration of the CD34+ cells, which include all of the hematopoietic progenitor cells, has improved the ability to determine how many cells are required for successful engraftment. Between 2 and 5×10^6 CD34+ cells/kg are adequate, and in some patients this goal may be reached in a single apheresis session.

If marrow is to be used, it is collected under general anesthesia, by repeated aspirations from both posterior iliac crests, and along the iliac crests laterally, in exactly the same way that is used for the collection of allogeneic marrow for transplantation. Usually on the order of 1000 mL of marrow is aspirated, containing between 1 and 3×10^{10} cells. The cells are then frozen.

The patient is then admitted for **high-dose chemotherapy,** which may contain any of a number of different combinations of drugs according to specific protocols (Table 22–8). Many ABMTx regimens include **total body irradiation** in addition to chemotherapy. The doses of drugs are chosen so as to result in total ablation of the marrow while avoiding lethal toxicity to other organs such as lung, liver, and heart. Within 1–4 days following chemotherapy, patients receive intravenous infusions of their marrow or PBSC or both and begin receiving daily injections of G-CSF or GM-CSF.

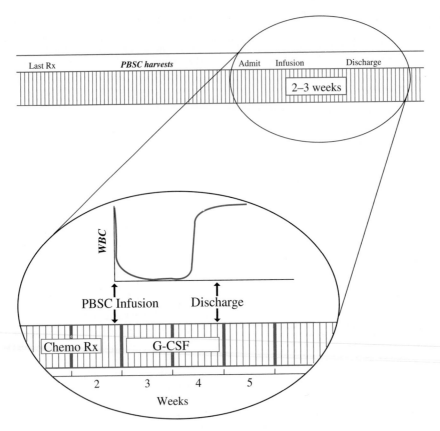

Figure 22–4. **Autologous marrow transplantation protocol.** The sequence of ABMTx involves collecting PBSCs on several occasions followed by marrow harvest. Then, after high-dose marrow ablative chemotherapy, the harvested marrow and PBSCs are used to transplant (reimplant) the patient's marrow.

Following reinfusion of the progenitor cells, there is a period of 5–10 days in which the patient is absolutely pancytopenic, with essentially no leukocytes, and dependent on platelet support. After this **latent period,** there is, under the influence of the myeloid growth factors, a rapid rise in the leukocyte count. Platelet recovery usually lags behind the white blood cells, and the patients may require platelet support for weeks to months, although the use of PBSC hastens platelet recovery.

The management of these patients is essentially the same as that of any patient receiving high-dose, marrow-ablative chemotherapy. They are **at high risk for severe infections and must receive intensive antibiotic coverage** (see Chapter 17). In addition, the chemotherapy may result in reversible **toxicity to other organs** that would not be seen with lower doses.

B. OUTCOME AND PROGNOSIS:

The ultimate outcome of ABMTx/PBSC therapy depends on three factors. First, there is a significant treat-

ment-related mortality, which is usually less than 10%. Second, and most likely, is the possibility that the patient's tumor could not be ablated completely by the chemotherapy and radiation. A fairly high percentage of patients relapse within the first 1–2 years. For most protocols in the treatment of high-grade non-Hodgkin's lymphomas, this is in the range of 30–50% of patients. Third, there is the possibility that the marrow and PBSC collections contain small numbers of tumor cells that will regrow. Since ABMTx/PBSC therapy involves the reinfusion of more than 10^{10} cells, and since even the most sensitive detection methods permit the identification of only about 1 tumor cell in 10^6 cells, it is possible that the patient can receive as many as 10^4 tumor cells even if they are undetectable. It has been shown in the case of non-Hodgkin's lymphoma that the risk of relapse is higher in patients who have such very small numbers of cells detectable in their stem cell collections.

Strategies for depleting these tumor cells, which in-

Table 22–8. Some typical chemotherapeutic regimens for lymphoma.

Regimen	Drug Dosage and Schedule
Single agent	
Cyclophosphamide or	100 PO qd
Chlorambucil	4–12 mg PO qd
Fludarabine	25 mg/m^2/IV days 1–5
CVP Repeated q3 weeks	
Cyclophosphamide	400 mg/m^2 PO days 1–5
Vincristine	1.4 mg/m^2 IV day 1
Prednisone	100 mg/m^2 PO days 1–5
CHOP Repeated q3 weeks	
Cyclophosphamide	750 mg/m^2 IV day 1
Adriamycin	50 mg/m^2 IV day 1
Vincristine	1.4 mg/m^2 IV day 1
Prednisone	100 mg PO days 1–5
Chemotherapy with autologous marrow support	
BCNU	112 mg/m^2 IV days 1–4
Cyclophosphamide	900 mg/m^2 IV q12h days 1–4
Etoposide (VP-16)	250 mg/m^2 IV q12h days 1–4
Infusion of autologous marrow cells	At least 2×10^6 CD34$^+$ cells/kg IV day 7

volve treating the marrow with **monoclonal antibodies, in vitro chemotherapy, or immunotoxins** ("purging"), have been evaluated but do not yet offer a consistently clear improvement in outcome. Recently, strategies for purification of the CD34$^+$ stem cells using immunoabsorptive columns based on the ability of monoclonal antibodies to bind to the CD34 antigen have entered clinical trials. There is hope that this procedure will simultaneously enrich for the desired stem cells and deplete unwanted tumor cells. It is striking that successful engraftment can be achieved by infusion of as few as 1 to 2×10^6 purified CD34$^+$ cells, with exactly the same engraftment kinetics as infusion of 10,000 times more unenriched marrow or blood cells.

The **prognosis** for the patient with relapsed or refractory non-Hodgkin's lymphoma who undergoes a modern ABMTx protocol is 30–50% long-term disease-free survival. Although far from perfect, this represents a significant improvement over conventional chemotherapy for this patient group.

Treatment Regimens for T-Cell Lymphomas

Early-stage **mycosis fungoides** with disease limited to the skin is best treated with topical therapy. Barely perceptible skin lesions (plaques, papules, or eczematous patches) will usually respond to topical steroids, alone. PUVA therapy (oral psoralen with UVA irradiation) or topical nitrogen mustard (mechlorethamine) applied as an aqueous solution or ointment will induce complete remission, lasting more than a year, in most patients with skin-limited disease. Hypersensitivity reactions are, however, seen in up to 50% of patients treated with mechlorethamine. If topical therapy doesn't work, total-skin electron-beam irradiation can be used, usually in combination with maintenance PUVA, interferon-α, or oral methotrexate to prevent rapid relapse.

Patients with **cutaneous tumors and nodal involvement** are treated with local-field electron beam and PUVA maintenance or, in the case of refractory or visceral disease, single-agent (methotrexate, 2-CdA, fludarabine, or pentostatin) or combination chemotherapy (EPOCH). Patients with **generalized erythroderma** should receive photophoresis, together with low-dose interferon-α or methotrexate when the response is poor. **Photophoresis** involves collecting the patient's leukocytes by leukopheresis after the oral administration of methoxypsoralen and then exposing them to UV light. When the treated leukocytes are reinfused they somehow stimulate a host response to the tumor cells and significant improvement in the patient's erythroderma. Photophoresis has also been used as an adjuvant to chemotherapy in Sezary cell leukemia patients.

LGL disease in otherwise asymptomatic patients may best be simply observed. Survivals can exceed 10 years. The principal indications for treatment are recurrent infections secondary to severe neutropenia and B symptoms. Patients may respond to prednisone alone or in combination with Cytoxan, or to low-dose oral methotrexate. Combination chemotherapy (CHOP-like regimen) has been used in patients with aggressive disease with only limited success.

BIBLIOGRAPHY

Diagnosis

Argatoff LH et al: Mantle cell lymphoma: A clinicopathologic study of 80 cases. Blood 1997;89:2067.

Catovsky D, Matutes E: Splenic lymphoma with circulating villous lymphocytes/splenic marginal-zone lymphoma. Semin Hematol 1999;36:184.

Coiffier B et al: Indolent nonfollicular lymphomas: Characteristics, treatment, and outcome. Semin Hematol 1999;36:198.

Frederico M et al: Prognosis of follicular lymphoma: A predictive model based on a retrospective analysis of 987 cases. Blood 2000;95:783.

Harris NL et al: A revised European-American classification of lymphoid neoplasms: A proposal from the international lymphoma study group. Blood 1994;84:1361.

Harris NL et al: The World Health Organization classification of hematological malignancies report of the clinical advisory committee meeting, Airlie House, Virginia, November 1997. Mod Pathol 2000;13:193.

Hiddeman W et al: Lymphoma classification: The gap between biology and clinical management is closing. Blood 1996; 88:4085.

Semenzato G et al: The lymphoproliferative disease of granular lymphocytes: Updated criteria for diagnosis. Blood 1997; 89:256.

Tilly H et al: Prognostic value of chromosomal abnormalities in follicular lymphoma. Blood 1994;84:1043.

Willis TG, Dyer MJS: The role of immunoglobulin translocations in the pathogenesis of B cell malignancies. Blood 2000; 96:808.

Zucca E et al: The gastric marginal zone B cell lymphoma of the MALT type. Blood 2000;96:410.

Therapy

Appelbaum FR: Treatment of aggressive non-Hodgkin's lymphoma with marrow transplantation. Marrow Transplant Rev 1993;3:1.

Armitage JO: Treatment of non-Hodgkin's lymphomas. N Engl J Med 1993;328:1023.

Fisher RI et al: Comparison of a standard regimen (CHOP) with three intensive chemotherapy regimens for advanced non-Hodgkin's lymphoma. N Engl J Med 1993;328:1002.

Pittaluga S et al: Clinical analysis of 670 cases in two trials of the European organization for the research and treatment of cancer lymphoma cooperative group subtyped according to the revised European-American classification of the lymphoid neoplasms: A comparison with the working formulation. Blood 1996;87:4358.

Press OW et al: A phase I/II trial of iodine 131-tositumomab (anti-CD20), etoposide, cyclophosphamide, and autologous stem cell transplantation for relapsed B-cell lymphomas. Blood 2000;96:2934.

Rowe JM et al: Recommended guidelines for the management of autologous and allogeneic bone marrow transplantation. Ann Intern Med 1994;120:143.

Shipp MA et al: A predictive model for aggressive non-Hodgkin's lymphoma: The international non-Hodgkin's lymphoma prognostic factors project. N Engl J Med 1993;329:987.

Steinbach G et al: Antibiotic treatment of gastric lymphoma of mucosa-associated lymphoid tissue. Ann Intern Med 1999; 131:88.

The non-Hodgkin's lymphoma classification project: A clinical evaluation of the international study group classification of non-Hodgkin's lymphoma. Blood 1997;89:3909.

The international non-Hodgkin's lymphoma prognostic factors project: A predictive model for aggressive non-Hodgkin's lymphoma. N Engl J Med 1993;329:987.

Verdonck LF et al: Comparison of CHOP chemotherapy with autologous bone marrow transplantation for slowly responding patients with aggressive non-Hodgkin's lymphoma. N Engl J Med 1995;332:1045.

Hodgkin's Disease

Hodgkin's disease is a distinct type of lymphoma that in many ways offers a paradigm for the diagnosis and treatment of hematologic malignancies. Accurate diagnosis and staging are critically important for successful treatment. The concept of staging is nowhere more clearly illustrated than in Hodgkin's disease. Clinical staging of the Hodgkin's disease patient provides both a strong predictor of prognosis and a foundation for the selection of a specific treatment regimen. In addition, treatment of Hodgkin's disease is based on solid principles of radiobiology and chemotherapy that serve as a model for all other treatment regimens. Because of this solid theoretical base, treatment of Hodgkin's disease has become very successful. Hodgkin's disease is one of the best examples of a malignancy that can be cured if diagnosed and managed well. However, despite our well-developed understanding of the clinical course, staging, and treatment of this disease, its cause remains unknown. Even the origin of the malignant cell is a source of controversy.

DIAGNOSIS & CLASSIFICATION

Like other lymphomas, **Hodgkin's disease** usually presents as an enlargement of the lymphoid organs, frequently accompanied by systemic symptoms such as fever, weight loss, fatigue, and so on. It is unique in several respects, however. Unlike the non-Hodgkin's lymphomas, the tumor masses largely comprise normal reactive T cells and are usually CD4 predominant, not a clone of malignant lymphocytes.

REED-STERNBERG CELLS & LYMPHOCYTIC/ HISTIOCYTIC (L&H) CELLS

The putative malignant cell is the **Reed-Sternberg cell,** a large, frequently binucleate cell that more closely resembles a macrophage-like cell than a lymphocyte. The relative number of the Reed-Sternberg cells may vary from very high to very low. In some cases only a very careful search will reveal the presence of these cells, without which the diagnosis cannot be made with certainty. The other cells found in the lesion are a diverse population of lymphocytes, eosinophils, and other reactive cells that, although they may represent by far most

of the cells in the lesion, are thought to be passive or at least secondary to the malignant process.

Reed-Sternberg cells have been difficult to study because they are present in small numbers and are difficult to separate from the tumor tissue, and because only very few cell lines have been established. Immunophenotyping studies of isolated Reed-Sternberg cells suggest that they are monoclonal B cells, though at least two phenotypically different cell lines have been identified. Despite many years of study, the mechanism by which Reed-Sternberg cells arise and their precise role in the malignant process remain obscure. In classical Hodgkin's lymphomas, Epstein-Barr virus (EBV) can be isolated from the Reed-Sternberg cell in approximately 50% of cases.

Because of the limitations of immunologic and genetic studies in this disease, diagnosis of Hodgkin's disease still depends on the pathologic interpretation of biopsy material. Diagnostic certainty requires the identification of Reed-Sternberg cells or, in the case of nodular lymphocyte predominant disease, "popcorn" or **L&H cells (lymphocytic or histiocytic cells (or both) of Lukes-Butler classification)** set in a diverse population of B and T lymphocytes, eosinophils, and other reactive cells. The overall histologic pattern of the tumor has a strong association with clinical course and can fall into one of five categories (Table 23–1).

Types of Hodgkin's Disease

Nodular lymphocyte predominant Hodgkin's lymphoma (NLPHL) is characterized histologically by a vague nodular pattern, rich in lymphocytes, containing a distinctive morphologic variant of the Reed-Sternberg cell, the so-called L&H (lymphocytic/histiocytic), or "popcorn" cell. These cells are surrounded by a collar of CD57+ T cells and large numbers of small polyclonal B cells. The phenotype of the "popcorn" cell resembles that of a B lymphocyte (CD15 and CD30−, CD19, 20, 22, and 45+). This form is relatively indolent and slow to spread, often resembling a low-grade non-Hodgkin's lymphoma.

The **more common histologic types** are nodular sclerosis, mixed cellularity, lymphocyte-depleted, and, the newly proposed, lymphocyte-rich classical Hodgkin's

Table 23–1. Histologic classification of Hodgkin's disease.

REAL Histologic Classification	Description	Frequency
Nodular/lymphocyte predominant	Nodular pattern with "popcorn" cells	4–5%
Lymphocyte-rich classical HL	Abundant mature lymphocytes, a few classical Reed-Sternberg cells	5–10%
Nodular sclerosis	Prominent fibrosis, mature lymphocytes, and Reed-Sternberg cells present	60–80%
Mixed cellularity	Both mature lymphocytes and Reed-Sternberg cells	15–30%
Lymphocyte-depleted	Predominantly large, poorly differentiated cells	< 1%

lymphoma. They share the common feature of the presence of classical or lacunar type Reed-Sternberg cells, both of which are monoclonal B cells with a distinct immunophenotype, CD15 and 30+, CD20 and 45−. Nodular sclerosis Hodgkin's disease is further characterized by variable amounts of collagenous connective tissue separating nodules of lymphocytes containing lacunar-type Reed-Sternberg cells. Depending on the number and degree of atypia of the Reed-Sternberg cells, **nodular sclerosis Hodgkin's lymphomas** can be subclassified as grade 1 or 2. **Grade 1 disease,** which makes up 75–85% of cases, has the best prognosis. **Mixed cellularity and lymphocyte-depleted Hodgkin's disease,** the other two histopathologic forms, carry the worst prognosis. They are characterized by fewer lymphocytes and relatively more classical bilobed Reed-Sternberg cells with prominent eosinophilic nucleoli. In some cases the predominant cells are difficult to distinguish from other poorly differentiated lymphomas or sarcomas.

CLINICAL FEATURES

The most common presentation of a Hodgkin's disease patient is the appearance of a painless or only slightly tender, rubbery swelling of a superficial **lymph node or a group of nodes** in a young adult. The tendency of Hodgkin's disease to first appear in a single node group in an otherwise healthy individual can make it difficult to distinguish from the lymphadenopathy associated with an infectious process. Nodes that are slightly tender are even more of a problem because tender nodes often accompany acute infections. In addition, Hodgkin's nodes can on occasion wax and wane in the same way as those associated with an infectious process. The diagnosis is obviously easier when the mass is large, presents in more than one area, and is associated with systemic symptoms (**B symptoms**) such as night sweats, fever, weight loss, pruritus, or fatigue.

The most **common areas of involvement in young patients** are the cervical, axillary, and mediastinal nodes. Extension to subdiaphragmatic nodes is seen in less than one-quarter of these patients if they seek medical attention without delay. Moreover, they are unlikely to have any involvement of liver, spleen, or other organs. Systemic symptoms are present in less than one-third of patients. Hodgkin's disease has an age-dependent incidence with a peak in young adults and another peak in the elderly. Unusual presentations, such as disease limited to the spleen or an extranodal site, are more common in the elderly. Moreover, whereas lymphocyte predominant and nodular sclerosis Hodgkin's disease are common in the younger age group, mixed cellularity and lymphocyte-depleted Hodgkin's disease are more often seen in patients 30 years or older.

The **incidence** of Hodgkin's disease has been linked to several factors, including environment, social status, infectious agents, and genetic propensity. It is slightly more common in men and has occurred as clustered cases in families, communities, and schools. It is also more common in developed countries. Patients who have had infectious mononucleosis or have a positive test for prior EBV infection have a threefold increased risk for developing the disease. There is also an increased incidence in individuals with occupational chemical exposures or immune deficiency states. These associations suggest an infectious cause, as well as a component of genetic susceptibility, which appears to be much more striking in Hodgkin's disease than in other lymphomas. Recent studies of identical twins have reinforced the fact that there is a genetic propensity to this disease with some yet undefined environmental or infectious process superimposed.

STAGING

Accurate staging is extremely important. The natural history of the disease suggests that it **arises in a single site and then spreads** from that site in an orderly and more or less predictable pattern from one lymphoid (usually nodal) site to contiguous lymphoid sites and from lymphoid sites to contiguous nonlymphoid sites. It is difficult to prove that this is always the case, and in some cases it clearly is not, but it is a useful concept that has led to a very successful strategy of staging and treatment. Thus, the **primary objective of staging** is to determine the current location of all the disease in the patient in order to plan a treatment that will address each of the involved areas and all contiguous sites of possible spread.

The staging of Hodgkin's disease is conceptually simple. One determines the location and extent of the disease, and then assigns a stage as outlined in Table 23–2. This staging does require a careful evaluation of the patient, including a full history, detailed physical examination, and several radiologic and laboratory studies.

History & Physical Examination

The **history** should document the timing and characteristics of the onset of the disease and the presence of systemic (B) symptoms, including weight loss, night sweats, low-grade fever, pruritus, and fatigue. On **physical examination,** all portions of the lymphoid organs should be carefully examined (Figure 23–1). Special attention should be paid to the lymphoid regions of the oral pharynx (Waldeyer's ring), the popliteal and epitrochlear regions, the subclavicular regions, as well as the more common axillary, anterior and posterior cervical, and inguinal regions.

Biopsy

A **biopsy** of the principal tumor mass or accessible enlarged node should be done, and the results reviewed with an experienced hematopathologist. It is not uncommon for the diagnosis of Hodgkin's disease to be confused or delayed by inadequate biopsy or too casual examination of a biopsy specimen. It is also common to find lymph nodes containing overt Hodgkin's disease

located adjacent to nodes that show only reactive hyperplasia. Therefore, biopsy specimens from more than one node should be taken if available. The presence of hepatomegaly suggests extension of the disease outside of the lymphatic system. Infiltration of the skin can result in generalized pruritus, appearance of subcutaneous nodular tumors, or in its most severe form, exfoliative dermatitis.

Radiologic Studies

Radiologic studies are important to accurate staging. A **routine chest x-ray** will reveal patients with bulky mediastinal disease. To more accurately detect lymph node involvement of the mediastinum and abdominal nodes, a **CT scan** of both thorax and abdomen should be performed. The CT scan is sensitive to lymph node enlargement or tissue invasion in the mediastinum, lung, and upper abdomen. To fully evaluate retroperitoneal nodes of the lower abdomen, **bipedal lymphangiography** can be performed. This technique will detect disease in nodes of near normal size that may be missed by CT scanning alone. Lymphangiography is unnecessary if the CT scan shows definite tumor involving the retroperitoneal nodes. It is also contraindicated in patients with extensive chest involvement owing to possible respiratory compromise. In selected patients, an **MRI** may be valuable in defining disease, especially disease involving non-lymphoid organs or residual disease in treated areas. A **technetium scan** may help define bony involvement in patients who complain of bone pain.

Laboratory Studies

The **laboratory evaluation** of the Hodgkin's disease patient should include a complete blood count, tests of renal and liver function (including alkaline phosphatase

Table 23–2. Staging system for Hodgkin's disease.

Stage	Description	Example
I	Involvement of a single lymphoid region or a single nonlymphoid site (I$_E$)	Nodes on one side of the neck only
II	Involvement of two or more regions on the same side of the diaphragm	Nodes in the neck and chest
III	Involvement of two or more regions on both sides of the diaphragm	Nodes in the neck and retroperitoneum or the spleen
IV	Spread of disease from lymphoid sites to nonlymphoid organs, involvement of more than one nonlymphoid organ	Nodes in the chest and infiltration of the marrow and lung
B	Each stage is further modified as B by the presence of fever, weight loss, or night sweats	Nodes in the retroperitoneum and groin with fever and night sweats (IIB)

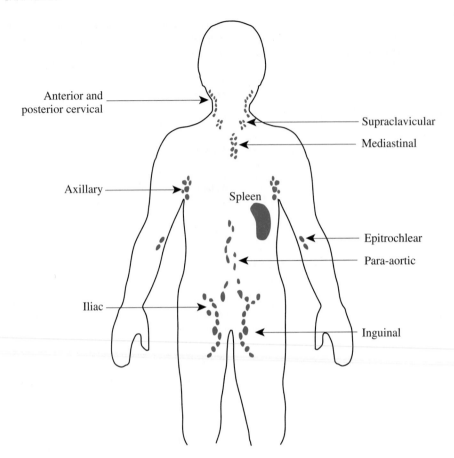

Figure 23–1. **The major regions of lymph nodes.** Because Hodgkin's disease usually spreads from one to another contiguous node region, it is important to define which regions are involved as a part of the staging process.

and lactic dehydrogenase [LDH] levels), a serum calcium, and bilateral iliac crest marrow aspirates and biopsies. These tests are especially important in evaluating disease extension outside of the lymphatic system. When anemia is present, **studies of iron supply** should be ordered to determine whether it is secondary to the inflammatory nature of the disease or results from marrow infiltration by tumor. A **marrow biopsy** may be helpful in the latter case. Even though the classic histologic patterns seen in lymph node biopsies are not reproduced in the marrow, it may be possible to identify Reed-Sternberg cells. Typically these cells are the size of a small megakaryocyte and contain two bean-shaped nuclei, each with a single large nucleolus. In some cases, Reed-Sternberg cells cannot be identified, but the normal marrow structure is disrupted by small noncaseating granulomata or patchy fibrous tissue.

Abnormalities of the granulocyte and lymphocyte counts may be observed. Some patients present with an eosinophilia or monocytosis, whereas others have an absolute lymphopenia. The latter is a bad prognostic sign and may be associated with lymphocyte-depleted Hodgkin's disease and a loss in **skin test responsiveness** (**anergy**). Older patients presenting with splenic disease can demonstrate thrombocytopenia or an autoimmune hemolytic anemia. In contrast to the non-Hodgkin's lymphomas, immunologic and gene rearrangement studies of blood cells cannot be used to either make the diagnosis or confirm the spread of the disease. All of the peripheral blood changes are reactive in nature.

Patients with abnormal liver chemistries or a suspicious lesion on CT should have a **guided needle biopsy** of the lesion or **laparoscopic liver biopsy.**

Staging Laparotomy

A staging laparotomy may be indicated in patients with clinical stage I or II disease. It is in this group of patients where successful treatment may be accomplished with radiotherapy limited to the areas of clinical disease and adjacent lymphoid areas. Undetected disease outside the treated areas will certainly result in relapse, however. The staging laparotomy allows the detection of occult abdominal node or organ involvement. One-third to one-half of patients who appear to have clinical stage I or II disease will be reclassified following staging laparotomy as stage III or IV. Patients with stage IA disease limited to the neck or mediastinum and those with stage I or IIA disease and lymphocyte predominant histology should be treated without a staging laparotomy. In these patients, salvage chemotherapy for recurrence is so effective that long-term survival is not compromised.

A well-performed **staging laparotomy should include** a biopsy of all of the abdominal node groups regardless of their size or appearance, splenectomy, and both a wedge biopsy and multiple needle biopsies of the liver. Every attempt should be made to locate and take a biopsy of any lymph node that appears suspicious on the lymphangiogram. Biopsy sites should be marked with clips. A flat plate of the abdomen during surgery can help ensure that all suspicious nodes are successfully identified. Although surgical mortality is extremely low (less than 0.5%), it is best to avoid the procedure if at all possible. In children less than 5 years of age, splenectomy is not indicated because of an increased risk of recurrent septicemia.

Adult patients should always be immunized preoperatively with *Haemophilus* and polyvalent pneumococcal vaccines. Moreover, the staging workup should have been exhaustive enough to assure the clinician that the laparotomy is absolutely necessary. For example, no patient should go to surgery who has not had studies of liver chemistries, blood and marrow evaluation, CT scan of the abdomen, and, if possible, bipedal lymphangiography. If disease can be shown to be present on both sides of the diaphragm or involve the liver or marrow, the patient can be staged clinically and does not need surgery.

Prognosis

The patient's prognosis and subsequent management are determined largely by the stage of the disease. The **number of node sites involved and the spread to nonlymphoid organs** are the strongest prognostic indicators. If a patient has disease isolated to a single node group, even an adverse histology will not significantly change the relatively good prognosis or the selection of therapy. There are, however, observations that do have an impact on prognosis. The most important of these is the presence of **B symptoms,** especially when fever and significant weight loss are both present.

Other **factors that suggest a poor prognosis** include bulky mediastinal tumor, a high LDH level, nonlymphoid organ involvement, severe marrow disease, and a poor response to initial radio- or chemotherapy.

THERAPY AND CLINICAL COURSE

The several possible combinations of histology, B symptoms, location of disease, and prognostic factors together with varying regimens of either radiotherapy or chemotherapy make it difficult to propose a rigid logic tree for the treatment of Hodgkin's disease. Nevertheless, there are some clear basic principles that guide the choice of therapy. It is well established that both radiotherapy and chemotherapy can cure Hodgkin's disease. The therapeutic goal, therefore, is to provide the highest cure rate in the shortest period with the least morbidity. This goal should be achievable in almost all patients with stage I or II disease and in a sizable majority of those with more advanced stage III or IV disease. Treatment failure most often results from either inaccurate staging or a suboptimal radio-/chemotherapy regimen.

Stages IA & IIA

Stages IA and IIA disease without bulky adenopathy are generally treated with high-energy radiation delivered to the involved areas and the adjacent uninvolved areas. Involved areas should receive a tumoricidal dose of 4000 cGy, whereas adjacent uninvolved areas are given 3600 cGy. Standard radiation ports include the **mantle** for patients with disease limited to the neck and the **inverted Y** for patients with disease limited to the lower abdominal or inguinal nodes (Figure 23–2). Additional treatment to the mediastinum and periaortic nodes is required for patients with mediastinal or upper abdominal involvement.

Patients with stages IA and IIA Hodgkin's disease localized above the diaphragm do extremely well with radiotherapy. The stage IA patient has a survival rate of better than 90% at 10+ years, whereas the stage IIA patient has a survival rate of better than 80%. Relatively few patients (less than 10%) present with disease localized below the diaphragm. Those with lymphocyte-predominant disease limited to the inguinal and lower abdominal node regions respond very well to the inverted Y radiotherapy approach.

Stage II

Patients with stage II disease and a large mediastinal mass have a relapse rate of at least 50% following radiotherapy alone. This is also true for chemotherapy alone, however. Therefore, patients with large mediastinal tumors are best approached with combined modality

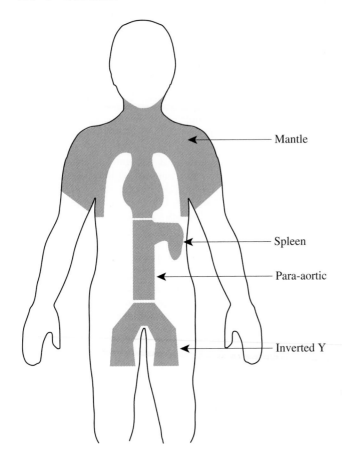

- Mantle

- Spleen

- Para-aortic

- Inverted Y

Figure 23–2. **Radiotherapy ports compared to the major lymph node regions.** These ports are designed to deliver targeted radiation while avoiding regions or organs such as the lung, marrow, spine, and gonads.

therapy; that is, initial treatment with chemotherapy followed by radiotherapy. Even then, a residual mediastinal abnormality is seen in 60–90% of these patients. Whether this is residual tumor or unresolved scar tissue can only be distinguished by watching and waiting. If, after therapy, the residual mass is stable and the patient has no B symptoms, it can be assumed to be a scar. If the mass increases in size, however, or the patient has a recurrence of B symptoms, the presence of resistant tumor is more likely. A gallium scan may be helpful to distinguish the two possibilities. If there is avid uptake of the gallium by the mass, it is likely that the disease is recurring. In very young patients, regeneration of the thymus can also result in high gallium uptake and mimic recurrent disease.

Side Effects & Complications of Radiation Therapy

Side effects of radiation therapy include nausea and fatigue, especially in patients receiving abdominal radiation. Transient hair loss over the areas of radiation is expected. Patients who receive mantle radiation may develop parotitis after the first or second treatment. When multiple areas are irradiated, marrow depression can occur. Generally, it is observed near the end of a prolonged course of therapy and is relatively mild with white blood cell counts of 1–2000/μL and platelet counts not below 50,000/μL. Neutropenia leading to sepsis is very unusual, and recovery from marrow depression occurs spontaneously without the need for growth factor treatment.

Long-term **complications** of radiation therapy include decreased salivary flow and hypothyroidism in patients who have received mantle therapy, pulmonary or cardiac complications if the mediastinal port is not well plotted, and loss of marrow reserve in those patients who receive extensive irradiation. The most important late complication of radiotherapy is the development of a second malignancy. The risk of post-therapy leukemia, non-Hodgkin's lymphoma, or tumors involving the genitourinary tract, lung, skin, or colon has been reported by some investigators to be as high as 10% during the first decade after treatment.

Stages IIIB & IVA/B

Stages IIIB and IVA or B patients should be treated with multidrug chemotherapy. The chemotherapy of Hodgkin's disease is particularly interesting because it was the first successful application of multiagent chemotherapy in which several different drugs were chosen for their partial effectiveness against the disease and for their nonoverlapping toxicities. Table 23–3 outlines some of the chemotherapeutic regimens currently used for Hodgkin's disease. The MOPP protocol (nitrogen mustard–vincristine-procarbazine-prednisone) was the first and is still widely used. Other combinations have been more recently used in order to decrease toxicity and increase efficacy. In particular, the ABVD regimen (Adriamycin-bleomycin-vinblastine-DTIC) does not appear to carry the increased risk of secondary leukemia associated with MOPP. The combination of MOPP with ABVD allows the use of two different non–cross-resistant regimens for patients who relapse after MOPP or whose disease is resistant to initial therapy.

The **key to effective chemotherapy** is to give full doses on a tight schedule. Dose reductions and delays should be avoided if at all possible. In those patients who develop myelosuppression after each cycle of drugs, it is important to try to continue with the maximum dose of drug and to use a growth factor such as granulocyte colony-stimulating factor to overcome the myelosuppression. Chemotherapy is carried out over 6–12 monthly cycles according to the tumor response. Radiologic studies of areas of known disease should be carried out after the fourth and sixth cycles. In those patients who respond rapidly and completely, therapy can be discontinued after the sixth cycle. If the disease is slow to respond or persistent, up to 12 cycles of therapy should be given.

The **response rate** to the MOPP regimen in patients with stages III and IV disease is better than 80% with a 60% disease-free survival at 10+ years. The combined MOPP/ABVD regimen may give as high as a 90% response rate with 75% disease-free survival at 10+ years. The combined regimen may place the patient at a disadvantage, however, for subsequent salvage therapy. **Maintenance chemotherapy or combined radiotherapy** is not recommended since it does not improve disease-free survival and can lead to an increased incidence of second malignancy. Maintenance therapy with interferon may be an exception, offering improved disease-free survival without the risk of second malignancy.

Table 23–3. Typical chemotherapeutic regimens for Hodgkin's disease.

Regimen	Dose and Schedule
MOPP	Repeat every 28 days for 6 months
Nitrogen mustard	6 mg/m^2 IV, days 1 and 8
Vincristine	1.4 mg/m^2 IV, days 1 and 8
Procarbazine	100 mg/m^2 PO, days 1–14
Prednisone	40 mg/m^2 PO, days 1–14
ABVD	Repeat every 28 days for 6 months
Adriamycin	25 mg/m^2 IV, days 1 and 15
Bleomycin	10 mg/m^2 IV, days 1 and 15
Vinblastine	10 mg/m^2 IV, days 1 and 15
DTIC	375 mg/m^2 IV, days 1 and 15
MOPP/ABVD	Alternating cycles of MOPP and ABVD
MOPP/ABV	Repeat every 28 days for 6 months
Nitrogen mustard	6 mg/m^2 IV, day 1
Vincristine	1.4 mg/m^2 IV, day 1
Procarbazine	100 mg/m^2 PO, days 1–7
Prednisone	40 mg/m^2 PO, days 1–14
Adriamycin	35 mg/m^2 IV, day 8
Bleomycin	10 mg/m^2 IV, day 8
Vinblastine	6 mg/m^2 IV, day 8

Stages IB–IIB & IIIA

Patients with stages IB–IIB and IIIA disease may be managed with varying regimens of radiotherapy and chemotherapy. The stage IB–IIB patient with only a single systemic symptom can be treated with radiotherapy alone with the expectation of a better than 80% 10-year survival. In patients with several B symptoms, the response is so poor, however, that chemotherapy should be used from the beginning. The expected response rate may fall below 50%, especially in patients with nodular sclerosis histology.

Patients with stage IIIA disease need to be very carefully staged to accurately identify the extent of node involvement. In the subset of patients who have disease above the diaphragm and surgically proven disease limited to upper abdominal nodes or the spleen, **total nodal irradiation** (ie, mantle plus para-aortic and inverted Y fields) can give an excellent therapeutic result. When the lower abdominal and iliac nodes are involved, either chemotherapy or a combined modality approach using three or four cycles of chemotherapy followed by total nodal or involved field irradiation should be used. The latter provides a better than 90% remission rate and an improved chance of disease-free survival.

Salvage Therapy

Patients must be carefully monitored after successful initial treatment. Relapse can occur at any time, even in stages IA and IIA patients, including late relapses in up to 15% of these patients. Patients with more advanced disease will relapse sooner and more frequently (Figure 23–3). There is still an excellent chance, however, to achieve a second remission and prolonged periods of disease-free survival. If the patient relapses more than 12 months after initial therapy, re-treatment with the same regimen will be successful 70–80% of the time and will result in a sustained remission. If relapse occurs sooner than 12 months, a different chemotherapy regimen should be instituted. For example, a MOPP-treated patient should be changed to the ABVD regimen. A response is seen about 50% of the time, with success depending a great deal on the presence of such factors as B symptoms, bulky disease, and adverse histologies.

All patients with relapsed Hodgkin's disease should be considered for **high-dose chemotherapy followed by autologous marrow transplantation.** Those with more responsive disease, lack of B symptoms, and a longer duration of remission are more likely to achieve long-term survival after this form of salvage therapy, but even unfavorable prognosis patients can benefit. A typical autologous transplant/chemotherapy regimen is described in Chapter 22. This approach has the potential of providing a better chance for long-term disease-free survival; 55–65% of patients appear to be disease-free after 3–5 years in recent series. The success rate is greatly influenced by patient selection, however. Older patients, patients who have been exposed to a large number of chemotherapy drugs with or without irradiation, and those who have poorly responsive tumor also tend to fail to respond to autologous marrow transplantation. Another distressing drawback of an autologous transplant is a reported incidence of secondary acute myeloid leukemia/myelodysplasia of 9–15% after 5–7 years.

Other possible salvage therapies for patients who are not candidates for or who fail autologous transplantation include single-agent vinblastine; combination chemotherapy with drugs such as etoposide, ifosfamide, and cisplatin; or, as recently reported, natural killer–activating monoclonal antibody. To date, none of these has shown great promise.

Complications of chemotherapy, the combined modalities of chemotherapy and radiotherapy, and autologous marrow transplantation include vital organ damage and prolonged immunosuppression. Radiation pneumonitis and pericarditis, together with drug-induced chronic restrictive pulmonary disease and myocardiopathy, increase in frequency with exposure to intensive chemo-/radiotherapy. The risk of a second malignancy is also present. This situation is most dra-

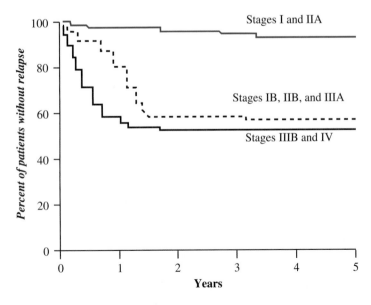

Figure 23–3. **Clinical stage and survival.** The influence of stage on the long-term survival of patients with Hodgkin's disease is greater than that of any other single prognostic factor.

matic for those patients who receive combined modality therapy at an early age or who receive an autologous transplant as salvage therapy. Another risk for the young patient is gonadal dysfunction following chemotherapy. Even a few treatment cycles with MOPP or MOPP/ABVD combinations will result in azoospermia in males secondary to irreversible damage to the testes. ABVD therapy has been recommended in young males because of its lower incidence of testicular damage. Young males should be offered sperm storage prior to beginning chemotherapy if they wish to ensure their ability to have children. Young women have less difficulty with ovarian failure following chemotherapy. Less than one-quarter of young women will become infertile, but more than 80% of women over the age of 30 will immediately enter menopause. Chemotherapy and radiotherapy in the treatment of Hodgkin's disease in young women have not been associated with teratogenicity.

Hodgkin's disease patients must be looked on as immunosuppressed individuals throughout their lives. Even with successful treatment, cellular immunity may not return to normal. Furthermore, most Hodgkin's disease patients will experience an episode of herpes zoster and may be at risk for disseminated vaccinia if exposed to a child with chickenpox. Patients who have had splenectomy are considered at risk for infections with encapsulated organisms, especially *Streptococcus pneumoniae* and *Haemophilus*. Up to 10% of young patients who have a splenectomy for the diagnosis of

Hodgkin's disease will experience at least one life-threatening episode of pneumococcal sepsis during the first 10 years after staging. It is essential that these patients be immunized to polyvalent pneumococcal vaccine prior to their staging and receive a periodic booster. If they experience an episode of sepsis, prophylaxis with oral antibiotics should be considered.

BIBLIOGRAPHY

Advani RH, Horning SJ: Treatment of early stage Hodgkin's disease. Semin Hematol 1999;36:270.

Aisenberg AC: Problems in Hodgkin's disease management. Blood 1999;93:761.

DeVita VT, Hubbard SM: Hodgkin's disease. N Engl J Med 1993;328:560.

Harris NL: Hodgkin's lymphomas: Classification, diagnosis, and grading. Semin Hematol 1999;36:220.

Hummel M et al: Hodgkin's disease with monoclonal and polyclonal populations of Reed-Sternberg cells. N Engl J Med 1995;333:901.

Mack TM et al: Concordance for Hodgkin's disease in identical twins suggesting genetic susceptibility to the young-adult form of the disease. N Engl J Med 1995;332:413.

Mauch PM: Controversies in the management of early stage Hodgkin's disease. Blood 1994;83:318.

Urba WJ, Longo DL: Hodgkin's disease. N Engl J Med 1992;326:678.

Yuen AR et al: Comparison between conventional salvage therapy and high dose therapy with autografting for recurrent or refractory Hodgkin's disease. Blood 1997;89:814.

Acute Lymphocytic Leukemia 24

Acute lymphocytic leukemia (**ALL**) is a disease that primarily affects children. It is the most common malignancy in children under 15 years of age. The diagnosis and treatment of ALL in children constitutes one of the great success stories of hematology. Like Hodgkin's disease, ALL has been approached with a combination of good science and perceptive clinical insights that has produced a high frequency of cures for a disease that was a tragedy for its victims. A good understanding of the principles of diagnosis and treatment of ALL serves as a model for the approach to all leukemias. Although the application of these principles to treat adult ALL is less likely to produce a cure, it is still the best approach to diagnosis and management.

CLASSIFICATION

The classification of ALL is based on a combination of morphologic (French-American-British [FAB]), immunologic, and genetic characteristics.

MORPHOLOGIC CHARACTERISTICS

Similar to the FAB classification of the acute myelogenous leukemias, ALL can be divided into three classes, L1, L2, and L3, from the morphologic appearance of lymphocytes in the peripheral blood and marrow (Figure 24–1).

With **L1 disease** the lymphocytes are uniformly small with round nuclei, little cytoplasm, and inconspicuous nucleoli. **L2 disease** consists of large heterogeneous cells with more cytoplasm, irregular nuclei, and prominent nucleoli, whereas **L3 disease** is characterized by large cells with abundant, deeply basophilic cytoplasm, round nuclei, and prominent nucleoli. As regards the **special stains** used in the FAB classification, ALL lymphoblasts usually show positive staining for periodic acid–Schiff (PAS) and terminal deoxynucleotide transferase (TdT) but are negative for esterase and peroxidase. The L1 form of ALL is more commonly seen in children, whereas the L2 form is more common in adults. Only the L3 classification has strong connections with the more modern immunologic and genetic classifications.

Immunologic Classification

The immunologic classification divides ALL into those cells derived from very early B-cell precursors (pre–B cells) and those from the more mature B- and T cells. The surface markers used in making this distinction as well as the relative frequency of the various subtypes are summarized in Table 24–1. A subset of ALL showing lineage infidelity can also be defined by immunologic studies. This condition is most frequently manifested by the expression of one or more myeloid markers, such as CD13 or CD33, together with the expected markers for ALL. This subgroup, now called **MY1 ALL,** is more common in adults (perhaps 10–20% of cases) than in children (5–10%). In adults, it may carry a poorer prognosis.

The immunologic classification may also be made genetically by studying the cells' **immunoglobulin gene rearrangements.** It is the most definitive method for determining whether the cell is of B- or T-cell origin. Rearrangement of immunoglobulin heavy chain genes, and to a lesser extent light chain genes, is seen in the vast majority of B-cell and pre–B cell ALL. At the same time, these cells will also show rearrangement of T-cell–receptor genes. In contrast, T-cell ALL will always show rearrangement of T-cell–receptor genes and only rarely concomitant rearrangements of immunoglobulin genes.

Genetic Classification

The third basis for the classification of ALL is the presence of a cytogenetic abnormality. These occur in a nonrandom fashion and are known to have considerable prognostic significance. The presence of cytogenetic abnormalities may be defined on two different levels. The first level is the presence of an abnormal amount of DNA in each cell. This condition is referred to as **DNA aneuploidy** and is easily detected by flow cytometry. **Hyperploidy** (the presence of an increased number of chromosomes per cell) is more common in children, where it defines a group with better prognosis. **Hypodiploidy** is very rare. Most cases present with a normal cellular DNA content. In these patients, how-

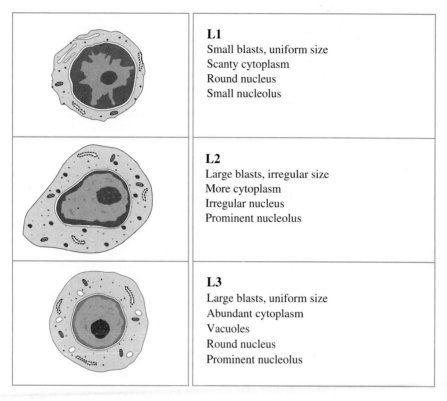

L1
Small blasts, uniform size
Scanty cytoplasm
Round nucleus
Small nucleolus

L2
Large blasts, irregular size
More cytoplasm
Irregular nucleus
Prominent nucleolus

L3
Large blasts, uniform size
Abundant cytoplasm
Vacuoles
Round nucleus
Prominent nucleolus

Figure 24–1. Morphologic types of ALL. There are three major morphologic types of ALL. The small cell type L1 is most common in children but also occurs in adults. The L2 and L3 forms are more common in adults and have a significantly worse prognosis.

ever, karyotype study will frequently demonstrate a structural abnormality of individual chromosomes.

Nonrandom translocations are the most common cytogenetic abnormality in children with ALL. They fall into several distinct subgroups. The t(8;14) translocation is highly correlated with B-cell ALL of the L3 morphology. The t(4;11) translocation has been associated with the MY1 ALL subgroup and a poorer prognosis. Approximately 5% of children and up to 30% of adults with ALL will have a t(9;22) translocation similar to the Philadelphia chromosome defect of chronic myelogenous leukemia (CML). Detailed mapping of the breakpoint cluster region (BCR) locus shows differences, however, between the Ph[1] positive ALL and CML. Both children and adults with t(9;22) have a very poor prognosis. Finally, the t(1;19) translocation is associated with pre–B cell, whereas the t(11;14) translocation is seen with T-cell ALL.

Table 24–1. Immunologic markers in ALL.

Phenotype	Characteristic Markers	Frequency (%)	
		Children	Adults
Pre–B	CD10+ (CALLA), sIg−	80–90	70–80
B-cell	CD10±, sIg+	0–5	5–10
T-cell	CD10−, sIg−, CD7+, CD5+, CD2+, CD6±, CD3±	10–20	10–20

CLINICAL FEATURES

There are actually two peaks in the incidence of ALL, one below 10 years of age and another, much smaller peak, above 50 years. In childhood, ALL is most frequently seen between 3 and 7 years of age, although the disease can occur in infants. Although the middle-aged adult is more likely to present with acute myeloid leukemia (AML), detailed immunologic and cytogenetic studies are necessary so as not to miss the occasional ALL patient.

The presenting symptoms and signs of ALL are similar in children and adults and do not differ significantly from those of any form of acute leukemia. The onset is usually abrupt with little or no history or prodromal symptoms. The **predominant signs and symptoms** are moderate to severe anemia, granulocytopenia, and thrombocytopenia. Patients report increasing weakness and easy fatigability. If the anemia is severe, they may experience shortness of breath and congestive heart failure. Severe thrombocytopenia is associated with the appearance of petechiae, especially over the lower extremities, and epistaxis. Bacterial infections such as otitis media, pharyngitis, or pneumonia may result from the granulocytopenia.

Some patients, especially children, complain of bone pain or have pain with bony pressure. Sternal tenderness is common. Asymptomatic **central nervous system (CNS)** involvement is likely to be present in most patients and is a major issue in the treatment of ALL. At the same time, symptoms and signs of CNS involvement are unusual. Only the occasional patient with advanced meningeal involvement will complain of headache, vomiting, or both. Most patients will have diffuse adenopathy on physical examination, although it is rarely so prominent as to be a presenting complaint. Both the adenopathy and meningeal involvement are more typical of the more mature B- and T-cell ALL phenotypes.

Laboratory Studies

The **key laboratory studies for diagnosing ALL** are the complete blood count, blood film and marrow aspirate for cell morphology, and both immunophenotyping and cytogenetic analyses. In addition, since the initial tumor burden is a significant factor in a patient's response to therapy and prognosis, laboratory and x-ray studies aimed at documenting the extent of tumor growth are important.

A. COMPLETE BLOOD COUNT (CBC):

The CBC is invariably abnormal in patients who present with ALL. The most striking finding is a high white blood cell count, consisting primarily of a uniform population of lymphoblasts. Counts in excess of $100,000/\mu L$, which are most often associated with T-cell ALL, can be seen (Table 24–2). At the same time, up to 30% of cases present with a normal or low total white blood cell count. Granulocytopenia is usually present and, in patients with very high lymphoblast counts, granulocytes may be undetectable. Anemia and thrombocytopenia are variable in degree but are nearly always present.

B. BLOOD FILM & MARROW ASPIRATE:

The marrow aspirate is usually diagnostic, showing massive replacement of normal marrow by the same uniform population of lymphoblasts. The marrow can be so packed that aspiration is unsuccessful and a

Table 24–2. Risk factors for acute lymphocytic leukemia.

Standard Risk	High Risk
Risk linearly related to WBC	WBC greater than $100,000/\mu L$[a]
Age 1–10 years	Less than 1 yr or > 10 yr (risk increases with age)
Females	Males[a]
None or asymptomatic CNS	Overt CNS involvement[a]
	Mediastinal mass[a]
	T-cell phenotype[a]
	Non-Caucasian

[a] These factors are probably not independent because they tend to be seen together.

Note: Of the risk factors listed, WBC and age are clearly independent and are by far the most significant.

biopsy is required. Rarely, the initial marrow may show hypo- or aplasia, suggesting an aplastic anemia. Usually, these patients will respond to glucocorticoid therapy with rising counts, thereby declaring themselves as having ALL.

Even the best hematologist or pathologist cannot always distinguish ALL from AML by cellular morphology alone. **Histochemical stains** (ie, peroxidase, combined esterase, PAS, and TDT stains) can be very helpful. The ALL blast should be peroxidase and esterase negative and PAS positive. Primitive blasts will show positive TdT staining. Histochemistry can be confusing or equivocal, however, especially in adults. A reliable distinction between ALL and AML depends much more on immunophenotyping and cytogenetics than on morphology or histochemistry.

C. Immunophenotyping & Genetic Analyses:

Immunogenetic studies are absolutely essential in distinguishing B- and T-cell ALL and in classifying the subtypes of ALL. Cytogenetics and immunophenotyping must be obtained early in the diagnostic workup when blasts are abundant. Once therapy is initiated, these studies may be difficult to perform or impossible to interpret.

D. Other Laboratory Abnormalities:

The other laboratory abnormalities that are associated with ALL include hypogammaglobulinemia, elevated lactic dehydrogenase (LDH) and uric acid levels, and a variety of electrolyte abnormalities such as hyperphosphatemia, hypocalcemia, and hyperkalemia. Both the hyperphosphatemia and hyperkalemia can worsen dramatically during initiation of therapy when large numbers of leukemic blasts are lysed.

E. Studies to Detect Tumor Growth:

Although the level of the peripheral blood count and the height of the LDH level provide a sense of the patient's tumor burden, a careful search should be made for node-based tumor masses. This search should include an **examination of the patient for lymphadenopathy and splenomegaly** and a **chest x-ray** to look for a mediastinal mass.

A large mediastinal mass is seen in up to 50% of cases of T-cell ALL. If a **biopsy** is done, it usually shows the presence of lymphocytes identical to those found in marrow and blood and most typical of the cell type seen in lymphoblastic lymphomas. In fact, some children will present initially with a mediastinal tumor, without evidence of leukemia in the blood or marrow. Since such patients will usually progress to overt ALL within a short period, T-cell ALL and T-cell lymphoblastic lymphoma are considered to be similar in terms of management and prognosis.

DIAGNOSIS

A diagnosis of ALL is usually **easily made in children.** It is the dominant form of acute leukemia. When children present with a very high peripheral lymphoblast count, coupled with modest adenopathy and splenomegaly, there is almost no chance that it can be confused with AML. Finally, histochemical stains and immunologic marker studies will confirm the diagnosis.

In adults where ALL is an unlikely diagnosis, it can be more difficult to distinguish ALL from AML. Immunologic marker studies are essential because morphology and histochemistry frequently do not clearly make the distinction. Moreover, in the occasional case, the final diagnosis will require gene rearrangement studies. This fact is especially true for the MY1 ALL subset and the occasional case of AML where blasts express at least one lymphoid marker, usually CD7. These individuals must be studied for their immunoglobulin gene and T-cell receptor gene rearrangement. In addition, cytogenetic studies will often reveal abnormalities typical of either ALL or AML.

Other forms of lymphoma, particularly hairy-cell leukemia, prolymphocytic leukemia, and Sezary cell leukemia, may be confused with ALL, occasionally. When the overall clinical picture of these diseases is considered, however, the morphology, clinical characteristics, and the presence of mature lymphoid markers should make the distinction (see Chapter 21). A few **nonlymphoid tumors** may be confused with ALL. Neuroblastoma and rhabdomyosarcoma in children and Ewing's sarcoma and small cell lung cancer in adults can have the morphologic appearance of ALL. In each case, however, immunologic markers should clearly show that these cells do not belong to either the lymphoid or myeloid lineages. Moreover, gene rearrangements typical of lymphoid cells will not be present.

Activated normal lymphoid cells can closely resemble leukemic lymphoblasts morphologically. Reactive lymphocytosis, as seen in conditions such as infectious mononucleosis or tuberculosis, can present with large numbers of atypical lymphocytes and to the less sophisticated eye be mistaken for ALL. If confusion arises, immunologic markers will also show that reactive lymphoblasts have a mature phenotype and frequently consist of different cell types. For example, the atypical lymphocytes of infectious mononucleosis are predominantly mature CD8 T cells. Genetic studies will always show that the gene rearrangements present in reactive lymphocytes are polyclonal, not monoclonal, thus ruling out leukemia.

THERAPY & CLINICAL COURSE

Soon after diagnosis, ALL must be treated with an intensive multidrug regimen that has a high probability of inducing remission. Several drugs have activity in this disease, and they are used in various combinations. Most institutions have treatment protocols in effect for this disease that use varying combinations, doses, and treatment schedules. The drugs commonly used to treat ALL are listed in Table 24–3.

Remission Induction Protocols

Remission induction protocols result in profound myelosuppression with a prolonged period of pancytopenia followed by regrowth of normal hematopoiesis. Treatment with filgrastim, 5 μg/kg/day beginning on day 2 of chemotherapy, can significantly shorten the period of neutropenia, without risk of impairing the remission rate. During the early recovery phase, it is frequently difficult to be certain of remission because of the presence of variable numbers of immature lymphoid cells. Thus, a follow-up examination of marrow should be done at 2–4 weeks with careful evaluation of immunologic markers to confirm remission. Nearly all children and more than 90% of adults will achieve remission with modern therapy.

Prophylactic Treatment of the CNS

Once remission has been achieved, it is important to treat **sites harboring previously undetected leukemic cells** that may have escaped eradication. The most common site is the CNS. Although overt CNS involvement is unusual at presentation, about 50% of patients will relapse in the CNS within 2 years if not specifically treated. Other sites include the testes and the ovary, although these are much less common. Therefore, a second requirement of therapy is the prophylactic treatment of the CNS.

Depending on the protocol, this may include **irra-diation** of the CNS or **intrathecal therapy,** most commonly with methotrexate. Cranial radiation (18 Gy for standard-risk patients and 25–28 Gy for high-risk patients) is very well tolerated by children. Long-term follow-up studies, however, have detected significant effects of cranial radiation on learning and intellectual functions. This result has led to increasing use of intrathecal chemotherapy as a substitute for irradiation. Boys must be followed with careful physical examination of the testes to detect any masses that may indicate relapse. If masses are suspected, this should be confirmed with biopsy and then treated with local irradiation followed by reinduction chemotherapy.

Maintenance Chemotherapy

After prophylactic CNS treatment, patients enter into a phase of maintenance chemotherapy. The details of this phase vary depending on the protocol. They may consist of continued administration of relatively low doses of agents such as 6-mercaptopurine and methotrexate or periodic "consolidation" treatments with higher doses of multiple agents. The total duration of treatment is usually 2–3 years.

Prognosis

More than 80% of children who achieve complete remission and finish 2–3 years of therapy will be cured of their disease. The prognosis in adults treated with the conventional ALL protocol is much worse—30–40% long-term survival. Patients who relapse 12 or more months following first remission will frequently achieve a second remission with a repeated course of conventional chemotherapy. Such remissions are usually shorter, however, than the first remission, and the overall prognosis after relapse is poor. Patients who relapse

Table 24–3. Chemotherapeutic regimens for ALL.

	Usual Dose and Route	Major Toxicities
Vincristine	2 mg/m^2 IV weekly	Neuropathy
Prednisone	40 mg/m^2 PO daily	Psychosis, hypertension, ulcer
Asparaginase	500 IU/m^2 IV daily × 10 days	Allergic reaction
Daunorubicin	30–60 mg/m^2 IV daily × 3 days	Myelosuppression, cardiotoxicity
Methotrexate	15–25 mg/m^2 various schedules	Myelosuppression
6-Mercaptopurine	90 mg/m^2 PO daily	Myelosuppression
Cyclophosphamide	100 mg/m^2 PO daily	Myelosuppression
Cytosine arabinoside	100 mg/m^2 IV or SC daily	Myelosuppression

during chemotherapy or within 6 months of first re-mission have a very poor prognosis. An improved out-come in adults, 40–50% survival rates, has been re-ported with aggressive chemotherapy, including CNS treatment, based on childhood protocols. The up-front CNS treatment reduced the rate of CNS relapse to less than 20% versus 50% in conventionally treated pa-tients.

Patients achieving long-term disease-free survival face some risk of a second malignancy, particularly gliomas. In addition, many patients will have decreased fertility, although to date there does not appear to be an increased incidence of birth defects in the offspring of ALL survivors.

Marrow Transplantation

All patients who relapse should be considered candi-dates for marrow transplantation as soon as they achieve second remission. If a matched, related donor is available, **allogeneic transplantation** offers the best chance of long-term disease control. If no match is available, then an **autologous transplant,** usually with purging of the marrow with anti-CD10 (CALLA) anti-bodies, is the best choice. Purging can be shown to achieve substantial kill of ALL cells by in vitro studies; however, improved clinical results have been difficult to demonstrate. The alternative is an allogeneic transplant from a matched, unrelated donor.

Ph[1] Positive ALL

In adults with Ph[1] positive ALL, there have been encouraging early results with treatment directed at inhibition of the BCR-ABL tyrosine kinase. The com-bination of these new drugs with conventional chemotherapy is being evaluated and may offer new ap-proaches to these very difficult cases.

BIBLIOGRAPHY

Coelan EA, McGuire EA: The biology and treatment of acute leukemia in adults. Blood 1995;85:1151.

Geissler K et al: Granulocyte colony-stimulating factor as an ad-junct to induction chemotherapy for adult acute lymphoblas-tic leukemia—A randomized phase-III study. Blood 1997; 90:590.

Hoelzer D et al: Improved outcome in adult B-cell acute lym-phoblastic leukemia. Blood 1996;87:495.

Pinkel D: Therapy of acute leukemia in children. Leukemia 1992; 6:127.

Pui CH, Behm FG, Crist WM: Clinical and biologic relevance of immunologic marker studies in childhood acute lymphoblas-tic leukemia. Blood 1993;82:343.

Zang M-J et al: Long-term follow-up of adults with acute lym-phoblastic leukemia in first remission treated with chemo-therapy or bone marrow transplantation. Ann Intern Med 1995;123:428.

Plasma Cell Disorders

Plasma cells are terminally differentiated cells of the B-lymphocyte lineage. They are thought of as cellular factories whose entire energy and synthetic capacity is devoted to producing a single antibody protein. They are normally incapable of dividing and are thought to have a relatively short life span of perhaps several weeks. Plasma cells are abundant both in the lymph nodes, where they are found predominantly in the medullar cords, and in the marrow. They have a distinctive morphology and are easily identified in the marrow (Figure 25–1).

The most common malignancy involving plasma cells is multiple myeloma. It is an interesting and instructive disease from the standpoint of diagnosis and pathophysiology; however, from the standpoint of therapy it is one of the most difficult of the hematologic malignancies.

■ THE BIOLOGY OF PLASMA CELL DISORDERS

After stimulation by specific antigen, the germinal center B cells differentiate to generate long-lived memory B cells on the one hand and plasma cells on the other (see Chapter 19). After then moving to the bone marrow, the plasma cell stops proliferating and manufactures large amounts (1 ng or more per cell) of the same antibody that was initially displayed on the surface of the B cell. The normal plasma cell lives only for several weeks or months. Therefore, to maintain the continued production of any antibody, new plasma cells need to be regenerated from programmed B-cell precursors.

The **creation of an immortalized malignant plasma cell line** appears to involve the translocation of the c-*myc* oncogene to the IgH locus. Two cellular substances have also been shown to regulate apoptosis in plasma cells and many other lymphoid cells. These substances are the **BCL-2 gene product** and **interleukin (IL)-6,** which have the effect of preventing apoptosis. Interestingly, both of these products have been shown to be markedly overproduced in malignant plasma cell disorders. Thus, multiple myeloma appears to be a classic example of a malignant disorder that results primarily from the failure of mature cells to die rather than from excessive proliferation of precursors. The result is a "piling up" of a clone of plasma cells and marked overproduction of a single antibody that appears in the plasma as an M-component (**M-protein**). Nearly 1 billion cells need to accumulate before sufficient M-protein is produced to be detected clinically. **Additional mutations** are seen later in the disease process and are associated with chemoresistance and tumor growth independent of IL-6. The most important of these are a mutation of the *ras* oncogene on chromosome 13 and a p53 mutation.

USE OF M-COMPONENT IN DIAGNOSIS & STAGING

The **M-component** is an easily measured, quantifiable tumor marker and as such has been used extensively to both diagnose and stage plasma cell disorders. By measuring the level of M-component in serum and estimating turnover rate of immunoglobulins, it is possible to use the M-component to estimate total body burden of malignant plasma cells. In addition, by making some assumptions about the rate of accumulation of the plasma cells, it is possible to estimate the amount of time that they have been accumulating and thus estimate the time of onset of the malignant process. These calculations have shown that it is very likely that the malignant event occurs 10 years before the onset of symptoms.

CELL LINEAGE AND POSSIBLE ETIOLOGY

Since the M-component is a highly specific marker, the lineage of cells belonging to the clone has been traced using **anti-idiotypic antibodies** that are specific for the M-component. Several such studies have detected increased numbers of malignant B cells extending all the way from the pre–B-cell stage through the entire B-cell differentiation pathway to the plasma cell. These observations establish that the myeloma cells are fully capable of differentiation and that malignant behavior results from their failure to die rather than their uncontrolled proliferation or failure to differentiate.

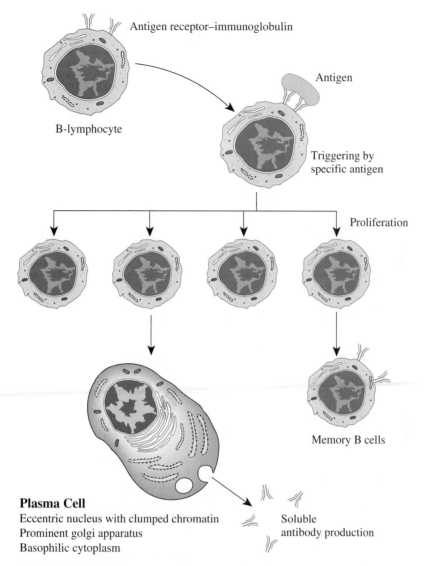

Figure 25–1. **Plasma cell differentiation and morphology.** B lymphocytes express on their surface a small sample of the antibody that serves as the receptor for specific antigen. When they encounter the antigen, they are stimulated to proliferate and differentiate, which leads to development of memory B cells and plasma cells. The plasma cell is highly specialized to produce and secrete large amounts of the same antibody.

An important **clue to the possible etiology** of plasma cell disorders comes from observations in the BALB/c mouse, which has a markedly increased propensity to develop myeloma. The malignant tendency is clearly amplified by chronic antigenic stimulation of the mice. In humans, M-components have been shown, in a few cases, to have antibody activity specific for an antigen known to have been encountered by the patient, such as HIV or bacterial polysaccharides. It is likely, therefore, that the oncogenic event that leads to malignant plasma cell disorders occurs in a very early B-cell precursor, perhaps as a result of both a genetic propensity and chronic antigenic stimulation. The resulting clone of cells continues to differentiate normally and reveals itself years later as a massive accumulation of plasma cells.

T-CELL ABNORMALITIES

In addition to the abnormalities of the B cells that lead to multiple myeloma, many patients will also have abnormalities in the T-cell compartment. CD4 T cells are decreased and there is a concomitant increase in CD8 T cells and sometimes NK cells. These changes may serve as additional explanations for the immune deficiency state that accompanies myeloma. Intriguing recent observations, however, of increased numbers of isotype- and idiotype-specific T cells in myeloma suggest a more active role for T cells in modulating B-cell function. There is some interest in the possible therapeutic exploitation of this by immunizing the patient (or a prospective marrow donor) with the patient's M-component in the hope of augmenting T-cell function against the malignant B cells.

INTERLEUKIN-6 AND VASCULAR ENDOTHELIAL GROWTH FACTOR (VEGF)

Recently, the role of the bone marrow microenvironment has been emphasized. The **growth of myeloma cells** appears to be highly dependent on **exogenous IL-6** produced by bone marrow stromal cells. The production of IL-6 by these cells is stimulated by the presence of the myeloma cells, perhaps mediated by transforming growth factor-β. This suggests a paracrine role for IL-6. Therapy with antibodies against IL-6 and its receptor is being studied. Another factor produced by marrow stem cells that appears to be important in the growth of myeloma cells is the **vascular endothelial growth factor** (**VEGF**). This suggests that increased angiogenesis may play a role in myeloma and that anti-angiogenic therapies may have a role. Initial results with trials of **thalidomide** have been very successful. Other potential mechanisms of action for thalidomide include inhibition of cytokine production, or a direct effect on myeloma cell growth. Thalidomide analogues and other immunomodulatory drugs are the subject of active study.

■ LABORATORY DIAGNOSIS OF MONOCLONAL GAMMOPATHY

All of the plasma cell disorders are characterized by an accumulation of a clone of plasma cells producing a homogeneous immunoglobulin product. This monoclonal gammopathy can be demonstrated either at the level of the soluble product in serum or at the cellular level.

M-COMPONENTS

The characteristic finding that unites all of the plasma cell disorders is the presence of an M-component. This component is present in serum of an increased level of immunoglobulin associated with a single band on electrophoresis, and reaction of that band with an antibody to a single immunoglobulin heavy chain and light chain forms the classic definition of an M-component (Figure 25–2).

Several cases exist in which unique properties of the M-component protein have an important **pathophysiologic role in the disease process.** For example, IgM M-components, because they are pentameric, and IgA M-components, which frequently dimerize, are much more likely to lead to hyperviscosity syndromes at lower concentrations than IgG M-components. Because M-components are antibodies, they sometimes have unusual binding properties that lead to problems, such as vitamin B_{12} deficiency, leukocyte or platelet dysfunction, and hemolytic anemia.

The M-component may not be a normal intact immunoglobulin in a significant number of plasma cell disorders (Table 25–1). Abnormal plasma cells can produce excess free light chains and, less frequently, free heavy chains or other immunoglobulin fragments. The different molecular weights of these proteins and their different solubilities can lead to various clinical syndromes. For example, low molecular weight fragments such as free light chains will pass though the glomerular basement membrane and accumulate in the kidney. High molecular weight M-components, such as IgM or dimeric IgA, will be largely confined to the vascular space and can be rapidly removed by plasmapheresis, whereas monomeric IgG will be widely distributed through the extravascular space and can be difficult to remove.

CLONAL PLASMA CELLS

When increased numbers of plasma cells are demonstrated in a marrow aspirate or tissue biopsy, it is diagnostically useful to determine if they are clonal. This situation is especially important when a serum M-component cannot be demonstrated or is present in low concentration. Because the plasma cell produces large amounts of immunoglobulin, it is possible to label the cells themselves with antibodies directed against immunoglobulin heavy and light chain classes. The antibody reagent staining of the plasma cell cytoplasm can be demonstrated in fixed tissue sections or on films. Each plasma cell produces only one antibody and, therefore, will label with only one heavy chain and one light chain reagent. Since a normal marrow contains plasma cells from many clones, however, cells will

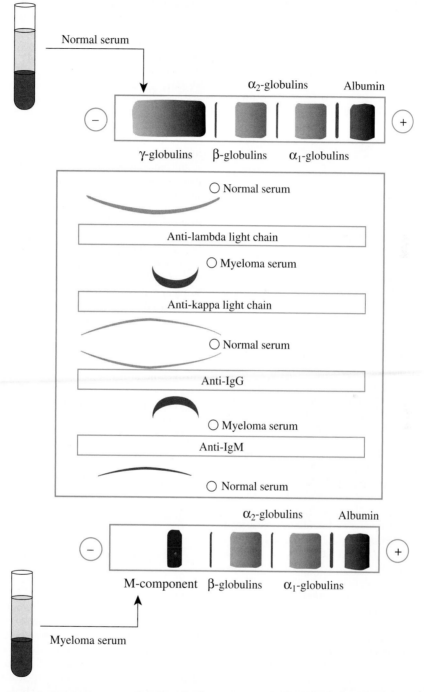

Figure 25–2. **Identification of an M-component.** Electrophoresis of normal serum results in a diffuse region of gamma globulins containing a large number of individual antibodies. Electrophoresis of a serum containing an M-component shows decreased levels of the normal diffuse gamma globulin and a prominent, electrophoretically homogeneous band. When tested with specific antibodies against light chains and heavy chains (immunoelectrophoresis), the M-component reacts with only one heavy chain and one light chain antibody, demonstrating immunologic homogeneity.

Table 25–1. Monoclonal proteins produced by plasma cell tumors.

Type	%
IgG	52
IgA	21
IgD	2
IgE	< 0.01
IgM (Waldenstrom's)	12
Light chain only	11
Heavy chain only	< 1
2 or more	0.5
None	1

be found that label with antibodies to IgG, IgA, and IgM, in order of decreasing frequency, and the normal ratio of κ light chain to λ light chain expressing plasma cells will be about 2:1. In the case of a monoclonal gammopathy, plasma cells that express only a single heavy chain and a single light chain will predominate. In addition, malignant plasma cells will sometimes show other abnormalities, such as multiple nuclei and globules, or even crystals of immunoglobulin, in their cytoplasm.

Chromosomal analysis has been less useful in the diagnosis of myeloma. Three translocations, t(4;14), t(14;16), and t(11;14), have only been described in myeloma samples but can be difficult to detect. Monosomy 13 and trisomies of chromosomes 3, 5, 7, 9, 11, 15, 19, and 21 occur frequently but are less specific. A deletion of 13q14, detected by interphase fluorescence in situ hybridization, is seen in up 50% of multiple myeloma patients at the time of presentation and is associated with a significantly poorer survival.

With evolution of the disease, **other cellular abnormalities** can be appreciated. Early on, the growth fraction of the malignant clone is low—less than 1% of the plasmablasts are dividing at any one time. This increases dramatically to levels greater than 20% with disease progression, especially when a patient relapses from chemotherapy. The latter is associated with **point mutations of the N-*ras* and K-*ras* oncogenes,** as well as a **point mutation of p53** in patients with extramedullary disease. **Plasma cell phenotype changes** include an initial loss of CD19 expression with CD56 overexpression, followed by CD38 expression and CD56 loss as the disease progresses.

■ MULTIPLE MYELOMA (PLASMA CELL MYELOMA)

CLINICAL FEATURES

Multiple myeloma accounts for 10–15% of hematologic neoplasms and about 1% of all cancer deaths. The most common clinical presentation of multiple myeloma is the recent onset of **unexplained back pain** or **normochromic, normocytic anemia** in an older patient. In recent times, however, up to 60% of new patients are first diagnosed when a **serum or urine M-component** is detected on routine laboratory testing. Approximately 70% of myeloma patients are over 60 years of age and 90% are over 50 years. The diagnosis is frequently missed on the first evaluation of the patient.

The diagnosis of multiple myeloma can easily be missed if the physician does not have a high degree of suspicion. It is important to **include myeloma in the differential diagnosis** of any older patient presenting with back pain or anemia even when the history suggests a possible cause for the pain such as recent stress or trauma. The diagnosis is also frequently delayed in patients who have another disease, such as osteo- or rheumatoid arthritis, which may cause bone pain, anemia, or both.

Less commonly, myeloma may present as an isolated mass lesion, the so-called **solitary plasmacytoma.** These lesions may be found in the skin, the gastrointestinal (GI) tract, the nasopharynx, and elsewhere. They are not clinically distinctive and can only be defined as plasmacytomas by biopsy. Most patients presenting with isolated plasmacytomas will be found to have multiple myeloma on further workup; rarely a patient will have an isolated tumor and can be treated with local radiotherapy.

Renal Manifestations & Hypercalcemia

Occasionally the myeloma patient will present with **acute renal failure** or sudden, symptomatic hypercalcemia. The cause of the **hypercalcemia** is primarily the rapid destruction of bone by osteoclast-activating factors secreted by the plasma cells. These factors include IL-1, tumor necrosis factor-β, and IL-6. The cause of the renal failure is multifactorial, including light chain deposition, dehydration, and hypercalcemia. **Amyloid nephropathy** with irreversible renal damage is less common. The patient with resistant disease, however, is at risk for recurrence of these problems. An episode of back pain requiring bed rest may result in return of hypercalcemia. Similarly, an acute infection with fever may result in enough dehydration to precipitate renal failure. With disease progression, renal failure can become a limiting factor in the design of an effective chemotherapy regimen.

Hematologic Manifestations

Myeloma patients have an increased susceptibility to infection secondary to the decreased rate of production of normal immunoglobulins, possibly because of dendritic cell dysfunction or a leukocyte abnormality induced by the M-component. The major hematologic manifestation of myeloma is **anemia,** owing to decreased erythropoiesis. The degree of anemia may be disproportionate to the degree of marrow involvement by plasma cells. Patients who have begun chemotherapy for the disease may have severe myelosuppression. Less commonly, the M-component may interfere with platelet function, leading to bleeding, or with leukocyte function, leading to recurrent infections.

Hyperviscosity of the blood, owing to large concentrations of IgG (usually greater than 100 grams per liter) or dimerization of IgA at lower concentrations, is sometimes seen in myeloma, although it is much more common in macroglobulinemia. It is markedly worsened by dehydration. The clinical manifestations are fatigue, headache, blurring or loss of vision, confusion, and ischemia. Measurement of serum viscosity will be at least three times normal before symptoms can be attributed to hyperviscosity. Treatment of this complication must be undertaken promptly with hydration, initiation of chemotherapy, and plasmapheresis.

Laboratory Studies

Any patient suspected of having a plasma cell disorder should have a quantitative measurement of serum immunoglobulins, electrophoresis of urine for light chains, a marrow aspirate and biopsy with immunologic labeling of plasma cells, a complete blood count (CBC), tests of kidney function, serum Ca^{2+}, albumin, and β_2-microglobulin, as well as x-rays of the skull and pelvis with careful inspection for excessive osteopenia or lytic lesions. Any area of localized bone pain should also be x-rayed.

A. HEMATOLOGIC STUDIES:

The CBC can provide important clues to the diagnosis of myeloma. As the disease advances, the patient will almost certainly develop a normocytic, normochromic anemia secondary to either infiltration of the marrow with plasma cells or renal damage. Since the distinction is important for managing the patient, any anemia should be fully evaluated with marrow, iron studies, and renal function measurements. Differential diagnosis of a marrow damage anemia from the anemias of re-

nal disease and inflammation is discussed in Chapters 3 and 4. In contrast to the early appearance of anemia, changes in granulocyte and platelet count occur much later and are usually associated with chemotherapy. In contrast to patients with B- and T-cell lymphomas, it is impossible to identify the malignant plasma cell line from studies of the peripheral blood. Plasma cells only circulate in very small numbers in patients with advanced disease. Rarely, patients will progress to plasma cell leukemia with increasing numbers of circulating clonal plasmablasts.

Another important clue from the CBC relates to the **amount and class of the patient's M-component.** As the level of this protein increases, there is an increased tendency for red blood cell rouleaux formation. This tendency can be visually appreciated on the peripheral blood film, and when pronounced, can produce a false elevation in the mean cell volume secondary to red blood cell agglutination. An **elevation of the sedimentation rate** to levels greater than 100 mm/hour (Westergren method) in an otherwise healthy individual is also suggestive of a plasma cell disorder, either benign monoclonal gammopathy or myeloma. With older populations, where the incidence of plasma cell disorders is much higher, a sedimentation rate can be a low-cost, high-yield screening test. At the same time, not all sedimentation rates greater than 100 mm/hour turn out to be myeloma. Collagen vascular disorders, infections, and other malignancies are also associated with very high sedimentation rates.

B. IMMUNOGLOBULIN STUDIES:

Ninety-five percent of patients will have an M-component, the most common being IgG. About 25% of patients will have an IgA or rarely an IgD or IgE M-component, whereas 20% of patients have only light chain detectable (Table 25–1). Both the amount and class of the protein are important in diagnosing myeloma (Table 25–2). The presence of a high level of serum or urine M-component (or both) or light chains, together with plasma cell infiltration of the marrow, is the major criterion for diagnosis. Even without evidence of other organ damage, the level of the patient's M-component will correlate with the tumor burden and will guide management decisions.

The **M-component may be first detected** on routine serum electrophoresis as a narrow peak that deforms the normal symmetry of immunoglobulin electrophoresis pattern (see Figure 25–2). Depending on the class of protein, the peak can appear at any point in the distribution of the immunoglobulins. The **quantity of M-component** can be derived from the electrophoretic pattern or by direct quantitation with an anti-immunoglobulin antibody. By combining antibodies to the various classes of immunoglobulin—both sin-

Table 25–2. Diagnostic criteria for multiple myeloma.

Major criteria

Marrow plasmacytosis (> 15%) with expression of a single heavy and light chain class of immunoglobulin

Serum M-component, > 35 g/L or IgG or > 20 g/L of IgA

Urinary light chain excretion > I g/24 h of a single class (κ or λ)

A biopsy-proven plasmacytoma

Minor criteria

A. Less than 15% plasma cells in the marrow but with predominance of one immunoglobulin light chain class.

B. An M-component quantitatively less than specified above.

Lytic bone lesions or unexplained osteopenia on x-ray

Depressed levels of normal (non–M-component) immunoglobulins

Unexplained normochromic, normocytic anemia

Serum β_2-microglobulin level of > 4 mg/L

Unexplained renal dysfunction

Unexplained hypercalcemia

Note: The diagnosis of myeloma requires at least one major and one minor criterion or at least three minor criteria including A and B.

gle immunoglobulin heavy- and light-chain forms—with electrophoresis (immunoelectrophoresis), it is possible to accurately quantitate the actual M-component.

Although the level of M-component provides the most important measure of tumor burden, serial measurements of the β_2-microglobulin level have also been used clinically to follow the progression of myeloma. β_2-**Microglobulin** is a protein that is shed as a part of the life cycle of all lymphocytes, including plasma cells. Levels greater than 4 mg/L suggest a major increase in the number of plasma cells, even when the M-component is not dramatically increased. In addition, when measured serially during chemotherapy, a rise in the β_2-microglobulin level may precede a rise in the M-component in relapsing patients. The **plasma cell–labeling index** (the number of plasma cells in DNA synthesis) has also been used to predict rate of progression. Patients who demonstrate a low labeling index and a normal β_2-microglobulin have a median survival of 6 years when treated with conventional chemotherapy.

C. Organ Function Studies:

Although involvement of other organs is considered as part of the minor criteria in the diagnosis of myeloma (see Table 25–1), evidence of organ damage is integral to both the staging and management of the patient. It is essential, therefore, that the patient be carefully evaluated for structural and functional defects of bone, kidney, and, to a lesser extent, other solid organs.

THERAPY AND CLINICAL COURSE

From the time of presentation with symptoms, the median survival of patients with myeloma left untreated is 6–12 months, and with treatment about 3 years. When myeloma is diagnosed before onset of symptoms, there may be additional years before the disease becomes symptomatic. Available therapeutic options result in considerable toxicity and offer only modest prolongation of life. For these reasons most physicians do not begin treatment of a patient with myeloma before the onset of symptoms. The asymptomatic patient should be followed up with quantitative serum immunoglobulins, CBC, and tests of renal function and serum calcium every 3–6 months, as well as periodic x-rays to determine the rate of progression of disease.

Mainstay Therapy

When clear signs of progression occur, or when the patient is symptomatic, therapy should be started. For most patients the mainstay therapy is **melphalan** 6–9 mg/m² daily and **prednisone** 40–60 mg/day given for 4–7 days and repeated every 4–6 weeks. To maximize effectiveness, the dose should be adjusted to produce a mild neutropenia, a granulocyte count of 1000–1500/μL, or a platelet count of around 100,000/μL. If the blood counts are slow to recover, the next course of therapy must be delayed and the dosage reduced. In the responding patient, a gradual decrease in the quantity of the M-component is observed. Although the disease can be controlled in about 50% of patients, only 10–15% will achieve a "complete" remission as judged by disappearance of the M-component.

Multidrug Regimens and Newer Therapies

Younger patients who can tolerate more aggressive therapy, and those patients who progress on standard therapy, can be offered one of several multidrug regimens. The most common are combinations of vincristine, doxorubicin, and dexamethasone (**VAD**) or the **M2 protocol** (vincristine, BCNU, melphalan, cyclophosphamide, and prednisone). Although these combinations can provide a more rapid induction response, they do not significantly prolong overall survival. Agents that inhibit multidrug resistance (verapamil and cyclosporine) have shown little effect in relapsed patients.

If disease control is achieved, chemotherapy is usually stopped and the patient followed up until there is evidence of progression. However, several clinical trials have reported promising results using maintenance therapy with **interferon-α** to prolong remissions. Here again, a modest prolongation of remission of 5–12 months does not translate into a prolonged survival.

Moreover, the small benefit provided by the interferon-α is achieved at a significant cost in terms of the patient's well-being.

Promising results with **thalidomide,** alone or in combination with chemotherapy, are being reported and this may prove to play a role in primary or maintenance therapy. In addition, **pamidronate,** originally used to control hypercalcemia and bone lesions in myeloma, is now showing an effect on survival, which suggests that new generations of bisphosponates may have a role in preventing progression of the disease as well as treating the skeletal complications.

High-Dose Chemotherapy and Transplantation

High-dose chemotherapy with peripheral blood stem cell rescue (**autologous transplantation**) for patients under age 65 years can result in a complete remission (disappearance of the serum M-component), together with a prolonged survival. To be successful, transplantation must be performed early in the course of the disease, before patients become refractory to chemotherapy. Patients who are least heavily pretreated and still have sensitive disease have the best result. Response rates to high-dose chemotherapy with stem cell rescue are seen in 80% of such patients as compared with 50–60% with conventional chemotherapy. Moreover, 50% of the transplant patients survive for 5 years or more, compared with 10% with conventional chemotherapy.

Peripheral blood collections of CD34⁺ progenitor cells are almost certainly contaminated with malignant plasma cell precursors, guaranteeing future relapse. To date, no known purging or purification method has been able to make the CD34⁺ stem cell population disease free. In younger patients with an HLA-matched sibling, allogeneic marrow transplantation has been performed with promising results. This approach can only be considered, however, in the relatively small number of patients who are under 50 years of age, and the effect on overall survival remains to be determined.

Pain Relief and Management of Complications

Among the hematologic malignancies, multiple myeloma stands out for its destructive action on bone resulting in severe pain and disability. Almost all patients, at various times during the course of their disease, will have severe and sometimes intractable pain. **Adequate pain relief** should be a very important aspect in caring for these patients, for whom the physician often has little else to offer. The bisphosphonate **pamidronate,** given in a dose of 90 mg as a 4-hour

intravenous infusion every 4 weeks for six or more cycles, can reduce the incidence of bone fractures, prevent hypercalcemia, and decrease the patient's bone pain.

Hypercalcemia and acute renal failure usually improve rapidly with treatment. Hemodialysis and plasmapheresis acutely, while waiting for chemotherapy to take effect, can help prevent irreversible renal damage. Patients with **mild hypercalcemia,** a corrected serum calcium level (corrected calcium level = patient's serum calcium + [the normal albumin level (4 grams per deciliter) − the measured serum albumin × 0.8 mg/dL]) of less than 12 mg/dL (3 mmol/L), can usually be managed with hydration, steroids, and antimyeloma chemotherapy. More **severe hypercalcemia,** levels of 12–14 mg/dL or higher, need to be treated as an emergency. Following aggressive hydration (3 or more liters of 0.9% saline over 12–24 hours) and a loop diuretic (furosemide 20–40 mg every 12 hours), pamidronate or calcitonin or both should be administered.

The **dose of the bisphosphonate pamidronate** is 60–90 mg, administered intravenously over 4–24 hours. The onset of effect is apparent within 3–4 days, with a maximal effect at 10 days. The duration of effect can persist for 7–30 days. Repeated doses are effective for intractable conditions. Recent data suggest that pamidronate may also slow the progression of the underlying disease and increase survival. **Calcitonin** is a peptide hormone that rapidly inhibits bone resorption and decreases renal calcium reabsorption, perhaps through its effect on parathormone secretion. It is administered in a dose of 4 IU/kg body weight, subcutaneously every 12 hours. The dosage can be increased to 8 IU/kg every 6–12 hours after a day or two if the response is unsatisfactory. Since tachyphylaxis is expected, calcitonin is only used to stabilize the patient until pamidronate takes effect.

■ SECONDARY MONOCLONAL GAMMOPATHY

A monoclonal gammopathy is occasionally observed as an incidental laboratory finding in patients who are asymptomatic or have another disorder. The **most common diseases associated with secondary monoclonal gammopathy** are autoimmune diseases, AIDS, chronic infections, carcinoma, and lymphoma. Rarely it is possible to demonstrate that the M-component is an antibody directed against some antigen involved in the underlying process, such as HIV. More often, the source of the M-component cannot be identified. Approximately 2–5% of patients with lymphoma or lymphocytic leukemia will have a detectable M-component, most commonly IgM. The **important clinical issue** is to determine if the patient has occult lymphoma, carcinoma, or multiple myeloma and if the patient is likely to develop overt myeloma in the future. These patients should undergo the same diagnostic evaluation as the patient suspected of myeloma, including CBC, marrow examination for clonal plasma cells, renal function studies, and x-ray examination for lytic bone lesions. In addition, such patients should be followed up at close intervals with quantitation of their M-component.

It is unusual for the M-component to increase in cases of secondary gammopathy. Although these patients may have increased plasma cells in their marrow, they are usually polyclonal. Anemia, or osteopenia that cannot be explained on the basis of the underlying disorder, should increase the level of suspicion that the patient may have myeloma rather than secondary gammopathy.

■ MONOCLONAL GAMMOPATHY OF UNDETERMINED SIGNIFICANCE (MGUS)

Many older patients with monoclonal gammopathy will, on complete evaluation, be found not to fit the criteria for multiple myeloma, nor to have any underlying disorder associated with secondary gammopathy. They usually have small M-components, less than 10% marrow plasmacytosis, no anemia, bone lesions, or renal dysfunction, and they are asymptomatic. When this group of patients was first recognized it was questioned whether they had a different disease, perhaps one that was not malignant because they frequently remain free from progression for many years. Recently, studies of herpesvirus 8 infestation of marrow dendritic cells have recovered virus in 25% of these patients. Whether HHV 8 plays an etiologic role is unclear. Long-term follow-up of many MGUS patients has, however, shown that up to 26% of patients will progress to overt multiple myeloma at a rate of about 0.8% per year. Since it is not possible to predict which patients will convert, all MGUS patients should be followed up yearly with measurements of serum and urine M-component. No treatment is advised until the onset of symptoms or clear progression in terms of increased M-component.

■ AMYLOIDOSIS

One of the complications of the plasma cell disorders is amyloidosis. This condition is a clinical syndrome caused by the accumulation in the tissues of large amounts of insoluble glycoprotein material. The source of the glycoprotein is usually degradation products of larger proteins that have in common the ability to form the β-pleated sheet conformation. Several such proteins can give rise to amyloid deposits in a variety of clinical settings. The one most likely to cause amyloid, however, in the patient with a plasma cell disorder is the immunoglobulin light chain. Patients with **overproduction of immunoglobulin light chains** are at risk for the gradual accumulation of amyloid deposits that can cause a variety of signs and symptoms. The λ light chain is more than twice as likely to give rise to this problem.

CLINICAL FEATURES

In some cases, amyloid is discovered during the workup of a patient with a known plasma cell disorder, either myeloma or secondary gammopathy. The more difficult diagnostic situation is the case in which a patient with previous unknown plasma cell disease presents with symptoms related to amyloidosis. It requires a high degree of suspicion to make the correct diagnosis. Common target organs for amyloidosis are the tongue, the heart, the kidney, the skin, the blood vessel walls, the nerves and supporting tissues, the synovium, the GI tract, the adrenals, and the spleen. Any patient presenting with unexplained nephrotic syndrome, cardiomyopathy, heart failure, arrhythmias, neuropathy, carpal tunnel syndrome, arthralgias, splenomegaly, impotence, vascular insufficiency, or ecchymoses should be suspected of having amyloidosis.

DIAGNOSIS

The best diagnostic test is a **biopsy of the rectal mucosa or subcutaneous fat** that should be stained with Congo Red and examined under a polarizing microscope. Amyloid deposits give a birefringent, green staining pattern that is diagnostic. If a patient has signs or symptoms in a region amenable to needle biopsy, it may be wiser to seek the diagnosis there. For example, biopsy of subcutaneous tissue, peripheral nerve, synovium, or marrow may show amyloid deposits if the tissue is involved.

Any patient found to have amyloid deposits should have a **thorough workup for a plasma cell disorder.** The patient may have a small M-component or only free light chains. Amyloidosis can also arise from the deposition of proteins unrelated to plasma cells. Thus, other causes, such as chronic infections, chronic inflammatory diseases, and carcinomas, must be sought as well (Table 25–3). A family history may reveal evidence of one of the familial forms of amyloid, especially in persons of Mediterranean heritage. Infrequently, no underlying cause for the amyloid may be found. In cases such as renal amyloidosis, it may be dif-

Table 25–3. Diseases associated with amyloidosis.

Classification	Diseases	Common Clinical Manifestations
Primary or Ig light chain associated	Multiple myeloma Secondary monoclonal gammopathy Lymphoma	Macroglossia, cardiomyopathy, hepatosplenomegaly, nephrotic syndrome, carpal tunnel syndrome, peripheral neuropathy, purpura, and ecchymoses
Secondary	Tuberculosis Hanson disease Bronchiectasis Osteomyelitis Inflammatory bowel disease Rheumatoid arthritis Carcinoma	Hepatosplenomegaly, nephrotic syndrome, adrenal insufficiency; all of the above
Familial	Familial Mediterranean fever Other familial syndromes	Neuropathy, orthostatic hypotension; all of the above
Associated with hemodialysis	Long-term hemodialysis	All of the above
Associated with aging	Alzheimer's disease	Dementia

ficult to tell if the amyloid deposits are the cause or the result of chronic renal failure.

THERAPY AND CLINICAL COURSE

Because of its insoluble nature, it is very difficult to remove amyloid deposits or to reverse their formation. Treatment of the underlying disease may slow or stop amyloid deposition with very slow improvement in symptoms. Patients with **cardiac or renal involvement** have a very poor prognosis, with median survival on the order of 6 months. Patients with **familial Mediterranean fever** respond well to colchicine therapy with improvement in symptoms related to amyloid as well as their basic symptoms. It is possible that colchicine specifically inhibits amyloid deposition, perhaps by interfering with macrophage function. The response to steroid therapy is usually disappointing. Thus, patients with amyloid related to a **plasma cell disorder** should be treated with melphalan and prednisone primarily. Colchicine can be considered a second line of therapy for these patients. Patients with **renal failure** have undergone renal transplantation with good results. The development of amyloid deposits in the new kidney may take many years.

HEAVY & LIGHT CHAIN DISEASES

As mentioned earlier, about 20% of patients with plasma cell disorders will make only **light chains.** Such

patients may have deposits of intact light chains, usually in the kidneys and other organs. These deposits are not amyloid and do not stain with Congo Red. They most commonly present with renal failure or nephrotic syndrome as the major clinical manifestation, and it may be very difficult to demonstrate light chains in either serum or urine. Usually increased numbers of plasma cells with the appropriate light chain expression can be demonstrated in the marrow, which is best thought of as part of the spectrum of myeloma. The approach to diagnosis and treatment is the same.

Similarly, but much less commonly, patients may produce only free **heavy chains** or fragments of heavy chains. The production of α chains is the most commonly reported, although free γ and μ chains have also been found in some patients. These abnormal proteins may be difficult to demonstrate in the serum and urine and may accumulate in the tissues in a manner analogous to the light chains. α-Heavy chain disease most often affects the GI tract. It may follow a course that more closely resembles a lymphoma affecting the gut-associated lymphoid tissue than a plasma cell disorder.

WALDENSTROM MACROGLOBULINEMIA

Although usually classified and discussed in connection with the plasma cell disorders, Waldenstrom macroglobulinemia can be more accurately thought of as a lymphoma. The only feature that it shares with the plasma cell disorders is the overproduction of immunoglobulin. Unlike myeloma, this condition is always of the IgM class. The presentation, diagnosis, staging, clinical course, and therapy of macroglobulinemia are similar to those of the other lymphomas. Unlike myeloma, it does not present with bone pain, renal failure, lytic lesions, or hypercalcemia. The major organ involvement in macroglobulinemia is the marrow and the lymphoid tissues.

CLINICAL FEATURES

Macroglobulinemia is more common in older patients (median age 60 years), who usually present with fatigue, weight loss, anemia, bleeding, lymphadenopathy, hepatosplenomegaly, and often symptoms related to hyperviscosity (ie, confusion, visual symptoms, and ischemia). Hyperviscosity may be suspected when the clinician observes clumping of red blood cells in the retinal veins, so-called sausage segmentation, and hemorrhages. The IgM M-component may give rise to syndromes associated with cold agglutinin hemolytic anemia, or cryoglobulinemia (ie, urticaria, Raynaud's syndrome, or ischemia).

DIAGNOSIS

Patients with macroglobulinemia will invariably have an IgM M-component, although it may not be quantitatively large. The pentameric nature of IgM may give rise to the hyperviscosity phenomenon at much lower concentrations than IgG or IgA. The typical M-component in this disorder is 10–30 grams per liter. The marrow characteristically contains increased numbers of mast cells, and an infiltrate of small lymphocytes with variable degrees of "plasmacytoid" features such as eccentric nuclei, basophilic cytoplasm, or a prominent Golgi apparatus. Such cells have been termed "**plymphocytes.**" These cells invariably express IgM, usually κ, and, unlike typical plasma cells, they have immunoglobulin both on their surface and in their cytoplasm. Patients sometimes have a lymphocytosis, and even when they do not, it is usually easy to demonstrate the presence of abnormal, clonal lymphocytes in the blood by immunologic or genetic techniques. This situation contrasts with myeloma, where plasma cells are only observed in the blood in the terminal phases of the disease.

Because of the higher molecular weight of the IgM, it is primarily confined to the vascular space and does not cause renal failure. Neuropathy and hyperviscosity are more often seen related to the M-component. Hyperviscosity syndrome should not be diagnosed unless the serum viscosity is measured to be at least three times normal.

Whenever possible, patients suspected of macroglobulinemia should have a biopsy of involved lymphoid tissues. A significant incidence of low-level IgM M-components exists in many lymphomas, and thus the patient should receive an evaluation identical to that performed in any patient with non-Hodgkin's lymphoma (see Chapter 22).

THERAPY

Patients with hyperviscosity should be treated promptly for this life-threatening complication. Hydration, with careful attention to the possibility of congestive heart failure, institution of chemotherapy, and plasmapheresis, will usually control the syndrome. Because the IgM protein is confined to the intravascular space, plasmapheresis can rapidly lower the concentration of M-component. For long-term control, it must be combined with cytotoxic chemotherapy directed at M-component production.

Patients who have relatively small M-components and mild or no symptoms should be observed closely with repeated quantitation of M-components in order to determine the rate of disease progression. Some patients may be followed up in this way for several years. Patients with progressive increase in their M-component or the onset of anemia and other symptoms should be treated with an alkylating agent, usually chlorambucil or cyclophosphamide, as single agents or combined with prednisone. The goal of therapy is to control the disease progression and to decrease the size of the M-component. The additional toxicity of multi-agent chemotherapy is difficult to justify in these older patients, and attempts to use more aggressive therapy have not had good results.

The median survival of these patients with this therapeutic approach is 5 years. Although the role of newer agents such as fludarabine has yet to be established, it is clear that some of these patients will respond.

BIBLIOGRAPHY

Diagnosis

Barlogie B, Alexanian R, Jagannath S: Plasma cell dyscrasias. JAMA 1993;268:2946.

Bataille R, Harousseau J: Multiple myeloma. N Engl J Med 1997; 336:1657.

Billadeau D, Quam L, Thomas W: Detection and quantitation of malignant cells in the peripheral blood of multiple myeloma patients. Blood 1992;80:1818.

Buxbaum J: Mechanisms of disease: Monoclonal immunoglobulin deposition. Amyloidosis, light chain deposition disease, and light and heavy chain deposition disease. Hematol Oncol Clin North Am 1992;6:323.

Hallek M, Bergsagel PL, Anderson KC: Multiple myeloma: Evidence for a multistep transformation process. Blood 1998; 91:3.

Kyle RA: Diagnostic criteria of multiple myeloma. Hematol Oncol Clin North Am 1992;6:347.

Zojer N et al: Deletion of 13q14 remains an independent adverse prognostic variable in multiple myeloma despite its frequent detection by interphase fluorescence in situ hybridization. Blood 2000;95:1925.

Therapy

Attal M et al: A prospective randomized trial of autologous bone marrow transplantation and chemotherapy in multiple myeloma. N Engl J Med 1996;335:91.

Berenson JR for the Myeloma Aredia Study Group: Efficacy of pamidronate in reducing skeletal events in patients with advanced multiple myeloma. N Engl J Med 1996;334:488.

Buckner CD et al: Marrow transplantation for malignant plasma cell disorders: Summary of the Seattle experience. Eur J Haematol 1989;43:186.

Gregory WM, Richards MA, Malpas JS: Combination chemotherapy versus melphalan and prednisone in the treatment of multiple myeloma: An overview of published trials. J Clin Oncol 1992;10:334.

Mandelli F et al: Maintenance treatment with recombinant interferon alpha 2b in patients with multiple myeloma responding to conventional induction chemotherapy. N Engl J Med 1990;322:1430.

Niesvizky R, Siegel D, Michaeli S: Biology and treatment of multiple myeloma. Blood Rev 1993;7:24.

Macrophage Disorders

Disorders of the monocyte/macrophage lineage can be broadly classified under the headings of benign or reactive histiocytosis, malignant histiocytosis, and the storage diseases. In naming these disorders, the term "histiocyte" is used interchangeably with "macrophage" to describe the tissue-bound phagocytic cells found throughout the body. The morphologic appearance of the tissue macrophage is key to the differential diagnosis of these disorders. For example, **reactive histiocytosis** is characterized by prominent monocytosis and tissue granulomatous reaction typical of the normal role of histiocytes in both the immune system and in host defense against infection. **The storage diseases** are a manifestation of genetic deficiencies of certain enzymes responsible for the degradation of carbohydrates and lipids. Even though these enzyme deficiencies presumably affect all the cells in the body, they are manifest primarily as an abnormality of macrophage morphology because of their prominent role in degrading cellular debris. Primary **malignancies of the tissue macrophages** are quite rare. Marrow and tissue invasion by erythrophagocytic histiocytes is a primary distinguishing feature.

THE NORMAL MONOCYTE-MACROPHAGE SYSTEM

As with the other hematopoietic cell lines, the monocyte-macrophage cell lineage arises from the common hematopoietic stem cell. Cell differentiation and maturation to form mature circulating monocytes is under the control of **granulocyte macrophage colony-stimulating factor (GM-CSF)**, **granulocyte colony-stimulating factor (G-CSF)**, and **monocytic colony-stimulating factor (M-CSF)**. The mechanism underlying the subsequent migration of monocytes into tissues and the formation of tissue histiocytes (alveolar macrophages, hepatic Kupffer cells, dermal Langerhans cells, marrow reticuloendothelial cells, etc) is not well understood. It is associated with distinct changes in cell surface antigen receptors and intracellular enzymes.

The monocyte-macrophage system has **three principal functions:** bacterial phagocytosis and killing, antigen presentation to T lymphocytes to initiate the immune reaction, and modulation of the inflammatory response. Monocytes also appear to play a role in coag-

ulation. They express ligand for P-Selectin on the cell surface and are incorporated into clots, where they play a role in fibrinolysis.

Phagocytosis and Bacterial Killing

Together with neutrophils, monocytes and macrophages actively phagocytize bacteria. With activation, these cells are then able to kill the ingested bacteria by superoxide generation. There are clear similarities and differences in the antimicrobial abilities of the monocyte and macrophage as compared with the neutrophil. For example, the tissue-based macrophage contains much less myeloperoxidase than either the circulating neutrophil or monocyte. These differences are in part responsible for the clinical manifestations of some infections. The formation of granulomas in patients with certain infections, such as tuberculosis, in part reflects the inability of the tissue macrophage to lyse the mycobacterium. Patients with chronic granulomatous disease are examples of having an inherited defect in the ability of the monocyte-macrophages to generate superoxide.

Role in Immunity

Monocytes and tissue macrophages play a key role in the initiation of the immune response. They process antigen and present it to T lymphocytes to initiate the subsequent proliferation of B lymphocytes and the production of antibody. Macrophages also release interleukin (IL)-1, which stimulates T lymphocytes to release several cytokines essential to the full immune response (Figure 26–1). This interaction is complex. The presentation of antigen involves a shared characteristic of the macrophage and T cell, the expression of both Class I and Class II major histocompatibility complex (MHC) molecules. The **Class I MHC molecules** are involved in CD8 T-cell interactions, whereas the **Class II MHC molecules** play a role in CD4 T-cell interactions (see Chapter 19).

Role in the Inflammatory Response

Monocytes and tissue macrophages also play a role in the inflammatory response by the release of cytokines

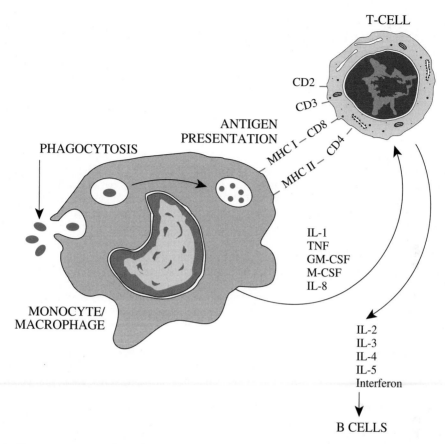

Figure 26–1. **Monocyte-macrophage function.** The normal monocyte-macrophage is capable of phagocytosis, that is, the killing of pathogens, and presentation of digested antigen to T cells to promote the full immune response. Monocytes also release several cytokines to stimulate the T-cell response and promote the inflammatory response.

such as GM-CSF, G-CSF, M-CSF, IL-1, IL-8, tumor necrosis factor, and the interferons. They can also secrete proteases such as tissue plasminogen activator, collagenase, and elastase. These enzymes play a role in the tissue structural changes associated with the inflammatory reaction.

CLINICAL FEATURES

Benign or reactive monocytosis is most often associated with a severe, prolonged inflammatory response, an immune disorder, or a lymphoproliferative disease state (Table 26–1). The host defense role of the monocyte can be of diagnostic value in the workup of the patient with a fever of undetermined origin. Subacute bacterial endocarditis, tuberculosis, Hodgkin's disease, and many of the collagen vascular diseases are frequently accompanied by a modest monocytosis, with counts of 500–1000/μL. In any of these situations,

the dominant clinical features are those of the primary illness.

Patients with **malignancies of the monocyte-macrophage lineage** can present either as a leukemic state or as a wasting illness with marked fever, weight loss, and pancytopenia secondary to organ infiltration with malignant histiocytes. A small percentage of **adult leukemias** demonstrate pure monocyte morphology (Chapter 17). Patients with relatively subacute courses will often present with a distinctive hypertrophy of the gums secondary to monocyte infiltration. Patients who present with a myeloproliferative disorder frequently demonstrate an increase in their absolute monocyte count. Chronic myelomonocytic leukemia is classified on the basis of the monocytosis in blood and marrow. The presentation of the patient with a myeloproliferative disorder with prominent monocytosis does not differ significantly from those patients where the count is not elevated (Chapter 18).

Table 26–1. Causes of reactive monocytosis.

Inflammatory diseases
Sarcoidosis
Bacterial infections
Subacute bacterial endocarditis
Tuberculosis
Sepsis with granulocytopenia
Syphilis
Autoimmune disorders
Systemic lupus erythematosus
Rheumatoid arthritis
Temporal arteritis
Polyarteritis
Ulcerative colitis/Crohn disease
Hemolytic anemia/ITP
Hematopoietic disorders
Lymphopoietic malignancies
Hodgkin's disease
Non-Hodgkin's lymphomas
Multiple myeloma
Aplastic/Hypoplastic anemias
Cyclical neutropenia

The storage diseases are typically diagnosed during childhood or early adult life based on distinctive abnormalities of the liver, spleen, bone, and central nervous system (CNS). Dramatic expansion of tissue macrophages produces marked hepatosplenomegaly in patients with Type I **Gaucher disease.** These patients also develop deformity of the ends of the long bones (**Erhlenmeyer flask deformity of the distal femur**), pathologic fractures, and aseptic necrosis of the femoral heads. They can also experience episodes of bone pain and swelling without clear radiologic findings.

Patients with Tay-Sachs disease, Niemann-Pick disease, and Type II or Type III Gaucher disease present in infancy with marked **neurologic abnormalities.** These abnormalities include a general failure to develop neurologically, blindness, deafness, and marked motor weakness or spasticity. A distinctive physical finding in infants with Tay-Sachs disease is the presence of cherry red spots in the retinas.

Laboratory Studies

A. COMPLETE BLOOD COUNT (CBC):

Diagnosis of a reactive monocytosis or leukemia may be made from the CBC. The normal absolute monocyte count is less than 500/μL. **Reactive monocytosis** is associated with modest increases in the absolute count to 500–1500/μL. Very high monocyte counts suggest an **acute leukemia or leukemoid reaction.**

Unfortunately, individual monocyte morphology is not very helpful in the differential diagnosis of a leukemoid reaction from a true leukemia. Even with special stains, immunophenotyping, and chromosomal analysis, it can be difficult to definitively separate the two conditions.

B. MARROW ASPIRATE, BIOPSY, AND OTHER TESTS:

Diagnosis of **malignant histiocytosis** or a **lipid storage disease** is usually made from the marrow aspirate, biopsy, or both. The key finding is invasion of the marrow structure by morphologically abnormal macrophages. In patients with **Gaucher disease,** the marrow is infiltrated with large macrophages whose cytoplasm is filled with a characteristic pinkish, striated material with a few vacuoles. This material is actually an insoluble glycolipid, **glucocerebroside.** The morphologic appearance of these cells is so unique that a good pathologist or hematologist can usually make the diagnosis from the marrow appearance. Patients with Gaucher disease also consistently show an increased **acid phosphatase activity in serum.** With increasing splenomegaly, most patients develop a normocytic, normochromic anemia or pancytopenia secondary to hypersplenism. **Patients who have had a splenectomy** typically show marked changes in red blood cell morphology including severe aniso- and poikilocytosis, nucleated red blood cells, and Howell-Jolly bodies.

Patients with **Niemann-Pick disease** can be diagnosed from the appearance of large, foamy macrophages in the marrow. The droplet-like material in these cells is **sphingomyelin.** Any confusion with Gaucher cells can be eliminated based on the pinkish staining quality with **periodic acid–Schiff stain** and by examining an unstained preparation by phase microscopy. The sphingomyelin droplets within the cells are birefringent under polarized light. Rarer, adult forms of Niemann-Pick disease may lack typical foam cells in the marrow but demonstrate histiocytes with a pale bluish cytoplasm (**sea-blue histiocytes**). This finding is also seen in patients with chronic myelogenous leukemia and myeloproliferative disorders.

DIAGNOSIS

The full classification of disorders of the monocyte-macrophage system is summarized in Table 26–2. Each of the major categories will be discussed separately.

Reactive & Leukemic Monocytosis

Any patient who presents with an absolute monocyte count greater than 500/μL must be considered as a candidate for a reactive or leukemic monocytosis. A full study of the hematopoietic profile with special

Table 26–2. Disorders of the monocyte-macrophage system.

Benign (reactive monocytosis)
Leukemic monocytosis
  Acute or subacute monocytic leukemia
  Myeloproliferative diseases
   Chronic myelo-monocytic leukemia
   Chronic myelogenous leukemia
   Myelodysplasias
Malignant histiocytosis
Lipid storage diseases
  Gaucher disease
  Niemann-Pick disease
  Tay-Sachs disease

---

stains, immunophenotyping, and chromosomal analysis will usually identify those patients who have a hematopoietic malignancy. This malignancy can take the form of an acute or subacute leukemia where the predominant cell form in circulation is an immature (**promonocyte**) or mature monocyte. Frequently, these patients have counts in excess of 10,000/μL. Patients with myeloproliferative disorders who demonstrate an absolute monocytosis as a component of their disease generally have much lower counts. In addition, most of these patients show distinctive chromosomal abnormalities (see Chapter 18).

Reactive monocytosis is seen in a wide spectrum of diseases. It is observed in association with lymphoproliferative disorders including both the non-Hodgkin's lymphomas and Hodgkin's disease. A wide array of collagen vascular diseases are accompanied by a modest monocytosis, including lupus erythematosus, temporal arteritis, polyarteritis nodosa, rheumatoid arthritis, ulcerative colitis, and Crohn disease. Several infections demonstrate monocytosis as a distinctive feature. This includes sarcoid, subacute bacterial endocarditis, syphilis, and tuberculosis. Patients who have cyclic neutropenia or are made neutropenic with chemotherapy can also demonstrate a significant monocytosis in the recovery phase.

Malignant Histiocytosis

Malignancy of the monocyte-macrophage line can present as a tissue-based disease with severe anemia, pancytopenia, hepatosplenomegaly, and lymphadenopathy. The course of the disease process is usually rapid with dramatic wasting, recurrent fevers, bone pain, and in some cases skin and soft tissue tumor infiltrates. The diagnostic finding of the most common form of malignant histiocytosis (**histiocytic medullary reticulosis [HMR]**) is the presence in the marrow aspirate or biopsy of macrophages that have ingested intact red blood cells (**erythrophagocytosis**). In addition, the histiocytes may be quite pleomorphic with immature nuclei containing one or more nucleoli. These cells are positive for both acid phosphatase and nonspecific esterase. HMR can be confused with other lymphomas such as Hodgkin's disease or even one of the non-Hodgkin's lymphomas.

Lipid Storage Disorders

A. GAUCHER DISEASE:

Gaucher disease is the most common of the lipid storage disorders. It is an autosomal recessive disease caused by a **defect in the production of the enzyme glucocerebrosidase.** This enzyme is required for the digestion of glycolipids in the lysosomes of all macrophages. When the enzyme is missing or defective, the extremely insoluble compound glucocerebroside accumulates within the cell's cytoplasm.

Gaucher disease is most **common in the Ashkenazi Jewish population,** whose heritage is largely from middle and northern Europe. Rarely, patients of Swedish heritage will have a predilection for the disease. It is estimated that the frequency of homozygotes in the Ashkenazi population is greater than 1 in 800. The most common mutations result in a decreased production of the enzyme that is encoded on the short arm of chromosome 1. The type of mutation will dictate the severity of the clinical manifestations, which range from severe disease presenting at infancy to almost asymptomatic forms diagnosed only in adults or the elderly.

1. Clinical subtypes—Three clinical subtypes of Gaucher disease have been identified. **Type I** is the most common, representing more than 99% of cases. It also has the most heterogeneous presentation, with disease limited to the macrophages of the spleen, marrow, and liver. **Type II** disease is much more severe, presenting in early infancy with fulminating neurologic symptoms and early death, usually within 18 months of life. **Type III** disease presents during childhood with neurologic symptoms. It has a much longer natural history.

Patients with Type I Gaucher disease commonly present with hepatosplenomegaly, bony abnormalities, anemia or pancytopenia or both, and progressive liver dysfunction. The presence in marrow of large numbers of the characteristic Gaucher cell is diagnostic. Other unique clinical findings are the development of the Erhlenmeyer flask deformity of the ends of long bones and the striking elevation of the serum acid phosphatase activity. It is also possible to directly test peripheral leukocytes for the level of β-glucosidase activity if there is any doubt about the diagnosis.

Gaucher-like cells may be seen in the elderly patient or individual who has a myeloproliferative or lymphoproliferative disorder. On occasion, a Gaucher-like cell may be observed in the marrow of an AIDS patient. This presence is not owing to a deficiency of β-glucosidase but rather reflects a marked increased uptake of cellular debris by the macrophages, producing an overstuffed cytoplasm.

2. Prenatal and genetic diagnosis—Since Gaucher disease is inherited, prenatal diagnosis by amniocentesis is possible by measuring β-glucosidase activity in harvested cells or by genetic analysis. There is a characteristic restriction length polymorphism associated with the most common mutation. Heterozygotes for Gaucher disease have one-half the normal enzyme levels and can be accurately diagnosed by genetic analysis. They do not have Gaucher cells in the marrow and are clinically normal.

B. NIEMANN-PICK DISEASE AND TAY-SACHS DISEASE:

Niemann-Pick and Tay-Sachs disease, which are the other less-common lipid storage diseases, also have a higher incidence in the Ashkenazi Jewish population. This suggests a common explanation for the balanced polymorphism of these glycolipid storage diseases. **Niemann-Pick disease** is characterized by the accumulation of sphingomyelin in the macrophage to produce the typical foam cells in marrow, lymph nodes, and other organs. Patients with **Tay-Sachs disease** show an accumulation of GM-2 ganglioside in the CNS. Both of these conditions generally present during infancy with severe neurologic dysfunction. Since there are no effective treatments available, genetic screening and genetic counseling are important for prevention.

THERAPY

Effective management obviously is dictated by the specific abnormality of the monocyte-macrophage system.

Reactive monocytosis is a sign of another disease process and will respond to the treatment of that disease. Acute and subacute monocytic leukemia is treated like other acute leukemias with ablative chemotherapy (see Chapter 17). Malignant histiocytosis (HMR) is usually a rapidly progressive disease that responds poorly to combination chemotherapy or radiotherapy. At best, chemotherapy is palliative.

Gaucher Disease

Until recently, the management of patients with Gaucher disease was limited to **splenectomy** for marked hypersplenism and **orthopedic procedures** such as hip replacements to provide symptomatic relief and maintain mobility. Although splenectomy may improve the patient's hematologic picture, it can be associated with a rapid worsening of liver and bone involvement, as macrophages in those sites take on the increased burden of dealing with the extra amounts of glucocerebroside.

This situation has now changed dramatically. The missing enzyme, β-glucosidase, has now been purified and made available as a pharmaceutical (**Ceredase**). Repeated intravenous infusion of the enzyme will result in a gradual regression of the signs and symptoms of Gaucher disease over a long period. Although it is safe, Ceredase use costs from $300,000 to $750,000 per year per patient. Recently the enzyme has become available as a recombinant product (**imiglucerase**), which may reduce the cost. It may eventually be possible to use gene implant therapy to correct the enzyme deficiency.

BIBLIOGRAPHY

Beutler E: Gaucher disease: New molecular approaches to diagnosis and treatment. Science 1992;256:794.

Beutler E: Lipid storage diseases. In: Beutler E et al (editors): *Hematology*, 6th ed. McGraw-Hill, 2001.

PART III

Disorders of Hemostasis

Normal Hemostasis

Any disruption of vascular endothelium is a potent stimulus to clot formation. As a localized process, this acts to seal the break in vascular continuity, limit blood loss, and set the stage for healing. Control of the reaction to prevent runaway thrombosis involves several counterbalancing mechanisms, including anticoagulant properties of intact endothelial cells, circulating inhibitors of activated coagulation factors, and production of fibrinolytic enzymes to dissolve the clot. Most abnormalities in hemostasis involve a defect in one or more of the integrated steps in this coagulation process. It is important, therefore, to understand the normal sequence of hemostasis.

Normal coagulation is best described according to its major components—vessel wall, platelet function, coagulation factor cascade, and clot inhibition/lysis.

VESSEL WALL

The normal endothelial cell lining of the vessel wall plays an **essential role in preventing thrombus formation.** First and foremost, it provides a physical barrier between circulating platelets and highly thrombogenic subendothelial connective tissue. In addition, endothelial cells are active metabolically in control of blood flow, platelet aggregation, and the coagulation cascade. They are a primary source for production of nitric oxide and prostacyclin, both of which are important in promoting smooth muscle relaxation and vessel dilatation. Disruption of the endothelial cell surface results in unopposed smooth muscle contraction and vessel spasm. This is an effective reflex to stem blood loss and sets the stage for thrombus formation.

When damaged, endothelial cells are capable of encouraging platelet adhesion, activation, and aggregation (Table 27–1). They are a source of **von Willebrand factor (vWF),** the essential cofactor for platelet adhe-

sion, and they contain an activation antigen, **granular membrane protein 140 (GMP 140),** that can be expressed on the cell surface. This is P-Selectin, which is the same activation antigen that is present in α granules of platelets. The primary role of **P-Selectin** on endothelial cells may be to encourage attachment of monocytes and granulocytes to the injury site.

On the other hand, normal endothelial cells adjacent to an injury site play a role in **limiting clot formation.** In the presence of thrombin, release of prostacyclin by normal endothelial cells increases dramatically to inhibit platelet activation and aggregation. Endothelial cells can also inhibit coagulation by promoting protein C activation and binding of thrombin to antithrombin III. Finally, they are a primary source of **tissue plasminogen activator (t-PA),** the principal physiologic fibrinolytic enzyme.

PLATELET FUNCTION

Normal circulating platelets resemble an oblong disk, measuring 2–4 μm on the long axis with a volume of 5–12 fL. They are essentially fragments of megakaryocyte cytoplasm. Although lacking a nucleus, the cytoplasm contains mitochondria for aerobic metabolism, glycogen stores for anaerobic glycolysis, and specific granules of importance in coagulation (Figure 27–1). Almost 20% of the platelet volume comprises these granules, whereas 25% of the protein in the platelet is actin and myosin needed for platelet contraction.

When stimulated by contact with subendothelial tissue, platelets adhere to the exposed collagen and undergo an immediate shape change with extension of pseudopods. **GPIa/IIa** is one of the platelet adhesion receptors (**integrins**) involved in collagen binding, but not the most important, since congenital absence of GPIa/IIa does not result in a significant bleeding ten-

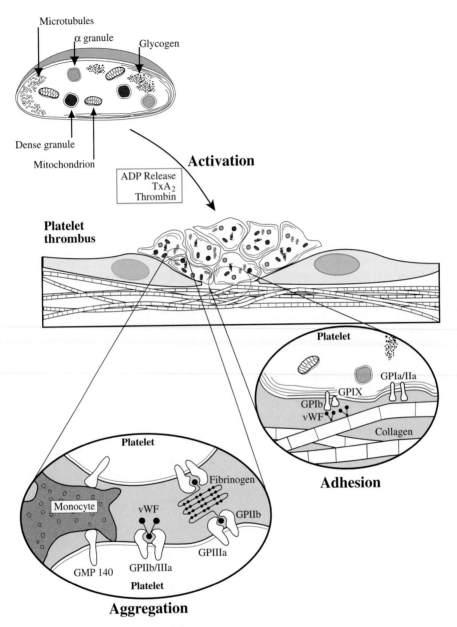

Figure 27–1. **Platelet activation and aggregation.** Platelet activation involves both a shape change with extension of pseudopods and a release reaction where the contents of intracellular granules are expelled from the platelet to stimulate activation of other platelets. Formation of a platelet thrombus at the site of injury requires both platelet adhesion and aggregation. Surface GPIa/IIa receptors bind directly to exposed collagen. GPIb and GPIIb/IIIa receptors interact with von Willebrand factor (vWF) to adhere to the subendothelial tissue. Aggregation involves the GIIb/IIIa receptor and fibrinogen as an essential cofactor. The expression of the α-granule receptor, GMP 140 (P-Selectin), binds to monocytes and incorporates them in the clot.

Table 27-1. Endothelial cell factors.

Procoagulant	Anticoagulant
Vessel contraction	**Platelet inhibition**
Coagulation factor production	Nitric oxide
Factor C inhibitor	Prostacyclin
Factor VIII	ADPase
HMW vWF	**Clot inhibition/lysis**
Fibronectin	Heparans
Activation antigen expression	Thrombomodulin
P-Selectin (GMP 140)	Tissue factor pathway inhibitor
	Plasminogen activator

dency. **GPIb/IX-V and GPIIb/IIIa (integrin $\alpha_{IIb}\beta_3$)** play far more important roles. GPIb/IX-V is the principal adhesion factor, while GPIIb/IIIa mediates aggregation. vWF is an essential cofactor for adhesion, binding connective tissue elements to the platelet via the platelet surface receptor GPIb/IX-V. This is followed by a conformational change in the GPIIb/IIIa receptor site and rapid aggregation of platelets on the surface to form a white (platelet) thrombus. **Fibrinogen** plays a key role in aggregation by its binding to GPIIb/IIIa receptors on adjacent platelets.

This first wave of aggregation is reversible, lasting a matter of minutes when the stimulus is weak. A second wave of aggregation is associated with degranulation and release of adenosine 5'-diphosphate (ADP) from dense granules, platelet factor 4 and β-thromboglobulin from the α-granules, and the generation of thromboxane A_2 and thrombin (Table 27–2). P-Selectin also appears on the platelet surface as α-granule contents are released. ADP, thrombin, and thromboxane A_2 provide a strong stimulus for **further platelet activation and aggregation.** Thrombin stimulates fibrinogen conversion to fibrin to stabilize the aggregate as a fibrin clot. Runaway platelet aggregation is inhibited by release of prostacyclin and nitric oxide by surrounding normal endothelial cells, deactivation of thrombin by antithrombin III, and degradation of ADP by a membrane-associated ADPase.

Several **other substances are released as a part of platelet degranulation** (see Figure 27–1). In addition to ADP, dense granules release serotonin and **ionized calcium,** an essential cofactor in both platelet aggregation and subsequent platelet contraction. Platelet factor 4 from the α-granule appears to bind heparin. Other α-granule contents include β-thromboglobulin, whose action is unknown, and clotting proteins, including fibrinogen, factors V and VIII, thrombospondin, and fibronectin. Chemotactic factor and platelet-derived growth factor are also released. Finally, platelet factor III on the surface of aggregated platelets serves as a proco-

agulant to facilitate factor X activation and conversion of prothrombin to thrombin. Surface activation helps protect the Xa-Va complex and thrombin from circulating inhibitors.

COAGULATION CASCADE

The cascade of interactions of the circulating clotting factors is shown in Figure 27–2. Viewed from a laboratory testing perspective, the cascade can be divided into intrinsic and extrinsic pathways. This situation fits the commonly used laboratory tests, the prothrombin time (PT) measurement for the extrinsic pathway,

Table 27-2. Platelet coagulant factors.

Activation antigens (integrins)
GPIa/IIa: collagen receptor
GPIb/IX-V: vWF receptor
GPIIb/IIIa: fibrinogen receptor
P-Selectin
Platelet-associated proteins
Specific
Platelet factors 3 and 4
β-thromboglobulin
Platelet-derived growth factor
Nonspecific (absorbed)
Fibrinogen
Plasma proteins (albumin, IgG)
vWF, other coagulation factors
Plasminogen
Reactive compounds
Biogenic amines
Serotonin
Histamine
Catecholamines
Adenine nucleotides (ADP, cyclic AMP)
Cations (CA++)
Thromboxane A_2

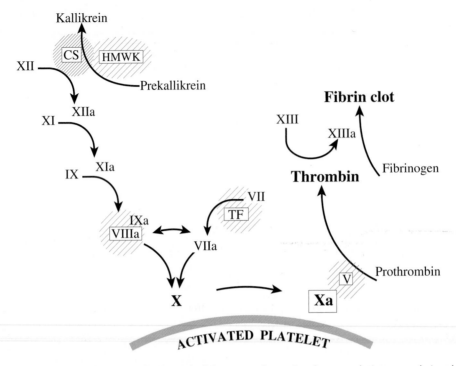

Figure 27–2. **The coagulation cascade.** From the laboratory viewpoint, the coagulation cascade involves both an intrinsic and extrinsic pathway. The intrinsic pathway is initiated by activation of factor XII (Hageman factor) by surface contact (CS), whereas the extrinsic pathway begins with the activation of factor VII by tissue microsomal lipoproteins (TF). Physiologically, the two pathways work together to provide maximum stimulation of factor X, which, in the presence of factor V, activates prothrombin to thrombin. The last step in the cascade is the activation of fibrinogen to fibrin clot with factor XIII acting as a clot-stabilizing factor.

and the partial thromboplastin time (PTT) for the intrinsic pathway. From a physiologic standpoint, however, the cascade may better be divided into four components: the extrinsic, or tissue factor (TF), system; the intrinsic, or Hageman factor-contact, system; activation of the common pathway; and the final formation of clot by thrombin.

Extrinsic, or Tissue Factor (TF), System

Activation of factor VII to VIIa by TF expressed by injured endothelial cells is, clinically, the most important initiator of coagulation. Once formed, TF-VIIa complex activates factor X both directly and by activation of factor IX (Figure 27–2). The TF-VIIa stimulus, however, is rapidly inhibited by **tissue factor pathway inhibitor** (**TFPI**). Sustained factor X activation, sufficient to form a stable clot, is dependent on continued activation of factors IX and VIII by thrombin. Factor

XI activation by thrombin also plays a role in sustaining the activation of factor IX.

Intrinsic, or Hageman Factor-Contact, System

Initiation of the intrinsic pathway, as measured in the laboratory by the PTT, involves activation of **factor XII** (**Hageman factor**) to XIIa, which then catalyzes the activation of factor XI. **Essential cofactors for this reaction** include presence of a contact surface, prekallikrein, and high-molecular-weight kininogen (HMWK). The rate of the reaction is further accelerated by XIIa, which encourages the formation of kallikrein and release of a kinin-free HMWK. Although this is a well-defined reaction in the laboratory, its clinical importance is unclear. Deficiencies in factor XII, prekallikrein, and HMWK prolong the PTT but are not associated with a clinical abnormality. Deficiencies of factors XI and XIII are as-

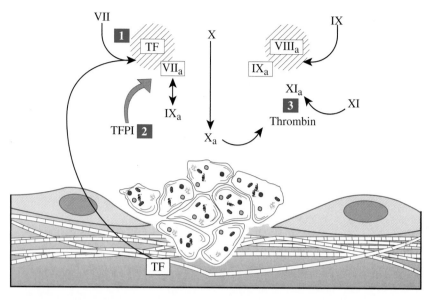

Figure 27–3. **Common pathway activation in vivo.** Tissue factor (TF) is the normal initiator of factor X activation (**1**). Its action is inhibited, however, by tissue factor pathway inhibitor (TFPI), which rapidly binds to the TF-factor VIIa-X complex (**2**). Continued formation of factor Xa, therefore, depends on an intact factor IXa-VIII pathway activated by factor XIa-thrombin (**3**).

sociated with abnormal bleeding, but only because of clot instability.

Activation of the Common Pathway

Factors IXa and VIIa are both highly active serine proteases. They are closely allied in the subsequent activation of the common pathway factors X and V (see Figure 27–2). The action of each requires the presence of a cofactor. Factor VIIIa is the essential cofactor for IXa, whereas microsomal lipoprotein derived from damaged tissue (TF) is cofactor for VIIa.

Rather than being two distinct physiologic systems, an intrinsic pathway and an extrinsic pathway, tissue factor-VIIa and factor IXa-VIIIa complex are highly integrated in vivo. In the presence of excess TF, factor VII activation of the common pathway reaches a maximum rate as illustrated by laboratory measurement of the PT. A normal PT is typically between 11 and 13 seconds. The most likely in vivo sequence of events for the common pathway activation of factor X is illustrated in Figure 27–3. TF is the most potent activator of factor VII, and it initiates clotting. The formation of the TF-factor VIIa-Xa complex is immediately inhibited, however, by tissue factor pathway inhibitor (TFPI) limiting the extent of factor X activation. Sustained Xa formation depends on an intact factor IXa-VIIIa pathway activated

by factor XIa with thrombin as a primary stimulus for the activation of factor XI. Since the level of TF at an injury site is usually limited, clot formation depends on an intact factor IXa pathway and adequate amounts of factor VIII. This situation helps explain why patients with hemophilia, either factor VIII or IX deficiency, demonstrate an abnormal bleeding tendency.

The final step in the common pathway involves both **platelet membrane surface** to support the reaction and **factor V** as an essential cofactor. Factor V greatly enhances activation of Xa, and a marked deficiency in factor V or a defect in the membrane binding of factor Xa-Va complex results in a bleeding tendency. Therefore, the importance of the platelet membrane both as a localizing site for the clotting sequence and as a facilitator of the common pathway sequence cannot be overemphasized.

Clot Formation

The Xa-Va complex enzymatically cleaves prothrombin to form thrombin. The amount of prothrombin in circulation is relatively large compared with other factors, providing an amplification of the final step of thrombin generation and cleavage of fibrinogen to produce a fibrin clot. Thrombin also amplifies the coagulation sequence by stimulating platelet activation to provide ad-

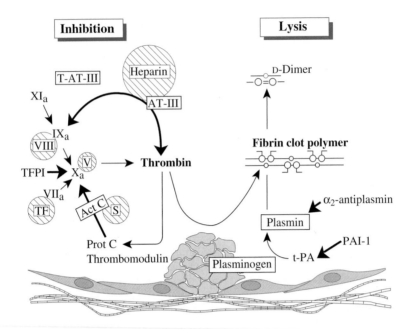

Figure 27–4. Clot inhibition and lysis. Clot size is controlled by inhibitors of platelet function and coagulation and by the fibrinolytic system. The most important inhibitors of the coagulation cascade are the thrombin-initiated activation of protein C, which, in the presence of protein S, enzymatically destroys factors V and VIIIa. Antithrombin III (AT-III) is another circulating inhibitor of thrombin and to a lesser extent factors Xa, IXa, and XIa. Tissue factor pathway inhibitor (TFPI) is a plasma and endothelial cell–bound inhibitor of Xa and the VIIa-TF complex. In terms of the fibrinolytic system, endothelial cells release a plasminogen activator (t-PA) that activates clot-bound plasminogen to plasmin. Plasmin breaks down the fibrin polymer, releasing several fibrin fragments including a cross-linked D-dimer fragment. Measurements of the D-dimer are used clinically to determine the rate of clot lysis.

ditional membrane surface for activation of factors X and V and, finally, by activating factors XI and XIII. Factor XIIIa is an active transamidase, which in the presence of calcium converts the gel-like fibrin clot to an insoluble fibrin polymer.

CLOT INHIBITION/LYSIS

The character of the thrombus is influenced by the type of vessel involved and the location. In major arteries, high blood flows tend to limit the growth of a thrombus on the vessel wall. As platelets aggregate on the surface they are dislodged and factors such as ADP, thromboxane A_2, and thrombin, which stimulate aggregation and clot formation, are rapidly dissipated. This situation limits the thrombus to the initial platelet aggregate, producing a so-called **white thrombus.** In contrast, clotting in smaller vessels or in the venous circuit where blood flow is much slower is characterized by maximum platelet aggregation and incorporation of other blood cells, including red blood cells in the final

fibrin clot. This condition produces a characteristic **"red thrombus."**

Size and stability of a newly formed clot are also influenced by several inhibitors of coagulation and by the fibrinolytic system. Inhibitors of platelet activation and aggregation are described in Chapter 34. **Direct inhibitors of the coagulation cascade** include protein C, protein S, antithrombin III, and TFPI. They are essential to the control of thrombus formation. A deficiency in any of these can set the stage for an increased tendency to thrombosis, especially in the venous circuit.

Thrombin binds to and is inactivated by the endothelial cell membrane surface protein, **thrombomodulin** (Figure 27–4). This transforms thrombin from a procoagulant into an enzyme that activates circulating protein C. **Activated protein C** then inhibits further clot formation by enzymatically cleaving factors Va and VIIIa. **Protein S** acts as a cofactor for activated protein C by helping overcome the protective effect of Xa-Va binding on the platelet membrane. **Antithrom-**

bin III is an inhibitor of serine protease enzymes and has activity against thrombin and activated factors Xa, IXa, and XIa. Activity of antithrombin III is dramatically enhanced by the presence of exogenous heparin and perhaps endothelial cell heparan.

TFPI is a protease inhibitor that binds Xa and the VIIa-TF complex in a two-step reaction that inhibits further VIIa-TF activation of factor X. It is found both in plasma and bound to the surface of the vascular endothelium. It is unclear whether TFPI deficiency can result in a hypercoaguable state. α_2-**Macroglobulin** is another protease inhibitor capable of complexing with enzymes such as trypsin, plasmin, and kallikrein. Its role clinically is not clear. α_1-**Antitrypsin and C1 esterase inhibitor** may also inhibit serine protease enzymes of the coagulation cascade.

The fibrinolytic system plays a key role in clot formation by localizing the thrombus to the site of injury and dissolving it as part of vessel healing to reestablish blood flow. With thrombus formation, circulating plasminogen is incorporated in the newly formed clot, bound to fibrin. Normal endothelial cells adjacent to the injury site can activate this bound plasminogen to plasmin by the release of t-PA. This is a highly regulated reaction so that thrombolysis is limited to the surface of the clot, thereby providing a sensitive control of thrombus size.

Excessive clot lysis and destruction of circulating fibrinogen is prevented in part by the specificity of the binding of t-PA to the plasminogen-fibrin complex. At least four other inhibitors of fibrinolysis also play a role. A glycoprotein, **plasminogen activator inhibitor-1 (PAI-1)**, is present in plasma at a concentration greater than the physiologic concentrations of t-PA released by endothelial cells. PAI-1 has a high affinity for and binds to any t-PA in circulation. In addition, escape of plasmin into circulation is prevented by its interaction with circulating α_2-**antiplasmin.** This is an extremely rapid and complete reaction and serves to prevent generalized fibrinogenolysis. Activation of intrinsic pathway factors XI and XIII are also involved in stabilizing clot. **Factor XIII** inhibits fibrinolysis by cross-linking fibrin chains and by binding α_2-antiplasmin to fibrin. **Factor XI** activation by thrombin mostly within the clot stimulates the activation of thrombin activatable fibrinolysis inhibitor (TAFI), resulting in the elimination of plasminogen binding sites on the clot surface. Thrombomodulin appears to further enhance this pathway.

By nature of the cross-linking process in fibrin clot formation, degradation results in a series of fragments with distinctive structure. The pattern of fibrin breakdown has been recognized in the development of laboratory tests of fibrin destruction. The most unique product is a fragment called the **D-dimer,** which consists of two cross-linked D moieties originating from two different fibrinogen molecules. Appearance of the D-dimer fragment in circulation is considered to be an indication of active clot turnover.

BIBLIOGRAPHY

Bick RL: *Disorders of Thrombosis Hemostasis: Clinical and Laboratory Practice.* ASCP Press, 1992.

Furie B, Furie BC: Molecular and cellular biology of blood coagulation. N Engl J Med 1992;326:800.

Goodnight SH, Hathaway WE: *Hemostasis & Thrombosis,* 2nd ed. McGraw-Hill, 2001.

Mann KG et al: Surface-dependent reactions of the vitamin K-dependent enzyme complexes. Blood 1990;76:1.

Rapaport SI: Blood coagulation and its alterations in hemorrhagic and thrombotic disorders. West J Med 1993;158:153.

Thompson AR, Harker LA: *Manual of Hemostasis and Thrombosis,* 3rd ed. FA Davis, 1983.

Clinical Approach to Bleeding Disorders

28

Evaluation of a patient for a bleeding tendency is a common routine in clinical medicine. It requires identification of key elements in the patient's history and physical examination and integration of these data with laboratory measurements and therapeutic maneuvers. Often the evaluation is part of the diagnosis and management of another illness, as for example the patient who bleeds excessively during or after surgery or who develops a coagulopathy as a part of a systemic illness. Therefore, successful diagnosis of a bleeding disorder very much depends on the skills of the clinician at the bedside.

CLINICAL EVALUATION

Important diagnostic information is provided by the clinical setting because of the clear associations between bleeding abnormalities and certain disease states. To uncover these relationships, the clinician needs to collect the following data:

- **Who:** The patient's age, sex, racial background, and family history of abnormal bleeding all are important.
- **When:** Any association with a disease state, trauma, surgery, or drug ingestion should be identified. In addition, details of the time of onset and course of the bleeding event are important.
- **Where:** The site or sites of bleeding, whether skin, mucous membranes, gastrointestinal (GI) tract, solid organ, joint, or muscle, need to be identified.
- **What:** The physical characteristics of the bleeding, especially the distinction between petechial (capillary) hemorrhage and the purpura, ecchymoses, and hematoma formation seen with larger vessel bleeding, need to be described.

Based on these data, it is often possible to target the **nature of the bleeding disorder.** Patients who have a hematologic malignancy or are undergoing high-dose chemotherapy are at risk for severe thrombocytopenia. In contrast, patients receiving warfarin can be expected to show an abnormality in the production of the vita-

min K–dependent coagulation factors. Liver disease patients are at risk for developing a multifactor deficiency state and, at times, a defect in fibrinogen structure and function. Finally, patients with severe sepsis can develop a consumptive coagulopathy.

As for the detection of a **congenital coagulopathy,** the absence of any complicating illness or anticoagulant drug exposure obviously directs the clinician's attention to the possibility of an inherited defect. In this situation, the patient's age, sex, and race and the characteristics of the onset and course of the bleeding can be major clues to the diagnosis.

LABORATORY STUDIES

Several laboratory tests are available to evaluate the coagulation pathways. Some of these tests, such as platelet function and assays for specific factor levels, require the expertise of a consultant hematologist and a reference laboratory. Others are available through the routine laboratory. It is the routine tests that every clinician should be able to use in evaluating a coagulation defect (Table 28–1). These tests include the platelet count, bleeding time (BT), prothrombin time (PT), activated partial thromboplastin time (aPTT), thrombin time (TT), assays for fibrinogen concentration and breakdown products, and measurements of inhibitor levels, including antithrombin III and α_2-antiplasmin levels.

A. PLATELET COUNT:

The platelet count can be estimated by inspecting a Wright's stained peripheral film. Normally, at least one platelet is seen for every 20 red blood cells. When the count is severely depressed to levels below 20,000/μL, it can be difficult to identify even a single platelet per high-power field.

An accurate measurement of platelet number can be obtained by light microscopy using a counting chamber and phase microscopy or from any of the available electronic blood cell counters. The normal platelet count should fall between 150,000 and 300,000/μL of whole blood. Falsely low levels can occur if platelets aggregate because of poor anticoagulation of the speci-

Table 28–1. Routine coagulation tests.

Test	Normal Values
Platelet count	150,000–300,000/μL
Bleeding time (BT) (template)	3–7 min
Prothrombin time (PT)	10–12 sec
Partial thromboplastin time (aPTT)	25–38 sec
Thrombin time (TT)	9–35 sec
Fibrinogen assay	
Healthy individuals	200–400 mg/dL
With severe illness	400–800 mg/dL
Fibrin/fibrinogen fragments	
Latex agglutination	0–11 (< 10 μg/mL)
D-Dimer assay	< 500 ng/mL
Antithrombin III level	80–120%
α_2-antiplasmin level	80–120%

men or the presence of an EDTA-sensitive antibody that causes platelet agglutination. Inspection of a stained film from the same blood specimen will usually reveal the platelet aggregates.

B. TEMPLATE BLEEDING TIME (BT):

The BT is used clinically to detect a significant defect in platelet function. A template apparatus (eg, Simplate, General Diagnostics, Warner Lambert Pharmaceuticals, Co.) should always be employed. To perform the technique, a blood pressure cuff is placed around the patient's upper arm and inflated to 40 mm Hg. The volar surface of the forearm is cleaned with alcohol and is air dried. The template is then pressed firmly against the skin and two 1-mm-deep × 10-mm-long incisions are made. A stopwatch is started, and at 30-second intervals the blood from each of the wounds is carefully blotted with filter paper without interfering with the wound itself. A normal BT should range from 3 to 7 minutes.

There is a **direct relationship between the platelet count and the BT** (Figure 28–1). With counts above 100,000/μL and normal platelet function, the BT should be less than 7 minutes. As the count falls below 100,000/μL, the BT lengthens, reaching levels of 20–30 minutes as it approaches 10,000/μL. This predictable relationship makes the determination unnecessary (and inappropriate) in the evaluation of thrombocytopenic patients.

The true value of the BT is to detect a functional defect in a patient with normal platelet count. Both uremia and aspirin therapy prolong the BT to values of 8–15 minutes. These can be highly variable, however,

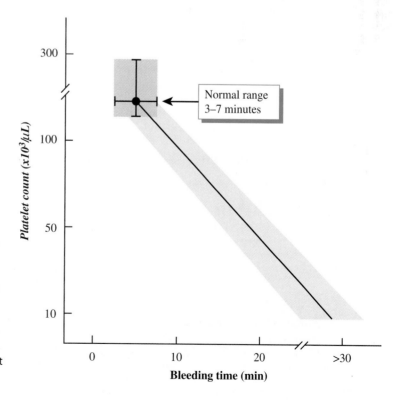

Figure 28–1. The effect of thrombocytopenia on the bleeding time (BT). Normal patients with platelet counts greater than 100,000/μL have a BT of between 3 and 7 minutes. As the platelet count falls below 100,000/μL, the BT becomes progressively longer, reaching values in excess of 25–30 minutes once the count falls below 10,000/μL.

and may not be detectable unless the BT is very carefully done. Some individuals are more sensitive to aspirin than others. At the same time, the BT is of great value in detecting patients with clinically significant von Willebrand disease, a congenital defect in the synthesis of von Willebrand factor (vWF). In this situation, the BT is often longer than 30 minutes.

C. PROTHROMBIN TIME (PT):

The PT provides a measure of the extrinsic and common pathways. Compared with the PTT, it is more sensitive to multiple deficiencies of the vitamin K–dependent liver factors. The assay is performed by adding back to citrated plasma both calcium ion and a commercial or human brain thromboplastin (Figure 28–2). This provides a strong stimulus to the activation of factor VII.

The PT can vary significantly depending on the **type of thromboplastin used.** Commercial thromboplastins generally give normal values of 10–12 seconds, which is somewhat shorter than results for a human brain thromboplastin. When the PT is used to monitor a patient receiving an oral warfarin, the sensitivity of the thromboplastin must be taken into account in interpreting the prolongation of the PT. This situation has led to the development of a standardized method of expressing the prolongation as an **international normalized ratio** (see Chapter 36).

As a screen for any single factor deficiency, the PT is most sensitive to a reduced level of factor VII. In patients with liver disease, the levels of the vitamin K–

dependent factors must be reduced by more than 50–60% to prolong the PT. As a general rule, a PT that is one and a half to two times the control value suggests reduced levels of factors to below 20% of normal. When the PT is greater than two times the control, factor levels are most likely below 10% of normal.

The **PT can also be prolonged** by large amounts of heparin in circulation and either a reduced level of fibrinogen (< 100 mg/dL) or the appearance of abnormal fibrinogen molecules or fragments in circulation. Finally, the PT may be prolonged if the blood specimen is stored too long prior to assay, owing to a breakdown of coagulation proteins.

D. ACTIVATED PARTIAL THROMBOPLASTIN TIME (aPTT):

The aPTT measures both the intrinsic and common pathways (ie, factors XII, XI, IX, VIII, X, and V). For this assay, citrated plasma is activated with a contact surface material such as kaolin, together with calcium ion and a phospholipid (Figure 28–3). Depending on the reagents, the normal aPTT can range from 25 to 38 seconds. Therefore, the clinician must be familiar with the normal range of times for local laboratories.

The **aPTT can be prolonged** by a deficiency of any of the factors in the intrinsic or common pathway, by the presence of a circulating inhibitor, or because of a fibrinogen abnormality. Factor deficiencies must be relatively severe—levels below 40% of normal, multiple, or both—to significantly prolong the aPTT. Al-

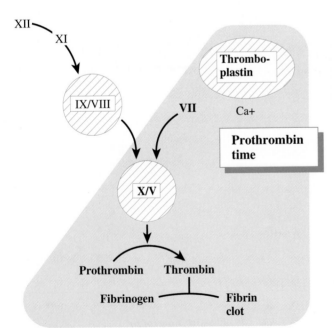

Figure 28–2. **The prothrombin time (PT).** Laboratory measurement of the PT is performed by adding a commercial or human brain thromboplastin and calcium ion to citrated plasma to activate the extrinsic pathway. The test detects deficiencies of factors VII, X, V, prothrombin, and fibrinogen. It is not sensitive to deficiencies of factors in the intrinsic pathway.

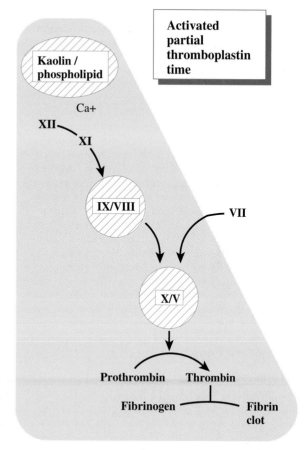

Figure 28–3. **The activated partial thromboplastin time (aPTT).** Laboratory measurement of the aPTT is performed by adding kaolin, phospholipid, and calcium ion to citrated plasma to activate the intrinsic pathway. This test can detect significant deficiencies in factors XII, XI, IX, VIII, X, V, prothrombin, and fibrinogen. It does not detect deficiencies in factor VII. The test is very sensitive to the presence of a circulating anticoagulant (eg, lupus anticoagulant or an antifactor VIII or IX antibody).

though it is somewhat less sensitive than PT to depressions of the vitamin K–dependent factors, it is more sensitive to the presence of a circulating anticoagulant, including heparin and the lupus anticoagulant (**antiphospholipid antibody**). To identify an anticoagulant, the laboratory can perform a repeated aPTT with a 1:1 mix of patient and normal plasma. While the admixture of normal plasma will partially or completely correct a prolonged aPTT secondary to a single factor deficiency (ie, factor VIII or IX deficiency), it will have little or no impact on the aPTT that is prolonged because of a high titer circulating anticoagulant.

E. THROMBIN TIME (TT):

The TT measures the last step in the common pathway, that is, conversion of fibrinogen to fibrin. It is performed by adding a dilute solution of bovine thrombin to citrated plasma. The normal control can be adjusted to give a TT of anywhere from 9 to 35 seconds, depending on the thrombin dilution. Prolonged TTs are seen in patients with decreased or abnormal fibrinogens and high levels of fibrin degradation products. Therefore, it is a

sensitive indicator of disseminated intravascular coagulation (DIC) and liver disease. In addition, even very small amounts of heparin in circulation can dramatically prolong the TT by directly inhibiting the added thrombin.

F. FIBRINOGEN ASSAYS:

The concentration of fibrinogen in plasma is best measured by a chemical or immunologic method where the ability of the fibrinogen to clot does not influence the assay. The normal fibrinogen concentration is 200–400 mg/dL. Fibrinogen is an acute phase reactant, however, and levels of 400–800 mg/dL are common in patients with acute, severe illness.

The level of functional fibrinogen can also be assayed. The **von Clauss kinetic assay** employs a dilute solution of plasma and an excess of thrombin to make fibrinogen the rate-limiting factor in the clotting reaction. The resulting clotting time in seconds is compared with a standard dilution curve to determine the concentration of clottable fibrinogen. This assay is very sensitive to the presence of inhibitors of fibrin formation such as dysfibrinogenemia or the presence of fibrin degradation products.

The presence of fibrin or fibrinogen fragments in serum can be measured directly by a **latex particle agglutination method.** Using latex particles coated with an antiserum to various fragments of fibrin or fibrinogen, it is also possible to semiquantitatively estimate the presence of these fragments. Although a normal individual will show 0 to 1+ agglutination (less than 10 μg/mL), a patient with DIC and marked breakdown of fibrin will be strongly positive, 3 to 4+ agglutination (greater than 10–40 μg/mL). A false-negative test may be observed, however, in some patients with consumptive coagulopathies if the antiserum is not sensitive to the smaller D and E fragments of degraded fibrin. Moreover, positive agglutination reactions are seen in patients with liver disease because of the production of abnormal fibrinogen molecules and elevated levels of immunoglobulins.

The **D-dimer test** for fibrin fragments uses a monoclonal antibody to the cross-linked D regions of degraded fibrin. This test is more specific for the appearance of split products secondary to fibrinolysis and should not detect abnormal fibrinogen molecules or fibrinogen fragments. Normal patients have D-dimer levels below 500 ng/mL, whereas DIC patients can have levels of several thousand ng/mL according to the severity of their illness.

G. TESTS OF FIBRINOLYSIS:

The **euglobulin lysis time** is a screening test for excessive fibrinolysis. It is performed using the plasma euglobulin fraction prepared from fresh, citrated platelet-poor plasma. After clot formation, the time for spontaneous lysis is measured; the normal euglobulin lysis time is from 60 to 300 minutes. It is shortened in conditions characterized by increased fibrinolysis—liver disease, after administration of tissue-type plasminogen activator, α_2-antiplasmin deficiency, plasminogen activator inhibitor (PAI-1) deficiency, or systemic hyperfibrinolysis. However, it is rarely shortened in patients with DIC.

Immunoassays for the levels of antithrombin III and α_2-antiplasmin in plasma can be of value in evaluating the patient with DIC. As the natural inhibitor of thrombin, **antithrombin III** is rapidly depleted whenever thrombin generation increases. The assay for the level of antithrombin III uses as a standard a dilution curve of normal plasma, so that a normal individual is expected to have an antithrombin III level of close to 100% (range 80–120%). A significant depletion is considered to be present whenever the level is below 60%. In situations of severe DIC, it is not unusual to see levels as low as 10–30%. **Antithrombin III deficiency** (levels of 40–60%) is also seen as an inherited family trait and has been correlated with an increased tendency to venous thrombosis.

α_2-**Antiplasmin** is the natural inhibitor of plasmin.

As plasminogen is activated to plasmin, α_2-antiplasmin binds to the plasmin and is rapidly removed from circulation. Thus, the level of α_2-antiplasmin in plasma can be used to evaluate the rate of plasmin generation in fibrinolysis. Like the antithrombin III assay, α_2-antiplasmin levels are measured as percent of normal (range 80–120%). Individuals with dramatically increased levels of fibrin turnover as a part of DIC will have levels well below 60% of normal.

Both antithrombin III and α_2-antiplasmin are produced by the liver. Although they are not vitamin K–dependent factors, severe liver disease is associated with reduced levels of both proteins. This can cause confusion in distinguishing between low-grade DIC and liver disease.

APPROACH TO THE PATIENT

Clinical evaluation of a bleeding patient can be defined as a five-step algorithm (Table 28–2). This also provides a basis for planning management, including the initial decisions regarding the administration of blood components.

Step 1: Is There a Problem With the Patient's Platelets?

Often as not, a platelet problem can be anticipated because of an **associated disease process.** Patients with damaged marrows secondary to aplastic anemia, a hematologic malignancy, or drug exposure (especially chemotherapy) can be expected to present with thrombocytopenia secondary to decreased platelet production. Severe thrombocytopenia secondary to increased destruction can accompany autoimmune and lymphoproliferative disorders (see Chapter 30). Abnormalities in platelet function can be inherited or result from drug exposure (see Chapter 31).

One clinical tip-off to a platelet abnormality is the appearance of **petechial hemorrhages.** Depending on the severity of the thrombocytopenia, they may be limited to the legs or arms or become widespread, involving virtually every organ. Severe thrombocytopenia and platelet functional defects also result in easy bruisability, mucous membrane bleeding, epistaxis, menometrorrhagia, and a tendency for small vessel oozing during surgery.

Screening laboratory tests for a suspected platelet defect include the platelet count and, in those patients with a normal platelet count, a BT to evaluate function. The tendency for abnormal bleeding in patients who are thrombocytopenic is not a simple reflection of the severity of the thrombocytopenia. Although an otherwise normal individual may show little in the way of bleeding until the platelet count falls to below 10,000/μL, patients with a malignancy, an obstetrical complication,

Table 28–2. Evaluation of the bleeding patient.

Step 1:	**Platelet problem?** Thrombocytopenia or a platelet functional defect	Platelet count Bleeding time
Step 2:	**Single factor deficiency?** Factor VII, VIII, IX, X, V, XI, fibrinogen	PT, aPTT
Step 3:	**Multiple factor deficiency?** Vitamin K deficiency, liver disease, warfarin Fibrinogen assay therapy	PT, aPTT, TT
Step 4:	**Circulating anticoagulant?** Heparin, factor VIII or IX antibody, lupus anticoagulant	aPTT with 1:1 mix TT Reptilase time

Step 5:	**Consumptive coagulopathy?**
	TTP, HUS, vasculitis, sepsis, obstetrical complication,
	  trauma, liver disease
		DIC screen:
		  Platelet count
		  PT, aPTT, TT, fibrinogen, antithrombin III, α_2-antiplas-
		  min, D-Dimer assay, blood film

or ongoing sepsis can demonstrate a severe bleeding when the platelet count falls below 20,000/µL. This drop may reflect a combination of thrombocytopenia and platelet dysfunction or an increased requirement for platelets because of endothelial cell damage. The latter possibility is most dramatically illustrated when patients undergo surgery or experience trauma. In this setting, abnormal bleeding can occur when the platelet count falls to below 50,000 or even 100,000/µL.

Clinically significant platelet dysfunction can be detected using the **BT.** The BT is at best a crude test, however, and should not be used as a routine screening test. This situation is especially true for preoperative patients where modest prolongations of the BT do not predict surgical bleeding. It is also difficult to get an accurate measurement when the patient is seriously ill. Patients who are septic, uremic, or receiving a drug that inhibits platelet function can be assumed to have some degree of platelet dysfunction. An attempt to quantitate this by doing a BT can be frustrating and can provide such conflicting data that it is useless. Therefore, the BT should be reserved for patients who have a bleeding history suggestive of an inherited defect in platelet function, as for example patients who may have clinically significant von Willebrand disease.

Step 2: Does the Patient Have an Inherited Coagulopathy, Single-Factor Deficiency?

An inherited coagulopathy may be suspected because of the clinical presentation. The patient with a severe factor deficiency, as for example the factor VIII or factor IX hemophiliac, will usually present with a history of repeated bleeding episodes beginning soon after birth and extending throughout childhood and adult life (see

Chapter 32). When the deficiency is less severe, the patient may report abnormal bleeding following trauma or surgery, an unexplained hemarthrosis, or muscle hematoma. In contrast to the patients with platelet defects, factor-deficient individuals have difficulties with purpura, hemarthrosis, hematomas, and large vessel bleeding, not petechial bleeding.

The **PT and aPTT** are the most valuable screening tests for detecting a single factor deficiency. They must be interpreted as a matched pair. If the PT is significantly prolonged and the aPTT is normal, the patient may have a factor VII deficiency. If the aPTT is very long although the PT is normal, an intrinsic pathway defect, especially factor VIII or factor IX deficiency, is most likely.

This interpretation of PT and aPTT values is only valid in patients with an appropriate clinical history who are not receiving an anticoagulant drug, and who do not have either liver disease or a consumptive coagulopathy. The PT is very sensitive to even modest depletions of the common pathway factors. Therefore, a long PT with a normal aPTT is typical of patients receiving warfarin therapy or who have liver disease. In contrast, the aPTT is more sensitive to heparin and circulating anticoagulants giving a long aPTT, while the PT is normal. These possibilities need to be excluded before concluding that a single-factor deficiency is present.

Step 3: Does the Patient Have a Deficiency of Several of the Vitamin K–Dependent Coagulation Factors?

Both **warfarin therapy** and **liver disease** typically produce multiple factor deficiencies involving the extrinsic and common pathways (see Chapter 33). Patients with severe liver disease can also demonstrate defects in the production of fibrinogen in terms of both the total amount and its functional characteristics. Therefore, it is important to look for any history of poor nutrition, vitamin K malabsorption, coumarin ingestion, or the symptoms and signs that would indicate worsening liver disease.

The **type of bleeding** may also be a clue. As with a single coagulation factor–deficiency state, petechial hemorrhages are not expected; patients usually show a combination of easy bruisability, widespread purpura, and mucous membrane/GI tract bleeding. The severe liver disease patient frequently presents with a dramatic upper GI bleed.

The **PT, aPTT, TT, and fibrinogen assays** are key laboratory tests for the identification of a multiple factor–deficiency state. As mentioned, the PT is very sensitive to modest reductions in the vitamin K–dependent factors, factors VII, IX, X, V, and prothrombin. The vitamin K–deficient patient would be expected to have a very long PT with a normal or slightly prolonged aPTT. Similarly, patients receiving warfarin or with early liver disease would be expected to have a prolonged PT and normal aPTT. In contrast, the patient with more severe liver disease can show prolongations of the PT, aPTT, and TT. The latter reflects the dysfibrinogenemia and buildup of fibrinogen and fibrin breakdown products that act as inhibitors of the TT. Finally, the very severe liver disease patient may also show a discrepancy between the von Clauss fibrinogen assay that detects clottable fibrinogen and an assay of total fibrinogen.

Step 4: Is There a Circulating Anticoagulant Present?

A circulating anticoagulant may explain the patient's bleeding tendency. Administration of **heparin** to prevent venous thrombosis or to maintain catheter patency is almost universal in severely ill patients cared for in intensive care units. This can get out of control, resulting in a prolonged aPTT and TT. It can also be responsible for the patient's bleeding problem.

Pathologic anticoagulants must also be considered. The lupus anticoagulant (antiphospholipid antibody) can occasionally cause a bleeding tendency, although it is more frequently associated with arterial thrombosis. When present, the lupus anticoagulant will usually prolong the aPTT to a greater extent than the PT. The spontaneous appearance of an antifactor VIII or IX antibody can also lead to severe abnormal bleeding. Here again, the aPTT will be preferentially prolonged.

Once considered, it is usually not difficult to confirm the **presence of a circulating anticoagulant.** The use of heparin therapeutically or in the maintenance of

vascular catheters can target heparin as the offending agent. In addition, in contrast to the other circulating anticoagulants, heparin has a dramatic impact on the TT, prolonging it to 60 seconds or more. The routine laboratory is also able to confirm the presence of heparin by neutralizing it with protamine, removing the heparin with an absorbent column, or performing a reptilase/TT.

Presence of a lupus anticoagulant or an antifactor VIII antibody may be confirmed by repeating the aPTT using a 1:1 mix of the patient's plasma and normal plasma. Patients with single or multiple coagulation factor deficiency states will show partial correction of the aPTT as normal plasma is added. There will be little or no correction of the aPTT in the patient with a circulating anticoagulant. This situation reflects the high titer of the anticoagulant that cannot be overcome by addition of a modest amount of normal plasma.

Step 5: Does the Patient Have a Consumptive Coagulopathy?

Depending on the disease process, patients can exhibit a high rate of platelet consumption or an activation of the entire coagulation cascade, DIC. Platelet thrombus formation is seen in conditions such as thrombotic thrombocytopenic purpura (TTP), hemolytic uremic syndrome (HUS), and in some patients with vasculitis. Patients with TTP, HUS, or vasculitis have symptoms and signs of multiple organ damage, especially kidney, brain, and skin damage secondary to small vessel obstruction. Thrombocytopenia is most severe in patients with TTP and less prominent in individuals with HUS or vasculitis. Red blood cell fragmentation is also a tip-off to the presence of one of these conditions.

A. DISSEMINATED INTRAVASCULAR COAGULATION (DIC):

Full-blown DIC is more common (see Chapter 34). It is most often seen in patients who have experienced major trauma, are septic, or who have an obstetrical complication. It is the coagulopathy of the critically ill patient. Clinically, these patients present with widespread bleeding, including purpura, oozing from needle puncture and catheter insertion sites, mucous membrane and GI bleeding, and severe bleeding with surgery.

Hospital laboratories usually offer a battery of coagulation **tests to screen for DIC.** This battery should include a platelet count, PT, aPTT, TT, fibrinogen assay, tests for fibrin fragments, a blood film examination for red blood cell fragmentation, and, if available, antithrombin III and α_2-antiplasmin levels. Together, these tests provide an overview of the major components of the coagulation cascade. The PT and aPTT measure the coagulation factor pathways. The TT, fibrinogen, fibrin breakdown products, antithrombin III, and α_2-antiplasmin assays provide information as to fibrinogen consumption, clot formation, and fibrinolysis. Finally, red blood cell fragmentation on the peripheral film can indicate the presence of a vasculitis and thrombus formation in arterial vessels.

DIC can be **confused with severe liver disease,** especially when it is relatively low grade. This condition reflects the fact that the liver is the major site of production of many of the coagulation factors, including fibrinogen, antithrombin III, and α_2-antiplasmin. It also plays a role in the removal of fibrin degradation products. It is important, therefore, to try to exclude significant liver disease as a part of the diagnosis of DIC.

DEFINITIVE DIAGNOSIS & MANAGEMENT

Routine evaluation of the patient is generally sufficient to plan the first steps in management. This is certainly true for life-threatening bleeds in critically ill patients. For example, severe thrombocytopenia or a platelet functional defect or both should be treated with platelet transfusions in the short-term emergency situation. Similarly, a single-factor deficiency can be effectively reversed by administering the appropriate purified factor or fresh frozen plasma. Treatment with vitamin K and fresh frozen plasma can also be effective in the patient with multiple deficiencies of vitamin K–dependent factors.

As for the DIC patient, effective therapy and survival depends on the clinician's ability to gain control of the clinical disorder that initiated the consumptive coagulopathy. Once the patient's condition is controlled, the DIC patient will respond well to the stepwise replacement of platelets, fibrinogen, and, if necessary, many of the coagulation factors.

Long-term management requires a definitive diagnosis of the patient's condition. This diagnosis may require the expertise of a consultant hematologist and a hemostasis reference laboratory. Several assays can be used to define platelet functional abnormalities and deficiencies in specific factors. It is also possible to identify and quantitate the presence of specific circulating anticoagulants.

BIBLIOGRAPHY

Bick RL: *Disorders of Thrombosis Hemostasis: Clinical and Laboratory Practice.* ASCP Press, 1992.

Goodnight SH, Hathaway WE: *Hemostasis & Thrombosis,* 2nd ed. McGraw-Hill, 2001.

Hoffman R et al: *Hematology: Basic Principles and Practice,* 1st ed. Churchill Livingstone, 1991.

Lind SE: The bleeding time does not predict surgical bleeding. Blood 1991;77:2547.

Owen CA: Historical account of tests of hemostasis. Am J Clin Pathol 1990;93:S3.

Rodgers RPC, Levin J: A critical reappraisal of the bleeding time. Semin Thromb Hemost 1990;16:1.

Thompson AR, Harker LA: *Manual of Hemostasis and Thrombosis,* 3rd ed. FA Davis, 1983.

Vascular Purpura

A vessel wall defect can result in abnormal bleeding despite an otherwise normal coagulation system. Since there are no reliable clinical tests of vascular integrity, diagnosis of an abnormality in vascular structure depends on a high level of suspicion. For example, multiple small telangiectasias on the lips can be a tip-off to the diagnosis of hereditary hemorrhagic telangiectasia. In patients with a normal platelet count and normal platelet function, presence of petechiae, purpura, or excessive bleeding after minor trauma or surgery raises the question of an underlying vascular defect.

NORMAL VESSEL FUNCTION

To maintain normal hemostasis, blood vessels must provide a leak-proof container that resists thrombus formation. As illustrated in Figure 29–1, there is an organized structure to the vessel wall that serves these functions. Endothelial cells that line the blood vessels provide much more than a simple barrier to prevent the escape of blood cells. The endothelial cell is very active metabolically, synthesizing several **mediators that help control the interaction between blood components and the vessel wall.** Some of these, such as prostacyclin (PGI_2), heparan sulfate, plasminogen activator, thrombomodulin, and ADPase, act to maintain blood in its fluid state by counteracting platelet activation, aggregation, and clot formation, whereas others are important in the **migration of leukocytes from circulation into tissues.** These are the integrins (β_1 and β_2), the selectins (ELAM, GMP 140, and leukocyte adhesion molecule [LAM]-1), and the Ig-like receptor, PECAM-1.

Endothelial cells also play a major role in **determining the structure and function of the subendothelium.** This role includes production of components of the subendothelial matrix (ie, elastin, laminin, thrombospondin, fibronectin, and several types of collagen). In addition, endothelial cells control vessel wall tone by continuously secreting prostacyclin and nitric oxide (endothelial-derived relaxing factor [EDRF]). These substances diffuse into the vessel wall and act as potent smooth muscle relaxants. Loss of nitric oxide production because of endothelial cell damage results in immediate vessel spasm. In addition, both prostacyclin and nitric oxide are also released into circulation where they suppress platelet activation.

Vessel Structure

Vessel structure **varies according to the location** in the circulatory system. Although most vessels are lined by a continuous layer of endothelial cells tightly bound to each other, fenestrated endothelium is seen in the sinusoids of the liver and spleen. This situation reflects the special transport needs of these organs.

The subendothelial structure of the vessel **also varies according to functional needs.** For example, larger arteries that must resist high intraluminal pressures have thick muscular walls with a well-defined internal elastic lamina. In the lower-pressure venous circuit, the concentration of smooth muscle cells, elastic tissue, and collagen fibers decreases proportionately.

The **reaction to injury also varies** according to the structure of the vessel. Larger vessels with thick muscular walls rapidly contract when injured to slow or stop blood flow and encourage thrombus formation. Veins and venules are more easily damaged and rely to a greater extent on platelet thrombus formation and activation of the coagulation cascade to seal breaks. In contrast, capillary disruption is associated with much less extensive bleeding, and repair may occur with little involvement of the coagulation system.

CLINICAL FEATURES

Clinical presentation may be enough to make the diagnosis. Clues to look for in the **history** include the clinical pattern of the bleeding, the relationship to minor trauma and drug ingestion, dietary habits, and symptoms or signs of systemic illness. Often, the patient is aware of factors that contribute to the abnormal bleeding and the characteristics of past bleeding episodes.

The **physical examination** by itself may be diagnostic. For example, an elderly patient with marked skin atrophy and multiple bluish-colored ecchymoses on the forearms and backs of the hands almost certainly has senile purpura. In the case of a congenital disorder of subcutaneous collagen, **Ehlers-Danlos syndrome,** the patient's skin lacks its normal resistance to

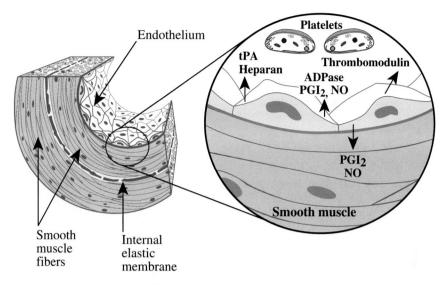

Figure 29–1. **Vessel wall structure and function.** Endothelial cells of the vessel wall play an important role in hemostasis. They produce inhibitors of platelet activation, including ADPase, prostacyclin (PGI_2), and nitric oxide. They also play a role in counteracting clot formation by providing thrombomodulin, heparan, and tissue plasminogen activator. Nitric oxide and prostacyclin produced by the endothelial cell are also important in determining vessel wall tone. When endothelial cells are damaged, the loss of nitric oxide production results in immediate vessel spasm secondary to unopposed smooth muscle contraction.

traction and can be easily pulled away from underlying structures. This condition places blood vessels at great risk for disruption even with minor trauma. Patients with **scurvy** (vitamin C deficiency) can also be identified from their unique physical appearance. First of all, the scurvy patient with abnormal bleeding wall almost always demonstrates marked weight loss and a gait disturbance. Bleeding manifestations include the unique trio of gum bleeding, widespread ecchymoses on the inner upper thighs (saddle distribution), and perifollicular hemorrhages.

Another clue to a vascular abnormality is the **nature of the purpuric lesion.** In patients with vasculitis, individual petechial or purpuric lesion may be slightly raised and firm, so-called **palpable purpura.** This may be immediately preceded by an urticarial lesion in patients with Henoch-Schönlein purpura. As vasculitic lesions resolve, they can leave an area of hyperpigmentation or an atrophic scar. Larger purpuric tumors of the skin are seen in AIDS patients who develop Kaposi's sarcomas and in patients with amyloid deposition in the skin. With amyloidosis, purpura is usually associated with plaques or papules of waxy-appearing skin. Furthermore, skin bleeding can be easily induced in the amyloidosis patient by pinching or stroking the skin. Finally, a careful examination of the mucous membranes is essential to look for the telangiectasia that characterizes patients with hereditary hemorrhagic telangiectasia.

Laboratory Studies

By definition, a patient with vascular purpura should have normal coagulation studies. Routine screening tests should be performed, including a measurement of the platelet count, prothrombin time, and activated partial thromboplastin time. More in-depth studies of platelet function may need to be ordered if the diagnosis is not clear from the patient's history and physical examination. Any attempt to provoke vascular hemorrhage with a test such as the tourniquet test is not recommended. The tourniquet test does not discriminate between vascular bleeding and defects in platelet function. Moreover, even a few moments of compression of venous return from an extremity can result in severe purpura in patients with a major vascular abnormality.

DIFFERENTIAL DIAGNOSIS

Simple bruising of exposed areas of the skin without other signs of abnormal bleeding is a very common complaint. It is seen frequently in fair-skinned women and may be worsened by aspirin ingestion. Some of these individuals actually have very mild von Willebrand disease. Many more appear, however, to have no identifiable defect in platelet function; they simply bruise very easily. In a similar fashion, appearance of a conjunctival hemorrhage brought on by coughing or development in the elderly of purpuric lesions over the lower extremities is best classified as **mechanical purpura;** that is, purpura resulting from increased mechanical stress to a vessel. It does not suggest an underlying vascular or coagulation factor defect.

STRUCTURAL ABNORMALITIES

Abnormalities in structure of the subcutaneous tissue are commonly associated with vascular purpura (Table 29–1). Senile purpura in the elderly patient is a direct result of atrophy of the skin and subcutaneous tissues. Purpura can also be seen in patients receiving prolonged steroid therapy as a result of collagen breakdown. Chronic venous stasis of the lower extremity is another common cause of purpura involving the lower extremities. **Pseudoxanthoma elasticum,** an inherited defect in the elastic fibers of the vessel wall, is associated with skin purpura, severe bleeding from the gastrointestinal (GI) and genitourinary tracts, excessive menstrual bleeding, and spontaneous retinal hemorrhages. These patients can be recognized from their characteristic yellowish xanthomalike skin lesions over the neck and axilla and angioid streaks in the retina. Patients with Ehlers-Danlos syndrome demonstrate abnormalities in the various types of collagen in the vessels and subcutaneous tissues. Because of this, the skin is so fragile that it bruises with the slightest trauma. These patients are easily identified because of their velvety, hyperextensible skin and hyperextensible joints.

More severe bleeding from several sites is more typical of patients with **vitamin C deficiency** and anatomic defects of vessels. The importance of vitamin C in collagen biosynthesis is dramatically illustrated in the scurvy patient. The pathognomonic lesion of scurvy has the appearance of perifollicular hemorrhages surrounding individual deformed, corkscrew-shaped hairs. Easy bruisability and the formation of widespread ecchymoses over the lower extremities, particularly the inner upper thigh (saddle distribution), is also seen, however. Bleeding gums and deep intramuscular and subperiosteal hemorrhages may also be present.

Congenital defects of the vessel wall will also result in an abnormal bleeding tendency. The autosomal dominant disorder, **hereditary hemorrhagic telangiectasia,** is the best example of such an abnormality. The underlying defect is a progressive degeneration of the vessel wall leading to development of widespread angiomatous lesions. On physical examination, these are most easily observed over lips and mucous membranes as small (1–3 mm in diameter), violaceous, nonpulsatile telangiectasias. They blanch with pressure and therefore should not be confused with petechiae. The number of lesions typically increases as the patient ages and this is associated with increased bleeding, especially epistaxis and GI bleeding. The disease is not limited to the skin and mucous membranes; all organs are involved. **Telangiectasias in lung and liver** can expand to form large arterial-venous fistulae. These lesions can lead to a life-threatening hemorrhage or present such an increased demand on cardiac output as to result in high output failure.

Vasculitis

Petechial and purpuric eruptions accompany several bacterial, viral, rickettsial, fungal, and parasitic infections (Table 29–2). A variety of lesions may be seen, including petechiae, discrete purpuric macules and papules, diffuse purpura, hemorrhagic bullae, and marked, widespread purpura with infarction of the skin (**purpura fulminans**). The mechanism involved is not simply damage to the endothelial cell lining. Often as not, there are multiple, simultaneous abnormalities of hemostasis, including thrombocytopenia, disseminated intravascular coagulation, immune-complex vasculitis, and septic emboli. For example, bacterial endocarditis patients will present with a mixture of lesions from simple petechiae to purpuric papules on palms and fingertips (**Osler's nodes**), hemorrhagic lesions of the retina (**Roth spots**), and evidence of immune vasculitis (proteinuria and red cells in the urine).

Sudden appearance of palpable purpura, often preceded by an urticarial rash, suggests a septic or aseptic vasculitis. When a purpuric rash is associated with fever, malaise, polyarthralgia, and colicky abdominal

Table 29–1. Causes of vascular purpura.

Structural abnormalities
Senile/steroid purpura
Pseudoxanthoma elasticum
Ehlers-Danlos syndrome
Scurvy
Hereditary hemorrhagic telangiectasia
Vasculitis
Henoch-Schönlein purpura
Bacterial sepsis
Polyarteritis
Dysproteinemias
Mixed cryoglobulinemia
Multiple myeloma
Waldenstrom macroglobulinemia
Benign hyperglobulinemic purpura
Amyloidosis

Table 29–2. Infectious purpura.

Bacterial
Endocarditis (acute and subacute)
Meningococcemia
Purpura fulminans
Gram-negative sepsis
Henoch-Schönlein purpura
Viral
Parvovirus
Rubella, varicella, roseola
Cytomegalovirus
Coxsackie B6
Herpes (HHV-6)
Hantaan virus
Hemorrhagic fevers
Rickettsial
Rocky mountain spotted fever

pain, a diagnosis of **Henoch-Schönlein purpura** can be made. This syndrome is most common in childhood and early adolescence, although it can also affect young adults. There is often a history of a recent upper respiratory infection suggesting a hypersensitivity reaction to a bacterium such as β-hemolytic streptococcus. The role of an autoimmune reaction is further supported by the appearance of an IgA-immune complex in the serum during the first several weeks of the illness. The vasculitis is not limited to the skin but involves other organs, such as the bowel and kidney. Hemorrhage into the bowel wall is responsible for the abdominal tenderness and colic and can result in a bowel intussusception as hemorrhagic segments of bowel are invaginated into normal segments of bowel. Bleeding from the GI tract can be significant, and in severe cases, bowel necrosis can occur. Renal involvement can also be significant, with hematuria, proteinuria, and transient renal failure. The histologic lesion resembles that of an IgA nephropathy.

Dysproteinemias

Several of the dysproteinemias may be associated with abnormal bleeding (see Table 29–1). **Mixed cryoglobulinemia** can produce a syndrome resembling Henoch-Schönlein purpura with nonthrombocytopenic vascular purpura, vasculitis, polyarthralgia, and nephritis. In patients with **multiple myeloma** or **Waldenstrom macroglobulinemia,** the development of an abnormal bleeding may be multifactorial. When the disease is severe, thrombocytopenia is usually the dominant problem. Other mechanisms may be involved, however, including coagulation factor deficiencies, interference with platelet function (**acquired von Willebrand dis-**

ease), interference with fibrin monomer aggregation, and the development of a vessel wall abnormality. Episodic purpura has also been reported in patients with **diffuse polyclonal hypergammaglobulinemia,** a rare condition that is typically seen in adult females. Most often, development of purpuric lesions over the lower extremities is preceded by localized tenderness or a burning sensation with or without an urticarial eruption. **Aseptic vasculitis** may be detected by biopsy. It may be associated with a collagen vascular disorder such as lupus erythematosus, rheumatoid arthritis, or sarcoidosis. However, patients can have no other apparent abnormality and are carried under the diagnosis of **benign hyperglobulinemic purpura.**

Patients with **amyloidosis** can demonstrate a significant bleeding tendency. Systemic amyloidosis has been associated with factor X deficiency on the basis of selective binding of the coagulation factor to the abnormal M protein. Amyloidosis of the skin is associated with vascular purpura. Typically, purpuric lesions are easily induced by gently pinching or stroking the involved skin areas. Moreover, these patients report the appearance of widespread purpura following minor trauma. Coughing or straining at stool can result in periorbital purpura by increasing hydrostatic pressure.

THERAPY AND CLINICAL COURSE

For those patients who complain of easy bruisability without an identifiable coagulation defect, there is little to offer in the way of treatment. They should be assured of the benign nature of the condition and cautioned against the use of aspirin and nonsteroidal analgesics. The same is true for the elderly patient with senile purpura. The patient should be counseled as to the cause of the purpura and should be urged to try to avoid even minor trauma to the hands, lower arms, and legs.

Conditions that do respond to therapy include vitamin C deficiency and in some instances the aseptic vasculitis of Henoch-Schönlein purpura. In the first case, just a few days of **oral ascorbic acid** (**vitamin C**) will correct the abnormal bleeding tendency. Patients with vasculitis can respond to **corticosteroid therapy** or, in the case of severe multiorgan disease, full **immunosuppressive therapy.**

Patients with hereditary hemorrhagic telangiectasia represent a major management dilemma. As the disease progresses, it is impossible to prevent continuous blood loss. Therefore, treatment must try to provide adequate iron supply to make up for the loss of blood. As discussed in Chapter 5, there are limits to the amount of iron that can be derived from any single route of iron administration. **Oral iron** to the point of GI intolerance will provide only 40–60 mg of iron per day, an amount sufficient to support a marrow production level of only two to three times normal. This situation is often not enough to make up for the amount of blood being lost from the GI tract. Somewhat higher marrow production can be attained by administering intravenous **iron dextran.** To promote maximum marrow production, the iron dextran should be given in doses of 1–2 grams intravenously at monthly intervals together with full oral iron therapy. This treatment will provide sufficient iron supply and delivery to the marrow to support production levels up to three to five times normal. If this does not make up for the blood loss, repeated red blood cell transfusion will be necessary.

BIBLIOGRAPHY

Beutler E et al: *Hematology,* 6th ed. McGraw-Hill, 2001.

Bick RL: *Disorders of Thrombosis Hemostasis: Clinical and Laboratory Practice.* ASCP Press, 1992.

Finder KA et al: Hypergammaglobulinemic purpura of Waldenstrom. J Am Acad Dermatol 1990;23:669.

Francis RB: Acquired purpura fulminans. Semin Thromb Hemost 1990;16:310.

Hoffman R et al: *Hematology: Basic Principles and Practice.* Churchill Livingstone, 1991.

Rainier SS, Sanchez RL: Vasculitis in children. Semin Dermatol 1992;11:48.

Thrombocytopenia

Normal hemostasis requires an adequate number of well-functioning platelets in circulation. Chances of bleeding increase as the platelet count falls. The overall risk to the patient depends, however, on the presence of other disease states. Although a normal individual can tolerate a platelet count less than 10,000/μL, an acutely ill patient is at risk for bleeding with platelet counts of 20,000–30,000/μL or even 100,000/μL if surgery is required. Thus, clinical evaluation must match the degree of thrombocytopenia to the disease state. This is also true in planning management.

NORMAL PLATELET KINETICS

The normal circulating platelet count is maintained within relatively narrow limits (150,000–450,000 platelets/μL in Northern Europeans and 90,000–300,000 platelets/μL in people of Mediterranean descent). The platelet volume is inversely related to the platelet count, so the mass of circulating platelets is the same for these two populations. Approximately one-third of platelets are sequestered in the spleen. Since a platelet has a lifespan of approximately 9–10 days, some 15,000–45,000 platelets/μL must be produced each day to maintain a steady state. New platelet production is the responsibility of the **megakaryocyte,** a very large multinucleated cell (10,750 fL) found in relatively small numbers in the marrow (0.1% of marrow cells). As with other hematopoietic cells, megakaryocytes are derived from the pluripotent stem cell under the control of growth factors such as interleukin (IL)-3, IL-6, granulocyte macrophage colony stimulating factor, IL-11, and a lineage-specific thrombopoietin (c-*Mpl* ligand).

Thrombopoietin (**TPO**) is by far the most important regulatory protein in the production of platelets. The gene for TPO is located on chromosome 3 (3q26-27). TPO mRNA is expressed in the liver, kidneys, and marrow stroma. It translates a 38-kDa protein that is heavily glycosylated to give a 90-kDa glycoprotein with a plasma half-life of 20–30 hours. The receptor for TPO is **c-*Mpl,*** which is present on both megakaryocytes and platelets. The normal plasma TPO level averages 100 pg/mL. Levels rise exponentially as the platelet count falls and then decline as the megakar-

yocyte and platelet mass increase (not just the platelet count). This helps explain why TPO levels and platelet production are not increased in patients with hypersplenism, since splenic pooling does not decrease the megakaryocyte/platelet mass. When TPO is absent, the marrow megakaryocyte mass is reduced by more than 80%.

Endogenous TPO is capable of stimulating megakaryocyte growth (proliferation and endomitosis), cytoplasmic maturation, and platelet release. Recombinant TPO stimulation of the marrow results in visible increases in both the number of megakaryocytes and the size and ploidy (**nuclearity**) of the individual cell by day 3, followed by a rise in the platelet count by day 5. It also results in the release of young platelets that are larger than normal and contain increased RNA, similar to the release of marrow reticulocytes in response to erythropoietin. Platelet production generally can increase by six- to eight-fold within 10 days in response to TPO or increased platelet destruction. Feedback regulation involves uptake and catabolism of TPO by platelets. Therefore, patients with idiopathic thrombocytopenic purpura (ITP) with maximum levels of platelet production will show normal TPO levels as the growth factor is cleared along with the platelets. The effect of TPO on platelet production can also be altered by abnormalities in the megakaryocyte receptor, postreceptor signaling, and TPO clearance.

CLINICAL FEATURES

There are no specific symptoms or unique clinical features that unerringly point to the presence of thrombocytopenia. Patients with very low platelet counts demonstrate significant bleeding from multiple sites including the nose, mucous membranes, gastrointestinal (GI) tract, skin, and vessel puncture sites. One sign that strongly suggests thrombocytopenia is the appearance of a **petechial rash** involving skin or mucous membranes. This condition is usually most pronounced over the lower extremities (increased hydrostatic pressure). Hemarthrosis and hematoma formation are not typical and usually indicate a coagulation factor defect.

Most often, diagnosis of thrombocytopenia is made from **laboratory measurement of the platelet count.**

With modern automated counters, even very low counts can be measured rapidly and accurately. Errors in measurement are limited to undercounting based on sample clotting or because of spontaneous platelet agglutination or binding to circulating white blood cells. Pseudothrombocytopenia is usually detected by the laboratory technologist on inspection of the blood film. There are three principal causes of pseudothrombocytopenia: EDTA-induced agglutination (owing to an IgM or IgG antibody), cold agglutinins, and platelet satellitism (platelet-leukocyte rosette formation).

Development of thrombocytopenia may often be anticipated by the clinician. For example, chemotherapy patients and patients with hematopoietic malignancies are at high risk for impaired platelet production. Septic patients can develop a consumptive thrombocytopenia secondary to activation of the coagulation sequence. Therefore, a careful evaluation of the overall clinical situation to look for an etiologic connection is essential. It is also important in judging the severity of the thrombocytopenia and the need for replacement therapy.

Laboratory Studies

Whenever the etiology of the thrombocytopenia is unclear, studies should be carried out to assess platelet production and destruction. A **marrow aspirate** or **biopsy** or both should be performed to look for a hematopoietic disease process, especially infiltration by a malignant cell line, and to evaluate the number and appearance of megakaryocytes. If available, a measurement of antibodies on the platelet surface can also be performed. The platelet-associated (antiplatelet) antibody assay (**PAIgG assay**) is very sensitive to the presence of IgG, IgM, complement, or all three on the platelet surface.

A strongly positive PAIgG assay in a patient with increased numbers of megakaryocytes in the marrow suggests (but does not prove) an autoimmune destruction defect such as ITP or autoimmune thrombocytopenia secondary to lupus erythematosus or a lymphoproliferative disorder. A weakly positive antiplatelet antibody test is not specific and may be observed in several situations including liver disease and sepsis and with various malignancies. In some of these settings, the thrombocytopenia is the product of several disease mechanisms, including a production defect, increased splenic pooling, and poor survival secondary to nonimmune destruction. Several **phase III assays that measure platelet glycoproteins and antibody binding to these glycoproteins** (GPIIb/IIIa and GPIX) have now been developed. They fall into three broad categories—immunoblot analysis, immunoprecipitation assays, and glycoprotein immobilization assays. While they may be less sensitive than the PAIgG assay, their specificity and positive predictive value for immune-related thrombocytopenia are better, approaching 80–90%.

A few laboratories also offer a test for the **antiplatelet IgG antibody associated with heparin-induced thrombocytopenia.** This is a technically difficult assay; the antibody can only be indirectly detected by measuring the release of serotonin or microparticles from platelets exposed to patient plasma and varying amounts of heparin. Moreover, appearance of the heparin-induced antibody can be evanescent. If the assay is not performed close to the time of the thrombocytopenic event, the antibody may not be detectable.

DIFFERENTIAL DIAGNOSIS

The diagnosis of thrombocytopenia is best organized according to the normal physiology of platelet production, distribution in circulation, and destruction. This protocol provides an overall classification that helps guide the differential diagnosis of specific disease states (Figure 30–1).

Production Disorders

A failure in platelet production can result from **marrow damage** where all aspects of normal hematopoiesis are depressed even to the point of marrow aplasia (**aplastic anemia**). Reductions in marrow megakaryocyte mass are seen in patients receiving radiation therapy or cancer chemotherapy, as a result of exposure to toxic chemicals such as benzene and insecticides, or as a complication of viral hepatitis. An effort should always be made to look for a reversible cause, especially exposure to common drugs such as thiazide diuretics, alcohol, and estrogens. Infiltration of marrow by a malignant process will also disrupt thrombopoiesis. Hematopoietic malignancies including multiple myeloma, the acute leukemias, lymphoma, and myelofibrosis frequently produce a platelet production defect. Metastatic carcinoma and Gaucher's disease are less likely causes. In the newborn, megakaryocyte hypoplasia is a complication of rubella infection during pregnancy or because of the use of thiazide diuretics by the mother. Congenital hypoplastic thrombocytopenia with absent radia (**TAR syndrome**) and Fanconi's syndrome are rarer causes of megakaryocyte hypoplasia. Otherwise unexplained amegakaryocytic thrombocytopenia may initially be confused clinically with ITP because of the severity of the thrombocytopenia. However, a failed response to standard ITP therapy, marrow morphology, and progression to pancytopenia, aplastic anemia, or leukemia confirm the diagnosis.

Reduced production of platelets can also result from an intrinsic **abnormality of the megakaryocyte.** In

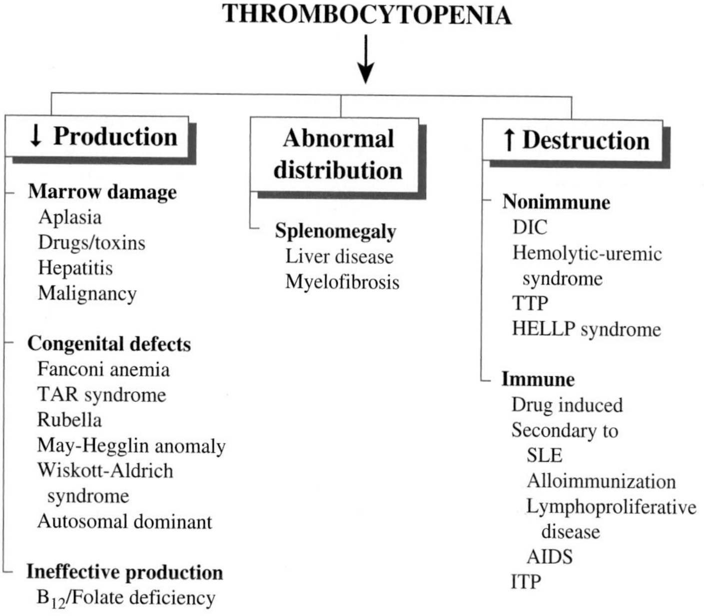

THROMBOCYTOPENIA

```
              ┌──────────────┬──────────────┐
    ┌─────────▼────────┐ ┌───▼────────┐ ┌───▼────────────┐
    │ ↓ Production     │ │ Abnormal   │ │ ↑ Destruction  │
    └──────────────────┘ │distribution│ └────────────────┘
                         └────────────┘
```

↓ Production

Marrow damage
Aplasia
Drugs/toxins
Hepatitis
Malignancy

Congenital defects
Fanconi anemia
TAR syndrome
Rubella
May-Hegglin anomaly
Wiskott-Aldrich
 syndrome
Autosomal dominant

Ineffective production
B$_{12}$/Folate deficiency

Abnormal distribution

Splenomegaly
Liver disease
Myelofibrosis

↑ Destruction

Nonimmune
DIC
Hemolytic-uremic
 syndrome
TTP
HELLP syndrome

Immune
Drug induced
Secondary to
 SLE
 Alloimmunization
 Lymphoproliferative
  disease
 AIDS
ITP

Figure 30–1. **Differential diagnosis of thrombocytopenia.** Evaluation of thrombocytopenia is best organized according to the apparent defect in platelet production, distribution, or destruction.

this situation, the marrow megakaryocyte mass is increased but formation of new platelets is reduced (**ineffective thrombopoiesis**). Several hereditary thrombocytopenias are characterized by ineffective platelet production, including May-Hegglin anomaly, Wiskott-Aldrich syndrome, and autosomal dominant thrombocytopenia. The patient with **May-Hegglin anomaly** typically has bizarre, giant platelets in circulation and **Döhle bodies** (basophilic inclusions) in white blood cells and platelets. Platelet production is variably ineffective; one-third of patients are significantly thrombocytopenic and at risk for bleeding. **Wiskott-Aldrich syndrome** is an X-linked disorder that presents with a combination of eczema, immune deficiency, and thrombocytopenia. Circulating platelets are smaller than normal, function poorly, and have a reduced survival. The latter, however, is not enough to explain the severity of the thrombocytopenia; ineffective thrombopoiesis is the principal abnormality. Finally, patients with **autosomal dominant thrombocytopenia** generally show increased megakaryocyte mass with ineffective production and in some cases the release of macrocytic platelets into circulation. Many of these patients have nerve deafness and nephritis (**Alport's syndrome**).

Ineffective thrombopoiesis is also seen in patients with vitamin B$_{12}$ or folate deficiency, including patients with alcoholism and defective folate metabolism. The defect is identical to the maturation defect seen in the red blood cell and white blood cell lines. Marrow megakaryocyte mass is increased, but effective platelet production is reduced. This failure in platelet production is rapidly reversed by appropriate vitamin therapy.

Disorders of Distribution

The total number of platelets available for hemostasis includes those in circulation and an exchangeable pool of platelets in the spleen. Normally, up to one-third of platelets are held within the spleen. With conditions that produce splenomegaly, this trapping can increase significantly. However, since platelets in the splenic pool continue to be in equilibrium with those in circulation, platelet survival is relatively normal and there is little risk of thrombocytopenia-related bleeding.

Splenomegaly by itself should not reduce the platelet count to below 40,000–50,000/μL. With lower counts, it is important to look for a concomitant defect in platelet production or destruction. For example, patients with lymphomas or autoimmune disease can demonstrate both increased splenic pooling and a reduced platelet survival secondary to an autoantibody. In this situation, splenectomy can be an effective therapy. In contrast, patients with advanced liver disease who demonstrate congestive splenomegaly without a reduction in platelet life span do not benefit from splenectomy. The bleeding tendency of the cirrhotic patient is a multifactorial problem where deficiencies in coagulation factors and abnormal fibrinolysis are more significant issues.

Patients with **advanced myelofibrosis** develop marked splenomegaly with extramedullary hematopoiesis. In this circumstance, the spleen becomes both a production and destruction organ, and it can be extremely difficult to determine the balance between the two. Patients may present with thrombocytopenia, suggesting a marked pooling/destruction defect, or a very high platelet count indicating excessive production. Furthermore, splenectomy can dramatically upset the balance, either by converting the thrombocytopenic patient to one with marked thrombocytosis or by further crippling platelet production to accentuate an already severe thrombocytopenia.

Nonimmune Destruction Disorders

Platelet consumption as a part of intravascular coagulation is seen in several clinical settings. When the entire coagulation pathway is activated, the process is referred to as **disseminated intravascular coagulation (DIC)**. It can be dramatic, with severe thrombocytopenia and marked prolongations of coagulation factor assays, or more "low grade," with little or no thrombocytopenia and less tendency for abnormal bleeding.

Platelet consumption also occurs as an isolated process (**platelet DIC**). Viral infections, bacteremia, malignancy, high-dose chemotherapy, and vasculitis regardless of etiology can result in sufficient endothelial cell damage to dramatically increase the rate of platelet use without full activation of the coagulation pathway. Basically, this is an accentuation of the normal vessel repair process, where platelets adhere to exposed nonendothelial surfaces and then aggregate with fibrinogen binding. With marked endothelial disruption, enough platelets will be consumed to result in thrombocytopenia. Vessel occlusion is not the rule but can occur with severe vasculitis. AIDS patients can develop a consumptive thrombocytopenia with organ damage secondary to arterial thrombosis.

Thrombotic thrombocytopenic purpura (TTP) and **hemolytic uremic syndrome (HUS)** are two overlapping syndromes characterized by nonimmune platelet consumption, platelet thrombus formation, and organ damage. The TTP syndrome complex includes fever, thrombocytopenia with an otherwise negative DIC screen, multiple small vessel occlusion involving both the kidney and central nervous system (CNS), and microangiopathic anemia with schistocyte formation. The presence of schistocytes on the peripheral blood smear is considered to be essential to the diagnosis. **Schistocytosis** results from mechanical fragmentation of red cells flowing past intrarteriolar platelet thrombi.

TTP can occur as a chronic, relapsing illness, on a familial basis, after chemotherapy (mitomycin C, pentostatin, gemcitabine cyclosporine) or bone marrow transplantation, with ticlopidine therapy, or as a post-partum complication. However, most cases occur sporadically and have no clear cause. The immediate mechanism behind the thrombotic thrombocytopenia would appear to be a deficiency in von Willebrand factor (vWF)–cleaving protease activity based on an inherited trait or, in the case of sporadic cases, an antibody directed at the enzyme. This results in the appearance in circulation of very large vWF multimers, which bind to platelets and stimulate aggregation. Although it has traditionally been thought to be a rare disorder, the incidence of TTP and TTP-related deaths appears to be on the rise in many communities. Whether this is a true increase or the result of a heightened awareness is unclear.

The syndrome of HUS is characterized by a severe nonimmune hemolytic anemia and renal failure, without CNS abnormalities, marked thrombocytopenia, or prominent schistocytosis. A similar underlying mechanism of small vessel platelet occlusion, nonautoimmune hemolysis, and the impairment of renal function makes it important, however, to consider both syndromes as a continuum (TTP-HUS) in the differential diagnosis. Pure HUS is more commonly seen in children and young adults in association with hemorrhagic colitis, secondary to verotoxin-producing enteric bacteria, especially the *Escherichia coli* serotype O157:H7. Food-borne outbreaks have resulted from ingestion of poorly cooked contaminated meat. One distinguishing laboratory feature may be the level of vWF-cleaving protease in plasma. TTP patients typically have low or undetectable levels, while classic HUS patients have normal levels.

Thrombocytopenia is a frequent complication in **pregnancy.** Mild thrombocytopenia (platelet counts greater than 70,000/μL), seen in 6–7% of women at gestation, is most often a physiological change, similar to the dilutional anemia of pregnancy. Thrombocytopenia in association with hypertension is observed in 1–2% of pregnancies, and as many as 50% of preeclamptic mothers will develop a DIC-like picture with severe thrombocytopenia, platelet counts of 20,000–40,000/μL, at the time of delivery. This is referred to as the **HELLP syndrome** and is recognized from the combination of red blood cell hemolysis (*H*), elevated liver enzymes (*EL*), and low platelet count (*LP*). Physiologically, it very much resembles TTP. Control of the patient's hypertension and completion of the delivery is usually enough to bring the process to a halt. However, some patients will go on to full-blown TTP-HUS following delivery. Postpartum TTP is a severe illness with a poor prognosis.

Autoimmune Thrombocytopenia

Thrombocytopenia is a common manifestation of autoimmune disease. A list of conditions associated with autoimmune destruction of platelets can be found in Table 30–1. The severity of the thrombocytopenia is highly variable. With some conditions the patient's platelet count falls to as low as 1000–2000/μL. In other patients, the ability of the megakaryocytes to increase platelet production results in a compensated state with platelet counts ranging from 20,000/μL to near normal levels.

Diagnosis of immune destruction can usually be made from the clinical presentation and demonstration of an **increase in marrow megakaryocyte number and ploidy.** Expansion of the megakaryocyte mass is taken as prima facie evidence that a high rate of platelet production is trying to compensate for a shortened survival of platelets in circulation. The more severe the thrombocytopenia, the easier the diagnosis, since the disparity between marrow megakaryocyte proliferation and platelet count is most pronounced. Diagnosis is more difficult when the thrombocytopenia is less severe and there is no obvious clinical condition to explain the finding. In this situation, an **assay for platelet-associated antibody, a measurement of platelet lifespan, or both** may be necessary to make the diagnosis.

Table 30–1. Types of autoimmune thrombocytopenia.

Neonatal thrombocytopenia
  Isoimmune
  Associated with maternal ITP
  Drug-related
Drug-induced (immunologic)
  Drug-dependent (haptens) quinidine, quinine, sedormid
  Drug-related sulfonamides, gold salts, antibiotics, etc
  Heparin-induced
Lymphoma/leukemia
Autoimmune disorders
  Lupus erythematosus
  Thyroiditis
  Colitis/ileitis
Infectious disease
  HIV infection
  Rubella, rubeola, and chickenpox in children
  Infectious mononucleosis
  Viral hepatitis
  Cytomegalovirus
  Lyme disease
  Sarcoidosis/histoplasmosis
Post-transfusion purpura
Marrow transplantation
Idiopathic (ITP)
  Acute ITP (? viral induced)
  Chronic ITP

A. NEONATAL THROMBOCYTOPENIA:

Neonates are at risk for thrombocytopenia either owing to alloimmune sensitization during pregnancy or as a result of maternal autoimmune thrombocytopenia (Figure 30–2). Alloimmune thrombocytopenia is associated with a high incidence of intracranial hemorrhage. Mothers who lack the PL[A-1] platelet antigen are at risk for alloimmunization when the fetus is PL[A-1] positive. Less commonly, other alloantigens (Baka, Bra) or class 1 HLA antigens are targets for sensitization. Most affected children are delivered without difficulty but soon after develop petechiae and purpuric lesions. The thrombocytopenia can be severe and, if left untreated, will persist for several weeks. If available, measurement of platelet-associated antibody and the specificity of antibody in the newborn's plasma to the PL[A-1] antigen can be diagnostic. Since only 2% of the population lacks the PL[A-1] platelet antigen, a demonstration that the mother's platelets are PL[A-1] negative also suggests alloimmunization.

Measurements of in utero fetal platelet counts by cordocentesis in women who are known to be PL[A-1] negative have shown counts below 20,000/μL before 24 weeks' gestation in 50% of affected children. Furthermore, for those with counts above 80,000/μL, repeated measurement demonstrated a fall of approximately 10,000/μL per gestation week, resulting in severe thrombocytopenia by the time of birth in most children. This is associated with a 10–20% chance of intracranial hemorrhage, a quarter of which occur while in utero. When there is a history of a previous birth complicated by alloimmunization and intracranial hemorrhage, chances of severe thrombocytopenia with hemorrhage are even higher. This has led to the recommendation to treat such mothers with intravenous immunoglobulin plus or minus steroids.

Children born to mothers with chronic autoimmune thrombocytopenic purpura (ITP) are also at risk for immune thrombocytopenia, since the mother's antibody crosses the placenta. However, the incidence of severe neonatal thrombocytopenia complicating maternal ITP is very low. Fewer than 12% of newborns of ITP mothers will have platelet counts below 50,000/μL and 5% or less have platelet counts below 20,000/μL. Intracranial hemorrhage or a life-threatening bleed is very uncommon, with a reported incidence of below 1%. The chance of being affected correlates to some degree with the severity of the mother's illness; very high levels of maternal platelet-associated IgG place the fetus at greatest risk. Therefore, these mothers need to be monitored during pregnancy and treated according to the severity of their thrombocytopenia to suppress antibody production. A history of severe neonatal thrombocytopenia in a sibling is another indicator of more severe disease.

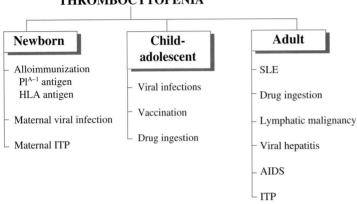

AUTOIMMUNE THROMBOCYTOPENIA

Newborn
- Alloimmunization
  PI^(A-1) antigen
  HLA antigen
- Maternal viral infection
- Maternal ITP

Child-adolescent
- Viral infections
- Vaccination
- Drug ingestion

Adult
- SLE
- Drug ingestion
- Lymphatic malignancy
- Viral hepatitis
- AIDS
- ITP

Figure 30–2. **Diagnosis of autoimmune thrombocytopenia.** The patient's age and clinical presentation can provide a basic structure for evaluating an autoimmune thrombocytopenia. The differential diagnosis for each age group is distinctly different.

B. POSTVIRAL THROMBOCYTOPENIA IN CHILDREN:

During childhood and adolescence, an abrupt onset of severe autoimmune thrombocytopenia most often is related to a recent viral infection. The incidence is highest before 10 years of age. The affected child presents 1–2 weeks after an infection such as rubella, rubeola, or chickenpox or a respiratory viral infection with petechial and purpuric lesions of the skin and mucous membranes. Immunization with live vaccine for measles, chickenpox, mumps, and smallpox can also act as an inciting event. When petechial and purpuric lesions are widespread, thrombocytopenia is usually severe, with counts less than 10,000/µL. The rest of the blood count is normal, although the number of activated lymphocytes in circulation may be increased. Examination of a marrow aspirate should reveal normal to increased numbers of megakaryocytes. Assays for platelet-associated antibody are usually positive, especially if performed when the thrombocytopenia is first detected.

Generally, the clinical presentation makes diagnosis of immune thrombocytopenia in children relatively easy. Absence of fever, organ damage that would suggest platelet thrombus formation, or an abnormal cell morphology of a hematologic malignancy rules out diagnoses such as sepsis (especially meningococcemia), TTP or HUS, or acute leukemia. When there is no evidence for any of these, bone marrow and platelet-associated antibody studies need not be performed before initiating intravenous immune globulin therapy. Additional testing can be reserved for those children who have failed therapy after 6–12 months or who are being considered for splenectomy. Drug-induced thrombocytopenia must be considered in any child taking a medication in the weeks preceding the fall in the platelet count. A good rule is to stop all medications immediately, even if the association is unlikely.

C. THROMBOCYTOPENIC PURPURA IN ADULTS:

Differential diagnosis of autoimmune thrombocytopenia in the adult begins with a careful history to identify any exposures to drugs, blood products, or viral infections (see Figure 30–2). As a corollary to neonatal thrombocytopenia, PL^(A-1)-negative adults can develop post-transfusion purpura following exposure to a blood product. In this situation, PL^(A-1) antigen contributed by the transfusion product in a soluble form transfers to the patient's PL^(A-1)-negative platelets, which results in the patient's immune system generating anti-PL^(A-1) antibodies that destroy the patient's own platelets. Although multiparous PL^(A-1)-negative women are at greatest risk, post-transfusion purpura has been reported in both men and women. Usually, a potent alloantibody with PL^(A-1) specificity is readily detected in the patient's plasma.

1. Association with drugs—Several drugs can produce an immune thrombocytopenia. Quinine, quinidine, and sedormid are the best known and have been studied extensively. Clinically, patients present with severe thrombocytopenia, with platelet counts below 20,000/µL. These drugs act as haptens to trigger antibody formation and then serve as obligate molecules for antibody binding to the platelet surface. At least for these drugs, the antibodies appear to reversibly bind by their FAB regions to platelet membrane GPIb/IX or GPIIb/IIIa receptors or both. This results in a conformational change and the exposure of a neoepitope, leading to antibody formation. Thrombocytopenia can also occur within hours of the first exposure to a drug because of pre-formed antibodies with reactivity against the suddenly exposed neoepitope. This has been reported with varying frequency with abciximab (ReoPro) therapy. Other drugs, such as alpha methyldopa, sulfonamides, and gold salts, also stimulate autoantibodies. They are not, however, obligate haptens in the resultant platelet destruction.

2. Association with heparin—The association of heparin with thrombocytopenia deserves special emphasis. In patients receiving heparin for more than 4–6 days, IgG antibodies to heparin-platelet factor 4 complex can form that are capable of binding to FC receptors on platelets. Moreover, heparin-induced antibodies are capable of inducing platelet activation, aggregation, and thrombus formation, which can result in severe tissue damage (loss of limbs, strokes, myocardial infarction) and unusual sites of thrombosis (adrenal, portal vein, skin). The incidence of **heparin-induced thrombocytopenia** (**HIT**) varies with the type of heparin used. Although 10–15% of patients receiving bovine heparin develop an antibody, fewer than 6% of patients receiving porcine heparin will.

The risk of developing HIT is related both to the dose of heparin and duration of therapy. Patients receiving full-dose heparin for more than 5 days or who receive heparin on more than one occasion should be closely monitored for the development of thrombocytopenia. Even a modest fall in the platelet count (50,000–150,000/μL) can signal the appearance of an antibody and mandate stopping the heparin. If heparin is continued, there is a significant risk of a major thromboembolic event. The risk varies with the clinical situation, reaching 40–50% in postoperative patients with high circulating levels of thrombin. Acute HIT can occur in patients restarted on heparin within 20 days of a prior exposure. The patient can appear to have an acute drug reaction with a sudden onset of severe dyspnea, shaking chills, diaphoresis, hypertension, and tachycardia. Such patients are at extreme risk of a fatal thromboembolism if heparin is continued.

3. AIDS/HIV infection—Thrombocytopenia is a common complication of HIV infection and may be the first manifestation of the disease. Early on, there is both impaired production and immune destruction of platelets secondary to immune complex binding to platelets. Megakaryocytes may be increased or decreased in number, platelet survival is significantly reduced, and platelet function is supernormal. Tests for antiplatelet antibodies are usually positive, with detection of IgG, IgM, and complement on the platelet surface. Although 10–20% of patients may experience a spontaneous remission, most behave like chronic ITP patients and require therapy with some combination of zidovudine (AZT), steroids, and immune globulin. As the disease progresses, platelet production fails and patients become resistant to therapy. This condition may relate to a direct infection of megakaryocytes by the virus, since megakaryocytes have CD4 on their surface.

Therefore, end-stage AIDS patients can show severe thrombocytopenia with a greater tendency for bleeding complications.

4. Lymphoproliferative and autoimmune disorders—Immune destruction of platelets is a common component of several lymphoproliferative and autoimmune disorders. Hodgkin's disease, non-Hodgkin's lymphoma, and chronic lymphocytic leukemia are associated with production of autoantibodies with platelet specificity. Autoimmune thrombocytopenia can complicate organ and marrow transplantation. It can also occur in nonmalignant situations when the immune system is stimulated as, for example, with infectious mononucleosis, histoplasmosis, sarcoidosis, viral infections, viral hepatitis, and Lyme disease.

Thrombocytopenia can be an early manifestation of autoimmune diseases, especially systemic lupus erythematosus, and may precede other symptoms and signs. It is important, therefore, to look for a history of arthralgia, arthritis, skin disease, unexplained pleurisy, hepatitis, or inflammatory bowel disease. Laboratory evaluation of any patient with autoimmune thrombocytopenia should include tests for rheumatoid factor, complement levels, and antinuclear antibodies including single- and double-stranded DNA. A search should also be made for other autoantibodies including red blood cell antibodies (Coombs' test), a circulating anticoagulant, and in patients with white blood cell counts of less than 4000/μL, antileukocyte antibodies.

D. IDIOPATHIC THROMBOCYTOPENIC PURPURA (ITP):

Thrombocytopenia unrelated to a drug, an infection, or autoimmune disease is generally classified as (**autoimmune**) **ITP.** This diagnosis can only be made by excluding all other causes of nonimmune and immune destruction. Similar to immune thrombocytopenia in children, it can be an acute disease in adults. However, most cases proceed to a chronic form of ITP where a continued high level of marrow platelet production is required to maintain a chronically low to near normal platelet count in the face of a shortened platelet life span.

ITP patients usually present because of **abnormal bleeding.** The site of the bleeding may vary, although petechial and purpuric lesions of the skin and mucous membranes are most typical. Some patients report increased bruising, recurrent epistaxis, or menorrhagia for some weeks or months prior to presentation. Typically, thrombocytopenia must be severe before bleeding becomes a problem. This condition reflects the fact that the high level of platelet production that occurs in these patients is associated with an output of platelets that demonstrate better than normal function. The latter provides some protection for the patient; ITP patients with platelet counts even as low as 2000/μL are usually not at great risk for a major organ or intracerebral bleed. Patients with chronic ITP generally show less severe thrombocytopenia, with platelet counts of 20,000–100,000/μL. The least severe of these can be very difficult to diagnose. Whereas severe autoimmune thrombocytopenia typically shows a normal or increased number of megakaryocytes with increased ploidy in the marrow, the least severe of the chronic ITP patients may have little or no expansion of the marrow megakaryocyte mass together with a relatively modest shortening of platelet life span. In this situation, assays for platelet-associated antibody or direct measurements of platelet life span may be the only way to make the diagnosis.

Studies of **platelet-associated immunoglobulins** in ITP patients show varying amounts of IgG, IgM, IgA, and complement on the platelet surface, although an increase in platelet-associated IgG is the most consistent finding. By phase III assays, the immunoglobulins show specificity for the platelet glycoproteins GP-Ib, -IIB, -IIIa, as well as the GP-IIb/IIIa complex. Interaction of the antibody with this site only rarely produces a functional abnormality, however. The principal effect is rapid removal and destruction of involved platelets. Measurements of platelet-associated antibody have a long and checkered history. When methods are compared, they appear to be highly variable in their sensi-

tivity and specificity. Moreover, extensive studies of these assays in thrombocytopenic patients have failed to show a unique ITP pattern. Because of this, the antiplatelet antibody assay has not become the gold standard for the diagnosis of ITP.

ITP patients can also have **unbound antibody in their plasma.** Studies of the effect of infusing plasma from ITP patients into normal subjects have demonstrated the destructive effect on platelets of this free antibody (Figure 30–3). Furthermore, platelet life span measurements using homologous and autologous platelets in ITP patients typically show dramatically shortened life spans. Platelet survivals in the most severely affected patients can be measured in hours rather than days, with destruction mainly in the spleen. With less severe ITP, radiolabeled homologous and autologous platelet survivals show a more variable picture. Some patients demonstrate only modest shortenings in platelet survival suggesting a subnormal rate of platelet production. This situation may indicate the presence of an antibody with enough specificity for the megakaryocyte to result in a suppression of megakaryocyte proliferation and platelet production. This inconsistency in the behavior of ITP autoantibodies is reflected in the patient's response to therapeutic platelet transfusions. Although most ITP patients receiving platelet transfusions rapidly destroy most of the product, up to

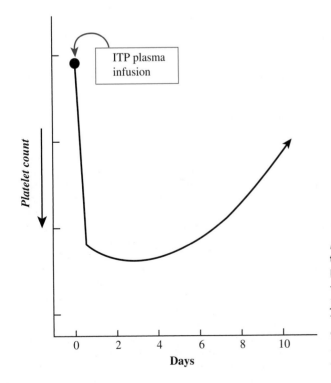

Figure 30–3. **Thrombocytopenia in response to an infusion of plasma from a patient with ITP.** Patients with ITP often have unbound antibody in their plasma that when infused into a normal subject will cause a sudden and dramatic thrombocytopenia. Platelets are rapidly cleared by reticuloendothelial cells of the spleen and liver. Over the next several days, antibody is cleared from circulation and new platelets are produced.

30% of patients can demonstrate near normal post-transfusion platelet increments and survivals.

THERAPY AND CLINICAL COURSE

As with the diagnosis, therapy should be planned according to the pathophysiologic defect, whether an abnormality of platelet production, distribution in circulation, or destruction. Management decisions may need to be made before the full workup is completed. In this case, they must be based on the clinician's best guess as to the disease process. Regardless of the cause of the thrombocytopenia, platelet transfusions are appropriate if the patient is experiencing a life-threatening hemorrhage or is bleeding into a closed space such as an intracranial hemorrhage. Long-term management usually requires other therapeutic maneuvers to either improve platelet production or decrease high levels of platelet destruction.

Production Disorders

A. PLATELET TRANSFUSION:

Platelet transfusions are a mainstay in the management of patients with platelet production disorders. Random donor platelets are separated from units of donated whole blood by centrifugation or from a single donor by cytapheresis (Chapter 37). A unit of apheresis platelets is equivalent to a random donor pool of 6–10 units. For patients who become alloimmunized to donor platelets, blood banks also provide HLA-matched single-donor platelets. Based on the patient's HLA type, donors can be selected for best fit for HLA identity. The more closely HLA-matched the platelets, the better chance they have of surviving in a multiply transfused, alloimmunized patient. Platelet crossmatching has also been used in some blood centers to predict compatibility. It may, in the right hands, be better than HLA-matching.

1. Tailoring therapy to the patient—Platelet transfusion therapy must be tailored to the severity of the thrombocytopenia, the presence of bleeding complications, and the patient's underlying disorder (Table 30–2). A normal individual can tolerate a platelet count of 5000–10,000/μL without difficulty. The uncomplicated patient undergoing chemotherapy does not need to have a prophylactic transfusion until the platelet count falls below 10,000/μL. At the same time, patients with sepsis, malignancy, leukemia, or complication of pregnancy are at risk for bleeding with platelet counts of 20,000–30,000/μL. Even higher platelet counts are needed when a patient requires surgery. For relatively minor procedures such as catheter insertions, biopsies, or lumbar puncture, the platelet

Table 30–2. Recommended platelet counts per μL to avoid bleeding.

Platelet Count	Clinical Condition
> 100,000	Major surgery
> 50,000	Trauma, minor surgery
> 20,000	Prevention of bleeding in patients with sepsis Leukemia, malignancy
> 5–10,000	Normal individuals
< 5000	ITP patients at low risk

count should be above 50,000/μL. If major surgery is required, the platelet count should, if possible, be increased to 100,000/μL to control bleeding. Maintenance transfusions of platelets during and after surgery may also be necessary if there is considerable platelet consumption. Therefore, platelet counts immediately after transfusion and at frequent intervals are important in planning for further platelet needs (Figure 30–4).

The **usual platelet transfusion order** is for a single unit of apheresis platelets or a pool of 4–8 units of random blood donor platelets. Hospitalized, uncomplicated chemotherapy patients requiring prophylactic platelet transfusions can be given fewer units (3-unit pool) at more frequent time intervals with a saving in the total number of units transfused. Random and single donor platelets are not type-specific to the recipient, other than ABO type. In fact, since they contain very few red blood cells, they do not even need to be ABO compatible. In Rh negative women of childbearing age, sufficient red blood cells are transfused to raise a risk of sensitizing the mother. Therefore, such women should receive Rh negative products or be treated with RhoGAM following transfusion.

2. HLA alloimmunization—Each unit of apheresis platelets or six units of random donor platelets (six-pack) should raise the platelet count in a normal size (70 kg) adult by ~50,000/μL (Figure 30–4). This condition assumes, of course, no problems with alloimmunization or an increased rate of destruction secondary to a complicating illness. If a patient is exposed repeatedly to platelet transfusions, HLA alloantibodies can develop that will effectively shorten the life span of transfused platelets. Usually, such antibodies will not appear before 1–2 months after exposure to blood products and are less likely to occur in immunosuppressed patients.

To detect HLA alloimmunization, a platelet count should be measured 1 hour after transfusion. If it is far below the expected increment, HLA sensitization is

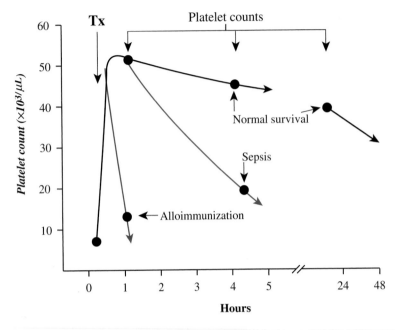

Figure 30–4. **Platelet transfusion therapy.** Transfusion of a single unit of pheresed platelets or a six-pack of random donor platelets should increase the platelet count by 50,000/μL. Post-transfusion platelet counts should be measured at 1, 4, and 24 hours to determine survival. Alloimmunized and septic patients will show dramatically reduced recoveries (a low count at 1 hour) or survivals or both.

possible. Such patients can be HLA-typed and transfused with single-donor HLA-matched platelets or cross-matched platelets. The diagnosis is likely if this produces a better increment at 1 hour. When HLA-matched or cross-matched platelets do not give a good result, a careful evaluation should be made to look for other causes of nonimmune or immune platelet destruction. Finally, to plan subsequent platelet transfusions, measurements of the platelet count need to be performed at intervals post-transfusion, usually at 4 and 24 hours (see Figure 30–4). More frequent measurements may be needed in the acutely ill patient who is consuming large amounts of platelets because of a vasculitis or DIC related to sepsis.

3. Adverse reactions—Adverse reactions associated with platelet transfusion are similar to those of other blood products. Immediate febrile reactions are most often the result of leukocyte-related cytokines in the platelet supernatant and may be ameliorated by using leukodepleted platelet concentrates (double spun or filtered) and by premedicating the patient. Bacterial contamination resulting in sepsis is somewhat more common than that seen with red cell transfusion, inasmuch as platelets are stored at room temperature. Despite routine testing, there is a small risk of transmission of non-A, non-B, non-C hepatitis. Routine testing for HIV and human T-cell leukemia virus-1 (HTLV-1) largely eliminates the risk for transmission of these viruses. Testing for cytomegalovirus (CMV) can be very important in patients undergoing transplantation. The

CMV-negative transplant patient should receive CMV-negative product.

4. Long-term management—Long-term management of the patient with a platelet production defect depends on the cause and the ability to reverse the production abnormality. For example, thrombocytopenia in the leukemic patient should reverse with effective control of the leukemia. In this situation, platelet transfusion support is only required during periods of ablative chemotherapy. Patients with irreversible marrow damage will require chronic platelet transfusions. Although this is technically feasible, the risk of alloimmunization is very high.

Patients with ineffective thrombopoiesis secondary to an intrinsic abnormality of megakaryocytes may be treated similarly to those with a production disorder when there is a bleeding episode. Ineffective thrombopoiesis associated with either vitamin B_{12} or folate deficiency should be immediately treated with appropriate vitamin therapy. Recovery of the platelet count to normal occurs within a matter of days, making platelet transfusion unnecessary in all but the most acute situations.

B. PLATELET GROWTH FACTORS:

Theoretically, platelet growth factors should be effective in decreasing the severity of thrombocytopenia and platelet transfusion requirement in any patient with a reversible thrombocytopenia secondary to a production defect, such as is seen with cancer chemotherapy. The therapeutic roles of IL-11 and recombinant thrombopoietin/*Mpl* ligand (**rHuTPO/PEG-rHuMGF**) in the treatment of disorders of platelet production have now been studied in several clinical trials. Based on a study of the ability of IL-11 (Neumega) to reduce the platelet transfusion requirements in breast cancer patients undergoing chemotherapy for metastatic disease, it has been approved for use by the US Food and Drug Administration. Its drawback, however, is the inflammatory reaction that accompanies treatment.

Also in cancer patients, PEG-rHuMGF in doses of 0.3 and 1.0 μg/kg/day resulted in a two- to sixfold rise in the platelet count, beginning on day 10 and peaking 2–12 days after the last injection. The thrombocytopenia associated with AIDS also responds to PEG-rHuMGF. The mechanism in primate and human studies appears to be a correction of the abnormal megakaryocyte apoptosis and ineffective platelet production caused by the HIV infection. Unfortunately, parallel studies in volunteer platelet donors, where it was used to increase the platelet harvest, demonstrated the appearance of neutralizing antibodies to the PEG-rHuMGF with cross-reactivity to native thrombopoietin. This has brought a halt to its clinical development. A study of rHuTPO given as a single dose of 0.3–2.4 μg/kg showed a platelet count rise of up to four times baseline. Early release of reticulated platelets and increases of platelet counts to levels of 1,000,000/μL or higher were not associated with changes in platelet function. Moreover, no major organ, hemostatic, or hematopoietic toxicities have been observed. Therefore, rHuTPO may hold more promise clinically.

Disorders of Distribution

Low platelet counts secondary to splenomegaly are generally not associated with abnormal bleeding. Therefore, platelet transfusions are not recommended. If the count falls to below 20,000–30,000/μL, the patient needs to be evaluated for a concomitant platelet production or destruction defect. The presence of one or the other of these will dictate therapy. If a production abnormality appears to be present, a trial of platelet transfusions can be attempted. Measurements of the platelet count 4 and 24 hours after transfusion can help predict the effectiveness of further transfusion therapy (see Figure 30–4). Patients with very large spleens will show a lower than normal increment following transfusion owing to the pooling of platelets in the spleen. Unless there is a significant component of increased destruction, however, the platelet count should remain relatively stable for the next 24 hours. When an immune destruction defect is present, little in the way of post-transfusion increment is observed, and the count quickly falls back to pretransfusion levels.

Patients with myelofibrosis can be a therapeutic dilemma. In the thrombocytopenic myelofibrotic patient, it can be very difficult to predict whether splenectomy will improve or worsen the patient's thrombocytopenia. In addition, in some patients the spleen is actually controlling a tendency to overproduction. A splenectomy in this type of patient will result in a rise in platelet counts in excess of 1 million/μL.

Destruction Disorders

Proper management of patients with platelet destruction disorders depends on the diagnosis. In those individuals who have nonimmune destruction as a part of DIC, the only effective therapy is the treatment of the underlying cause of the DIC (see Chapter 34). If the primary condition can be corrected, coagulation factors and platelet count will recover on their own. Similar to patients with DIC, patients with TTP or HUS should only receive platelet transfusions for life-threatening bleeding. With these conditions, potential harm from platelet transfusions is of even greater concern; they may lead to increased thrombosis and organ damage secondary to marked platelet aggregation and activation.

A. MANAGEMENT OF PATIENTS WITH TTP, HUS, OR HELLP:

The recommended therapy for **TTP-HUS** is plasmapheresis with plasma exchange. High-dose steroid therapy is also given, although the evidence for its effectiveness is poor. **HUS** patients will usually require dialysis until renal function recovers. Speed is essential. The earlier the diagnosis and the sooner the plasma exchange is initiated, the better the response. Patients who have progressed to coma and severe renal failure have a very poor prognosis. Other parameters of disease activity, including the severity of the anemia and thrombocytopenia, or the elevation of the lactic dehydrogenase level (LDH), are poor initial predictors of outcome. However, a rapid rise in the platelet count and fall in the LDH within the first 3 days of plasma exchange does predict recovery.

The response of **TTP** patients to plasma exchange can be distressingly slow, requiring frequent, even daily, treatments over several weeks. Furthermore, the duration of therapy must be determined by trial and error. Once a response is attained, the frequency of the treatments should be gradually decreased and the patient closely observed for exacerbation/relapse of disease. As long as plasma exchange appears to have a beneficial effect, it should be continued, even if the patient shows only a partial response. Some patients may evolve into a chronic, smoldering form of the disease with continued thrombocytopenia but without progressive organ damage. In this case, they are indistinguishable from chronic ITP patients. Plasmapheresis and plasma infusions have had a major positive impact on overall prognosis. Most patients caught early in their disease will now survive, whereas in the past TTP was a fatal illness. Up to 20% of idiopathic TTP patients do relapse at least once within 5 years and another 25% will demonstrate decreased renal function (creatinine clearance below 40 mL/minute).

HELLP syndrome presents a somewhat different therapeutic challenge. Most often, the disease process ends with delivery of the fetus. However, some women will continue to exhibit HELLP or will convert to a TTP-like syndrome postpartum. They should receive aggressive pheresis with cryopoor plasma exchange. Response will be poor if there is any organ damage. Women who develop HELLP syndrome or TTP during or after pregnancy should consider termination of future pregnancies. If the decision is made to go ahead with a pregnancy, the woman should continue to receive aspirin and Persantin as prophylaxis.

The treatment of TTP/HUS/HELLP is empiric; the mechanism of action of plasma infusions or plasma exchange or both is not fully understood. One explanation is that a missing plasma factor, vWF-cleaving protease, is being replaced. Plasma infusions may be all that is required in patients with chronic relapsing TTP, which is characterized by high plasma levels of unusually large multimers of vWF secondary to the cleaving enzyme deficiency. At the same time, the more common acute single-episode TTP appears to be associated with an IgG autoantibody against the vWF-cleaving protease enzyme. These patients respond best to plasma pheresis using **cryopoor plasma** (the supernatant fraction of plasma after preparation of cryoprecipitate), which contains lower levels of the larger-molecular-weight vWF fractions, for the plasma exchange. The underlying defect in HUS is even less well understood; HUS patients do not appear to have abnormalities in vWF-cleaving protease. Children with diarrhea-associated HUS generally recover spontaneously without the need for pheresis.

B. NEONATAL THROMBOCYTOPENIA:

Treatment of autoimmune thrombocytopenia must be disease-specific. When mild, neonatal thrombocytopenia, whether isoimmune or associated with maternal ITP, does not require therapy. For severe thrombocytopenia, an infusion of immunoglobulin in a dose of 400 mg/kg body weight, given daily for up to 5 days, is the therapy of choice. Its immediate effect is to bind to the antibody to form an idiotype–anti-idiotype dimer and prevent binding to its antigen. Platelet transfusions for neonatal thrombocytopenia should be reserved for children with evidence of intracranial hemorrhage. PL^{A-1}-negative platelets obtained from the mother can be highly effective in treating isoimmune thrombocytopenia. The maternal platelets should be washed prior to transfusion to avoid further supply of anti-PL^{A-1} antibody to the child.

Newborns of mothers with autoimmune thrombocytopenia should have daily platelet counts for the first 4 days after birth. In addition, any newborn with a platelet count below 50,000/μL should have ultrasound brain imaging to rule out intracranial hemorrhage. Newborns with platelet counts below 20,000/μL should be treated with intravenous gammaglobulin. If there is evidence of intracranial hemorrhage, combined gammaglobulin/prednisone therapy is indicated.

C. AUTOIMMUNE THROMBOCYTOPENIA IN CHILDREN:

In children who develop an autoimmune thrombocytopenia following viral illness, severe thrombocytopenia is usually self-limited, lasting less than 1–2 weeks. If the platelet count is above 30,000/μL and there is little in the way of mucocutaneous bleeding, the child can simply be observed. More than 90% of these children will recover completely. Any child with a count below 10,000/μL or below 20,000/μL with mucous membrane or life-threatening bleeding should be hospitalized and treated with intravenous immune globulin, 1 gram per kilogram on day 1 and 400 mg/kg/day for the next 2–5 days, together with high-dose oral or parenteral glucocorticoid. Splenectomy should be reserved for the child who continues to have marked thrombocytopenia with abnormal bleeding for more than a year. Emergency splenectomy is only appropriate if the child is experiencing a life-threatening hemorrhage. More than 70% will achieve a sustained remission after splenectomy, but not without a future risk of fatal bacterial sepsis.

D. DRUG-INDUCED THROMBOCYTOPENIA:

In patients with autoimmune thrombocytopenia secondary to drug ingestion, the most important management step is to discontinue the drug. Corticosteroid therapy may speed recovery in patients with an ITP-like picture, such as may be seen in patients reacting to sulfamethoxazole. To prevent a life-threatening thromboembolic event in patients with HIT, all heparin, including the small amounts used in line maintenance, must be stopped immediately as soon as the platelet count begins to fall even modestly. Any delay, such as waiting for an antibody assay of a further fall in the platelet count, puts the patient at high risk. The rate of recovery will then depend both on the clearance rate of the drug and the ability of the marrow megakaryocytes to proliferate and increase platelet production. Even when the platelet count is very low, bleeding is unlikely and patients can be allowed to recover on their own. If continued anticoagulation is required, the patient should be switched to a non-reacting thrombin inhibitor, such as danaparoid, Lepirudin, or argatroban (see Chapter 36).

The treatment of thromboembolic complications in patients with HIT can be especially difficult. Oral anticoagulants should never be used. The immediate reduction in protein C levels with initiation of warfarin therapy can lead to severe thrombotic disease, including massive skin necrosis and limb gangrene secondary to widespread small vein thrombosis ("venous limb gangrene syndrome"). Furthermore, low-molecular-weight heparin cannot be substituted; there is 100% cross-reactivity with the heparin antibody. Danaparoid, a mixture of heparan sulfate, dermatan sulfate, and chondroitin sulfate, has less than 10% cross-reactivity and is currently the drug of choice for patients with known or suspected heparin-associated thrombocytopenia (see Chapter 36).

E. AIDS-ASSOCIATED THROMBOCYTOPENIA:

HIV-infected patients who develop thrombocytopenia early in their disease can be treated with AZT. Approximately 60% of patients will show a response, and up to 50% will have a long-lasting improvement in their platelet counts. The effect is not immediate; it can take up to 1–2 months before the platelet count improves. In those patients who do not respond, splenectomy can help in more than 85% of the cases. Splenectomy is only effective, however, if done early in the course of disease, whereas the marrow megakaryocyte mass can still compensate for the increased rate of platelet destruction.

Corticosteroids, intravenous immune globulin, and intravenous anti-D have also been used in AIDS patients. Although corticosteroids have a positive effect, long-term treatment runs the risk of encouraging opportunistic infection. Intravenous immune globulin can give a good response, but the relapse rate is high and thus requires repeated treatment. In patients who are Rh positive, anti-D therapy seems to be more effective but is limited by how low the hemoglobin can be permitted to fall. With disease progression, HIV-infected patients develop a platelet production defect that only responds to platelet transfusion therapy. AIDS patients who develop a consumptive thrombocytopenia with organ damage may benefit from plasmapheresis.

F. ADULT AUTOIMMUNE THROMBOCYTOPENIA:

Thrombocytopenia secondary to autoimmune disease is best treated by controlling the systemic illness. For patients with **Hodgkin's and non-Hodgkin's lymphomas,** this treatment involves combinations of **radiation therapy, chemotherapy, and marrow transplantation.** The immune destruction of platelets that occurs as a complication of an infectious disease will usually resolve as the infection is controlled. **Corticosteroids** may be used occasionally on a short-term basis to treat patients with very low platelet counts. This condition is most often an issue in patients with infectious mononucleosis who develop severe thrombocytopenia.

Severe autoimmune thrombocytopenia (ITP) with bleeding manifestations in adults should be treated as a medical emergency with high-dose corticosteroids, prednisone 1–2 mg/kg body weight, daily or 1 gram of methylprednisolone by intravenous infusion, given daily for the first 3 days (Figure 30–5). If there is clinical evidence of intracranial hemorrhage, the patient should also be given intravenous immunoglobulin and platelet transfusions at least every 8–12 hours, regardless of the effect on the platelet count. Several patients who receive platelet transfusions will show a relatively normal post-transfusion increment and reasonable survival. However, even when there is no post-transfusion increment, sufficient numbers of the transfused platelets may survive to improve hemostasis.

High-dose corticosteroid therapy should be continued until the platelet count rises in excess of 50,000/μL. It can then be tapered rapidly as the platelet count enters the normal range. Some adults do not respond to prednisone and go on to develop chronic ITP. In this circumstance, high-dose corticosteroid therapy cannot be continued for prolonged periods. These patients are candidates for **intravenous immunoglobulin** given in a dose of 1 gram per kilogram intravenously over 6–8 hours on each of 2 days or after the first day 400 mg/kg daily for 5 days. Intravenous anti-D IgG can be used in Rh+ patients, especially those who have not had splenectomy. The recommended initial dose is 50 μg/kg given over 3–5 minutes intravenously in patients with hemoglobins of greater than 10 grams per deciliter and 25–40 μg/kg when anemia is a concern. A substantial increase in platelet count within 1–3 days, peaking at 7–14 days, and lasting for up to a month, is seen in responsive patients. The dosage and timing of subsequent treatments, if needed, depend on the clinical response to the first dose. Since anti-D's therapeutic effect involves Fc receptor blockade by sensitized red blood cells, extravascular hemolysis with a fall in the hemoglobin level is an anticipated event. The hemoglobin decrease by 2 weeks after treatment should be around 2 grams per deciliter, although decreases of 4–6 grams per deciliter are seen in 3–4% of patients. Immediate intravascular hemolysis with hemoglobinemia, hemoglobinuria, and reversible renal impairment has been rarely observed.

Response to therapy—Up to 80% of children have a good response to intravenous immune globulin therapy by itself, even to the point of achieving a normal

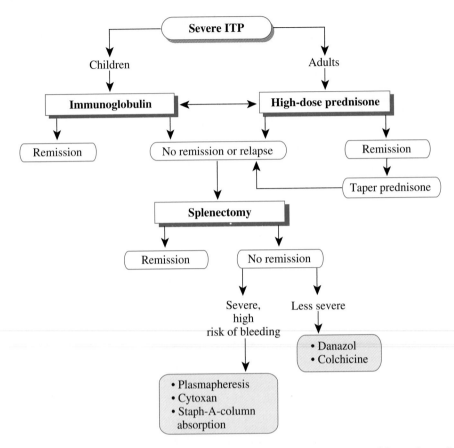

Figure 30–5. Treatment of severe autoimmune thrombocytopenia. Management of the patient with ITP begins with high-dose corticosteroid, immune globulin therapy, or both. Splenectomy, chemotherapy, plasmapheresis, and staph-A column absorption are indicated when there is little or no response.

platelet count. About half of these patients will have a sustained response, whereas the others will require repeated therapy for recurrent thrombocytopenia. The prolonged effect of immunoglobulin therapy is related to induction of T-cell suppression and down-regulation of B-cell autoantibody production. Adults are less likely to respond to immunoglobulin. However, those who do respond and then relapse can be expected to have an excellent response to splenectomy.

If ITP persists for more than 3–4 months, it is extremely unlikely that the patient will spontaneously recover. In this case, splenectomy should be considered if the platelet count is below 10,000–20,000/µL. Approximately 75–80% of patients will achieve a permanent remission after splenectomy. However, the platelet count is maintained by a continued increased level of marrow production that compensates for the shortened platelet life span. These patients are at risk for thrombocytopenic episodes later in life. If splenec-

tomy is recommended for a patient with chronic ITP, it is extremely important to immunize with pneumococcal, meningococcal, and *Haemophilus influenzae* vaccines prior to surgery to reduce the risk of postsplenectomy sepsis. In children less than 5 years of age, postsplenectomy prophylactic antibiotic therapy may also be advisable.

Refractory thrombocytopenia after therapeutic trials of prednisone, intravenous immunoglobulin, and splenectomy is uncommon. If the patient fails all therapy and is at risk for a severe, life-threatening bleed, **intravenous cyclophosphamide,** given as a 1-gram bolus on one to three occasions, may reduce the level of antiplatelet antibody. **Plasmapheresis** and **extracorporeal absorption of IgG using an antistaphylococcal protein-A-silica column** may be worth trying if the patient is experiencing a life-threatening bleeding. High-dose dexamethasone therapy has also been used but without much success.

With less-severe chronic ITP, drugs such as **colchicine** and **danazol** have been reported to increase the platelet count. Colchicine must be given in doses of 0.6–1.2 mg four times a day by mouth for up to 2 months before an effect is seen. This drug can produce severe GI side effects. Danazol is given in a dose of 200 mg two to four times a day by mouth. As many as 50% of patients will respond to danazol, with an improvement in platelet count within 2–6 weeks. A new and novel therapy, anti-CD40 ligand, is currently under study. **CD40** is a B-cell antigen that binds to a T-cell ligand to augment antibody production. The rationale for anti-CD40 ligand therapy is, therefore, to suppress antibody production without impairing other aspects of immune competency. Finally, since some ITP patients appear to have a simultaneous failure in platelet production, thrombopoietin therapy may play a role. This needs to be studied.

Management of **chronic ITP in pregnancy** deserves special attention. Most women can be managed throughout their pregnancy with no medication, modest amounts of **prednisone,** or intermittent use of **intravenous immunoglobulin.** To avoid the side effects of prednisone therapy, high-dose intravenous immunoglobulin, 1 gram per kilogram (prepregnant weight) given on a schedule of once a month or in severe cases as often as every week, is effective in two-thirds of women. In those cases where the thrombocytopenia is severe, higher-dose steroid therapy, 0.5–1 mg/kg prednisone per day together with weekly intravenous immunoglobulin, during the last 2–3 weeks of pregnancy, may be needed to prevent maternal bleeding. Even with severe ITP in the mother, most children are born with normal platelet counts. Less than 4% will have a platelet count below 20,000/μL and less than 1% will exhibit a bleeding complication. Neonatal platelet counts may continue to fall for 7 or more days following delivery. Therefore, children at risk should have their platelet counts checked every 2–3 days until the count rises.

Despite the low incidence of bleeding complications in children born to ITP mothers, prophylactic Caesarean section is still recommended by some obstetricians to decrease the chance of intracranial hemorrhage. There is no good evidence that Caesarean section is significantly better in protecting the child. Moreover, this approach actually increases the risk of serious maternal bleeding and often requires platelet transfusion support. Although the risk for the fetus reflects the severity of the mother's ITP, this relationship is not a hard-and-fast rule. A child with severe thrombocytopenia and bleeding complications may be born to a mother with apparently mild disease. This misfortune cannot be predicted by assays of maternal platelet-associated antibody. In addition, attempts to anticipate the problem by measuring a scalp vein platelet count immediately after rupture of the membranes have proved unreliable.

BIBLIOGRAPHY

Pathophysiology

Basser RL et al: Thrombopoietic effects of pegylated recombinant human megakaryocyte growth and development factor in patients with advanced cancer. Lancet 1996;348:1279.

Fannuchi M et al: Effects of polyethylene glycol-conjugated recombinant human megakaryocyte growth and development factor on platelet counts after chemotherapy for lung cancer. N Engl J Med 1997;336:404.

Kaushansky K: Thrombopoietin: The primary regulator of platelet production. Blood 1995;86:419.

Kunicki TJ, Newman PJ: The molecular immunology of human platelet proteins. Blood 1992;80:1386.

Tomer A, Hanson SR, Harker LA: Autologous platelet kinetics in patients with severe thrombocytopenia: Discrimination between disorders of production and destruction. J Lab Clin Med 1990;118:546.

Autoimmune Thrombocytopenia

Ballem PJ et al: Kinetic studies of the mechanism of thrombocytopenia in patients with human immunodeficiency virus infection. N Engl J Med 1992;327:1779.

Ballem PJ et al: Mechanisms of thrombocytopenia in chronic autoimmune thrombocytopenic purpura: Evidence of both impaired platelet production and increased platelet clearance. J Clin Invest 1987;80:33.

Bussel JB et al: Fetal alloimmune thrombocytopenia. N Engl J Med 1997;337:22.

Crowther MA et al: Thrombocytopenia in pregnancy: Diagnosis, pathogenesis, and management. Blood Rev 1996;10:8.

George JN: Platelet IgG: Measurement, interpretation, and clinical significance. Prog Hemost Thromb 1991;10:97.

George JN et al: Idiopathic thrombocytopenic purpura: A practice guideline developed by explicit methods for the American Society of Hematology. Blood 1996;88:3.

Gill KK, Kelton JG: Management of idiopathic thrombocytopenic purpura in pregnancy. Semin Hematol 2000;37:275.

Scadden DY, Zon LI, Groopman JE: Pathophysiology and management of HIV-associated hematologic disorders. Blood 1989;74:1455.

Warkentin TE: Clinical presentation of heparin-induced thrombocytopenia. Semin Hematol 1998;35:9.

Warner M, Kelton JG: Laboratory investigation of immune thrombocytopenia. Clin Pathol 1997;50:5.

TTP

Furlan M et al: Von Willebrand factor-cleaving protease in thrombotic thrombocytopenic purpura and hemolytic-uremic syndrome. N Engl J Med 1989;339:1578.

Shumak KH et al: Late relapses in patients successfully treated for thrombotic thrombocytopenic purpura. Ann Intern Med 1995;122:569.

Torok TJ, Holman RC, Chorba TL: Increasing mortality from thrombotic thrombocytopenic purpura in the United States: Analysis of national mortality data. Am J Hematol 1995;50:84.

Tsai H, Lian EC: Antibodies to von Willebrand factor-cleaving enzyme in acute thrombotic thrombocytopenic purpura. N Engl J Med 1989;339:1585.

Therapy

Ahn YS et al: Long-term danazol therapy in autoimmune thrombocytopenia: Unmaintained remission and age-dependent response in women. Ann Intern Med 1989;111:723.

Berchtold P, McMillan R: Therapy of chronic idiopathic thrombocytopenic purpura in adults. Blood 1989;74:2309.

Beutler E: Platelet transfusions: The 20,000/μL trigger. Blood 1993; 81:1411.

Bussel JB et al: Intravenous anti-D treatment of immune thrombocytopenic purpura: Analysis of efficacy, toxicity, and mechanism of effect. Blood 1991;77:1884.

George JN: How I treat patients with thrombotic thrombocytopenic purpura-hemolytic uremic syndrome. Blood 2000; 96:1223.

Gernsheimer T et al: Mechanisms of response to treatment in autoimmune thrombocytopenic purpura. N Engl J Med 1989; 320:974.

Law C et al: High dose intravenous immune globulin and the response to splenectomy in patients with immune thrombocytopenic purpura. N Engl J Med 1997;336:1494.

McMillan R: Therapy for adults with refractory chronic immune thrombocytopenic purpura. Ann Intern Med 1997;126:307.

O'Malley CJ et al: Administration of pegylated recombinant human megakaryocyte growth and development factor to humans stimulates the production of functional platelets that show no evidence of in vivo activation. Blood 1996;88:3288.

Scaradavou A et al: Intravenous anti-D treatment of immune thrombocytopenic purpura. Blood 1997;89:2689.

Slichter SJ: Platelet transfusions a constantly evolving therapy. Thromb Haemost 1991;66:178.

Snyder HW et al: Experience with protein A-immunoadsorption in treatment-resistant adult immune thrombocytopenic purpura. Blood 1992;79:2237.

Taaning E, Skibsted L: The frequency of platelet alloantibodies in pregnant women and the occurrence and management of neonatal alloimmune thrombocytopenic purpura. Obstet Gynecol Surv 1990;45:521.

Vadhan-Raj S et al: Stimulation of megakaryocyte and platelet production by a single dose of recombinant human thrombopoietin in patients with cancer. Ann Intern Med 1997;126:673.

Platelet Dysfunction

An abnormality in platelet function can result in bleeding even when the platelet count is normal. Although most platelet function disorders are associated with a relatively mild bleeding tendency, awareness of these conditions can be important in the overall clinical management of the patient.

NORMAL PLATELET FUNCTION

The steps involved in platelet adhesion, aggregation, and subsequent clot formation are illustrated in Figure 31–1. Important elements of the system include the vessel wall, functional components of the platelet, and both **von Willebrand factor (vWF)** and fibrinogen. The ability of the vessel to contract and the condition of the subendothelial connective tissue are both important elements. Reflex contraction of the vessel reduces flow and encourages adhesion of platelets to exposed collagen. Loss of this reflex because of a distortion in vessel anatomy or an underlying collagen defect will interfere with normal platelet thrombus formation.

Platelet adhesion, activation, and aggregation play pivotal roles in platelet thrombus formation. A defect in any of these, including the expression of the GPIb or GPIIb/IIIa receptor, release of α-granule or dense granule contents, thromboxane A_2 synthesis, nucleotide metabolism, or the expression of factor V receptors, will result in a functional defect. In addition, both vWF and fibrinogen are essential to platelet adhesion, aggregation, and clot formation. vWF is required for the initial adhesion of platelets to subendothelial connective tissue, bridging collagen to the GPIb surface receptor of the platelet. Fibrinogen and vWF act as cofactors in platelet aggregation by interacting with both the GPIb and GPIIb/IIIa receptors.

Endothelial cells appear to be the primary source of plasma vWF. Initially, a propolypeptide is produced and stored as a dimer in the Weibel-Palade bodies of the endothelial cells. A portion of the peptide is then removed, and dimers are linked by disulfide bonds to form **multimers** of varying sizes. These multimeric forms are released into circulation, where they serve both as a cofactor in platelet adhesion/aggregation and as a carrier for factor VIII. The latter is important in determining the clearance rate of factor VIII from cir-

culation. The size distribution of multimeric forms of vWF is an important determinant of platelet function; larger multimeric vWF is associated with improved platelet function.

Megakaryocytes also manufacture vWF and incorporate it in the α-granules of mature platelets. The multimers within α-granules are even larger than those seen in circulation and are referred to as **unusually large vWF (ULvWF)**. This platelet vWF appears on the surface as platelets change shape and release their α-granule contents. It binds to the GPIIb/IIIa complex to encourage platelet aggregation in collaboration with fibrinogen.

CLINICAL FEATURES

As with thrombocytopenia, there are no specific symptoms or signs that indicate a platelet functional defect. Inherited defects are rare and are characterized by a relatively mild bleeding tendency. von Willebrand disease (vWD) is an exception to this rule, since some types are associated with severe and even fatal bleeding.

Patients with platelet functional defects generally present with easy bruisability, mucocutaneous bleeding of a purpuric nature, and bleeding from the genitourinary (often severe menorrhagia) and GI tracts rather than the petechial bleeding that characterizes thrombocytopenia. It is not unusual for the bleeding tendency to escape detection until aggravated by another abnormality. For example, the defect may first be suspected because of excessive bleeding following minor surgery or a dental extraction or unusual mucocutaneous bleeding with administration of anticoagulants or a platelet inhibitor such as aspirin. Therefore, a history of unusual bleeding, a family history suggestive of a congenital abnormality, and clinical picture can provide important clues.

Laboratory Studies

A. BLEEDING TIME (BT) AND TESTS FOR FACTOR DEFICIENCIES:

The BT has traditionally been used as a screening test for the presence of a platelet functional defect. If performed carefully in a well-standardized manner (see

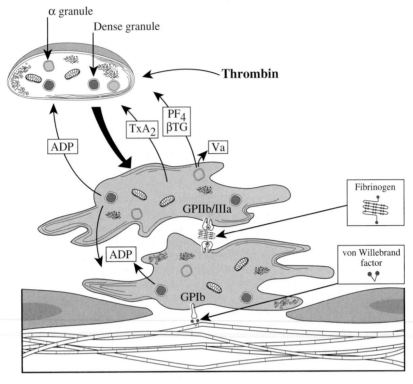

α granule

Dense granule

Thrombin

PF$_4$
βTG

TxA$_2$

ADP

Va

GPIIb/IIIa

Fibrinogen

ADP

von Willebrand
factor

GPIb

Figure 31–1. **Normal platelet function.** Important elements in platelet adhesion and aggregation include a platelet shape change; adhesion to subendothelial collagen; aggregation of activated platelets; and release of ADP, thromboxane A$_2$ (TxA$_2$), platelet factor 4 (PF4), and β-thromboglobulin (βTG) to stimulate further platelet activation and aggregation. Thrombin acts as a platelet activator to accelerate the process. von Willebrand factor is essential to the adhesion of the GPIb receptor to collagen, whereas fibrinogen is an essential cofactor in the GPIIb/IIIa aggregation process.

Chapter 28), the BT correlates with both platelet number and function. With platelet counts greater than 100,000/μL, the BT should be less than 8 minutes. As the count falls below this level, the BT lengthens, reaching times of 20–25 minutes when the count falls to 10,000/μL. Patients with functional defects, such as severe vWD, show BTs in excess of 20 minutes with a normal platelet count. Patients with an acquired functional defect secondary to aspirin therapy or uremia show more modest prolongations of the BT (8–20 minutes).

A prolonged BT can result from a severe defect in the coagulation cascade; the hemophiliac may have a prolonged BT if the test incision is disturbed. This situation reflects the instability of the platelet thrombus. It is important, therefore, to screen for factor deficiencies with measurements of the activated partial thromboplastin time (**aPTT**), prothrombin time (**PT**), **thrombin time, and fibrinogen concentration.** With exception of severe

vWD, these tests should be normal in patients with platelet functional defects. Severe vWD patients with low factor VIII levels can show a modest prolongation of the aPTT.

B. Complete Blood Count (CBC) and Blood Film:

A CBC with examination of the blood film can also be helpful. The CBC can provide evidence of hematopoietic disease, especially a myeloproliferative disorder where high numbers of circulating platelets are associated with abnormal function. Platelet morphology can help in diagnosing disorders such as Bernard-Soulier syndrome and α-granule deficiency.

C. Measurements of Platelet Activation/Aggregation:

Direct measurements of platelet activation/aggregation are possible using an aggregometer or flow cytometry. The **aggregometer** provides a graphic display of the wave of platelet aggregation seen in response to agonists such as ADP, epinephrine, collagen, or ristocetin (Figure 31–2). Specific functional defects respond differently to these agonists. For example, patients with vWD show decreased or absent aggregation with ristocetin, whereas other disorders demonstrate poor responses to ADP, epinephrine, and collagen.

D. FLOW CYTOMETRY:

A flow cytometry method employs fluorescent tagged monoclonal antibodies that specifically bind to activated but not resting platelets (Table 31–1). It can accurately detect levels and conformational changes of key activation/aggregation antigens, including GPIb, GPIIb/IIIa, P-Selectin (GMP 140 or S12), fibrinogen binding, and factor Va binding. Whole blood assays by flow cytometry can be used in the diagnosis of congenital deficiencies of surface antigens, storage pool disease, and platelet dysfunction following extracorporeal circulation. In the future, flow cytometry may also be useful in the clinical monitoring of the GPIIb/IIIa receptor

Table 31–1. Flow cytometry activation/aggregation assays.

Activation assays
GPIb expression
GPIIb/IIIa levels, conformational change with activation, and fibrinogen binding
P-Selectin (GMP 140 or S12) expression
Factor Va binding
Aggregation assays
Hyper-/hyporeactivity to agonists: ADP and thrombin

antagonists. From a research standpoint, the technique has been extremely valuable in studies of platelet activation/aggregation in patients with vascular disease, after extracorporeal circulation, and following cytokine stimulation. These measurements must be performed by a specialized coagulation laboratory since they are difficult to standardize and interpret.

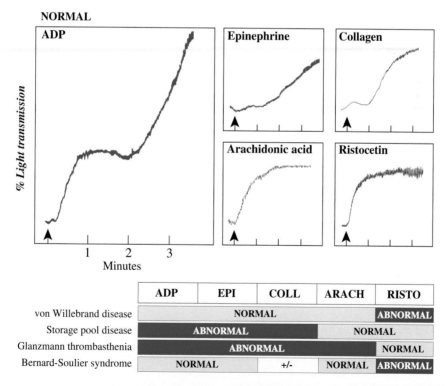

Figure 31–2. **Aggregometer studies in patients with congenital disorders of platelet function. Upper panels:** The normal pattern of aggregation to ADP, epinephrine, collagen, arachidonic acid, and ristocetin. von Willebrand disease can be identified because of an abnormal ristocetin aggregation pattern. This condition is distinctly different from patterns seen with storage pool disease, Glanzmann thrombasthenia, and Bernard-Soulier syndrome.

E. Assays for von Willebrand Factor (vWF):

Full evaluation of the patient with vWD requires several other tests, including assays for factor VIII activity, vWF antigen, vWF activity, and vWF multimer pattern by agarose gel electrophoresis. Together with the patient's bleeding history, family history, and BT, these assays permit the classification of vWD into one of several clinically important subtypes.

F. Research Assays:

Several research assays have been used to identify platelet structural abnormalities. For example, the absence of dense or α-granules can be detected by **electron microscopy**. Platelet α-granule content deficiency can also be confirmed by a direct **measurement of platelet factor 4 and β-thromboglobulin by radioimmunoassay**. Similarly, **thromboxane B$_2$**, the end product of thromboxane metabolism, can be measured to assess platelet metabolism, whereas direct measurements of **dense granule ADP and ATP** will differentiate storage pool deficiency from aspirin-induced cyclooxygenase deficiency.

DIFFERENTIAL DIAGNOSIS

Diagnosis of a platelet abnormality requires a high level of suspicion and a lot of detective work. Acquired functional abnormalities are clearly the most common abnormality. vWD leads the category of congenital disorders, in terms of both incidence and severity. Therefore, initial evaluation should look for a disorder in these two areas.

Acquired Abnormalities of Platelet Function

Abnormal platelet function occurs in three clinical settings—in association with hematopoietic disease, as a part of a systemic illness, or as a result of drug therapy. Often, the relationship is so strong that the mere presence of a specific drug or clinical condition is enough to make the diagnosis.

A. Myeloproliferative Disease:

Patients with myeloproliferative disorders (ie, polycythemia vera, myeloid metaplasia, chronic myelogenous leukemia) frequently exhibit abnormal platelet function. Some of these patients have very high platelet counts and demonstrate both abnormal bleeding and a tendency for arterial or venous thrombosis. Although the height of the platelet count alone does not correlate with the bleeding or thrombotic tendency, thrombocytosis in excess of 1 million/μL is considered to be a risk factor. In patients with polycythemia vera, expansion of the total blood volume and an increase in blood viscosity may contribute.

Other laboratory findings can be quite variable. The BT may be prolonged, but is a poor predictor of abnormal bleeding. Perhaps the most consistent laboratory abnormalities are defects in epinephrine-induced aggregation and dense and alpha granule function. An acquired form of vWD secondary to a loss of higher molecular-weight vWF multimers may also be observed.

B. Dysproteinemia:

Abnormal platelet function, including defects in adhesion, aggregation, and procoagulant activity, are observed in patients with dysproteinemias. Almost one-third of patients with Waldenstrom macroglobulinemia or IgA myeloma will have a demonstrable defect; IgG multiple myeloma patients are less commonly affected. The level (concentration) of the M protein spike appears to correlate with the abnormalities in platelet function. Fibrinogen breakdown fragments can also interfere with platelet function. This condition is illustrated by the functional defect that appears in patients with disseminated intravascular coagulation (DIC) and fibrin/fibrinogen breakdown. Fibrin fragments impair both fibrin polymerization and platelet aggregation. Of course, failure of platelet thrombus formation in the DIC patient is usually multifactorial, with thrombocytopenia, hypofibrinogenemia, and a loss of dense and α-granule function secondary to platelet activation all playing a role.

C. Cardiopulmonary Bypass:

Cardiopulmonary bypass and to a lesser degree hemodialysis produce a platelet functional defect. During bypass, platelets show progressive activation and a loss of α-granule contents. The aggregation response to ADP decreases and the BT becomes prolonged. This situation is a reversible defect; platelet function returns to normal within 12–36 hours following surgery.

D. Uremia:

Uremic patients consistently show a defect in platelet function that correlates with the severity of the uremia and anemia. It would appear that the uncleared metabolic product **guanidinosuccinic acid** acts as an inhibitor of platelet function by inducing endothelial cell nitric oxide (NO) release. Platelet adhesion, activation, and aggregation are abnormal, and thromboxane A$_2$ generation is decreased.

Most patients with severe uremia have a prolonged BT in excess of 30 minutes. This condition is corrected by hemodialysis. It may also relate to the patient's anemia, since the BT shortens with either transfusion or erythropoietin therapy. For acute bleeding episodes, DDAVP therapy can improve platelet function transiently. Infusion of conjugated estrogens (0.6 mg/kg/day) for 5 days will also shorten the BT. The improvement takes a day or more to appear and can last for up to 2 weeks. The mechanism of the conjugated estrogen effect appears to be the normalization of plasma levels of NO metabolites.

E. LIVER DISEASE:

In general, the most likely cause of hemorrhage in a liver disease patient is a discrete defect, such as bleeding varices or a gastric/duodenal ulcer, which needs to be treated directly and effectively. If, however, the patient has widespread bleeding, including ecchymoses and oozing from intravenous sites, a coagulopathy should be considered. Patients with liver disease have a multi-faceted defect in coagulation. Thrombocytopenia related to hypersplenism and a failed thrombopoietin response is common. Platelet dysfunction, secondary to high levels of circulating fibrin degradation products, further increases the bleeding tendency. In addition, reduced production of factor VII (principal cause of the prolonged PT in liver disease patients) and DIC with increased fibrinolysis add to the coagulopathy. Management of the liver disease patient must address each of these abnormalities (see Chapter 33).

F. DRUG INHIBITION:

Several drugs also affect platelet function (Table 31–2). In the case of **aspirin and the nonsteroidal anti-inflammatory (NSAID)** drugs, the impact on platelet function is well recognized. Aspirin is a powerful in-

Table 31–2. Drugs that inhibit platelet function.

Strong association
 Aspirin (aspirin compounds)
 Ticlopidine
 Abciximab (ReoPro)
 Nonsteroidal anti-inflammatory drugs
  Naproxen, ibuprofen, indomethacin, phenylbutazone, piroxicam, sulfinpyrazone
Antibiotics
 Penicillin—carbenicillin, penicillin G, ampicillin, ticarcillin, nafcillin, azlocillin, mezlocillin
 Cephalosporins—moxalactam, cefotaxime
 Nitrofurantoin
 Volume expanders
  Dextran, hydroxyethyl starch
 Heparin; fibrinolytic agents
Weak association
 Oncologic drugs
  BCNU, daunorubicin, mithramycin
 Cardiovascular drugs
  Beta blockers, calcium-channel blockers, nitroglycerin, nitroprusside, quinidine
 Alcohol

hibitor of platelet thromboxane A_2 synthesis through its irreversible deactivation of cyclo-oxygenase. NSAID drugs (indomethacin, ibuprofen, sulfinpyrazone, etc) also inhibit platelet function, but the effect is reversible and short-lived. From the clinical viewpoint, these agents are weak inhibitors of platelet function and are usually not associated with severe clinical bleeding. However, they will contribute to bleeding when other aggravating factors, such as other anticoagulants, a GI disorder, or surgery, are present. Certain **foods and food additives** (vitamins C and E, omega-3 fatty acids, Chinese black tree fungus) can also inhibit platelet function.

The impact of **antibiotics** on platelet function can be a major contributor to hemorrhage in critically ill patients. The penicillins, including carbenicillin, penicillin G, ticarcillin, ampicillin, nafcillin, and to a lesser extent mezlocillin, interfere with both platelet adhesion and platelet activation/aggregation. These drugs bind to the platelet membrane and interfere with vWF binding and the response of platelets to agonists such as ADP and epinephrine. Significant clinical bleeding can occur in the critically ill patient receiving one of these antibiotics. Without other aggravating factors, however, they will not cause a severe bleeding tendency. Platelet dysfunction has also been reported with selected **cephalosporins,** including moxalactam and cefotaxime. Most other antibiotics in this class do not produce a defect.

Volume expanders, such as the neutral polysaccharide dextran, can interfere with platelet aggregation and procoagulant activity when infused in large amounts. This result can be a significant disadvantage in the trauma or surgical setting when a dextran solution is being used for blood pressure support. At the same time, it has been used to prevent platelet thrombosis. Hydroxyethyl starch, a more popular volume expander, is less likely to interfere with platelet function but will cause a detectable defect if given in doses in excess of 2 liters of the 6% solution. Many other drugs have been reported to cause platelet dysfunction occasionally. This list includes several cardiovascular drugs, alcohol, and several of the oncologic drugs (see Table 31–2). The mechanisms involved have not been clearly defined.

Congenital Disorders of Platelet Function

vWD is the most common inherited abnormality of platelet function. All other disorders, including Bernard-Soulier syndrome, Glanzmann thrombasthenia, dense and α-granule deficiencies, and disorders of secretory and procoagulant activities, are rare. These defects can be grouped according to the functional defect. **Bernard-Soulier syndrome** is a disorder of adhesion, whereas

Glanzmann thrombasthenia is characterized by defective aggregation. The other defects are classified as disorders of granule secretion and platelet metabolism.

A. BERNARD-SOULIER SYNDROME:

Bernard-Soulier syndrome is an autosomal recessive defect in the expression of the GPIb-IX-V platelet membrane receptor. This defect effectively interferes with the platelet's ability to bind vWF and adhere to subendothelial connective tissue. It also produces an aggregation defect characterized by abnormal ristocetin aggregation (see Figure 31–2). Although this is similar to vWD, the abnormal aggregation response is not corrected by the addition of vWF.

Clinically, Bernard-Soulier patients present in childhood with epistaxis, mucocutaneous bleeding, and purpura, although the severity varies. Typically, the BT is in excess of 20 minutes in the presence of a normal to slightly reduced platelet count. Platelets are large, with some forms greater than 20 μm in diameter. However, the absence of Döhle bodies and the abnormal aggregation response to ristocetin clearly separates Bernard-Soulier syndrome from May-Hegglin anomaly.

B. GLANZMANN THROMBASTHENIA:

Glanzmann thrombasthenia is an inherited disorder of platelet aggregation. It is a very rare, autosomal recessive bleeding disorder that usually presents in infancy with mucocutaneous bleeding. Platelet count and platelet morphology are both normal. However, platelets fail to aggregate with any of the usual agonists—ADP, collagen, epinephrine, or thrombin (see Figure 31–2). The response to ristocetin is normal or somewhat impaired. The cause of this defect is a qualitative or quantitative deficiency in platelet surface GPIIb/IIIa, which is the platelet receptor required for platelet-platelet interaction.

Abnormal platelet function with clinical bleeding is also seen in patients with inherited defects in dense and α-granules (storage pool deficiencies). α-**Granule deficiency (gray platelet syndrome)** imparts a relatively mild bleeding tendency. The presence of the abnormality is often first recognized from the appearance of the patient's platelets on the Wright's stained blood film. The platelets lack their normal staining quality, appear gray in color, and are larger than normal. Patients with dense granule deficiency present with a somewhat more severe bleeding tendency. Often, the defect is associated with a congenital developmental defect, such as Chediak-Higashi syndrome, Hermansky-Pudlak syndrome, congenital hypoplastic thrombocytopenia with absent radia, or Wiskott-Aldrich syndrome. The characteristic laboratory abnormality is a failure in the second wave of platelet aggregation (see Figure 31–2). This situation reflects failure of the platelet to play its full role in

platelet-platelet interaction by releasing granule contents or activating the arachidonate pathway.

Poor platelet function owing to **abnormal platelet metabolism** has also been described. In some patients there appears to be a defect in thromboxane A_2 generation or in the aggregation response to thromboxane A_2 and other platelet agonists. Other patients have a deficiency in cyclo-oxygenase similar to the acquired defect seen with aspirin therapy. Platelet morphology and granule content are normal in these conditions, and the bleeding tendency tends to be mild unless the patient is exposed to a platelet-inhibitory drug such as aspirin.

Several conditions in patients with defects in the second wave of platelet aggregation but normal dense granule morphology are lumped together as "**platelet secretion/release defects.**" Many of these appear to have signaling abnormalities such as poor Ca^{++} mobilization or protein kinase C activation. Finally, a **defect in platelet procoagulant activity,** specifically the ability of the platelet surface to bind factor Va, can result in a bleeding diathesis. In this situation, routine studies of platelet function, including platelet aggregation studies, are within normal limits. This condition is an exceedingly rare cause of platelet dysfunction and can only be diagnosed by studying the role of platelets in prothrombin and factor X activation.

C. VON WILLEBRAND DISEASE (vWD):

vWD is inherited as an autosomal dominant trait with an estimated prevalence of from 1/100 to 3/100,000 individuals. However, severe vWD with a history of life-threatening bleeding is seen in fewer than five individuals per million population in Western countries. In the case of type 1 vWD, 40% of involved family members carry the allele for vWD but have normal vWF levels. As with the other platelet functional defects, symptomatic vWD patients usually present with mucocutaneous bleeding, especially epistaxis, easy bruising, excessive menses, and gingival and GI bleeding. Patients with very low factor VIII levels can exhibit hemarthroses and deep tissue bleeds. Often, presence of the disorder is not appreciated until an aggravating factor such as trauma or surgery is present.

vWD is **inherited as either an autosomal dominant or recessive trait.** Frequently there is a strong family history of abnormal and excessive bleeding. However, penetrance and expression of the mutant gene is highly variable. Even though autosomal dominant parents transmit the abnormal gene to 50% of their children, symptomatic disease is seen in only 30–40% of offspring. Patients with a single recessive gene are typically asymptomatic but can show abnormal vWF antigen and activity levels. Double heterozygote offspring, born to parents who both carry a defective gene, exhibit severe disease (type 3 vWD). Rarely, acquired vWD can be seen in patients with lympho-myeloproliferative or immunologic disease states secondary to autoantibodies directed at vWF.

1. Diagnosis—Diagnosis of vWD requires a high level of clinical suspicion and the skilled use of the laboratory. When the patient is critically ill and receiving several drugs and blood products, it is virtually impossible to make an accurate diagnosis. If vWD is considered to be a contributing factor to such a patient's bleeding, it should be empirically treated and the laboratory evaluation postponed until the patient is clinically stable and has not received either blood products or drugs for several weeks.

2. Screening laboratory tests and other tests—Screening laboratory evaluation for vWD should include measurements of BT, platelet count, PT, and aPTT. Patients with mild type 1 vWD will generally have normal studies. With more severe disease, the BT is prolonged, ranging from 15 to more than 30 minutes, whereas the platelet count is normal. Patients with severe deficiencies of vWF or defective binding of factor VIII to vWF will have a prolonged aPTT secondary to low levels of factor VIII in plasma. Specific assays of vWF levels and function are then necessary to confirm the diagnosis.

Full evaluation of vWD patients requires measurements of factor VIII coagulant activity (VIII:C), von Willebrand factor antigen (vWF:Ag), vWF activity (ristocetin cofactor activity), and vWF multimer size using agarose gel electrophoresis. Factor VIII activity is measured from the ability of dilutions of patient plasma to correct the prolonged aPTT of VIII-deficient plasma. VWF:Ag is quantitated by enzyme-linked immunosorbent assay or immunoassay, whereas activity (function) is measured by mixing different concentrations of ristocetin with patient plasma and normal platelets in an aggregometer. The vWF activity level will be proportional to or lower than the vWF:Ag level according to the subtype of vWF disease. vWF multimer analysis is of diagnostic importance in the classification of type 2 vWD variants (Table 31–3). The classification of vWD is important in planning clinical management.

3. Type 1 disease—Type 1 vWD is the most common variant, making up 80% of observed cases. It represents a quantitative defect in plasma vWF levels. Clinical severity of the disease is quite variable, but does correlate with the overall reduction in the plasma levels of vWF and factor VIII. In symptomatic patients, vWF:Ag and vWF activity are usually reduced to below 50% of normal. Blood type O patients normally demonstrate low normal vWF levels and should not be automatically diagnosed as mild type 1 vWD. Since vWF is the carrier protein for factor VIII in circulation, factor VIII levels will be significantly reduced in patients with severe type 1 disease, resulting in a prolongation of the aPTT. Analysis of vWF multimers shows a normal pattern.

Type 1 vWD appears to result from a **defect in vWF release from the Weibel-Palade bodies of the endothelial cells;** platelet and endothelial stores vWF are normal in most patients. This is supported clinically by the observation that type 1 vWD patients demonstrate a release of vWF from endothelial cells with the administration of desmopressin (DDAVP). Furthermore, vWF behaves as an acute phase reactant. Pregnancy and inflammatory states can artificially increase vWF levels, even to the point of masking the diagnosis of mild type 1 vWD.

Table 31–3. Characteristics of von Willebrand disease subtypes.

	Type 1	Type 2A	2B	2M	2N	Type 3
Vwf: RCoF[a]	Decreased	Markedly decreased	Normal to slightly decreased			Absent
vWF: Ag	Decreased	Decreased	Normal to slightly decreased			Absent
Factor VIII:C	Decreased	Decreased	Normal to decreased		Markedly decreased	Absent
RIPA[b]	Slightly decreased	Decreased	Normal/increased		Slightly decreased	Absent
Multimeric structure	Normal	Larger multimers absent			Normal	Absent

[a] Ristocetin cofactor activity.
[b] Ristocetin-induced platelet aggregation.

4. Type 2 disease—Type 2 vWD is characterized by a qualitative defect in plasma vWF. This can involve a reduction in the larger vWF multimers (types 2A and 2B vWD) or variable changes in vWF:Ag and factor VIII binding (types 2M and 2N vWD). The absence of the larger multimers results in a disproportionate decrease in the vWF activity (ristocetin cofactor activity) when compared with vWF:Ag. Factor VIII activity is less likely to be reduced in types 2A, B, and M vWD but is severely affected with type 2N disease.

Type 2A vWD patients have an absence of high- and intermediate-molecular-weight multimers of vWF in plasma. This is a heterogenous group of patients, based on at least two observed defects: production of vWF (which is susceptible to proteolysis) and increased destruction prior to cellular secretion. Some patients are still capable of releasing larger multimers into circulation when stimulated by DDAVP. Others show little or no response. Type 2A patients have a moderately severe bleeding tendency.

Type 2B vWD patients have an abnormal vWF with increased affinity for the platelet GPIb/IX receptor. Loading of the larger multimers of vWF onto platelets results in an apparent decrease in the plasma levels of high and intermediate vWF multimers, similar to type 2A vWD. At the same time, because of the excess vWF on the platelet surface, studies of vWF activity (ie, ristocetin-induced platelet aggregation [(RIPA]) will demonstrate an increased tendency to platelet aggregation. Clinically, excess vWF on platelet surfaces can lead to platelet aggregation in circulation, aggregate removal, and thrombocytopenia. Furthermore, pregnancy, inflammation, or DDAVP administration can, by increasing vWF release, worsen the thrombocytopenia. Despite the tendency to platelet aggregation, these patients have a bleeding tendency, not thrombotic disease.

Platelet-type vWD deserves special comment since it presents with many of the characteristics of type 2B vWD. However, increased binding of vWF multimers in platelet-type vWD is caused by a defect in the platelet GP1b receptor, not the patient's vWF. This is an important distinction when it comes to therapy. Platelet-type vWD patients require platelet transfusions as well as vWF replacement to correct their bleeding diathesis.

Type 2M vWD is characterized by a normal pattern of vWF multimers in plasma but a disproportionate decrease in vWF activity as compared with vWF:Ag. This is the result of the production of an abnormal vWF molecule with a decreased affinity for the platelet GP1b/IX receptor. Many of these patients will get a therapeutic response from DDAVP, whereas others require vWF replacement.

Type 2N vWD patients demonstrate a defect in factor VIII binding to vWF. Measurements of vWF activity and antigen are both normal, as is the analysis of the vWF multimeric pattern. Factor VIII activity levels are decreased, similar to a mild hemophilia A patient. Type 2N disease should be considered in the differential whenever a female patient presents with a low factor VIII level or female members of the patient's family are affected.

5. Type 3 disease—Type 3 vWD is characterized by a virtual absence of circulating vWF:Ag and very low levels of factor VIII:C (3–10% of normal). These patients experience severe bleeding with hemarthroses and muscle hematomas reminiscent of the hemophilia A or B patient. However, unlike classical hemophilia, their bleeding times are very prolonged. Inheritance of type 3 disease is still unclear. Patients may be double heterozygotes or homozygous for an abnormal gene. Parents are usually normal, which suggests an autosomal recessive pattern.

Finally, **acquired forms** of vWD have been described in association with myeloproliferative diseases, B-cell lymphomas, hypothyroidism, inherited connective tissue diseases such as Ehlers-Danlos syndrome, and congenital cardiac defects. About one-third of reported cases have been in association with a monoclonal gammopathy of uncertain significance (MGUS). A von Willebrand disease–like picture may also be seen in patients with inhibitors to factor VIII:C. In some of these conditions, there is a decrease in the larger vWF multimers (myeloproliferative disorders), in others an inhibition of vWF function secondary to a circulating inhibitor (lymphomas and MGUS), and in others a general depression in the levels of vWF and factor VIII (hypothyroidism).

THERAPY AND CLINICAL COURSE

Abnormalities in platelet function are often first appreciated as a complication of an acute illness or surgery. In this clinical setting, several aggravating factors may play a role in determining the severity of the bleeding tendency. Consequently, this is not a time when an accurate diagnosis can be made, and treatment should address as many potential contributing factors as possible. This list includes discontinuing drugs that inhibit platelet function, empirically replacing vWF and, according to the severity of the patient's bleeding, transfusing normal platelets. Although this approach lacks precision, it is effective. Both acquired and congenital disorders of platelet function can be acutely reversed in order to control severe clinical bleeding.

Long-term management of a platelet functional defect should be based on an accurate diagnosis. Patients with congenital defects should be counseled to avoid drugs that can aggravate the functional abnormality and cause bleeding. Obviously, aspirin and the nonsteroidal analgesics are prime offenders. vWD and thrombasthenia patients demonstrate significant prolongations of the bleeding time with aspirin ingestion and are at greater risk for clinical bleeding. These patients should also be well educated regarding the nature of their abnormality and should carry identification or wear a warning bracelet. This protocol can be invaluable as a guide to appropriate transfusion therapy in an emergency situation.

As a general principle, the **nature of the functional abnormality** will guide the choice of therapy. For example, the vWD patient who lacks normal amounts of vWF will respond to agents that increase plasma vWF levels. In this situation, the platelet is essentially normal once the vWF abnormality is corrected. In contrast, patients with congenital defects of platelet receptor expression, granule content, or platelet metabolism will require transfusion of normal platelets. As for the acquired abnormalities of platelet function, the truth lies somewhere in between. There is clinical evidence that patients with acquired defects secondary to drug ingestion, uremia, and liver disease will respond to DDAVP, vWF replacement, or both. These data suggest that an increase in plasma vWF levels may in part compensate for a platelet-based defect.

DDAVP (Desmopressin)

DDAVP is a synthetic analogue of the antidiuretic hormone, vasopressin. When given intravenously, it stimulates a release of vWF from endothelial cells to produce an immediate rise in plasma vWF and factor VIII:C. This enhances platelet function and in some types of vWD shortens the bleeding time. Its impact on factor VIII levels has been used to manage patients with mild hemophilia A who are undergoing minor surgery. Platelet functional abnormalities seen with drug ingestion, uremia, and liver disease may also improve, perhaps because of the release of very large vWF multimers. In uremic patients, erythropoietin therapy has now been reported to significantly decrease their bleeding tendency, making DDAVP less popular.

The success in treating the vWD patient depends on the disease type. Patients with milder type 1 vWD show an excellent response, with a shortening of the BT and a rise in vWF and factor VIII:C levels. Many of the patients with type 2A or 2M disease also have a good response to DDAVP, although the BT does not normalize and the effect is relatively short lived. Patients with type 2N vWD usually do not respond, although a therapeutic trial may identify the occasional patient who can be managed through minor surgery or a bleeding episode with DDAVP alone. Type 3 vWD patients will not respond to the drug, since these patients lack endothelial stores of vWF. Both vWF and

factor VIII must be provided to reliably correct the defect in both type 2N and type 3 patients.

DDAVP is contraindicated in patients with type 2B and platelet-type vWD. With both defects, stimulation of vWF release can cause an increase in platelet aggregation and a worsening of the patient's thrombocytopenia. In the type 2B patients, the abnormality in platelet function and the thrombocytopenia relates to the production of an abnormal vWF multimer. Therefore, effective treatment for such patients includes both vWF replacement and platelet transfusions.

DDAVP formulations include both **intravenous and intranasal preparations.** DDAVP is administered intravenously in a dose of 0.3 μg/kg. It should be diluted in 30–50 mL of saline and infused over 10–20 minutes to minimize side effects, especially the tachycardia and hypotension. Like its parent compound, DDAVP will cause headache, lightheadedness, nausea, and facial flushing in patients, especially when given rapidly. The drug also has a mild antidiuretic effect that can lead to water intoxication if the patient receives multiple treatments and large volumes of parenteral fluids. A highly concentrated nasal spray can be self-administered in women with type 1 vWD in the management of menorrhagia. It can also be effective in controlling the bleeding associated with tooth extractions or minor surgery in vWD and mild hemophilia A patients. A 300-μg dose of intranasal DDAVP (Stimate nasal spray), administered by the application of 100 μL of a 1.5 mg/mL solution to each nostril, will increase the vWF level, on the average, three- to fourfold.

DDAVP therapy is most effective in treating mild bleeding episodes or in preventing bleeding during minor surgery. Its **drawback** is the short-lived nature of its effect. The improvement in the bleeding time and vWF level is limited to 12–24 hours. Moreover, the response to repeated doses can vary because of the development of tachyphylaxis. Most patients respond to two or three doses at 24-hour intervals, but some will require 48–72 hours between doses to recover. In those situations where control of the patient's bleeding tendency is very important, as for example following major surgery, DDAVP alone will be inadequate and vWF replacement is recommended.

von Willebrand Factor (vWF)

vWF replacement can be achieved by the transfusion of fresh plasma or plasma concentrates containing the vWF-VIII complex. Cryoprecipitate is a readily available and effective concentrate. Similar to DDAVP therapy, it results in an immediate shortening of the BT, which correlates with the infusion of the larger vWF multimers. Improvement in the BT can be relatively short-lived, however. Both it and the vWF:Ag levels de-

Table 31–4. Concentrate/cryoprecipitate dosing in von Willebrand disease.

		Major Bleed, Major Surgery	Less Severe Bleed, Minor Surgery
Severe, types 1 and 3 patients (vWF-VIII < 20%)	Day 1–2	30–40 U/kg[a]	20 U/kg
	Day 3–7	10–20 U/kg	10 U/kg
	> Day 8	5–10 U/kg	
Milder, type 1 patients	Day 1–2	20–30 U/kg	10 U/kg
	Day 3–7	5–10 U/kg	5 U/kg

[a] A "unit" of cryoprecipitate (the precipitate harvested from a unit of whole blood) = 100 U of factor VIII activity. Therefore, a 70-kg severe type 1 vWD patient with a major bleed would receive 20–30 "units" of cryoprecipitate per day (70 kg × 30–40 U/kg = 20–30 "units" of cryoprecipitate).

cay rapidly over the 6–12 hours after infusion. At the same time, factor VIII:C levels rise over the next 24 hours, out of proportion to the amount administered. This rise in the factor VIII level appears to impart a protective effect. Improvement in the patient's bleeding tendency lasts longer than indicated by either the BT or vWF level per se.

The **dosage schedule for cryoprecipitate** is highly empirical (Table 31–4). Patients with severe type 1 or type 3 disease should be managed like a severe hemophilia A patient. In both situations, vWF and factor VIII levels are less than 10%. To control their bleeding tendency, factor VIII:C must be increased in excess of 50–70% for a major surgical operation and 30–50% for minor surgery or less severe bleeding. For patients with less severe type 1 vWD, a combination of DDAVP and smaller amounts of cryoprecipitate is recommended. Just how much vWF factor must be given and the duration of therapy depend on the patient's clinical course. When cryoprecipitate is unavailable, one of the newer commercial forms of **factor VIII/vWF concentrate** may be substituted. However, the concentrate must contain the larger vWF multimers to be effective. Preparations rich in vWF include Humate P and Alphanate. A dose of 50 factor VIII U/kg every 12 hours will usually be sufficient. One advantage to these preparations is that they provide a product that carries less risk of viral transmission.

Because of their very low levels of vWF:Ag and factor VIII, type 3 vWD patients run the risk of developing antibodies to vWF after transfusion of any of these plasma products. Once this has occurred, the patient is at risk for an anaphylactoid reaction and subsequent vWF infusions are much less effective. **Antihistamines and steroids** can blunt the anaphylactoid reaction; **intravenous immunoglobulin** given at doses of 1 gram per kilogram per day for 2–3 days may transiently decrease the level of the anti-vWF antibody. Platelet transfusions can be used to treat patients who have developed alloantibodies.

Other Agents

Other drugs of value in managing vWD patients include **Premarin,** and the fibrinolytic inhibitor, **epsilon aminocaproic acid (EACA)**. Estrogens appear to increase the production of vWF by endothelial cells. During normal pregnancy, vWD patients can normalize their vWF:Ag and factor VIII:C levels, although their bleeding times usually stay prolonged. A positive effect on platelet function has also been observed in uremic patients given Premarin. EACA has been used in both hemophiliacs and patients with vWD to prevent bleeding associated with minor surgery, especially dental extractions. It is given to adults in a dose of 3–4 grams every 4–6 hours either intravenously or by mouth beginning just prior to the procedure and continuing for up to 5–7 days. **Intravenous IgG** may provide a sustained therapeutic effect on the bleeding tendency in patients with MGUS and acquired vWD.

BIBLIOGRAPHY

Acquired Platelet Function Defects

Bick LB: Platelet function defects: A clinical review. Semin Thromb Hemost 1992;18:167.

Federici AB et al: Treatment of acquired von Willebrand syndrome in patients with monoclonal gammopathy of uncertain experience: Comparison of three different therapeutic approaches. Blood 1998;92:2707.

George JN, Shattil SJ: The clinical importance of acquired abnormalities of platelet function. N Engl J Med 1991;324:27.

Michelson AD: Flow cytometry: A clinical test of platelet function. Blood 1996;87:4925.

Noris M, Remuzzi G: Uremic bleeding: Closing the circle after 30 years of controversies. Blood 1999;94:2569.

Sattler FR et al: Impaired hemostasis caused by beta-lactam antibiotics. Am J Surg 1988;155:30.

Weigert AL, Schafer AI: Uremic bleeding: Pathogenesis and therapy. Am J Med Sci 1998;316:94.

Woodman RC, Harker LA: Bleeding complications associated with cardiopulmonary bypass. Blood 1990;76:1680.

von Willebrand Disease

Ginsburg D, Bowie EJW: Molecular genetics of von Willebrand disease. Blood 1992;79:2507.

Rick ME: Diagnosis and management of von Willebrand's syndrome. Med Clin North Am 1994;78:609.

Sadler JE: A revised classification of von Willebrand disease. Thromb Hemost 1994;71:520.

Sadler JE, Gralnick HR: Commentary: A new classification for von Willebrand disease. Blood 1994;84:676.

Therapy

Hanna WT et al: The use of intermediate and high purity factor VIII products in the treatment of von Willebrand disease. Thromb Hemost 1994;71:173.

Mannucci PM: Desmopressin (DDAVP) in the treatment of bleeding disorders: The first 20 years. Blood 1997;90:2515.

Mannucci PM: Hemostatic drugs. N Engl J Med 1998;339:245.

Mannucci PM et al: Comparison of four virus-inactivated plasma concentrates for treatment of severe von Willebrand disease. Blood 1992;79:3130.

Rose EH, Aledort LM: Nasal spray desmopressin (DDAVP) for mild hemophilia A and von Willebrand disease. Ann Intern Med 1991;114:563.

Scott JP, Montgomery RR: Therapy of von Willebrand disease. Semin Thromb Hemost 1993;19:37.

Hemophilia and Other Intrinsic Pathway Defects

32

Defects in the intrinsic pathway are associated with a significant bleeding tendency. The sex-linked recessive disorders, hemophilia A and B, are the principal examples of this type of abnormality. A marked reduction in either factor VIII or IX is associated with spontaneous and excessive hemorrhage, especially hemarthroses and muscle hematomas. A deficiency in factor XI, another intrinsic pathway coagulation factor, can result in a less severe bleeding tendency.

THE NORMAL INTRINSIC PATHWAY

Interactions of the coagulation factors involved in the intrinsic pathway are illustrated in Figure 32–1. The initial activation stimulus is surface contact activation of **factor XII** (**Hageman factor**) to produce XIIa. This reaction is facilitated by the presence of high-molecular-weight kininogen and the conversion of prekallikrein to the active protease, kallikrein. Although this first step is extremely important in the laboratory measurement of the intrinsic pathway, the partial thromboplastin time (PTT), it is not associated with a clinical bleeding tendency.

Factor XIIa activates factor XI, which in turn activates **factor IX** (**Christmas factor**). Factor IXa then catalyzes the cleavage of factor X. The reaction between factors IXa and X is facilitated by binding both factors by calcium bridges to a phospholipid surface such as the surface of an activated platelet. This reaction requires presence of activated factor VIII as a cofactor to achieve a maximum reaction rate. Factor IX is a single-chain glycoprotein produced in the liver as one of the vitamin K–dependent factors. Its activation by factor XIa involves a cleavage of two successive internal peptide bonds to form a two-chain serine protease. Factor VIII appears to be synthesized by the liver and perhaps by lymphoid tissue under control of a single X-linked gene. It circulates as a procoagulant attached to von Willebrand factor (vWF). The latter relationship is extremely important. When the vWF level is reduced, factor VIII is more rapidly cleared from plasma, effectively reducing the activity level. In order to participate

as a cofactor in the activation of factor X, factor VIII must first be cleaved by thrombin to form factor VIIIa.

CLINICAL FEATURES

A severe deficiency of either factor VIII or IX results in a major bleeding disorder, clinically known as **hemophilia A** (**VIII deficiency**) or **hemophilia B** (**IX deficiency**). Even though hemophilia is a relatively rare disorder (1 per 5000 male births for hemophilia A and 1 per 30,000 male births for hemophilia B), descriptions of hemophilia as a sex-linked bleeding disorder can be traced back to biblical times. In part, this situation reflects the fact that the severe hemophiliac experiences major bleeds that start soon after birth and recur at frequent intervals during childhood. Moreover, once the hemophilia mutation appears in a family, it is sustained through successive generations with little variation in expression. At the same time, hemophilia can present as a new spontaneous mutation, usually in the maternal gamete, in approximately one-third of cases.

Hemophilia A

The molecular basis of hemophilia A has now been defined. The factor VIII gene is a very large, 186-kb gene on the X chromosome. Almost half of the patients with hemophilia A exhibit an inversion of a major portion of the VIII gene with a resultant failure in factor VIII production. The remainder show various point mutations, insertions, and deletions that may involve as little as one base pair to the entire gene. The most severe hemophiliacs generally have an inversion or deletion of major portions of the X chromosome genome and very low levels of factor VIII antigen and activity, usually less than 1%. Other mutations, including stop codon and point mutations and minor deletions, result in milder disease. In some of these patients, reduction in the factor VIII level is less pronounced, whereas in others a functionally abnormal protein is produced. The latter can be demonstrated by showing a discrepancy between the immunologic measurement of factor VIII

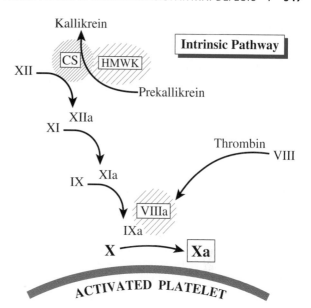

Figure 32–1. **The intrinsic pathway.** The intrinsic pathway as measured by the PTT assay is initiated by surface contact (CS) (kaolin) with facilitation by high-molecular-weight kininogen (HMWK) and its conversion of prekallikrein to the active protease, kallikrein. This stimulus converts factor XII to XIIa, which in turn activates factor XI to XIa and factor IX to IXa. Factor IXa then catalyzes cleavage of factor X. This reaction is facilitated by both binding of factor X to activated platelet surface and the presence of factor VIIIa in response to thrombin activation of factor VIII.

antigen (protein) and the coagulation assay of factor VIII activity.

As a rule of thumb, **clinical severity** of the patient's bleeding disorder is best **correlated with the factor VIII activity level.** Severe hemophiliacs have factor VIII activity levels less than 1% of normal (less than 0.01 U/mL) and are usually diagnosed during childhood because of frequent, spontaneous hemorrhages into joints, muscles, and vital organs. They require frequent treatment with factor VIII replacement and even then are at risk of developing a progressive, deforming arthropathy.

Even a level of detectable factor VIII activity of 1–5% of normal is enough to reduce the severity of the disease. These patients are at increased risk of hemorrhage with surgery or trauma but have much less difficulty with spontaneous hemarthroses or hematomas. Patients with factor levels greater than 6% are only mildly affected and may go undiagnosed well into adult life. They are at risk, however, for excessive bleeding with a major surgical procedure. Women carriers can also be at risk with surgery. Lyonization of the X chromosome is not purely random and can result in low levels of factor VIII or IX.

An inherited **combined deficiency of factors V and VIII,** due in most cases to a single mutation on the long arm of chromosome 18, is associated with a moderate bleeding defect. The gene mutation appears to result in a defect in the transport of V and VIII from the endoplasmic reticulum to the golgi. Factor V and VIII levels are 5–30% of normal. Patients who simultaneously inherit factor V Leiden may also have milder disease.

Hemophilia B

Hemophilia B patients have a similar clinical spectrum of disease. Factor IX levels of less than 1% are associated with severe bleeding, whereas more moderate disease is seen in patients with levels of 1–5%. Patients with factor IX levels of between 5% and 40% generally have very mild disease. This situation reflects the similarity in genetic transmission. Hemophilia B can result from several genetic mutations including deletions, point mutations, and frame shift defects involving the factor IX gene on the long arm of the X chromosome. Most patients show an absence of factor IX activity because of a functionally abnormal protein; less commonly there is an absence of both factor IX antigen and activity. One rare mutation (FIX Leyden) produces a hemophilia B picture in children that resolves at puberty as factor IX production increases.

The most characteristic clinical manifestation of the hemophilias is the **bleeding into the large joints of the upper and lower extremities.** This condition usually begins once the affected child reaches the toddler stage and then increases in frequency as the child becomes more active. Often, one or two joints become the principal targets of repeated hemarthroses. With time, this situation can result in a chronic synovitis, destruction of cartilage and bone, and a progressive flexion contracture. Bleeding into muscle (iliopsoas, gastrocnemius, and flexor muscles of the arm) or soft tissues with the formation of large spreading hematomas is also common. Damage to muscles results in further muscle atrophy and contractures.

Other bleeding manifestations include hematuria, intracranial hemorrhage, mucous membrane bleeding, and prolonged bleeding following minor trauma or surgery. Milder hemophiliacs may not be detected until surgery is performed or the patient has a dental extraction. Usually, the procedure is completed without evidence of unusual bleeding. However, within a few hours, the surgical wound or tooth socket begins to ooze, wound healing is disrupted, and blood flows into surrounding tissues. Hematoma formation in the pharyngeal and retropharyngeal areas can threaten the patency of the airway and present a medical emergency.

Large subperiosteal or muscle bleeds can on occasion lead to the formation of a **hemophilic pseudotumor.** These are cyst-like structures containing serosanguinous or dark brown viscous material bound to a fibrous membrane. Over time, pseudotumors expand and impinge on adjacent structures. Those that arise from a subperiosteal bleed, usually involving the pelvis or femurs, erode bone to form large cystic lesions.

Acquired Factor VIII or IX Inhibitors

Severe hemophilia patients are at risk for developing a factor VIII or, less commonly in the case of hemophilia B, a factor IX inhibitor, usually with the first 20–30 exposures to replacement therapy. Historically, up to 20% of hemophiliac children receiving fresh frozen plasma (FFP) and cryoprecipitate developed an inhibitor by age 10 years. Unfortunately, this problem has not been solved by the arrival of the high-purity concentrates and recombinant factor VIII. In general, factor VIII inhibitor patients fall equally into one of two groups according to the level of inhibitor. **High responders** demonstrate a marked inhibitor response after any factor infusion, reaching levels that cannot be neutralized by replacement therapy. The response is typical of induction of an alloantibody, and the patient is at risk for an anamnestic response when re-exposed to factor antigen. In contrast, **low responders** develop relatively low levels of inhibitor that are constant despite repeated exposure to factor VIII.

A **severe hemophilia-like syndrome** can occur in genetically normal individuals secondary to the appearance of an acquired autoantibody to either factor VIII or IX. These antibodies are in effect circulating anticoagulants. They bind to the factor and result in a loss of coagulant activity. Inhibitor patients are usually middle-aged or older and present with a history of sudden onset of severe, spontaneous hemorrhage involving skin, mucous membranes, muscles, and vital organs, rather than hemarthroses. Bleeding into the tongue and retropharynx can threaten the airway, whereas severe muscle bleeding can be highly destructive. Even though the inhibitor is an autoantibody against factor VIII or IX, there is only occasionally other evidence of autoimmune disease. About 7% of patients develop their inhibitor in the postpartum period.

Viral Infections in the Hemophiliac

Viral hepatitis and HIV infection progressing to AIDS can result from the repeated exposure to clotting factor concentrates. It is estimated that 80% or more of severe hemophiliacs over age 10 years were infected with HIV, hepatitis B virus (HBV), and hepatitis C virus (HCV) during the early 1980s. With the advent of highly purified factor VIII products, younger patients are at far lower, even negligible, risk. Coinfection with HIV and HCV promotes viral replication and progression of the patient's liver disease. The presence of HIV increases risk of liver failure by 21-fold in HCV-infected hemophiliacs. There is also a higher incidence of hepatocellular carcinoma in this group.

HIV transmission to sexual partners is a major concern. Safe sex practices are essential and, if an HIV-positive hemophiliac chooses to have children, the couple should be urged to adopt or use sperm from a healthy donor. Even so, up to 15% of female sexual partners will become infected. Once this occurs, there is a significant risk of transmission to the newborn.

Factor XI Deficiency

The only other intrinsic pathway defect associated with a bleeding tendency is **factor XI deficiency (Rosenthal's disease).** It is inherited as an autosomal recessive trait and, therefore, affects males and females equally. It is much rarer than either hemophilia A or B, affecting primarily Jews of Ashkenazi descent from Eastern Europe. Generally, the bleeding tendency if present at all is quite mild and may only be picked up following a surgical procedure. Hematomas and hemarthroses are very unusual, even in those patients with factor XI levels of less than 5%.

Laboratory Studies

A. PARTIAL THROMBOPLASTIN TIME (PTT) AND PROTHROMBIN TIME (PT):

Severe hemophilia A or B patients have a prolonged PTT and whole blood clotting time. With milder disease, the PTT may be only a few seconds longer than normal. Since the extrinsic pathway and platelet function are intact, the prothrombin time (PT) is normal. Thus, a **discrepancy between the PTT and PT** is enough to focus attention on the intrinsic pathway, that is, factor VIII, IX, or XI deficiency.

B. TESTS FOR FACTOR DEFICIENCIES:

As a part of the initial workup, it is also important to distinguish a factor deficiency from the presence of an inhibitor. This process is routinely done by performing a 1:1 mix of patient plasma and normal plasma to determine whether the prolonged PTT can be corrected. The classic hemophilia A patient with a deficiency in factor VIII activity but no circulating VIII inhibitor will show a partial to complete correction of the PTT when normal plasma is added to the reaction mixture. In contrast, a patient with a factor VIII inhibitor or lupus anticoagulant will not correct. Patients who develop spontaneous factor VIII inhibitors can be a diagnostic challenge. It is essential that other nonspecific inhibitors, heparin and lupus anticoagulants, be quickly excluded. This involves a **factor VIII assay and inhibitor quantitation using the Bethesda assay** to titer the inhibitor.

The full characterization of factor VIII or IX deficiency requires both an **immunologic measurement of the level of factor antigen** (VIII:AG) and an **assay of coagulant activity** (VIII:C). The measurement of the activity level as a percent of normal provides a guide to the severity of the patient's illness. In the evaluation of the less severe hemophilia A patient, a measurement of vWF is important to distinguish classic hemophilia from von Willebrand disease (vWD) (see Chapter 31). Type 1 and Type 2N vWD patients demonstrate factor VIII levels of 10–50% of normal. Type 2N vWD should be considered whenever a female shows factor VIII levels below 50% or the pattern of inheritance is unusual, or both.

C. Tests to Detect Carriers of Hemophilia A or B:

Accurate detection of carriers of hemophilia A or B in a family is required for genetic counseling and prenatal diagnosis. As illustrated in Figure 32–2, sisters of a hemophilia patient have a 50/50 chance of carrying the abnormal gene. In addition, all of the female children of a parent with hemophilia will be obligate carriers. These individuals may be identified by **measuring the factor VIII or IX activity level.** If the level is below the lower limits of normal, the individual almost certainly is a carrier. However, there can be considerable overlap of factor activity levels of carriers with the normal range—0.6 to 1.5 factor VIII or IX U/mL. Therefore, the **factor antigen level** should also be measured and compared with the activity level. If there is a mismatch (ie, antigen level is higher than activity), the individual in question is most likely a carrier for an abnormally functioning factor protein.

D. Clinical Genetic Testing:

Clinical genetic testing is becoming more available. A **DNA test for the intron 22 inversion,** which is found in 45% of severe factor VIII hemophiliacs, is now offered commercially. This test should only be performed in patients who have factor VIII activities of less than 1%. **Direct DNA sequence screening** is required in the other 55% of patients who have milder disease secondary to point mutations or deletions. In the occasional patient where a point mutation cannot be identified, potential female carriers can still be identified by **linkage analysis,** that is, demonstration of gene sequence differences between the subject's two X chromosomes. The same is true for factor IX deficiency diagnosis. Direct DNA testing or linkage analysis performed on chorionic villus biopsy material can then be used for prenatal diagnosis. This will not, of course, identify a proband with a new mutation, which is true for up to one-third of children born with hemophilia.

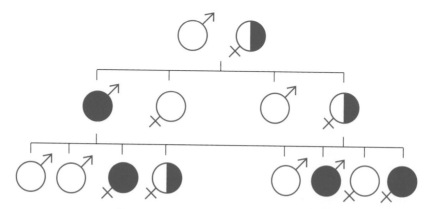

Figure 32–2. **The sex-linked inheritance pattern of hemophilia.** Children of a female hemophilia A or B carrier will have a 50/50 chance of inheriting the abnormal gene. All of the involved male children will have clinical disease, whereas female children will be asymptomatic carriers. As for the children of a male hemophiliac, all of the girls will be carriers.

THERAPY AND CLINICAL COURSE

Appropriate treatment obviously depends on knowing whether the patient has hemophilia A or B and the severity of the factor deficiency. It is also of great value to know the details of the patient's past clinical course. This knowledge can provide another measure of severity and usually produces a wealth of information as to the patient's and family's understanding of the illness and its management.

General Principles

When a hemophilia family is identified, every attempt should be made to develop an ongoing relationship with one of the regional comprehensive hemophilia centers. These centers are funded to provide a comprehensive approach to the medical and social needs of the hemophilia patient. The centers sponsor teams of experienced nurses, social workers, physical therapists, dentists, genetic counselors, and orthopedic surgeons with leadership from pediatric and adult hematologists. They provide a wide spectrum of services from medical consultation to assistance with managing school situations, guidance in vocational training, and assistance in employment. Most centers offer a semiannual clinic visit for the patient to meet with the comprehensive care team and for screening for evidence of complicating viral infections such as HIV, HBV, and HCV; for the appearance of a factor VIII or IX inhibitor; and for changes in cellular immunity. A comprehensive center can also assist the primary care physician in the day-to-day management of a hemophilia patient and provide up-to-date information on available therapeutic products.

Guidelines for Bleeding Management

The overriding principle of good management of a hemophilia bleed is **rapid and effective factor replacement.** With the exception of minor lacerations, which can be controlled locally, factor VIII or IX, whichever is appropriate, should be given for any episode of bleeding, regardless of location. **Prophylactic therapy** is generally reserved for situations of anticipated bleeding as with surgery or high-risk physical activities. However, with increased safety of recombinant factors VIII and IX, long-term prophylaxis can be a reasonable approach in patients with severe disease. Administration of 25–40 U/kg three times a week of recombinant factor VIII (or IX in hemophilia B) is enough to increase the plasma factor levels to greater than 1% and prevent most spontaneous hemarthroses. Another approach to prophylaxis, now under investigation, is early treatment of any joint bleed to factor levels of 60–80% of normal for several days to a week.

The adult hemophiliac patient is usually very sensitive to the **onset of a bleed.** Often there is an aura of mild discomfort localized to the muscle or joint that becomes increasingly painful over the next hour. This stage is followed by progressive swelling, constant severe pain, and limitation of motion of the muscle or joint. However, the severity of the bleed can be significantly reduced if factor VIII or factor IX treatment is begun immediately. To prevent tissue damage, any bleed into a muscle or joint must be stopped as soon as possible. If bleeding is not stopped, the structure of the muscle will be disrupted, resulting in severe scarring and loss of function. Recurrent hemarthroses result in destruction of cartilage and bone, synovial proliferation, and scarring. With time, joint function is lost and the patient develops a crippling deformity. Therefore, the best management of the hemophilia patient is **self-infusion of factor** as soon as a bleeding episode is suspected. This self-infusion will minimize the extent of the bleed and will also reduce the amount of factor needed for treatment (Tables 32–1 and 32–2). If a hemarthrosis goes untreated for several hours or a large muscle hematoma forms, the initial dose of factor must be increased significantly and replacement maintained for several days or longer when extensive rehabilitation is required.

A. CENTRAL NERVOUS SYSTEM BLEEDING AFTER HEAD TRAUMA:

Central nervous system bleeding following head trauma is another situation where treatment must begin immediately. The home treatment patient should administer sufficient factor to increase the factor VIII level to 100% of normal as soon as possible after an injury to the head or face. The patient presenting to the emergency room should be treated with factor VIII before one proceeds with the diagnostic workup. This treatment will prevent a fatal bleeding episode during the time required for history, physical examination, and CT scanning. Furthermore, no attempt should be made to perform a lumbar puncture without prior treatment with factor VIII. Tables 32–1 and 32–2 summarize the recommendations for factors VIII and IX replacement therapy.

B. INTERNAL BLEEDING OF THE CHEST AND ABDOMEN:

Bleeding involving the internal structures of the chest and abdomen can be difficult to diagnose. In the young child, the only indication of a bleed into a large muscle group such as the iliopsoas may be vague abdominal pain or a decrease in physical activity. To avoid severe destruction of muscle or the development of a pseudotumor, the patient should be evaluated with a CT scan. Watchful waiting or suboptimal factor replacement is not recommended.

Table 32–1. Factor VIII replacement therapy.

	Initial Dose (U/kg)	Maintenance (U/kg)
Hemarthrosis[a]		
At onset	10	Repeat only if needed
Fully developed	20	10–20 q 12 h for several days
Muscle hematoma	20–30	20 q 12 h for several days
Mouth bleeds	20–30	20 q 12 h for several days
(tongue laceration; postdental procedure)		Add EACA
Major surgery/tissue damage	50	20–30 q 8–12 h or as a continuous infusion
(major trauma; possible intracranial bleed; potential airway obstruction; severe abdominal pain)		(3–4 U/kg/h) for 5–7 days
Dental prophylaxis		
Severe hemophiliac	20	10–20 q 12 h for 1–2 days plus EACA for 7 days
Milder hemophiliac		EACA and DDAVP

[a] Studies are under way to look at more aggressive therapy, 30–40 U/kg for up to 1 week.

C. MUCOUS MEMBRANE BLEEDING:

Mucous membrane bleeding can be a recurrent problem with hemophiliacs. Treatment can vary according to the site and cause. Epistaxis can be controlled by packing or cautery. However, the clot that forms is often very friable and unstable, leading to recurrent bleeding. In this situation, factor replacement may be necessary. Any tongue or mouth laceration in the young child must be treated immediately with specific factor, and therapy will need to be continued over several days to avoid rebleeding. Uncontrolled bleeding into the soft tissues of the mouth can result in airway obstruction if blood tracks into the retropharyngeal area.

D. BLEEDING AFTER A DENTAL EXTRACTION:

Bleeding following a dental extraction can be prevented by using prophylactic therapy with factor VIII or IX or, in the less severe hemophiliac, by pretreatment with DDAVP, an antifibrinolytic agent such as epsilon aminocaproic acid (EACA), or both. EACA works by stabilizing the clot that normally forms immediately following extraction. If the original clot can be maintained to permit normal healing, factor therapy is unnecessary. This process is also true for very minor surgical procedures. However, most patients undergoing even minor surgery should be prepared with appropriate factor therapy.

Table 32–2. Factor IX replacement therapy.

	Initial Dose (U/kg)	Maintenance (U/kg)
Hemarthrosis		
At onset/minor bleed	20 FIX or 15 mL FFP	Repeat only if needed
Fully developed	30–60 FIX	20 q 24 h for several days
Muscle hematoma		
Minor bleed	20–30 FIX or 15 mL FFP	20 FIX or 10–15 mL FFP q 24 h
Severe bleed	30–50 FIX	30 q 24 h for 5–7 days
Major surgery/tissue damage	60–100 FIX	40–60 q 24 h for 5–7 days
Intracranial bleed	80–100 FIX	60–80 q 24 h for 5–7 days
Dental prophylaxis	10–20 FIX or 15 mL FFP	20 FIX q 12 h for 1–2 days

E. Hematuria:

Hematuria, both microscopic and macroscopic, is a common problem. The course is usually self-limited and can be managed with bedrest, increased fluid intake, and prednisone, 50 mg/day for 3 days. Factor therapy for several days will be needed in patients with gross hematuria. It may also be necessary to evaluate the patient for an unrelated renal cause of hematuria. Gastrointestinal (GI) bleeding is much less common. If it occurs, the patient should be fully evaluated for GI disease. Simple lacerations can usually be controlled with local measures; factor therapy to achieve factor levels greater than 50% is indicated any time a laceration requires suturing. Severe hemophiliacs should receive factor prior to a tetanus shot.

F. Major Surgery in Hemophilia A Patients:

Whenever major surgery is necessary in a patient with hemophilia A, the factor VIII level must be brought to near normal. In addition, repeated doses should be given every 8–12 hours or the patient should receive a continuous infusion dose of 3–4 U/kg/hour, to avoid any significant period of low factor VIII levels. Therapy must be continued for up to 2 weeks to avoid a postoperative bleed that can disrupt wound healing. Longer periods of therapy may be required in patients who undergo bone or joint surgery or who have a pseudotumor excised. In this situation, 4–6 weeks of replacement therapy may be needed. Periodic measurements of factor VIII levels in surgery patients can help in therapy planning. These measurements provide evidence of effective therapy and can also help avoid overuse of factor VIII during the postoperative period.

G. Treatment of Hemophilia B:

The recommended dosage schedules for the treatment of hemophilia B are summarized in Table 32–2. Guidelines for managing the hemophilia B patient do not differ a great deal from those for hemophilia A patients. However, the therapeutic products available for treating hemophilia B are different. Patients with milder disease and less-severe bleeds can be treated with recombinant or purified FIX concentrate, or fresh frozen plasma. Recombinant/purified product is essential for patients undergoing major surgery and those with major traumatic injuries or liver disease. **FIX-prothrombin complex concentrates (FIX-PCC)** are also available for more severe bleeding. However, FIX-PCC preparations carry an increased risk of thrombotic complications. As a part of the preparation of PCCs, some of the clotting factors are activated, thereby setting the stage for thrombosis or even disseminated intravascular coagulation (DIC). This risk appears to be greatest in patients undergoing orthopedic procedures.

Acquired Inhibitors

Management of the hemophilia A patient with an inhibitor will vary according to whether the patient is a high or low responder. The factor VIII inhibitor should always be titered. Using a modification of the PTT called the **Bethesda assay,** it is possible to measure units of inhibitor per milliliter of plasma. Low responders have titers less than 5–10 Bethesda U/mL and do not show anamnestic responses to factor VIII concentrates, whereas the high responders can have titers of several thousand Bethesda units. It is also important to question the patient regarding a previous anamnestic response to factor VIII therapy.

Patients in the low-responder category can usually be managed with **factor VIII concentrates.** Larger initial and maintenance doses of factor VIII are required and frequent assays of factor VIII levels are essential to guide therapy. When the titer of the factor VIII inhibitor exceeds 10 Bethesda units (high responder category), treatment with factor VIII concentrates alone is not feasible. Faced with this dilemma, it is best to try to manage the patient conservatively without replacement therapy for minor bleeding episodes. Major, life-threatening bleeds can be controlled by treatment with either **porcine factor VIII,** one of the **unactivated prothrombin complex concentrates** (Konyne-80, Proplex T, or Profilnine SD), an **activated PCC** (Autoplex T, FEIBA), or **recombinant factor VIIa** (NovoSeven). These therapies have associated risks that must be taken into account. Treatment with porcine factor VIII can stimulate an antibody to the animal protein; treatment with PCCs runs the risk of initiating DIC or widespread thrombosis. Recombinant factor VIIa is the better choice, although it may not be as reliable as factor VIII therapy. An alternative approach is to induce immune tolerance with large daily doses of **factor VIII** given for a year or more. While this is extremely expensive, it is actually more cost-effective over the long run for the 60–80% of children who develop tolerance.

Severe hemophilia B patients are also at risk for developing a factor IX inhibitor. They need to be evaluated in the same manner as the factor VIII inhibitor patients. A **modified Bethesda assay** can be used to quantitate the inhibitor level. Usually, the factor IX inhibitor patients can be managed acutely using a FIX-PCC. Attempts to induce immune tolerance are usually not successful, due to a high risk of anaphylactic reactions with the administration of large doses of FIX concentrate and the development of nephrotic syndrome.

Patients who develop an autoantibody to factor VIII or IX without a past history of hemophilia A or B can present with life-threatening hemorrhage and exhibit very high inhibitor levels in excess of several thousand Bethesda units. In this case, treatment with **factor VIIa** or **porcine factor VIII** or, in the case of a factor IX inhibitor, **factor VIIa** or **an activated PCC** will be required. If the acute bleeding can be controlled, most patients will respond to prednisone (50–80 mg/day) or, in the case of higher titer inhibitors, combined with oral cyclophosphamide (100–200 mg/day). **Intravenous gammaglobulin therapy** has also been reported to be of value in several anecdotal reports. Spontaneous improvement with a decrease in the antibody level and a recovery of factor coagulant activity may be observed over a period of months; this is true for most women with postpartum factor VIII inhibitors.

THERAPEUTIC PREPARATIONS

Major progress is being made in developing safe, effective products for treating hemophilia A and B. Since it is a time of great change, it is important to be aware of the various products available. It is also important to check on whether a new agent has been released. Hemophilia patients follow the development and availability of new products very closely and will want to be treated with the safest product regardless of cost.

Hemophilia A

Products available for treating hemophilia A include DDAVP, FFP, cryoprecipitate, purified factor VIII concentrates, and recombinant factor VIII. For patients with a factor VIII inhibitor and a life-threatening bleed, a purified preparation of porcine factor VIII is available. Recombinant activated factor VII (Novo-Seven) is now the preferred product for the treatment of inhibitor patients.

A. DDAVP:

DDAVP is an arginine vasopressin analogue that can cause the rapid release of vWF from endothelial cells. Since vWF is the carrier protein for factor VIII, DDAVP can increase the circulating level of factor VIII by two- to tenfold in the milder hemophiliac. Severe hemophiliacs will not respond. Its effectiveness must be defined for each patient by measuring the factor VIII level after administration. If it does work, it can be used quite successfully for managing minor bleeding episodes or for preparing the patient for minor surgery or dental work.

An intravenous dose of 0.3 µg/kg (up to 20 µg) of DDAVP infused slowly over 20–30 minutes is the same as recommended for the treatment of Type 1 vWD. Alternatively, DDAVP can be given subcutaneously in a dose of 0.4 µg/kg. When it works, the factor VIII level will, on the average, increase three- to four-fold within

30 minutes of injection. It can then be repeated at 12- to 24-hour intervals, although there is a significant risk of tachyphylaxis after the first few doses. A new **intranasal spray form of DDAVP (Stimate)** given in a dose of 300 µg (150 µg in children) may be equally effective. Side effects include flushing, headache, tachycardia, nausea, and abdominal cramping. In patients who are receiving hyponatremic intravenous fluids, there is a risk of water intoxication secondary to the antidiuretic effect of repeated injections.

B. FRESH FROZEN PLASMA (FFP):

FFP contains the same factor VIII and IX concentrations as normal plasma, that is, 1 unit of VIII or IX activity per milliliter of plasma. Therefore, the normal FFP unit contains 200–300 units of factors VIII and IX. When transfused, each unit of FFP can be expected to increase a patient's factor VIII level by 5–10%. Since very large volumes of FFP will need to be transfused to achieve factor levels better than 50% of normal, FFP has a very limited use in an emergency situation. Its only advantage is that it is usually readily available.

C. CRYOPRECIPITATE:

Cryoprecipitate prepared from flash frozen fresh plasma contains high levels of factor VIII, vWF, and fibrinogen. This is a relatively low-cost product that is prepared by transfusion centers as a blood component. A cryoprecipitate "unit" prepared from a single unit of donated blood will contain from 80 to 150 units of factor VIII in a small volume (30-fold concentrated compared with FFP). In a 75-kg patient who needs an initial treatment dose of 20 U/kg (total dose 1500 units), infusion of 10–15 cryoprecipitate "units" should provide an adequate treatment dose. A postinfusion measurement of factor VIII will help confirm the success of the treatment. With any of the factor VIII preparations, the measured factor VIII level following transfusion is usually 30% lower than the calculated response.

Complications of FFP and cryoprecipitate therapy include allergic reactions, immunosuppression, and viral infections. Allergic reactions include urticaria, bronchospasm, and anaphylaxis. Before the development of purified and recombinant products, most severe hemophiliacs became infected with hepatitis A, B, and C. Prior to the introduction of HIV testing in 1985, most patients were also exposed to HIV. The combination of HCV and HIV can result in severe hepatitis that is poorly responsive to interferon therapy. Up to 20% of HBV-infected hemophiliacs are chronic antigen carriers.

D. PURIFIED FACTOR VIII:

Purified factor VIII concentrates containing known amounts of factor VIII are also available. Since they are easier to store and prepare for infusion, they are preferred by most patients. Dosing can also be easier because they are assayed for factor VIII content. Several purification processes have been used to decrease the risk of viral transmission including heat treatment, solvent-detergent treatment, and, most recently, immunoaffinity purification using mouse monoclonal antibodies (Table 32–3). Current products that have been tested for purity include the very high purity products—Hemophil M and Monoclate P, and the intermediate/high-purity products—Alphanate, Profilate OSD, Koate HP, and Humate-P. Koate HP, Alphanate, and Humate-P also contain high-molecular-weight multimers of vWF, making them more effective for the treatment of Types 1 and 2 vWF patients. Affinity-purified VIII is capable of initiating an allergic reaction secondary to small amounts of mouse protein in the final product. The newest preparation, Kogenate FS, is nearly albumin free, which may further improve its safety.

E. RECOMBINANT FACTOR VIII:

Recombinant factor VIII is commercially produced using mammalian cells transfected with factor VIII complementary DNA. It appears to be biologically identical to human factor VIII and has proved both safe and effective in clinical trials. Compared with cryoprecipitate or purified concentrates, **Recombinate** (**Bioclate**) and **Kogenate** (**Helixate**) are equally efficacious, although considerably more expensive. Despite the costs, recom-

binant factor VIII is recommended for mild hemophiliacs who are HIV negative and have the occasional need for factor therapy. Severe adult hemophiliacs can be given either recombinant or, to reduce the cost, purified product, recognizing that there is still a potential risk of transmitting an as yet unrecognized infectious agent.

An understanding of the pharmacokinetics of a factor VIII infusion is important. Dosage recommendations in Table 32–3 are general guidelines that need to be modified according to the character of the bleed and the patient's measured response. Replacement of factor VIII to achieve a 100% plasma factor level will require an initial infusion of 50–60 U/kg (3500–4000 units in a 70-kg patient). Since the half-life of factor VIII is approximately 12 hours, repeated infusions of 25–30 U/kg every 12 hours will be needed to keep the plasma factor VIII level above 50%. When lower doses (20–30 U/kg) are used, mean postinfusion plasma levels will fall between 30% and 50% (for each unit per kilogram infused the plasma VIII level will rise ~2%).

Based on studies of previously untreated patients, it is estimated that 30–35% of patients exposed to factor VIII concentrate or recombinant product will develop **inhibitor antibodies** after only a few days of treatment (on average 10–12 days of exposure). One-third or more of these are low-titer, less than 5 Bethesda units, and some will disappear spontaneously. For long-term management, it is possible to reduce inhibitor levels by inducing immune tolerance. The strategy involves de-

Table 32–3. Factor VIII concentrates.

Brand Name	Preparation Method to Inactivate Viruses
Factor VIII: Ultrapure recombinant	
Recombinate	Affinity purified
Kogenate	Affinity purified
Factor VIII: High purity from human plasma	
Monoclate P	Affinity purified
Hemofil M	Affinity purified
Coagulation FVIII (American Red Cross)	Affinity purified
	Affinity purified
Factor VIII: Intermediate/high purity from plasma	
Alphanate	Solvent-detergent, heat
Koate HP	Solvent-detergent
Profilate OSD	Solvent-detergent
Humate-P	Pasteurized
Beriate	Pasteurized
Immunate	Vapor heated
Porcine Factor VIII	
Hyate C	None (no report of virus transmission)

sensitizing the patient's immune system to factor VIII by administering large, frequent doses of factor VIII protein over a prolonged period. Regimens of 25–50 U/kg or less of factor VIII, given daily or every other day, have been successful. Lower-titer inhibitors generally respond within 6 months, while higher-titer antibodies may take 12–40 months or never respond. Subsequently, the patient must have maintenance therapy of factor VIII concentrate given three times a week.

New recombinant preparations (ReFacto, Kogenate FS) that may be less immunogenic have become available. Whether this will reduce the incidence of inhibitor formation or allergic reactions still needs to be determined. The use of Refacto, a product where the heavily glycosylated B domain has been deleted, gives the same clinical response but, because of a difference in phospholipid binding, a lower than expected correction of the PTT.

F. Porcine Factor VIII:

Porcine factor VIII (Hyate C) is available for treating patients with factor VIII inhibitors. A dosage of 50–400 U/kg every 8–12 hours, guided by measurements of the factor VIII level, is recommended. It is usually effective in patients with human factor VIII inhibitors, unless the inhibitor level is extremely high. If an attempt is made to use Hyate C on more than one occasion, it is possible to induce an **antiporcine factor VIII antibody.** If this occurs, an otherwise resistant patient may, in the case of a life-threatening bleed, be treated with combinations of **activated PCC** (Autoplex T or FEIBA VH), **immunosuppressive chemotherapy, pheresis using an immunoabsorptive (Staph A) column,** and **recombinant factor VIIa.** The latter uses the extrinsic pathway to initiate successful clotting. It holds many advantages over porcine VIII and the other therapies and is now, after extensive clinical trials, nearing approval for use as first-line therapy in inhibitor patients.

G. Recombinant Factor VIIa:

At higher than normal concentrations, factor VIIa will facilitate the conversion of factor X to Xa and the generation of thrombins, even when factors VIII or IX or both are absent or a high-titer inhibitor is present. **Recombinant VIIa (NovoSeven)** is now available for the treatment of patients with factor VIII or IX inhibitors. A growing experience with the treatment of inhibitor patients has led to the current US Food and Drug Administration recommendation of a dose of 90 µg/kg IV every 2 hours until hemostasis is achieved, followed by an extra dose after 3–6 hours. Pulse doses appear to be preferable to continuous infusions of factor VIIa. Recombinant factor VIIa has also been used to control

bleeding during surgery and in cases of multiple trauma. Laboratory monitoring will demonstrate a shortening of the activated PTT, but this does not appear to correlate with the clinical control of hemostasis. Factor VII-deficient patients can be managed with a lower dose, 25–30 µg/kg, with redosing according to PT results. The risk of serious side effects, including widespread thrombosis or DIC, appears to be very low, although the experience to date is still limited.

H. Antifibrinolytics:

Antifibrinolytic agents can be helpful in controlling milder bleeding episodes, especially those associated with dental procedures. In effect, these agents enhance hemostasis by stabilizing the clot and discouraging rebleeding. **EACA (Amicar)**, is available for clinical use. EACA is given in a dose of 4 grams every 4–6 hours orally or by slow infusion for up to 7 days. It is well tolerated.

Hemophilia B

Several products are available for treating hemophilia B patients. **FFP** or **solvent/detergent-treated plasma (S/D plasma)** can be used for the patient with milder disease or a minor bleeding episode. Purified factor IX from plasma include AlphaNine SD and Mononine and the recombinant product Benefix. Commercially prepared **FIX-PCCs** Konyne 80, Proplex T, Profilnine, and Bebulin VH are available for the treatment of more severe bleeding episodes (Table 32–4).

Treatment with FFP or S/D plasma requires the administration of an **adequate dose** (see Table 32–2). To successfully treat a hemophilia B patient with a hemarthrosis or muscle hematoma with FFP, a dose of at least 15 mL/kg or approximately 1200 mL of FFP has to be given. This dose represents a major volume and cardiovascular challenge for the patient. If bleeding is controlled and no further treatment is necessary, FFP therapy will do the job. As with the use of FFP in hemophilia A, allergic reactions are common.

A purified factor IX concentrate, FIX-PCC, or recombinant IX must be employed for more **severe bleeds or prolonged treatment** over several days. Dosing recommendations are similar to those for factor VIII concentrates (see Table 32–2). However, the pharmacokinetics of factor IX are different. Because of its smaller molecular weight of 56,000 as compared with 330,000 for factor VIII, factor IX is not restricted to the intravascular space, giving it a volume of distribution of nearly twice that of factor VIII. Therefore, in order to achieve a 100% plasma level, a dose of 100 U/kg (7000 units in a 70-kg patient) needs to be administered. At the same time, factor IX has a half-life of 24 hours, so repeated infusions of 50 U/kg every

Table 32–4. Factor IX concentrates.

Brand Name	Preparation Method to Inactivate Viruses
Factor IX: recombinant	
BeneFIX	Affinity purified
Factor IX: purified concentration (factors IX, low levels II and X)	
AlphaNine SD	Solvent-detergent, nanofiltered
Mononine	Affinity purified, ultrafiltration
Factor IX: complex concentrates (factors IX, II, and X)	
Konyne 80	Dry heat
Proplex T	Dry heat
Profilnine SD	Solvent-detergent
Bebulin VH	Vapor heated
Factor IX: activated complex (all factors)	
Autoplex T	Dry heat
FEIBA VH	Vapor heated

24 hours are sufficient to keep the factor IX plasma level above 50%. Like factor VIII recommendations, doses of 30–50 U/kg will generally give mean IX levels of 20–30%, which is adequate for less-severe bleeds.

Recombinant or purified factor IX preparations are preferred for the treatment of the **uncomplicated hemophilia B** patient. Recombinant IX concentrate gives a somewhat lower plasma level of factor IX, about 20% lower when compared with the affinity-purified product. FIX-PCC concentrates will also work. However, if repeated doses of FIX-PCC are to be given to a patient, the problem of precipitating DIC or thrombosis by way of factor activation during preparation must be considered. The patient should be closely monitored, especially the levels of antithrombin III. Periodic infusions of FFP or AT-III concentrate (Thrombate III) should be given if the AT-III level is found to be low. Activated FIX-PCCs that contain purposely activated factors (Autoplex T and FEIBA VH) are available for treatment of patients with factor IX inhibitors. The dose is similar to the use of FIX-PCC. Once approved, factor VIIa is likely to be the therapy of choice for factor IX inhibitor patients.

Gene Therapy

Hemophilia is the ideal disease for gene therapy. Techniques are now under development to introduce the factor VIII gene into hepatocytes, fibroblasts, and endothelial cells using adeno-associated viral vectors. Stable expression of even a small number of gene-transfected cells would make a major difference; an increase in factor VIII or IX level of only a few percent would significantly reduce the clinical severity of the disease.

BIBLIOGRAPHY

Diagnosis

Brettler DB: Inhibitors of factor VIII and IX. Haemophilia 1995;1 (Suppl 1):35.

Hilgartner MW, Pochedly C: *Hemophilia in the Child and Adult,* 2nd ed. Raven Press, 1989.

Hoyer LW: Hemophilia A. N Engl J Med 1994;330:38.

Kessler CM: Proceedings of a symposium: Acquired factor VIII inhibitors in the nonhemophiliac: Historical perspectives, current therapies, and future approaches. Am J Med 1991; 91:5A.

Sadler JE: Recombinant DNA methods in hemophilia A: Carrier detection and prenatal diagnosis. Semin Thromb Hemost 1990;16:341.

Therapy

Berntorp E: Methods of haemophilia care delivery: Regular prophylaxis versus episodic treatment. Haemophilia 1995; 1(Suppl 1):3.

Bloom AL: Progress in the clinical management of haemophilia. Thromb Haemost 1991;66:166.

Furie B, Limentani SA, Rosenfield CG: A practical guide to the evaluation and treatment of hemophilia. Blood 1994;84:3.

Hedner U: Novoseven as a universal hemostatic agent. Blood Coagul Fibrinolysis 2000;11:107.

Kasper CK: *Recent Advances in Hemophilia Care.* Alan R. Liss, 1990.

Kasper CK et al: Hemophilia in the 1990s: Principles of management and improved access to care. Semin Thromb Hemost 1992;18:1.

Kenet G et al: Treatment of inhibitor patients with rFVIIa: Continuous infusion protocols as compared to a single, large, dose. Haemophilia 2000;6:279.

Kim HC et al: Purified factor IX using monoclonal immunoaffinity technique: Clinical trials in hemophilia B and comparison to prothrombin complex concentrates. Blood 1992;79:568.

Lee CA: Management of patients with HIV and/or hepatitis. Haemophilia 1995;1(Suppl 1):26.

Limentani SA et al: Recombinant blood clotting proteins for hemophilia therapy. Semin Thromb Hemost 1993;19:62.

Lozier JN, Brinkhous KM: Gene therapy and the hemophilias. JAMA 1994;271:47.

Shaffer LG, Phillips MD: Successful treatment of acquired hemophilia with oral immunosuppressive therapy. Ann Intern Med 1997;127:206.

Extrinsic and Common Pathway Coagulopathies

33

An abnormality in the extrinsic or common pathways can result in a significant bleeding tendency. Inherited deficiencies of a single coagulation factor, including factors VII, V, X, and prothrombin, are rare. More commonly, bleeding results from deficiencies in several factors. This situation reflects that they are mostly vitamin K–dependent factors produced by the liver, so liver disease or poor vitamin K intake can be expected to produce a multifactor abnormality.

THE NORMAL EXTRINSIC & COMMON PATHWAYS

Interactions of the factors involved in the extrinsic and common pathways are illustrated in Figures 33–1 and 33–2. The extrinsic pathway begins with activation of factor VII by **tissue factor,** that is, microsomal lipoproteins derived from damaged tissue. In the presence of excess tissue factor, factor VII activation provides a potent stimulus for the activation of factor X to Xa. With lower tissue factor levels, factor VIIa is inhibited by tissue factor pathway inhibitor, and further factor X activation depends on the intrinsic pathway, the activation of factor IX (VIII) by thrombin and factor XIa (see Chapter 27).

By definition, the common pathway (see Figure 33–2) involves Xa activation of prothrombin to form thrombin and the subsequent thrombin conversion of fibrinogen to fibrin clot. Activation of X to Xa and its interaction with prothrombin requires the presence of surface membrane and factor V. A major deficiency in any one of these elements, including the availability of platelet membrane, factor VII, X, V, or fibrinogen, can impair clotting and result in a bleeding tendency.

CLINICAL FEATURES

A single deficiency in any of these coagulation factors can be asymptomatic or produce a bleeding tendency ranging from easy bruising, epistaxis, and menorrhagia to severe hemophilia-type bleeding with major mucous membrane bleeding, hemarthroses, and hematoma formation. The latter is only seen in patients who have factor levels below 1–2%.

■ 1. CONGENITAL ABNORMALITIES

Hereditary deficiency of factor VII is a very rare autosomal recessive disease with highly variable clinical severity. Only homozygote patients have low enough factor VII levels to have symptomatic bleeding. These patients are easily recognized from their unique laboratory pattern of a prolonged prothrombin time (PT) but normal partial thromboplastin time (PTT) (Table 33–1).

Congenital deficiencies in factors X, V, and prothrombin are also inherited as autosomal recessive traits. They are all quite rare. Since all of these factors are part of the common pathway, patients with severe disease demonstrate prolongations of both the PT and PTT. Patients with congenital factor V deficiency may have a prolonged bleeding time because of the relationship between factor V and platelet function in supporting clot formation.

Congenital abnormalities in fibrinogen production will obviously interfere with the final step in the common pathway. Decreased levels of fibrinogen, either hypofibrinogenemia or afibrinogenemia, are relatively rare conditions inherited as autosomal recessive traits. Patients with afibrinogenemia have a severe bleeding diathesis with both spontaneous and posttraumatic bleeding. Since the bleeding can begin during the first few days of life, this condition may be initially confused with hemophilia. Hypofibrinogenemic patients usually do not have spontaneous bleeding but may have difficulty with surgery. Severe bleeding can be anticipated in patients with plasma fibrinogen levels below 50 mg/dL.

Dysfibrinogenemia

A more common defect is the **production of an abnormal fibrinogen.** The normal fibrinogen molecule is a 340-kDa glycoprotein composed of three pairs of polypeptide chains referred to as α, β, and γ. Fibrino-

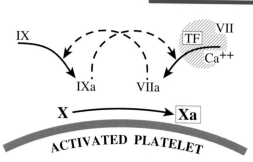

Extrinsic pathway

Figure 33–1. **The extrinsic pathway.** The extrinsic pathway is initiated by release of microsomal lipoproteins (tissue factor) from damaged tissue. This tissue factor (TF) activates factor VII, which plays a role in the activation of factors X and IX. With high levels of TF, factor X activation reaches a maximum rate. With lower levels, the interaction with factor IX is increasingly important.

gen is synthesized in the liver under the control of three genes, one for each chain, on chromosome 4. Mutations in one or another of these genes can impair the normal polymerization of the fibrinopeptides to form insoluble fibrin, resulting in a dysfibrinogenemia. More than 300 different mutations producing dysfunctional and, at times, reduced amounts of fibrinogen have now been reported. Many of these mutations are inherited as autosomal dominant traits.

The clinical presentation of dysfibrinogenemia is highly variable. Patients who demonstrate both a reduced amount and a dysfunctional fibrinogen (**hypodysfibrinogenemia**) usually exhibit excessive bleeding. This is also true for a few families who are homozygous for dysfibrinogenemia. Most dysfibrinogenemic patients, however, appear to be heterozygotes for the trait and, although they have abnormal coagulation tests, do not have a bleeding tendency. Overall, roughly 60% of dysfibrinogenemias are clinically silent, whereas the remainder can present with either a bleeding diathesis or a thrombotic tendency, in equal measure. A small number of dysfibrinogenemias have been associated with spontaneous abortion and poor wound healing.

Factor XIII Deficiency

Stability of fibrin clot is also hemostatically important. **Factor XIII (fibrin-stabilizing factor) deficiency** is a rare autosomal recessive disorder with an estimated prevalence of 1 in 5 million. Patients present at birth with persistent umbilical cord stump or circumcision bleeding. Adult patients demonstrate a severe bleeding diathesis, characterized by recurrent soft tissue bleeding, poor wound healing, and a high incidence of intracranial hemorrhage. Typically, the bleeding is somewhat delayed based on the role of factor XIII in stabilizing the fibrin clot. Blood clots form but are weak and unable to maintain hemostasis. Fetal loss in women with factor XIII deficiency can approach 100%, suggesting a critical role for the factor in maintaining pregnancy.

Figure 33–2. **The common pathway.** Both the intrinsic and extrinsic pathways stimulate the common pathway. Factor X is activated to Xa, which then stimulates the conversion of prothrombin to thrombin. This step is facilitated by the presence of both platelet surface membrane and factor V. Generation of thrombin and its action on fibrinogen are amplification steps in the formation of fibrin clot. Thrombin further amplifies coagulation by stimulating platelet activation and by activating factor XIII to stabilize fibrin polymer.

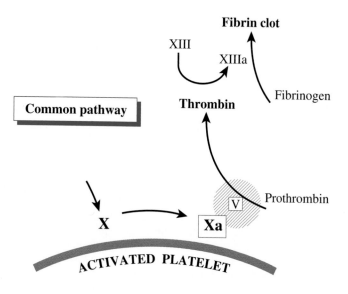

Common pathway

Table 33–1. Prothrombin time and partial thromboplastin time patterns with disease.

Defect	PT	PTT	PTT 1:1 mix
Extrinsic pathway			
Factor VII deficiency	Prolonged	Normal	—
Intrinsic pathway			
Factor VIII, IX, or XI deficiency	Normal	Prolonged	Shortens
Lupus anticoagulant	Usually normal	Prolonged	No correction
Anti-VIII or -IX antibody	Normal	Prolonged	No correction
Common pathway			
Congenital deficiencies			
Factor X, V, or prothrombin	Prolonged	Prolonged	Shortens
Hypo-/dysfibrinogenemia	Prolonged	Prolonged	Shortens
Liver disease/vitamin K deficiency			
Mild	Prolonged	Normal	—
Severe	Prolonged	Prolonged	Shortens
Anticoagulants			
Heparin therapy	Normal	Prolonged	—
Warfarin therapy	Prolonged	Normal	—
Heparin/coumarin overdose	Prolonged	Prolonged	—

Laboratory Studies

The first step in evaluating the extrinsic and common pathways is the measurement of both a **PT** and **PTT.** As summarized in Table 33–1, comparison of these two measurements can separate a congenital factor VII deficiency from a factor deficiency in the common pathway. Since both tests require normal fibrinogen function, hypo- or dysfibrinogenemia will prolong both the PT and PTT. Definitive diagnosis of a single coagulation factor deficiency requires **specific factor assays** for VII, X, V, and prothrombin. Diagnosis of hypo- or dysfibrinogenemia requires **assays of fibrinogen concentration and function.**

The PT and PTT assays are discussed in Chapter 28. Evaluation of fibrinogen involves measurements of both fibrinogen concentration and function. The most accurate measurement of total fibrinogen protein is provided by **immunoassay** or a **protein precipitation technique.** Although this approach will give a good measure of total fibrinogen, it does not provide information regarding the ability of the fibrinogen to polymerize to form fibrin. A functional assay, such as the **von Clauss assay,** provides a measure of clottable fibrinogen. This method uses thrombin to convert fibrinogen to fibrin, followed by measurement of the amount of fibrin in the clot. A dysfibrinogenemia should be suspected whenever there is a significant difference between the amount of fibrinogen measured immunochemically versus that measured by the thrombin clot (von Clauss) technique. **Other screening tests for fibrinogen dysfunction** include the thrombin time

(TT) and whole blood clotting time using a venom enzyme such as reptilase. Both are sensitive to fibrinogen dysfunction. Definitive diagnosis and subclassification of a dysfibrinogenemia requires **fibrinopeptide chain analysis by SDS polyacrylamide gel electrophoresis and amino acid sequencing.**

Factor XIII deficiency should be considered in a patient with a severe bleeding diathesis who has otherwise normal coagulation screening tests, including PT, PTT, fibrinogen level, platelet count, and bleeding time. **Clot dissolution in 1% monochloroacetic acid** can be used as a screen. Definitive diagnosis requires quantitating factor XIII activity by **radiolabeled putrescine incorporation into dimethylated casein.** Patients at risk for severe hemorrhage have factor XIII levels of close to 1%. Heterozygotes (factor XIII levels of around 50%) usually exhibit no bleeding tendency.

■ 2. ACQUIRED ABNORMALITIES

Differential diagnosis of an acquired coagulation defect involving the extrinsic or common pathway has to be done at bedside. The patient's disease history, nutritional status, and drug history must be carefully defined and integrated with the laboratory studies. If the PT is very prolonged but the PTT is normal, a congenital deficiency in factor VII is most likely (see Table 33–1). More often, however, the discordance between the two measurements is less marked. This situation is compatible with a multiple factor deficiency state secondary to hepatocellular disease, a nutritional deficiency of vitamin K, or treatment with warfarin. Basically, the PT is a more sensitive measure of modest reductions in multiple common pathway factors than the PTT.

A more balanced prolongation of the PT and PTT is seen in patients with **severe liver disease.** In addition to greater reductions in the vitamin K–dependent factors produced by the liver, abnormal fibrinogen molecules and fibrin degradation products appear and act as inhibitors of the two assays. In this circumstance, the PTT and a measurement of the TT are more sensitive to the fibrinogen abnormalities. Prolongations of the PT and PTT are also seen in patients with **disseminated intravascular coagulation** (**DIC**). This condition results from a combination of factor consumption, severe hypofibrinogenemia, and fibrinolysis with the appearance of fibrin degradation products.

The clinician must always be alert to the potential impact of **anticoagulant drugs** on these pathways. The coumarin family of drugs inhibits vitamin K reductase and interferes with carboxylation of glutamyl residues of prothrombin and factors VII, IX, and X. The most sensitive factor is factor VII because of its short half-life. This half-life can result in a prolongation of the PT with little or no effect on the PTT. Heparin also interferes with the common pathway by blocking the activation of fibrinogen by thrombin. Heparin at therapeutic levels will prolong the PTT with little effect on the PT.

Less common causes of a defect in the common pathway are listed in Table 33–2. Vitamin K–dependent factor deficiencies can result from the ingestion of drugs that interfere with vitamin K absorption. Cholestyramine binds bile acids and interrupts the absorption of fat-soluble vitamins. Use of excessive doses of vitamin E or A can also interfere with the absorption or metabolism of vitamin K. Salicylate overdose affects vitamin K metabolism and prolongs the PT. Finally, both cefamandole and cefoperazone can interfere with the intrahepatic metabolism of vitamin K. Severe malabsorption can result in a rapid depletion of vitamin K over a matter of days. Vitamin K deficiency is often seen in patients with small bowel disease such as bacterial overgrowth, short bowel syndrome, sprue, and regional enteritis.

Acquired deficiencies of single factors are rare. A deficiency in factor VII has been described in patients with homocystinuria, whereas low prothrombin levels have been reported in patients with lupus erythematosus. Patients with amyloidosis can develop a factor X deficiency owing to binding of factor X to the amyloid. Finally, factor IX levels as well as antithrombin III levels can fall because of urinary loss in patients with nephrotic syndrome.

Table 33–2. Acquired deficiencies of common pathway factors.

Reduced vitamin K intake
Hemorrhagic disease of newborn
Poor diet (lack of leafy vegetables)
Malabsorption
Pancreatitis
Small bowel disease
Biliary obstruction
Vitamin A or E administration
Drug ingestion
Cholestyramine
Mineral oil
Antibiotics
Abnormal metabolism
Hepatocellular disease
Protein-calorie malnutrition
Drug ingestion
Salicylates
Hydantoins
Antibiotics
Superwarfarins (rodenticides)
Other mechanisms
Amyloidosis: factor X binding
Nephrotic syndrome: factor IX and antithrombin III loss
Lupus erythematosus: antiprothrombin antibody
Homocystinuria: factor VII deficiency

Laboratory Studies

The laboratory evaluation of a possible acquired defect must be guided by the clinical picture. If a patient obviously has liver disease or is receiving an anticoagulant drug, a single test of the **PT** and **PTT** may be satisfactory. Since the PT is the most sensitive measure of a common pathway abnormality, this test is frequently used as a screening test to rule out disease or drug effects. In fact, many clinicians include the PT as a routine part of their evaluation of liver function.

In severely ill patients who demonstrate an abnormal bleeding tendency or who are at risk for bleeding, a **full evaluation of the extrinsic and common pathways,** together with measurements of fibrinogen concentration and fibrin turnover (**fibrinolysis**), is in order. Most laboratories offer a panel of tests for this evaluation. At a minimum, this panel should include a PT, PTT, TT, an assay of fibrinogen concentration, and a measurement of fibrin degradation products (split products, D-dimer, or both). Other valuable tests for evaluating the rate of clot formation and dissolution are the **antithrombin III** and α_2**-antiplasmin levels.** The interpretation of these tests is discussed in Chapter 34.

THERAPY

The treatment of a single-factor–deficiency state depends on the severity of the bleeding. The therapeutic objective is to replace enough of the missing factor to maintain a level sufficient to control bleeding and permit healing. This approach is similar to that for treating the patient with hemophilia.

Congenital Abnormalities

Most patients with factor VII deficiency can be treated with infusions of **fresh frozen plasma** (**FFP**). Patients with factor VII levels less than 1% will require treatment with a **prothrombin complex concentrate** (**PCC**) or, better, **affinity purified factor VII.**

Deficiencies in factors X, V, and prothrombin are generally treated with FFP or **detergent/solvent plasma** (**D/S plasma**) for any but the most severe bleeding episodes. FFP is basically flash frozen plasma harvested from a unit of donated blood. D/S plasma is FFP treated with the solvent tri- (*n*-butyl) phosphate and the detergent Triton X-100 to remove lipid-envelope viruses. Several units from different donors are pooled for transfusion. The concentration of the vitamin K–dependent factors in FFP is approximately the same as that of normal plasma in vivo. Therefore, to obtain a significant increase in the level of any factor, a considerable volume of FFP must be infused. As a rule of thumb, at least 4–6 units of FFP are needed to attain a 20–30% increase in any missing factor level. This level represents a considerable volume of plasma (800–1200 mL) and presents a significant cardiovascular challenge to the patient. Moreover, the duration of effectiveness of this replacement therapy depends on the turnover time of each factor (Figure 33–3). This protocol means that repeated infusion of FFP will be needed to maintain a factor level.

For a severe bleeder, several PCCs are commercially available (Table 33–3). The advantage of these products is that factor levels of 50% or higher can be achieved without the risk of volume overload. The disadvantages of PCCs are the risk of transmission of hepatitis B and C and the induction of widespread thrombosis, thromboembolism, and DIC. It is also important to recognize the variation in factor levels in the several products. The preferred product to treat patients with factor VII deficiency is **Proplex T** because of its high level of factor VII.

Most patients with dysfibrinogenemia have no clinical disease and, therefore, do not require therapy. For those who are symptomatic or are at risk for bleeding with surgery, plasma fibrinogen levels can be replaced with **cryoprecipitate.** To increase the fibrinogen level by at least 100 mg/dL in the average-sized adult, 10–12 units of cryoprecipitate should be infused, followed by 2–3 units each day (fibrinogen is catabolized at a rate of 25% per day). Patients with a thrombotic tendency will require long-term anticoagulation.

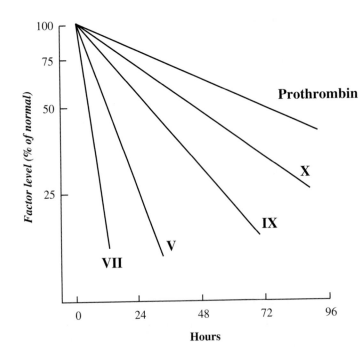

Figure 33–3. Coagulation factor turnover. Factors IX, X, and prothrombin have biological half-lives after transfusion of 24–72 hours. In contrast, factor V has a half-life of approximately 12 hours and factor VII a very short half-life of 2–5 hours. The shorter the turnover time of a factor, the more frequently the patient will need a repeated infusion of FFP.

Table 33–3. Prothrombin complex concentrates.

	Factor Levels (U/100 Units Factor IX)		
	Prothrombin	*Factor VII*	*Factor X*
Proplex T (Baxter Hyland)	50	400	50
Konyne-HT (Cutter)	100	20	140
Profilnine-HT (Alpha)	150	11	60
Bebulin VH	120	13	140

Factor XIII–deficient patients can be treated with FFP, cryoprecipitate, or a plasma-derived factor XIII concentrate—**Fibrogammin P.** Acute hemorrhage should be treated with an infusion of 50–75 U/kg body weight; prophylaxis is possible using intravenous injections of 10–20 U/kg at 4- to 6-week intervals depending on the patient's preinfusion plasma factor XIII level. Factor XIII has a long circulating half-life of 7–12 days, and adequate hemostasis is achieved with even very low plasma concentrations (1–3%).

Acquired Abnormalities

A. VITAMIN K DEFICIENCY:

Patients with vitamin K deficiency should be treated with oral or parenteral vitamin K according to the cause of the deficiency state. Simple dietary deficiency can easily be corrected with a daily oral supplement of 5–10 mg. Patients with severe malabsorption or a defect in vitamin K metabolism should receive 5–10 mg of vitamin K subcutaneously daily.

In the case of warfarin therapy, vitamin K administration (vitamin K_1 at a dose of 1–2 mg intravenously or 5–10 mg subcutaneously) can reverse the warfarin effect within 6–12 hours. If the effect must be reversed more rapidly, as in the case of a severe bleeding episode or emergency surgery, the patient should be given 4–6 units of FFP every 6–12 hours until the PT normalizes. In the patient who has ingested a rodenticide containing one of the long-acting warfarin congeners, a 50–100 mg dose of vitamin K or more by mouth will need to be given daily for extended periods. FFP will be required if the patient is acutely bleeding.

B. LIVER DISEASE:

Treatment of a patient with liver disease can be very difficult, since bleeding is usually multifactorial. There is often a vascular lesion such as bleeding varices, gastritis, or peptic ulcer that must be controlled locally. If the liver dysfunction is mild and associated with a poor diet, vitamin K therapy may improve factor production and shorten the PT and PTT. More likely, however, it will be ineffective.

The results of the **coagulation test profile should drive the approach to therapy.** First and foremost, the platelet count should be maintained at levels close to 100,000/μL by repeated transfusions of random donor platelets. The higher count is necessary to counteract the platelet function defect seen with liver disease. This can be difficult, however, since patients with advanced liver disease respond poorly to platelet transfusions. They not only have high rates of platelet destruction but also trap platelets in their enlarged spleens.

Next, if the fibrinogen level is less than 125 mg/dL, the patient should receive a transfusion with 10 units of cryoprecipitate, and the fibrinogen level should be monitored to determine the need for additional cryoprecipitate. Third, if the PT and PTT are both prolonged, the patient should receive FFP. Since the principal defect may be a reduced production of factor VII, a transfusion of 2 units of FFP, raising the factor VII level by 5–10%, will shorten the PT and may have a positive clinical effect. Attempts to normalize the PT and PTT must be discouraged. This would require the repeated infusion of large volumes of FFP, resulting in marked fluid overload. Finally, packed red blood cell transfusions should be given as required to maintain a hematocrit of ~30%.

Since abnormal fibrinolysis can be a significant factor in the bleeding diathesis of the liver disease patient, a trial of an antifibrinolytic, such as **epsilon aminocaproic acid (EACA)** or tranexamic acid, may be beneficial. EACA should be given as a bolus intravenously, 4–5 grams in the first hour, followed by a continuous infusion of 1 gram per hour for 8 hours. Maintenance is possible using an oral dose of 4 grams of EACA every 4 hours. **Tranexamic acid** is initiated with a 10 mg/kg intravenous bolus, followed by 10 mg/kg intravenously, every 6–8 hours.

BIBLIOGRAPHY

Alperin JB: Coagulopathy caused by vitamin K deficiency in critically ill, hospitalized patients. JAMA 1987;258:1916.

Beutler E et al: *Hematology,* 6th ed. McGraw-Hill, 2001.

Colman RW et al: *Hemostasis and Thrombosis: Basic Principles and Clinical Practice,* 2nd ed. JB Lippincott, 1987.

Dodd R: The risk of transfusion-transmitted infection. N Engl J Med 1992;327:419.

Horowitz B et al: Solvent/detergent-treated plasma: A virus-inactivated substitute for fresh frozen plasma. Blood 1992;79:826.

Kasper C: *Recent Advances in Hemophilia Care.* Alan R. Liss, 1990.

Lipsky JJ: Antibiotic-associated hypoprothrombinaemia. J Antimicrob Chem 1988;21:281.

Mannucci PM: Hemostatic drugs. N Engl J Med 1998;339:245.

Consumptive Coagulopathies

Widespread activation of the coagulation pathways can occur as a part of a systemic illness. When severe, it presents as acute disseminated intravascular coagulation (DIC) with life-threatening intravascular clotting and fibrinolysis. This can result in sufficient platelet and coagulation factor depletion to cause severe bleeding. Other conditions are associated with lower-grade DIC or a process that is limited to platelet thrombus formation (**platelet DIC**). In the latter case, organ damage can be the dominant abnormality. Therefore, it is important to be able to recognize the presence and nature of the DIC because it will help diagnose the illness, prevent organ damage, and manage the patient's bleeding tendency.

THROMBOSIS & THROMBOLYSIS

Thrombus formation is a highly controlled process, where platelet activation, aggregation, and subsequent clot formation are under delicate control. Normal endothelial cells adjacent to a site of injury are responsible for limiting platelet activation and aggregation by releasing prostacyclin and nitric oxide and by degradation of ADP by a membrane-associated ADPase (Figure 34–1). **Tissue factor pathway inhibitor** (**TFPI**) limits activation of factor X by binding to the TF-VIIa-Xa complex. At the same time, circulating thrombin is inactivated by **antithrombin III,** a specific protease inhibitor. This reaction is facilitated by heparin-like molecules produced by endothelial cells. In addition, thrombomodulin binding of thrombin effectively down-regulates thrombin activity by preventing the activation of factor V. Both protein C and protein S are cofactors in this reaction.

Formation of the fibrin clot is also carefully controlled. **Tissue plasminogen activator** (**t-PA**) produced by the endothelial cells activates plasminogen incorporated in the clot to the active protease, plasmin. The reaction is supported by the activation of protein C, which down-regulates circulating t-PA inhibitors. The end result is localized fibrinolysis and remodeling of the clot. Runaway fibrinolysis and destruction of fibrinogen is prevented by a circulating inhibitor of plasmin, α_2-antiplasmin, and thrombin activatable fibrinolysis inhibitor (TAFI).

An understanding of these interactions provides a framework for the diagnosis of a consumptive coagulopathy. Normal individuals maintain levels of platelets and coagulation factors within relatively narrow normal limits. When the coagulation pathways are strongly activated, the number of circulating platelets and the level of individual factors decrease according to the severity of the consumptive process. In addition, increased fibrinolysis and consumption of specific inhibitors are by definition integral to the concept of a consumptive coagulopathy.

CLINICAL FEATURES

A consumptive coagulopathy may present with symptoms and signs of organ damage secondary to microvascular thrombosis or as an abnormal bleeding tendency. Often the pattern of the coagulopathy is characteristic of the underlying systemic illness. For example, patients with widespread malignancy are at increased risk for thromboembolic disease and chronic low-grade DIC. In contrast, septic patients or women with an abruptio placentae or amniotic fluid embolism will more often demonstrate acute, severe DIC and a bleeding diathesis. It is extremely important, therefore, to evaluate the patient for both thrombotic and hemorrhagic manifestations typical of DIC (Table 34–1).

Thrombosis of the microvasculature is characterized by multifocal neurologic signs, skin infarction, acute renal shutdown, acute respiratory distress syndrome, and bowel infarction. Marked reductions in coagulation factors and platelets result in a combination of petechial hemorrhages and widespread purpura, mucous membrane bleeding, oozing around central lines and venipuncture sites, gastrointestinal (GI) and genitourinary bleeding, and intracerebral hemorrhage. In some patients, intravascular fibrin deposition results in red blood cell fragmentation and sufficient hemolysis to produce an anemia.

The importance of the clinical setting cannot be overemphasized. The common association of platelet consumption or DIC with severe, systemic illnesses should be enough to stimulate a full evaluation of the coagulation pathways as a part of the patient's management. This situation is certainly true if the patient ex-

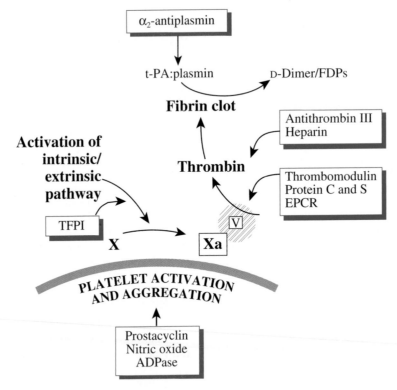

Figure 34–1. **Thrombosis and thrombolysis.** The rush to fibrin clot formation in a consumptive coagulopathy is counteracted by several inhibitors. Endothelial cells release prostacyclin, nitric oxide, and ADPase to inhibit platelet activation and aggregation. Tissue factor pathway inhibitor (TFPI) inhibits factor X activation by binding to the TF-VIIa-Xa complex. In addition, thrombomodulin produced by endothelial cells binds thrombin and down-regulates activation of factor V. Protein C and protein S are cofactors in this reaction. Antithrombin III also inhibits thrombin by using heparin-like molecules produced by the endothelial cells to facilitate the reaction. Finally, fibrin clot can be rapidly dissolved by the t-PA–driven plasmin system. The rate of fibrinolysis is assessed from the level of α_2-antiplasmin, the inhibitor of plasmin, and D-dimer/FDP levels.

Table 34–1. Signs and symptoms of consumptive coagulopathies.

Microvascular thrombosis	
Neurologic	Convulsions, delirium, coma, multifocal cortical infarction
Pulmonary	Hypoxemia, acute respiratory distress syndrome
Renal	Oliguria, uremia, renal shutdown
Gastrointestinal	Mucosal ulceration, bowel infarction
Skin	Skin infarction, digital gangrene
Bleeding manifestations	
Neurologic	Hemorrhagic infarction, massive intracerebral bleeding
Pulmonary	Pulmonary hemorrhage
Renal	Hematuria
Gastrointestinal	Mucous membrane and intestinal bleeding
Skin	Petechiae, purpura, epistaxis, generalized oozing from venipuncture sites and wounds

hibits any signs of unexplained organ failure or an abnormal bleeding tendency.

Laboratory Studies

To properly evaluate a patient for DIC, a battery of **coagulation tests** should be ordered, including at a minimum a platelet count, prothrombin time (PT), partial thromboplastin time (PTT), thrombin time (TT), fibrinogen assay, test(s) for fibrin split products, and both antithrombin III and α_2-antiplasmin levels. The **blood film** should be examined for red blood cell fragmentation and any abnormal cell forms. By performing these tests at one time, it is possible to get the truest picture of the balance between coagulation factor consumption and fibrinolysis. The DIC picture can change very rapidly. Therefore, when tests are drawn at separate times, it will be difficult to interpret the results.

The diagnosis of DIC cannot be made from any single observation or laboratory measurement. Rather, it is based on the concordance of the right clinical setting and laboratory evidence of aggressive coagulation and fibrinolysis. In patients with **high-grade DIC,** the consumption of coagulation factors exceeds production capacity and there is a decline in the levels of key coagulation factors, especially platelets and fibrinogen. This condition is assessed clinically with **measurements of platelet count, PT, PTT, and fibrinogen.** Usually there is a balanced reduction in coagulation factors in that the platelet count falls to below 50–100,000/μL, both the PT and PTT are modestly prolonged, and the fibrinogen level falls below 100 mg/dL. The more severe the DIC, the lower the platelet count and fibrinogen level. In patients with **low-grade DIC,** increased production levels of platelets and coagulation factors may be sufficient to compensate for the consumption. This increase makes the diagnosis more difficult. In fact, chronic low-grade DIC may only be diagnosed with **radiolabeled turnover studies of platelets and fibrinogen.**

The **fibrinolytic component of DIC** is assessed by measurements of the TT, circulating fibrin split products, and the antithrombin III and α_2-antiplasmin levels. Two assays are commonly used to detect fibrin split products, the **latex agglutination measurement of fibrin(ogen) degradation products (FDPs)** and the D-**dimer assay for fibrin split products.** Both assays should be performed for maximum sensitivity and specificity. The latex agglutination assay for FDPs is extremely sensitive but not as specific for fibrin breakdown. The D-dimer test is specific for fibrin clot lysis but less sensitive (Figure 34–2). The TT can be used as another indicator of active fibrinolysis; high levels of split products in circulation will prolong the TT. Used together, these tests should identify most patients with DIC.

Assays for antithrombin III and α_2-antiplasmin provide valuable information regarding **severity of the DIC.** As the specific inhibitor of thrombin, **antithrombin III** is progressively depleted with high levels of thrombin activation. Similarly, α_2-**antiplasmin** as the inhibitor of plasmin is depleted with increased rates of fibrinolysis. Depressions of both antithrombin III and α_2-antiplasmin to below 40–50% of normal suggest severe, ongoing DIC. Normal levels of both inhibitors suggest consumption limited to platelets, low-grade DIC, or recovery from a time-limited episode of DIC. In the latter case, antithrombin III and α_2-antiplasmin levels recover quickly once the stimulus for intravascular coagulation is removed and fibrinolysis ceases. Since α_2-antiplasmin has a somewhat faster recovery, a disparity can exist between the two levels, that is, an antithrombin III level below 40–50% and an α_2-antiplasmin level approaching normal. This situation typifies the patient who had a discrete DIC episode some 12–24 hours before the evaluation. By 48 hours after a limited DIC episode, both levels should be back to normal.

DIFFERENTIAL DIAGNOSIS

The differential diagnosis of a severe consumptive coagulopathy is relatively straightforward. **DIC resulting in abnormal bleeding** because of thrombocytopenia and hypofibrinogenemia is easily recognized from both the clinical setting and the pattern of laboratory abnormalities. It most often accompanies a severe systemic illness (Table 34–2). Sepsis, shock, a crush injury or surgical trauma, widespread malignancy, hemorrhagic pancreatitis, or an obstetric complication such as eclampsia, intrauterine fetal death, amniotic fluid embolism, or abruptio placentae are **common clinical settings** where DIC occurs with some frequency. They represent situations where there is a major vascular injury (release of endotoxin, hypotension), a release into circulation of a specific protease (trypsin in patients with pancreatitis), or release of a cellular thromboplastin (tissue injury from trauma or surgery, amniotic fluid embolism). Presence of any one of these conditions should raise the possibility of DIC, whereas the detection of the typical laboratory profile of DIC should alert the clinician to the presence and severity of the illness.

Isolated platelet consumption (platelet DIC) is seen in patients with vascular disorders such as vasculitis, hemolytic uremic syndrome (HUS), and thrombotic thrombocytopenic purpura (TTP). Usually, these patients present with symptoms and signs of organ damage, renal failure from glomerular thrombosis, skin infarction, and multifocal brain infarction. Red blood cell hemolysis owing to fragmentation by platelet and

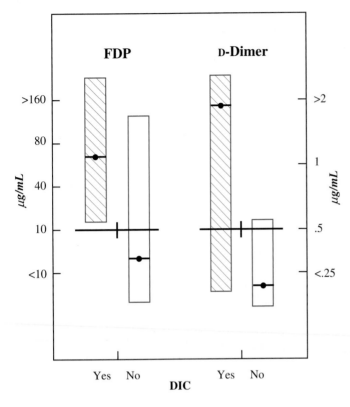

Figure 34–2. **FDP and D-dimer levels in patients with DIC.** Measurement of the FDP level is very sensitive to the presence of fibrinolysis in patients with DIC. It lacks specificity, however. Patients with liver disease and other systemic illnesses can have FDP levels well above 10 μg/mL. However, the D-dimer assay is more specific but somewhat less sensitive. Levels in excess of 1 μg/mL (1000 ng/mL) are only seen in patients with severe DIC. The D-dimer assay can fall within the normal range in patients with less severe disease.

fibrin thrombi is common in platelet DIC and is most marked in patients with HUS. Bleeding is not a major manifestation unless the platelet count falls to below 20,000/μL.

Association With Multidrug Chemotherapy or Marrow Transplantation

A high level of platelet consumption is also seen in patients who receive multidrug chemotherapy or undergo marrow transplantation. In this situation, drug-related endothelial cell damage may well be responsible for an increased use of platelets. Platelet counts are the last to recover following chemotherapy or transplantation, and it is difficult to attain good post-transfusion increments of platelets for several weeks after therapy. Platelets are rapidly consumed in these patients even in the absence of sepsis or an autoimmune process.

Organ Damage Versus an Atypical Clinical Presentation

When a patient presents with evidence of **organ damage** typical of vasculitis, TTP, or HUS, it can be assumed that the thrombocytopenia is the result of platelet DIC. However, when the **clinical presentation is atypical,** diagnosis of platelet DIC can be difficult and only approached by ruling out other possible causes of thrombocytopenia, including defects in platelet production (loss of megakaryocytes from the marrow) and immune destruction (autoimmune disorders and idiopathic thrombocytopenic purpura). This situation requires a marrow aspirate and biopsy for the presence of megakaryocytes and a measurement of platelet-associated immunoglobulin (antiplatelet antibody). The clinician must also look for clinical evidence of an autoimmune process including heparin-induced thrombocytopenia.

Association With Severe Sepsis

Severe sepsis is often accompanied by a consumptive coagulopathy. With septic shock, the onset and severity of the coagulation abnormalities can be dramatic, resulting in both a bleeding diathesis and life-threatening organ damage secondary to widespread thrombus formation. Bacteria are capable of activating both the extrinsic and intrinsic pathways. Gram-positive bacteria can induce tissue factor (TF) expression to drive factor VII activation, and TF levels in sepsis patients have been shown to be markedly elevated. Activation of the intrinsic pathway by direct binding of contact factors

Table 34–2. Diseases associated with consumptive coagulopathies.

Platelet consumption
 Vasculitis
 Thrombotic thrombocytopenic purpura
 Hemolytic uremic syndrome
 Intravascular prosthetic devices
 Postchemotherapy
Disseminated intravascular coagulation
 High-grade DIC
  Septicemia
  Acute promyelocytic leukemia
  Transfusion reaction (ABO mismatch)
  Crush injury
  Hemorrhagic pancreatitis
  Obstetric complications (eclampsia, abruptio placentae,
   amniotic fluid embolism)
  Snake venoms
  Prothrombin complex concentrate (PCC) administration
 Low-grade DIC
  Metastatic malignancy
  Vasculitis
  Chronic inflammatory disorders
  Paroxysmal nocturnal hemoglobinemia
  Giant hemangiomas
  Eclampsia
  Retained fetus syndrome

(kallikrein, high-molecular-weight kininogen, and factors XI and XII) to the surface of bacteria has also been implicated in both coagulation factor consumption, and because of release of bradykinin, septic shock. The marked fibrinolysis that accompanies activation of the coagulation pathways adds to the problem. Rapid depletion of fibrinogen, platelets, and coagulation factors contributes to the bleeding tendency, while eventual exhaustion of plasminogen and plasmin levels makes possible widespread fibrin deposition and vascular/organ damage.

Low-Grade DIC

Low-grade DIC is even harder to diagnose. Although most patients with malignancy have some degree of DIC, often this is not severe enough to lead to organ damage or abnormal bleeding. Moreover, routine coagulation tests do not show a pattern typical of platelet and coagulation-factor consumption and fibrinolysis. Many patients fall somewhere in the middle. Their laboratory studies are abnormal, including slight reductions in the platelet count; modest prolongations of PT, PTT, and TT; and a fibrinogen measurement that is lower than expected for the patient's disease state. It is important to remember that fibrinogen is an acute phase reactant and tends to increase to levels in excess of 600 mg/dL in patients with inflammatory illness and malignancy. A fibrinogen level of 200–300 mg/dL in such a patient must be regarded as a lower than expected level. The D-dimer assay provides perhaps the most sensitive and specific assay for low-grade DIC in these patients.

Significant Liver Disease

Confusion can arise when significant liver disease is present. The production of many of the coagulation factors, fibrinogen, and both antithrombin III and α_2-antiplasmin depends on normal liver function. Moreover, clearance of FDPs and D-dimer fragments is liver dependent. Therefore, even in the absence of DIC, it is possible to see thrombocytopenia (hypersplenism), prolongation of the PT and PTT (decreased production of the vitamin K–dependent factors), hypo- and dysfibrinogenemia (decreased hepatic protein synthesis), TT prolongation and accumulation of FDPs and D-dimers (decreased clearance of split products), and modest depressions of antithrombin III and α_2-antiplasmin (poor hepatocellular function). Patients with severe liver disease can also have a component of low-grade DIC that magnifies the issue.

THERAPY AND CLINICAL COURSE

The overriding principle in the treatment of DIC is effective management of the underlying illness. For those conditions where there is rapid, effective therapy, eg, bacterial sepsis, acute promyelocytic leukemia, or an obstetric complication, immediate treatment is the most important first step. This treatment will remove the cause of the DIC and allow the normal production capacity of the marrow and liver to correct the deficiencies of individual coagulation factors. Any attempt to replace coagulation factors by blood component transfusion without treating the basic illness runs the risk of adding fuel to the DIC fire and may not clearly benefit the patient.

Transfusions for Severe DIC

If the patient presents with severe DIC and a life-threatening bleed, treatment of the basic illness and the replacement of coagulation factors go hand in hand. As soon as the therapy for the systemic illness is begun, these patients need to have aggressive transfusion with platelets, cryoprecipitate, and fresh frozen plasma (FFP) in that order of importance. Platelet transfusions offer the best chance of gaining control of the patient's microvascular bleeding, especially when it is manifest as widespread skin, mucous membrane, GI, and vital organ bleeding.

Replacement of fibrinogen by transfusing cryoprecipitate is also important. In the patient with a fibrinogen level below 50 mg/dL, bleeding is hard to control without transfusions of sufficient cryoprecipitate to raise the fibrinogen level to above 100–200 mg/dL. In a 70-kg patient with a total blood volume of 5 liters (plasma volume of approximately 3 liters), transfusion of 10–12 units of cryoprecipitate should raise the fibrinogen level above 100 mg/dL. However, since it is hard to predict the result of a single transfusion, repeated measurements of the plasma fibrinogen should be used to guide therapy. Correction of other factor deficiencies is less critical. If the PT and PTT are very long, the patient can be given 4–6 units of FFP, which is sufficient FFP to increase the common pathway coagulation factors by 30%. This treatment will also help to increase the plasma fibrinogen.

Treatment of Severe Sepsis & Septic Shock

Several attempts have been made to inhibit coagulation and fibrinolysis in severe sepsis and septic shock patients. Both TFPI and antithrombin III have been shown to inhibit thrombin formation and ameliorate the coagulopathy, though it is unclear that either has a significant effect on overall survival. Other potential inhibitors under investigation include C1 inhibitor, thrombomodulin, proteins C and S, and C4b-binding protein. None are ready for widespread clinical use.

Treatment of Less-Severe DIC

When the DIC is less severe and the patient does not demonstrate a severe bleeding tendency, therapy of the primary illness should be initiated and factor replacement withheld. Once the stimulus is removed, normal marrow and liver production capacities for platelets and coagulation factors will correct the laboratory abnormalities within 24–48 hours. Anticoagulation with heparin is not recommended for treating DIC. Exceptions to this rule include children who develop widespread skin and digit necrosis (purpura fulminans) and adults with acute promyelocytic leukemia. In the latter case, moderate-dose heparin (500 U/hour) can be used during the period of induction chemotherapy in an attempt to block the thromboplastic action of leukemic cell lysis.

Treatment of Platelet DIC

Treatment of patients with platelet DIC (vasculitis, TTP, or HUS) involves using several additional therapeutic modalities. For patients who present with thrombocytopenia without signs of organ damage, **prednisone** in a dose of 100–200 mg per day orally or **methylprednisolone** 0.75/kg intravenously (IV) every 12 hours may be effective as much as 50% of the time. Patients with TTP or HUS and symptoms and signs of organ damage should be treated with high-dose methylprednisolone IV and **plasmapheresis with cryo-poor FFP (or D/S plasma) exchange,** 3–4 liters daily for at least 3–5 consecutive days (see Chapter 30). Although it is clear that plasmapheresis can be effective in halting organ damage, especially the central nervous system findings, it is still unclear how the treatment works. It has been proposed that the pheresis may remove a platelet aggregating factor (an unusually large von Willebrand factor form), whereas the prednisone interrupts an autoimmune process.

Patients with HUS may have a somewhat better prognosis, including a high expectation for recovery of renal function. Multiple relapses requiring **corticosteroids and repeated plasmapheresis** are not unusual and may continue for several months. In the completely refractory patient, immunosuppressive therapy and splenectomy have on occasion been effective. **Platelet DIC** patients should not receive platelet transfusions or antiplatelet agents unless there is CT scan evidence of a large intracerebral bleed. Infusion of platelets can lead to accelerated organ damage, and drugs that inhibit platelet function can lead to more severe bleeding.

BIBLIOGRAPHY

Bell WR, Braine HG, Ness PM, et al: Improved survival in thrombotic thrombocytopenic purpura–hemolytic uremic syndrome. N Engl J Med 1991;325:398.

Bick RL: Disseminated intravascular coagulation and related syndromes: A clinical review. Semin Thromb Hemost 1988; 14:299.

Carr JM: Disseminated intravascular coagulation in cirrhosis. Hepatology 1989;10:103.

Carr JM, McKinney M, McDonagh J: Diagnosis of disseminated intravascular coagulation, role of {sc}d-dimer. AJCP 1989; 91:280.

Colman RW, Rubin RW: Disseminated intravascular coagulation due to malignancy. Semin Oncol 1990;17:172.

Feinstein DI: Treatment of disseminated intravascular coagulation. Semin Thromb Hemost 1988;14:351.

Lusher JM: Thrombogenicity associated with factor IX complex concentrates. Semin Hematol 1991;28:3.

Rock GA et al: Comparison of plasma exchange with plasma infusion in the treatment of thrombotic thrombocytopenic purpura. N Engl J Med 1991;325:393.

Tallman MS, Kwaan HC: Reassessing the hemostatic disorder associated with acute promyelocytic leukemia. Blood 1992; 79:543.

Tapper H, Herwald H: Modulation of hemostatic mechanisms in bacterial infectious disease. Blood 2000;96:2329.

Thrombotic Disorders

Abnormal thrombus formation and thromboembolism can occur secondary to a wide variety of diseases or as a primary hypercoagulable state. The pathophysiologic basis for thrombotic disease includes abnormalities of blood vessels or blood flow, excessive production of thromboplastic substances as with localized tissue necrosis, and inherited abnormalities of coagulation factors. Thus, clinical evaluation of a patient with thrombotic disease involves both a search for a clinical condition that is known for its association with thrombosis or thromboembolism and laboratory evaluation of the anticoagulant and fibrinolytic pathways.

NORMAL CONTROL OF THROMBOSIS

Thrombus formation is normally limited by several physiologic systems. Excessive platelet aggregation is inhibited by rapid dissipation of platelet stimulatory substances such as ADP, thromboxane A_2, and thrombin from the site of thrombosis and direct platelet inhibition by ADPase, prostacyclin, and nitric oxide produced by adjacent normal endothelial cells. Together, these inhibitors limit the size of the platelet thrombus and activation of coagulation by platelets.

Fibrin clot formation is also controlled by several mechanisms, including antithrombin III (AT-III) inhibition of thrombin, endothelial protein receptor/ thrombomodulin-driven protein C/S inactivation of factors Va and VIIIa, tissue factor pathway inhibition, and fibrinolysis. As shown in Figure 35–1, tissue factor pathway inhibitor (TFPI) stops factor Xa activation of prothrombin by binding to the TF-factor VIIa-Xa complex. This process acts to limit the procoagulant effect of tissue factor (TF). Once thrombin is bound to thrombomodulin, it can no longer interact with fibrinogen or activate platelets. Circulating AT-III also avidly binds to thrombin and other serine proteases in the coagulation cascade to neutralize their activity. This reaction is facilitated by heparin-like substances on the endothelial surface, just as heparin therapy acts via the AT-III mechanism.

Protein C activation via its interaction with endothelial protein C receptor (EPCR) and the thrombin/thrombomodulin complex is another important pathway. EPCR binding appears to play a role in

larger vessels, whereas the thrombomodulin pathway is most active in the microcirculation. Activated protein C (APC) with protein S serving as a cofactor then destroys factors Va and VIIIa to inhibit the further formation of thrombin. Another important clot-controlling mechanism is **fibrinolysis.** Tissue plasminogen activator (t-PA) produced by endothelial cells activates the plasminogen incorporated in the fibrin clot to form the serine protease, plasmin. This reaction is kept specific for fibrin clot by the high affinity of plasminogen activator for fibrin. Fibrinolysis is regulated by the circulating plasminogen-activator inhibitor (PAI-1) that counteracts the action of t-PA and the plasmin inhibitors—α_2-antiplasmin and α_2-macroglobulin. Thrombin activatable fibrinolysis inhibitor (TAFI) also tends to suppress fibrinolysis by removing carboxy-terminal lysine residues from fibrin to limit plasmin binding to fibrin clot.

A **hypercoagulable state** can occur because of a defect in any of these normal anticoagulant mechanisms. The most common genetic risk factors are APC resistance secondary to a point mutation of the factor V gene and prothrombin gene mutation G20210A resulting in increased levels of prothrombin (factor II). AT-III, protein C and protein S deficiency states, and hyperhomocysteinemia are also associated with an abnormal thrombotic tendency. Increased levels of factors VIII, XI, IX, and fibrinogen have also been implicated in both venous and arterial thrombosis. A decreased level of t-PA or increased level of TAFI or PAI-1 may also result in a thrombotic tendency. At the same time, venous thrombosis and thromboembolism occur most frequently in association with vessel injury and certain disease states. Coagulation defects responsible for arterial thrombosis include elevations in fibrinogen and levels of the t-PA (antigen)/PAI-1 complex, hyperhomocysteinemia, platelet function defects (the PI^{a2} polymorphism of GPIIIa), and the appearance of an antiphospholipid antibody (lupus anticoagulant).

CLINICAL FEATURES

An abnormal thrombotic tendency can present with symptoms and signs of venous thrombosis, pulmonary embolism (PE), or occlusion of an arterial vessel.

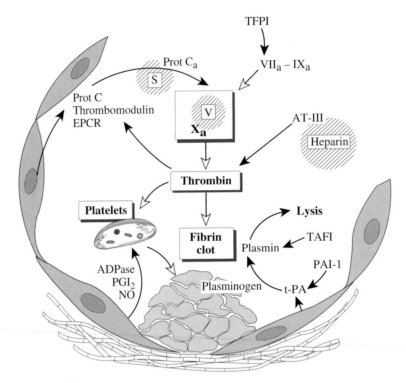

Figure 35–1. **Normal control of thrombosis.** Thrombus formation is controlled at several points. Platelet aggregation is inhibited by ADPase, prostacyclin (PGI_2), and nitric oxide (NO) released by adjacent normal endothelial cells. Tissue factor pathway inhibitor (TFPI) binds to TF-factor VIIa-Xa complex to suppress further tissue factor driving clotting. Fibrin clot formation is also controlled by direct inhibition by antithrombin III (AT-III) and protein C inactivation of factors V and VIII. The latter is stimulated by the interaction of thrombin with thrombomodulin and facilitated by protein S. Finally, the size of the fibrin clot is controlled by fibrinolysis. Endothelial cells release t-PA, which interacts with plasminogen incorporated in the clot to generate plasmin and break down the fibrin polymer.

Deep Venous Thrombosis (DVT)

Thrombosis involving the deep veins of the leg presenting as pain and swelling of an extremity is perhaps the most common clinical scenario and also one of the most difficult to diagnose. Deep venous thrombosis is often accompanied by an inflammatory response with tenderness, warmth, and erythema of the extremity, which makes it difficult to distinguish from other inflammatory disorders such as cellulitis; inflammation of a muscle, tendon, or bone; or a traumatic rupture of a popliteal cyst or muscle. Moreover, since the physical examination may not clearly separate these conditions, skilled use of tests such as impedance plethysmography, Doppler ultrasound, and contrast venography may be required to diagnose the condition.

Venous Thromboembolism

The estimated incidence of venous thromboembolism is 117 per 100,000 people each year, although it increases markedly with age to more than 900 per 100,000 for people age 85 or older. DVT with thromboembolism can occur with little warning. Thrombi form in the deep venous system of the thigh and pelvis in patients with malignancies or in otherwise normal individuals following trauma or surgery. This scenario carries a relatively high risk of embolization and in some cases death. Pregnant women have a fivefold higher risk of thromboembolism than nonpregnant women of the same age. It is very important, therefore, for the clinician to be alert to the risk of thrombosis and thromboembolism in certain clinical conditions.

Venous thrombosis is less common in other locations. Superficial veins of the legs and arms can thrombose because of trauma or because of irritation by an intravenous infusion, or as a complication of varicose veins. As long as the deep venous system is not involved, there is little risk of thromboembolism. Thrombosis of the subclavian or external jugular veins is not uncommon in patients with in-dwelling catheters. Spontaneous thrombosis of the subclavian, axillary, or brachial veins usually is the result of strenuous exercise with or without an anatomical defect such as thoracic outlet obstruction. Upper extremity thrombosis is rarely seen in patients with inherited hypercoagulable state. Thrombosis of the renal, hepatic, or mesenteric veins can occur in specific clinical situations. Renal vein thrombosis is associated with nephrotic syndrome and may be in part related to interference with the AT-III or protein C pathways (or both). Hepatic vein thrombosis is seen in patients with advanced cirrhosis or paroxysmal nocturnal hemoglobinuria (PNH), and after trauma or surgery.

Arterial Thrombosis or Thromboembolism

An arterial thrombosis or thromboembolism is easier to diagnose. Acute occlusion of an arterial vessel is recognized from the symptoms and signs of severe organ ischemia. In the case of the central nervous system, the patient manifests symptoms and signs of a stroke. With occlusion of a coronary artery, patients develop myocardial ischemia and infarction. Peripheral artery occlusions can also result from thrombosis or thromboembolism. Mural thrombi form in the heart in patients with atrial fibrillation or following anterior wall infarctions. These are innately unstable and will shed fragments of clot, which can occlude distal arterial vessels. The brain and kidney are at greatest risk of thromboembolic damage from a cardiac site. Less frequently, a large fragment will occlude a major vessel to an extremity. Thromboembolism can also occur as a result of a severely diseased vessel. Platelet and fibrin thrombi form on the surface of atheromatous plaques, break loose, and embolize to the distal branches of the involved vessel. This scenario is common in patients with atherosclerosis of carotid and coronary artery vessels. In some patients, the embolus will actually consist of atheromatous material that breaks loose from the surface of the vessel's so-called cholesterol emboli.

Importance of a Rapid, Accurate Diagnosis

The importance of a rapid and accurate diagnosis of thrombotic and thromboembolic disease cannot be overemphasized. Pulmonary thromboembolism can be prevented in patients with DVT with appropriate anticoagulant therapy. Therefore, every effort should be made to study patients at risk for venous thrombosis and to take preventive steps in high-risk patients.

Rapid diagnosis and therapy in patients with arterial thrombosis or thromboembolism is the most important component of good management. Fibrinolytic therapy of patients with coronary artery thrombosis can be extremely effective if delivered with minimal delay. Most patients treated with t-PA or streptokinase within 4 hours of the onset of their chest pain demonstrate clot lysis and reduced myocardial injury. In the patient with evidence of cerebral thrombosis or thromboembolism, accurate diagnosis is essential to defining prognosis and planning management. Thrombolysis can also be effective in thrombotic strokes if the patient is seen within the first 1–2 hours.

Laboratory Studies

Laboratory evaluation of a patient with thrombotic disease varies according to the presentation. Tests appropriate for diagnosing a DVT are not the same as those used for arterial thromboembolism. Moreover, laboratory evaluation of the anticoagulant pathways is only appropriate in certain clinical settings.

A. DETECTION OF A VENOUS THROMBUS:

Only three clinical studies—impedance plethysmography, Doppler ultrasound study, and contrast venography—can be used to detect a DVT. From the viewpoints of necessary expertise and cost-effectiveness, plethysmography is the easiest to perform and interpret and also the cheapest. The other studies cost more, require greater skill, and in the case of contrast venography, carry some risk of complications.

1. Impedance plethysmography—Impedance plethysmography will detect occlusive thrombi in the vessels of the thigh or pelvis in patients with symptomatic thrombophlebitis. The test involves inducing temporary venous congestion by inflation and deflation of a thigh blood pressure cuff to look for an impairment of venous drainage from the affected leg. Sensitivity and specificity are improved by repeating the measurement over several days. The method is insensitive to venous thrombosis limited to the calf, and measurements are compromised when there is a defect in arterial flow, an anatomic abnormality of the deep venous system, or venous obstruction from a mass in the abdomen. It is the least invasive test for the detection of iliac vein thrombosis in pregnant women. However, a false-positive result is common during the third trimester owing to compression of the pelvic vessels by the gravid uterus. If this test is used, the patient should be tested in the lateral recumbent position.

2. Compression ultrasonography—Compression ultrasonography (B-mode and Doppler) can also be used to detect major thrombi in the thigh. It will accurately detect a total occlusion or major partial obstruction that produces a compensatory increase in flow rates around the obstruction. In the hands of an experienced ultrasound operator, this method is as good as or better than impedance plethysmography for detecting major thrombi in the thigh. However, both tests have a sensitivity of less than 40%, with a specificity of better than 95% in patients with documented pulmonary emboli. This reflects the accuracy of the method and the fact that not all emboli originate in the leg veins. Just like plethysmography, ultrasound is even less sensitive in detecting thrombi in the calf. It cannot be used to rule out iliac vein thrombosis during pregnancy. Sensitivity of both plethysmography and ultrasound can be improved by repeating the studies over several days. A recent study of 405 patients suspected of having a first-episode DVT showed that a normal repeated ultrasound after 5–7 days effectively excluded clinically important thromboembolic disease.

As with any screening test, the positive and negative predictive values of compression ultrasound depend on the pretest probability. While the sensitivity of ultrasound is very poor in asymptomatic patients, certain clinical features will increase the likelihood of an abnormal finding. Patients can be classified as having a low, intermediate, or high **pretest probability** when one or more of the following clinical findings are present: a cancer diagnosis; paralysis or immobilization; lower leg cast; unilateral leg or calf swelling; unilateral pitting edema; and tenderness along the distribution of the deep venous system. High probability patients, those who have several of these features, will test positive better than 60% of the time.

3. Contrast venography—Contrast venography is the most definitive method for detecting deep venous thrombotic disease of the lower extremity. It involves the injection of contrast material into a superficial vein on the dorsal surface of the foot to visualize the deep venous system of the calf and thigh. When performed by an expert radiologist, thrombi can be detected as filling defects in major veins, often with evidence of abnormal collateral flow around the obstruction. Major distortions in the venous anatomy can also be defined in patients with chronic disease. When this method is done well, the entire venous anatomy of the leg is visualized. The technique is not without its complications, however. Patients can develop phlebitis from the dye.

B. DIAGNOSIS OF A PULMONARY EMBOLISM:

PE cannot be reliably diagnosed from the history, physical examination, or routine studies of lung anatomy and function such as the chest x-ray and measurement of the arterial PO_2.

1. Ventilation/perfusion lung scan—Whenever one suspects PE, it is essential to obtain a ventilation/perfusion lung scan. If one compares the distribution of an injected isotope to that of an inhaled isotope, it is possible to identify localized areas of perfusion/ventilation mismatch. If a section of lung appears to have an abnormality in blood flow but normal ventilation, there is a high probability of a pulmonary embolus. A matched perfusion/ventilation defect usually results from scarring or consolidation and is often seen in patients with pre-existing lung disease. Lung scans can be safely performed during pregnancy. Radiation exposure to the fetus is minimal, but this can be further reduced by restricting ventilation scanning to those patients who have an abnormal perfusion scan.

Lung scans should be read by the radiologist as high probability, nondiagnostic (this includes older terms, such as intermediate, low probability, and indeterminate), or normal. Overall, the lung scan has a sensitivity of only 41% but a specificity of 97%. When the scan shows more than one wedge-shaped, segmental perfusion defect without a matched ventilation defect in a patient with a normal chest x-ray, the probability of PE is greater than 80% (positive predictive value). At the other extreme, a completely normal ventilation/perfusion lung scan virtually excludes a major pulmonary embolus. However, many scans are equivocal and are read as nondiagnostic scans. In such patients, there is still a significant probability of a pulmonary embolus, depending on the pretest probability. If it is high, a nondiagnostic scan is associated with a 40–70% incidence of pulmonary embolus. When clinical suspicion is low, a nondiagnostic scan is associated with a 5–30% incidence of disease.

2. Pulmonary angiography—Management of the patient with an equivocal scan requires judgment on the part of the clinician. If it is important to confirm the diagnosis, pulmonary angiography can be performed. This test requires the expertise of either a cardiopulmonary specialist with experience in right heart catheterization or a skilled radiologist. The technique should be reserved for the patient who is a diagnostic dilemma or is at a high risk of bleeding if exposed to anticoagulant therapy. Patients who have a documented **DVT** by ultrasound do not need angiography even if the lung scan is negative, since they will need to be treated regardless. At the same time, the sensitivity of compression ultrasonography in detecting a peripheral thrombus in patients without clinical leg findings is very low. Less than 30% of patients who exhibit an embolism following surgery or as a complication of their congestive failure or cancer will have a positive test if they have a negative physical examination.

3. Spiral CT scan with contrast—Spiral CT scan with contrast can be used as an alternative to angiography. However, its sensitivity is greatest for proximal emboli in the great vessels of the lung. If it is positive, it is definitive. If negative, angiography is better at detecting distal emboli. Pulmonary angiography can also be of great value in diagnosing patients with multiple small pulmonary emboli that result in pulmonary hypertension. In this situation, the lung scan will generally be indeterminate.

4. Transthoracic echocardiography—Transthoracic echocardiography has been used as both a diagnostic and prognostic tool. Even when the patient shows no clinical symptoms/signs of hypotension, hypoxia, or congestive heart failure, a transthoracic echocardiogram can show signs of right heart hemodynamic strain. Findings include hypokinesis of the mid-right ventricular wall with normal contraction of the apex, and with massive emboli, right heart dilatation, tricuspid regurgitation, and bulging of the intraventricular septum into the left ventricle. The mismatch of normal apex contraction and mid-right ventricular wall hypokinesis has been promoted as an indication for thrombolytic therapy because of its relatively poor prognosis. A high troponin level in patients with right ventricular strain suggests severe dysfunction and can be used as another reason for immediate thrombolysis.

5. Other laboratory abnormalities—Other laboratory abnormalities associated with PE include elevated lactic dehydrogenase and bilirubin levels and an acute right axis shift on the electrocardiogram. These are not sensitive tests and typically require a relatively massive embolus.

6. Measurement of the D-dimer level—A measurement of the D-dimer level in plasma can help rule out a pulmonary embolus. Since most patients with a pulmonary embolus show an increase in their D-dimer level, a normal D-dimer level rules against an embolus. Elevated values are less specific.

The sensitivity and specificity of the D-dimer test varies with the method. Enzyme-linked immunosorbent assays (ELISA) are the most accurate but can take several days to perform. Although overly sensitive and less specific, a negative D-dimer test (less than 500 ng/mL) together with a negative impedance plethysmography or ultrasound examination in patients who present with a low pretest probability of a DVT has a negative predictive value of 98.5% (96–99.6%). At the same time, patients with an intermediate or high pretest probability for a pulmonary embolus can present with a normal D-dimer level, especially by the latex agglutination method. Furthermore, a negative D-dimer result in hospitalized patients and cancer patients cannot be used to exclude thrombotic disease, and a positive D-dimer test is not specific enough to discriminate between trauma, liver disease, disseminated intravascular coagulation (DIC), and thrombotic disease.

7. Guidelines for the diagnostic workup—Given this panoply of tests, how should one proceed with the diagnostic workup? The following is a list of proposed guidelines:

- The **lung scan and ultrasound are still the most useful first studies** in the evaluation of any patient who is suspected of having thromboembolic disease. Pre-existing lung disease will interfere with the lung scan. Absence of clinical findings of a proximal DVT will decrease the sensitivity but not specificity of the ultrasound.

- If the **lung scan is high probability or the ultrasound positive** (or both) in a patient with a high or intermediate clinical suspicion of an embolus, the patient should be treated with full-dose heparin. Furthermore, when the scan shows clot involving more than one-third of the lungs, a transthoracic echocardiogram should be performed to look for right ventricular hypokinesis. If it is present, peripheral thrombolysis with recombinant tissue-type plasminogen activator (rt-PA) should be considered to restore pulmonary blood flow.

- If the **lung scan is normal, the ultrasound negative, and the D-dimer less than 500 ng/mL** in a patient with a low to intermediate pretest suspicion of embolism, the patient does not need treatment. A second normal ultrasound study within the next week further reduces the likelihood of a significant DVT. However, since there is still a very small chance of thromboembolic disease, the patient should be followed up and studies repeated if symptoms recur or worsen. When the pretest suspicion is high, spiral CT scan, transthoracic echocardiography or, for the most definitive answer, pulmonary angiography should be considered. The patient has as much as a 40% chance of having a pulmonary embolus.

- If the **lung scan is read as nondiagnostic** (intermediate or low probability) in a patient with a negative ultrasound and a low pretest suspicion of pulmonary embolus, the probability of an embolus is low. A normal D-dimer test will further reduce the likelihood of disease. If the clinical suspicion is intermediate or high, 30–60% of patients will have had a pulmonary embolus. This makes the predictive value of the lung scan no better than a flip of a coin. Further study, preferably pulmonary angiography, is required to rule out disease.

These guidelines emphasize the importance of the pretest suspicion of disease in guiding testing and therapy. Since the symptoms and signs of PE are not specific, it is a test of the clinician's diagnostic skill to provide the pretest probability. As much as anything, the clinical setting should be taken into account. Most sudden life-threatening emboli occur in patients undergoing orthopedic (hip or knee operations) or neurosurgery, with prolonged bed rest following trauma, and in those individuals who have had a previous DVT or embolism. Therefore, the level of suspicion should be higher in these situations and should drive a more aggressive workup.

C. DIAGNOSIS OF AN ARTERIAL THROMBUS:

The evaluation of a patient with an arterial thrombus or thromboembolism includes studies of the occluded vessel and a search for a potential embolic source. A Doppler flow study can be used to locate and define the extent of blockage in patients with occlusions of extremity vessels. However, arteriography is almost always required to prepare the patient for surgery, whether thrombectomy or vessel bypass grafting.

Doppler flow studies can also be used to define patency of the carotid vessels and detect atherosclerotic narrowing in patients with cerebral artery thrombosis or thromboembolism. Common sites for atheromas are the junction of the vertebral and basilar arteries, the internal carotid arteries at the level of the carotid sinus, and the bifurcation in the middle cerebral artery. Atheromatous plaques promote thrombus formation at the site and can be a source for both cholesterol and platelet emboli. In patients with neurologic defects, a **CT scan** or **MRI** can help define the site and extent of disease. These studies are also important as guides to therapy by distinguishing between a cerebral infarction secondary to an embolus and a hemorrhagic stroke.

All patients with thromboembolic disease should be evaluated for a **cardiac source for the emboli.** Mitral valve disease and atrial fibrillation are associated with an increased risk for thrombus formation in the left atrium with subsequent embolization. Even without valvular disease, paroxysmal atrial fibrillation and atrial fibrillation associated with chamber dilatation and heart failure can result in thromboembolism. Mural thrombus formation in patients following acute anterior wall myocardial infarction is another potential source for emboli. If one of these is present, **echocardiography** can be used to document the mural thrombus. However, sensitivity of the measurement is poor and should not be used to rule out a cardiac source for emboli. The decision for anticoagulation must be based on the relative risk of embolization with each condition.

Coronary artery thrombosis is the most common clinical example of arterial thrombosis secondary to atherosclerosis and plaque rupture. Clinical presentation together with electrocardiograph signs of ischemia and infarction are enough to make the diagnosis and initiate thrombolytic therapy. The key role of platelets and coagulation in infarction has also been recognized in the recommendations for the use of aspirin and anticoagulants in management of patients with coronary artery disease. Since **anticoagulant therapy** cannot by itself prevent occlusion in a patient with a severe stenotic lesion, a full workup of the patient with coronary artery disease requires **coronary angiography leading to either angioplasty or bypass grafting.**

D. COAGULATION STUDIES:

The standard laboratory coagulation tests are primarily designed to detect the patient with a bleeding tendency. For example, the prothrombin time (PT) and partial thromboplastin time (PTT) are used to detect coagulation factor deficiencies. There are no comparable screening tests for a hypercoagulable state. Certainly, a shortening of the PT or PTT cannot be equated to a thrombotic tendency. Laboratory measurements that are important in the **evaluation of a patient with thrombotic disease** are listed in Table 35–1. They can be roughly divided into risk factors for arterial thrombosis versus those that lead to venous thrombotic disease. Elevated homocysteine levels are associated with both arterial and venous disease. Several markers of prothrombotic activity are available, including prothrombin fragment 1.2, thrombin antithrombin complex, D-dimer, and soluble fibrin polymer. Several studies have now shown elevated levels of these markers in thrombophilic patients. However, they are not yet in clinical use.

The clinical setting is an important guide for evaluating a hypercoagulable state. Conditions commonly associated with an **increased thrombotic tendency** are listed in Table 35–2. This list includes conditions where there is an abnormality in platelet number or

Table 35–1. Risk factors in thromboembolic disease.

Arterial	Venous
Fibrinogen level	Factor V Leiden/APCR
Factor VIII and XIIa levels	Hyperprothrombinemia
vWF antigen level	Antithrombin III deficiency
t-PA:ag/PAI-I level	Protein C and protein S deficiency
Platelet function/Pl^{a2} phenotype	Dysfibrinogenemia
Lp (a) level	Factor XII deficiency
Hyperhomocysteinemia	Increased levels of factors XI, IX, VIII, fibrinogen
Antiphospholipid antibody	Hyperhomocysteinemia
? Factor V Leiden/ prothrombin gene mutation	

Table 35–2. Conditions associated with a thrombotic tendency.

Platelet abnormalities
Thrombocytosis/myeloproliferative disorders
Diabetes mellitus
Hyperlipidemia
Heparin-induced thrombocytopenia
Lupus anticoagulant
Blood vessel defects
Venous disease/stasis/immobilization
Atherosclerosis/myocardial infarction
Atrial fibrillation
Prosthetic surfaces
Hyperviscosity
TTP/HUS/vasculitis
Systemic illness/coagulopathies
Trauma/long bone fractures
Orthopedic or major surgery
Malignancy
Pregnancy/oral contraceptives
Nephrotic syndrome
Infusion of prothrombin complex concentrates
Fat embolism
Sickle cell disease

---

function, endothelial cell function, blood flow, or the activation of the coagulation pathways. Laboratory findings in most of these conditions are nonspecific and not diagnostic. Routine coagulation screening tests are generally normal. One exception to this rule is the patient with a platelet count in excess of 1 million per milliliter. Thrombocytosis is associated with abnormal thrombosis, although the reverse is also true; these patients can present with an abnormal bleeding tendency owing to platelet dysfunction.

1. Assays used for an inherited hypercoagulable state—Laboratory testing is of greater value in the di-

Table 35–3. Inherited hypercoagulable states.

Factor V Leiden
Prothrombin gene mutation
Antithrombin III deficiency
Protein C and protein S deficiency
Fibrinolytic system defects
  Tissue plasminogen activator (t-PA) deficiency
  Plasminogen activator inhibitor (PAI) excess
  Abnormal plasminogen
  Hypoplasminogenemia
Dysfibrinogenemia
Factor XII deficiency
Hyperhomocysteinemia

---

agnosis of patients with an inherited hypercoagulable state (Table 35–3). A deficiency in one of the inhibitors of coagulation can result in a thromboembolic tendency (see Figure 35–1). Therefore, when the clinical presentation is appropriate, specific assays can be ordered to screen for factor V-APC resistance (factor V Leiden), presence of an antiphospholipid antibody (lupus anticoagulant), and deficiencies of factor XII, AT-III, protein C, protein S, t-PA, plasminogen levels (and activity), and fibrinogen function.

Available assays vary in their ease of performance and accuracy. **Factor V Leiden** can be measured indirectly using a modification of the PTT. This functional assay compares PTT times with and without the addition of a standardized amount of APC. A ratio (PTT with APC divided by the PTT without APC) of less than 1.8–2.0 indicates presence of the trait. A DNA-based assay, which avoids problems with the functional assay, is also available.

The **assay for antithrombin III** (AT-III) is excellent. It is a functional assay based on heparin-dependent inhibition of thrombin or factor Xa. Furthermore, the ranges of normal and heterozygote AT-III values do not overlap, making this a highly sensitive and specific test. In contrast, **assays for proteins C and S** are less accurate and there is considerable overlap of normal and heterozygote levels. To make matters worse, oral anticoagulants and liver disease will give a false-positive result by lowering the synthesis of both proteins C and S. In order to detect the different phenotypes of factors C and S deficiency, most laboratories do both total antigen and functional assays. However, in the case of protein S the functional assay is so unreliable that only the antigen measurement is useful.

The **PTT** can be used to screen for a **lupus anticoagulant immunoglobulin inhibitor** (**antiphospholipid antibody**). To confirm the presence of an inhibitor and rule out a coagulation factor deficiency, a 1:1 mixing study with pooled normal human plasma is performed. Antiphospholipid antibodies can also be measured by **ELISA** with much less assay variability.

Factor XII (**Hageman factor**) **deficiency** can be recognized from the dramatic prolongation of the PTT without evidence of a bleeding tendency. Factor XII together with high molecular weight, kininogen, and prekallikrein have an added role in activating the fibrinolytic system and maintaining vasodilatation. Failure in the latter systems may well contribute to the thrombotic tendency.

DIFFERENTIAL DIAGNOSIS

The diagnostic workup begins with the evaluation of the disease state that is associated with the thrombotic tendency. Often as not, the clinical situation is enough to define the proximate cause of the thrombosis. When a patient presents with a coronary artery thrombosis, the relationship of the thrombosis to localized atherosclerosis is so strong that a workup of the coagulation pathways is unnecessary. Similarly, the elderly patient with a thrombotic stroke is almost certainly an example of either local vessel thrombosis or embolization from a cardiac source. This situation is not true, however, for a young patient with a stroke where a lupus anticoagulant may be the cause of the thrombosis. Recurrent venous thrombosis or a strong family history of thrombotic disease should also stimulate a more extensive coagulation workup.

The **pathophysiology of the thrombotic tendency** associated with a specific disease state can be quite complex (see Table 35–2 and Figure 35–1). Hypercoagulability can result from a defect in one or several components of hemostasis. A patient with severe venous stasis, or hyperviscosity, can develop a thrombotic tendency even when the coagulation system and inhibitor levels are normal. Myeloproliferative disorders, especially polycythemia vera, essential thrombocytosis, and PNH, are associated with an increased incidence of thrombophlebitis, PE, and arterial occlusions. Patients with these conditions are also at risk for thrombosis of splenic, hepatic, portal, and mesenteric vessels. A common cause of hepatic vein thrombosis (Budd-Chiari syndrome) is the myeloproliferative disorder PNH. The pathogenesis of the thrombosis in these patients is not clear. Both the thrombocytosis and an abnormality in platelet function may play a role. Increased activation and aggregation of platelets has been postulated as a cause for the hypercoagulable state. Other conditions where platelet function may contribute to both a thrombotic tendency and accelerated atherosclerosis are the hyperlipidemias, hyperhomocystinemia, and diabetes mellitus. One-third or more of patients presenting with a stroke early in life will be heterozygous for hyperhomocystinemia.

Patients With Certain Malignancies

Patients with certain malignancies can demonstrate a marked thrombotic tendency. Adenocarcinomas of the pancreas, colon, stomach, and ovaries are the leading tumors associated with thromboembolic events. In fact, these malignancies can first present with a single or multiple episodes of DVT or migratory superficial thrombophlebitis. Overall, patients who present with primary thrombophlebitis show a 25–30% incidence of recurrence, and 20% of these will turn out to have cancer. The pathogenesis of the thrombotic tendency appears to relate to a combination of release of procoagulant factor(s) by the tumor, endothelial damage by tumor invasion, and blood stasis. Laboratory testing

may show no abnormalities, or some combination of thrombocytosis, elevation of the fibrinogen level, and low-grade DIC. In the latter case, it is assumed that the tumor must be a thromboplastic stimulus to coagulation. Chemotherapy and the placement of central venous catheters are also associated with an increased risk of thromboembolism.

Pregnancy and Oral Contraceptive Use

Pregnancy and oral contraceptive use have been reported to increase the risk of thrombosis. Similar to the malignancy model, several factors may play a role during **pregnancy.** This list includes vascular obstruction by the uterus, changes in blood rheology, increases in fibrinogen and coagulation factor levels, depression of the fibrinolytic system, and activation of the coagulation cascade at the uteroplacental interface. The risk of PE is highest during the third trimester and immediate postpartum period and is a leading cause of maternal death.

Factor V Leiden women are at increased risk of DVT during pregnancy and may also be at increased risk for second-trimester miscarriages. AT-III–deficient women have an increased incidence of prepartum thromboembolic disease, whereas individuals deficient in proteins C and S have more postpartum disease. Complications of pregnancy such as advanced age, hypertension, or placental disorders (eg, abruptio placentae) can also increase the thrombotic tendency and even produce full-blown DIC (see Chapter 34).

The association of **oral contraceptives** with thrombosis and thromboembolism also appears to be multifactorial. Since low-dose estrogen contraceptive pills have been introduced, the incidence has decreased significantly. However, women who smoke, have a history of migraine headaches, or are factor V Leiden heterozygotes are at increased risk (30-fold) for venous thrombosis, PE, and cerebrovascular thrombosis. At the same time, there appears to be less of a relationship between the use of estrogen at the time of menopause and the occurrence of thrombosis.

Nephrotic Syndrome Patients

Nephrotic syndrome patients are at risk for thromboembolic disease including renal vein thrombosis. The explanation for this is unclear. It has been attributed to lower than normal levels of AT-III or protein C secondary to renal loss of the coagulation protein, factor XII deficiency, platelet hyperactivity, abnormal fibrinolytic activity, and higher than normal levels of other coagulation factors. Hyperlipidemia and hypoalbuminemia have also been proposed as possible etiologic factors.

Primary Hypercoagulable States

Inherited defects in coagulation factors or the fibrinolytic system can set the stage for a thrombotic tendency (see Table 35–3). Generally, these patients have a fixed abnormality but a variable incidence of thrombotic disease. This situation may reflect the need for a second insult to initiate a thrombotic event. A family history of thrombotic disease is a strong predictor of recurrent disease in other family members. A primary hypercoagulable state can be identified in up to 70% of patients with a strong family history of thromboembolic disease, but in less than 15% of patients without such a history. The relative prevalences of the various congenital defects in DVT patients are shown in Table 35–4. Indications for a full evaluation for an inherited defect include the following:

- Presentation before age 50 without a predisposing factor
- Recurrent thrombotic events
- A strong family history of thromboembolic disease
- A life-threatening thromboembolic event
- Thromboembolism during pregnancy or while taking estrogen

Any testing for a primary hypercoagulable state must take into account the overall clinical picture. As a routine, patients should be tested for factor V Leiden; the 20210 AG prothrombin gene mutation; hyperhomocysteinemia; and deficiencies in AT-III, proteins C and S, and antiphospholipid antibodies. At the same time, a full battery of coagulation screening tests should be performed. This will avoid missing a coagulation abnormality that explains lower than normal levels of any of these factors. For example, a patient with liver disease or DIC will demonstrate deficiencies in AT-III, protein C, protein S, and abnormalities in the fibrinolytic system secondary to defects in coagulation factor production or excessive factor consumption (or both).

Table 35–4. Prevalence of hypercoagulable states in DVT patients.

Factor V Leiden	12–40%
Hyperhomocysteinemia	10–20%
Prothrombin gene mutation	6–18%
AT-III, protein S, and protein C	5–15%
Antiphospholipid antibody	10–20%

A. FACTOR V LEIDEN:

APC resistance secondary to the factor V G1691A mutation (Arg506Gln or Leiden mutation) on chromosome 1 has been detected in 20–60% of adult patients with a strong family history of thromboembolic disease. The prevalence of the gene mutation in the general population is about 1–7%, with a wide range for different ethnic groups. Allele prevalence can be as low as 0.5–2% for Hispanic, African, and Asian populations to as high as 3–5% in Northern Europeans and 14% in Greeks. Some patients with APC resistance do not appear to have the factor V Leiden mutation for reasons that are not clear, although at least one patient has been reported with an anti-APC antibody. These individuals are still at increased risk of thromboembolic disease. Lifelong risk of thrombosis depends on the patient's age; the presence of contributing factors such as surgery, trauma, pregnancy, and so on; and whether the patient is hetero- or homozygous for the abnormal gene. Homozygous individuals generally have a strong family history and are liable for thromboembolism at a young age. Heterozygous factor V Leiden deficiency, by itself, increases the risk of a primary DVT by at the most four- to sixfold, not enough to pose a significant lifelong risk of thromboembolic disease. Cerebral vein thrombosis is more common in carriers of the Leiden mutation. Women with the factor V mutation run an increased risk of recurrent fetal loss. Recent studies have implicated APC resistance as a risk factor for arterial thrombosis, particularly stroke in children and myocardial infarction in women. Coinheritance of AT-III, protein C, or protein S deficiency dramatically increases the risk of thrombosis. Patients with high plasma homocysteine levels are also at greater risk, a 20- to 30-fold increase in the risk of a primary DVT. The risk of recurrent DVT is also influenced by coinheritance of factor V Leiden and the G20210A prothrombin gene mutation, increasing the risk of recurrent DVT sufficient to consider long-term anticoagulation. The same is true for other combinations.

B. PROTHROMBIN GENE MUTATION:

Prothrombin is translated by a 21-kb gene located on chromosome 11. A point mutation in the 3′-untranslated region produces a genotype, G20210A, which is associated with higher than normal prothrombin levels and an increased incidence of recurrent thrombosis. This genotype can be detected in 18% of patients with strong family histories of thromboembolism. Furthermore, patients with recurrent DVTs in the Leiden Thrombophilia Study showed a 6.2% frequency for G20210A mutation, whereas the genotype is seen in only 1–2% of normal individuals. Women with the mutation also appear to more susceptible to cerebral vein thrombosis, especially if they use oral contraceptives.

C. ANTITHROMBIN III (AT-III) DEFICIENCY:

AT-III deficiency is inherited as an autosomal dominant trait, with an estimated frequency of 1 per 1000–5000 individuals. Typically, a heterozygote patient has an AT-III level of between 40% and 70% of normal. Two types of AT-III deficiency can be defined from measurements of antigen and activity levels. **Type 1** patients have low levels of both antigen and activity, whereas **Type 2** patients have low activity but normal antigen levels. AT-III–deficient individuals tend to have recurrent DVT and PE, although not all heterozygotes appear to have difficulty. Unusual sites, such as the cavernous sinus or brachial or mesenteric vein, may be involved. The onset of disease is often associated with factors that promote thrombosis in normal individuals, including venostasis, trauma, pregnancy, and the use of oral contraceptives. Although the trait increases the risk of thrombosis 20-fold, only 4% of patients with a clinical diagnosis of primary hypercoagulable state will be AT-III deficient.

D. PROTEINS C AND S DEFICIENCY:

Protein C and protein S deficiencies demonstrate a similar clinical pattern. **Protein C deficiency** is inherited as autosomal dominant or recessive genotype, and the heterozygote patient generally has a protein C level that is only slightly lower than normal. In fact, overlap of heterozygote protein C levels with normal values is so great that it makes diagnosis difficult. Diagnosis of **protein S deficiency** is even more difficult. The assay for protein S activity is so poor that diagnosis must be based on the S-antigen measurement, where again there is significant overlap with normal values.

Proteins C and S deficiencies increase the risk of recurrent venous thrombotic disease usually beginning in the second or third decade of life. Approximately 50% of protein C heterozygotes will develop a thrombosis without a predisposing event by age 50 years. However, just like AT-III deficiency, the incidence of disease in any family can be highly variable and may require a contributing factor. The incidence of thromboembolic disease in various families with protein S deficiency is also highly variable. Carriers of the protein S gene Gly295 - Val mutation show a very high incidence of clinical disease, odds ratio of nearly 20, whereas other family cohorts are much lower.

Compared with factor V Leiden, protein C and S deficiencies are far less common. All together, hereditary deficiencies of AT-III, protein C, and protein S are responsible for no more than 10–20% of patients with a primary hypercoagulable state.

E. HYPERHOMOCYSTEINEMIA:

Excess levels of homocysteine in plasma can be thrombogenic. **Marked hyperhomocysteinemia** (plasma homocysteine levels of greater than 100 μmol/L) is observed in children who are homozygous for a deficiency in cystathionine β-synthase, a rare defect seen in only 1 in 200,000 births. These children demonstrate severe mental retardation, lens and skeletal defects, and a high incidence of both atherosclerotic and thromboembolic disease at an early age.

Moderately elevated levels of plasma homocysteine (16–100 μmol/L) are seen in individuals who are heterozygous for an enzyme defect (cystathionine β-synthase, methylenetetrahydrofolate reductase), who have a deficiency of folic acid, pyridoxine (vitamin B_6), or vitamin B_{12}, or all of these. The normal metabolic pathways of homocysteine (Figure 35–2) include its conversion to methionine by the acceptance of a methyl group from N-5-methyltetrahydrofolate and transulfuration to cystathionine and cysteine. The former reaction is folate and vitamin B_{12} dependent, whereas the conversion to cystathionine is pyridoxine dependent. Therefore, nutritional deficiencies can result in slightly elevated plasma homocysteine levels, 10–16 μmol/liter. In addition, approximately 5% of the general population (38% of French-Canadians) exhibit a thermolabile methylenetetrahydrofolate reductase variant that is only 50% active. This is another cause of hyperhomocysteinemia, with homozygous individuals being at increased risk for venous thrombosis.

There can be **significant overlap of normal and abnormal serum homocysteine levels.** Patients who are heterozygous for an enzyme defect, most often cystathionine β-synthase, or are vitamin deficient can present with fasting homocysteine levels that are only 1–2 μmol/L higher than normal. The presence of an enzyme or vitamin defect can be revealed with oral methionine loading (0.10 grams per kilogram) and pre- and post-load plasma homocysteine measurements. Patients with an underlying enzymatic defect will show an exaggerated and irreversible increase in plasma homocysteine levels with methionine loading, whereas the exaggerated response in folate-deficient patients can be corrected with folate supplementation.

Mild to moderate hyperhomocysteinemia is considered to be an independent risk factor for both coronary artery and peripheral vascular disease, as well as for venous thrombosis. It may account for up to 10% of initial DVT events in young adults, especially young women. It is also a major risk factor for thrombotic strokes in younger individuals. End stage renal disease patients routinely show plasma homocysteine levels of 20–30 μmol/L, not correctable with folate supplementation. This may play a role in the increased pace of atherosclerosis in these patients. Hyperhomocysteine-

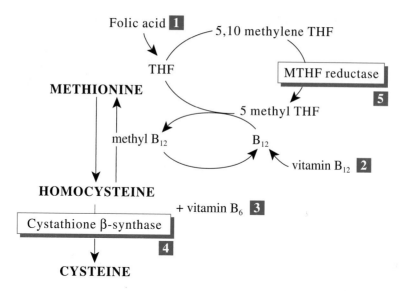

Figure 35–2. **The methionine-homocysteine metabolic pathway.** Deficiencies of folic (**1**), vitamin B$_{12}$ (**2**), or vitamin B$_6$ (**3**) can result in slight elevations of the plasma homocysteinemia, which are readily reversed with vitamin therapy. Patients with homozygous cystathione β-synthase (**4**) or MTHFR (**5**) deficiency exhibit marked hyperhomocysteinemia, thrombotic episodes at an early age, and severe neurological deficits. Patients heterozygous for either enzyme defect have minimally elevated homocysteine levels and may only be detected with methionine loading.

mia in an individual who is heterozygous for factor V Leiden may further increase the risk of thromboembolic disease and fetal loss secondary to placental infarction, although this is still somewhat controversial. Retrospective case-control studies have shown a strong correlation between the plasma homocysteine level and the risk of death from coronary artery disease and stroke. However, data from more recent prospective studies are less conclusive. The mechanism behind homocysteine toxicity is thought to involve direct damage to endothelial cells, resulting in heightened platelet adhesion, loss of the thrombolytic function, and smooth muscle proliferation.

F. COAGULATION PATHWAY FACTORS:

A higher risk of thrombosis has been reported in patients with elevated levels of one or more coagulation factors, including factors XI, VIII, IX, and perhaps VII. The mechanism of action may involve the generation of higher than normal thrombin levels, leading to generation of TAFI and, as a result, fibrinolytic-resistant fibrin clot. The PI^{a2} polymorphism of GPIIIa is associated with a modest increased risk for coronary artery disease.

G. DYSFIBRINOGENEMIAS:

Hypercoagulability has also been reported in patients with elevated fibrinogen levels and fibrinogen functional defects (dysfibrinogenemias). The plasma fibrinogen level, by itself, is an independent risk factor for coronary artery disease and acute myocardial infarction. In fact, it is as good a predictor as the low-density lipoprotein (LDL) cholesterol or high-density lipoprotein (HDL) level. Approximately 20% of patients who present with a dysfibrinogenemia will demonstrate a thrombotic tendency and, less frequently, an increased incidence of spontaneous abortion or poor wound healing. Apparent mechanisms include impaired thrombin binding that allows excess thrombin to circulate and initiate clotting and defective plasminogen activation.

H. IMPAIRED FIBRINOLYSIS:

Any defect in the functional capacity of plasminogen or the endothelial cell release of t-PA can result in a tendency to arterial and venous thrombotic disease. Furthermore, an increase in the circulating inhibitors of the plasminogen pathway (PAI-1 and TAFI) may be associated with a thrombotic tendency. Both t-PA and PAI-1 are now felt to be markers for future cardiovascular disease in otherwise normal populations. High normal bound t-PA/PAI-1 levels increase the risk of myocardial infarction by 1.5- to 3-fold. The best correlation is with the t-PA antigen level, a surrogate marker for PAI-1 activity. In addition, fibrinogen, t-PA:ag, and LDL cholesterol are independent risk factors, so additive abnormalities such as a high normal fibrinogen together with a high LDL cholesterol will increase the risk of myocardial infarction tenfold.

I. ANTIPHOSPHOLIPID ANTIBODIES:

An increased tendency to both venous and arterial thrombosis

Lupus

platelet defect. Recurrent pregnancy loss with placent... thrombosis has been associated with a decrease in annexin V levels.

The **initial tip-off to the presence of a lupus anticoagulant** is a prolongation of the PTT or, rarely, the PT that does not correct with a 1:1 mix with normal plasma. This reflects the fact that the antibody inhibits the activity of phospholipid/prothrombin complex in the PTT reaction. The failure of normal plasma to at least partially correct the PTT or PT rules out a coagulation factor deficiency state. The sensitivity of the PTT test depends a great deal on the type of phospholipid used to initiate clotting. Antiphospholipid/anticardiolipin antibodies can also be detected by immunoelectrophoresis. A quick ELISA method is now available to determine the titer and isotype of antiprothrombin antibodies. Low-titer antiphospholipid antibodies can appear as a transient event in a myriad of clinical settings. Therefore, repeated antibody measurements should be performed over 6–8 weeks before making the diagnosis of "antiphospholipid syndrome."

Clinical studies of patients with lupus anticoagulants have shown an **increased propensity to thrombosis,** with 30% of patients experiencing one or more thrombotic events during their lifetime. Isolated venous thrombosis or thromboembolism make up two-thirds of the cases; cerebral thrombosis accounts for the other third. Coronary artery occlusion is rare. Up to 20% of patients presenting with a venous thromboembolism not associated with other disease, surgery, or trauma

will demonstrate antiphospholipid antibodies. Patients can also present with "catastrophic antiphospholipid syndrome" characterized by multiorgan failure secondary to widespread small vessel thrombosis, thrombocytopenia, acute respiratory distress syndrome, DIC, and, on occasion, an autoimmune hemolytic anemia. Bacte... be triggering events for ... d antibod... ...d or early

...y artery oc... ...ic polymor... ...ong as that ...erhomocys... ...sk factor for ...ave been as... ...nary events, ...tic polymor... ...glycoprotein ...n reported to ...ixfold. Fibri... ...ase in t-PA/ ...a risk factor. ...IIa, as well as the appearance of an an... ...anticardiolipin antibody, may be associated with arterial thrombosis (Table 35–2). There is now strong evidence that **hs-CRP** (high sensitivity CRP—an assay that detects CRP levels in the normal range) predicts a higher incidence of coronary occlusion. Moreover, the combination of a high hs-CRP level and increased total cholesterol/HDL cholesterol ratio is associated with a 5- to 10-fold increased risk of a future coronary event, much greater than either risk factor alone. A high fibrinogen or factor VIII level also correlates with a modest increase in the risk of myocardial infarction.

PRINCIPLES OF MANAGEMENT

Good management depends on accurate diagnosis. Both the choice and duration of therapy differ greatly according to the nature of the thrombotic disease. As a general rule, patients with venous thrombosis or cardiac mural thrombi should immediately receive intravenous heparin and then change to full-dose warfarin therapy. In contrast, patients at risk for coronary artery or cerebrovascular thrombosis are best managed with a platelet inhibitor such as aspirin or ticlopidine (see Chapter 36).

Venous Thrombosis

The best management of thromboembolic disease is prevention. This begins with a careful assessment of risk factors for DVT, including patient age; prior episodes of DVT or PE; paralysis; long bone fractures; malignancy; obesity; congestive heart failure; estrogen use; and the presence of a primary hypercoagulable state. It also recognizes the thromboembolic potential of trauma and surgery, especially orthopedic and neurosurgery. Hip and knee replacement surgery in patients who do not receive prophylaxis is associated with a greater than 50% incidence of DVT and a 6% fatal PE rate. This is reduced to less than 10% for DVT and less than 0.2% for PE by prophylaxis with low-molecular-weight heparin (LMWH) or low-dose coumadin. Elastic stockings or intermittent pneumatic compression of the lower legs can also help reduce the incidence of DVT. Patients with a history of prior episodes of DVT or PE, or a hypercoagulable state, must receive prophylaxis, preferably with LMWH.

A. LOCATION AND EXTENT OF THE THROMBOTIC DISEASE:

In managing patients with a venous thrombosis, the location and extent of the thrombotic disease is a major guide to planning therapy. When the thrombus is limited to superficial veins of the leg or the deep veins of the calf, there is little risk of a pulmonary embolus. These patients can be managed with simple bed rest, a nonsteroidal anti-inflammatory drug, and support hose. At the same time, patients with symptomatic calf DVTs are at risk of developing chronic venous insufficiency and it can, therefore, be of benefit to treat. The availability of LMWH makes it feasible to give these patients 10–14 days of therapy at home, avoiding a costly hospitalization.

When the thrombus resides in the deep veins of the thigh, full-dose anticoagulation, first with heparin (full-dose, intravenous heparin in hospital, or, in the case of an ideal home situation, LMWH (Enoxaparin 1 mg/kg twice a day subcutaneously) for 10–14 days and then warfarin to an international normalized ratio (INR) of 2 to 3, for 6 months is recommended, unless there is a high risk of major hemorrhage. The incidence of recurrent thrombosis and PE is highest during the first 6–12 months, but the risk of a second DVT continues to be high for years. The length of the initial course of anticoagulation makes a difference. In trials comparing 6 weeks with 6 months of warfarin therapy, the rate of recurrence was reduced by 50% when anticoagulation was maintained for 6 months. Furthermore, this improvement was sustained for more than 5 years after therapy. In a randomized study of first-episode idiopathic venous thromboembolism treated with warfarin to an INR of 2.0 to 3.0 for 3 months or indefinitely (more than a year), continuous therapy resulted in a 95% reduction in recurrence compared with a 27% per patient year recurrence rate in the untreated group.

However, prolonged anticoagulation is associated with a risk of a major bleeding episode of up to 3% per year. Trials of low-dose warfarin therapy are currently under way to answer the question of whether protection can be offered while minimizing the risk of hemorrhage.

B. ABSENCE OF A SPECIFIC CAUSE:

In the absence of a specific cause (trauma, cancer, etc) or a primary hypercoagulable state, including factor V Leiden trait, approximately 20% of patients will develop a second DVT within 3–5 years after discontinuing anticoagulation. Factor V Leiden heterozygotes have been reported to have a fourfold risk of recurrent disease; 40% will develop a DVT within 3–5 years. However, other investigators have reported no increased risk of thrombosis recurrence in this group of patients. Regardless, the risk is not high enough to recommend lifelong anticoagulation, since chronic warfarin therapy is associated with a 10–15% lifetime risk of a fatal bleed. For patients who have had a second episode of thromboembolism, long-term anticoagulation is recommended unless the other risk factors increase the chance of a major hemorrhage, since the chance of life-threatening thromboembolism is much higher. Aspirin therapy in these patients is not recommended because it only adds to the risk of an anticoagulant-associated gastrointestinal bleed.

C. PREGNANCY:

Oral anticoagulants must be avoided in the treatment of venous thrombosis during pregnancy because of their teratogenic potential. Unfractionated heparin and LMWH are both safe, since they do not cross the placenta. LMWH therapy may also be efficacious in the treatment of women with microvascular thrombosis and recurrent miscarriages. Caution must be exercised in the use of epidural anesthesia at delivery when women are receiving heparin therapy.

D. ILEOFEMORAL THROMBOSIS:

Thrombolytic therapy has been used in patients with ileofemoral thrombosis, where the risk of postphlebitic venous insufficiency is extremely high. Unfortunately, only streptokinase is approved for peripheral use. It is effective less than 25% of the time, most likely because the thrombosis completely occludes the vein, preventing the drug from reaching the clot surface. Catheter-delivered urokinase can be more effective in this situation. Even when lysis is successful and venous patency is restored, there is no evidence that it will prevent chronic venous insufficiency. This may reflect the suggestion that the deep vein valves are irreversibly damaged early in the course of the thrombosis.

Pulmonary Embolism (PE)

The initial therapeutic approach to a pulmonary embolus will depend on the patient's hemodynamic status. Hemodynamically unstable patients with massive or multiple pulmonary emboli should receive thrombolytic therapy (rt-PA 100 mg infused over 2 hours) followed by full-dose unfractionated heparin for 10–14 days. Embolectomy can be life-saving in the patient with a large saddle embolus. Hemodynamically stable patients who demonstrate right ventricular hypokinesis on echocardiogram should also be considered for thrombolysis. The window of opportunity for thrombolysis is quite long. Patients will demonstrate a therapeutic response for up to 14 days. There is now good evidence that mortality is reduced and recovery is accelerated when thrombolytics are used in patients with large clot burdens. Otherwise, all patients who present with a high probability of PE, a positive lung scan, or ultrasound evidence of a DVT (or all three) should receive heparin for 10–14 days followed by oral anticoagulation to an INR of 2 to 3 for at least 6 months. If the patient is clinically stable, the hospitalization may be shortened by substituting LMWH, given as home therapy, after several days.

A. CARDIAC THROMBOEMBOLIC DISEASE:

Patients with unexplained atrial fibrillation or, even more important, atrial fibrillation with valvular disease, a dilated atrium, and evidence of heart failure or a previous embolus should receive moderate-dose warfarin therapy indefinitely. Patients with acute anterior wall infarctions who because of a wall motion abnormality are likely to form a mural thrombus need to receive warfarin for 2–3 months, after which there is little risk of embolism. Chronic anticoagulation is indicated in patients with artificial heart valves and dilated myocardiopathies, where mural thrombus formation is likely. Acute anticoagulation of patients with unstable angina with heparin and aspirin can reduce the incidence of acute myocardial infarction and death by 33%. Recent studies show a slight advantage of LMWH over unfractionated heparin, as well as a lower cost and a reduction in bleeding complications.

B. DISEASE-RELATED THROMBOSIS:

Patients with malignancy and thromboembolic disease can be resistant to therapy. Chronic warfarin therapy alone may not control the thrombotic tendency, and patients may require continuous heparinization with LMWH or the placement of a vena caval filter. Low-dose warfarin therapy (1 mg/day) should be used to reduce the incidence of catheter-related thrombosis. Thrombotic disease during pregnancy is another special situation. Warfarin therapy during the first trimester of pregnancy can be teratogenic. Near term, warfarin can increase the risk of hemorrhage, especially during delivery. Therefore, heparin is the preferred anticoagulant.

C. VENA CAVAL FILTERS:

In patients who fail anticoagulant therapy or have an absolute contraindication to anticoagulation, the placement of a vena caval filter can be used to prevent recurrent pulmonary emboli. Five different filters (two types of Greenfield filter, the bird's nest filter, the Simon nitinol filter, and the Vena Tech filter) are commonly available. They compare well in terms of efficacy, reducing the incidence of PE to less than 4% (median follow-up in most study series was 12–18 months). Filters are not more effective than long-term anticoagulation. However, anticoagulation combined with a vena caval filter may provide greater protection. Complications include insertion site (20–40%) and inferior vena caval thrombosis, tilting or migration of the filter, damage to the wall of the inferior vena cava, and filter fracture.

Primary Hypercoagulable States

Management of the patient with a primary hypercoagulable state presents additional problems. First, the incidence of thromboembolic disease in patients with one of these conditions varies so much that therapy should only be considered for patients who exhibit a strong thrombotic tendency. Heterozygous factor V Leiden patients without a history of thromboembolism have a normal life expectancy and a low to normal risk of future thromboembolism. This is also true for family members of patients with clinical disease. They need not receive chronic anticoagulation therapy. High-risk patients, who should be considered for lifelong anticoagulation, include those who have had more than one spontaneous thrombosis or a life-threatening thromboembolism and any individual who is a double heterozygote. Asymptomatic carriers of factor V Leiden, an antiphospholipid antibody, or an AT-III, protein C, or protein S defect should, however, always receive vigorous prophylaxis in situations that predispose them to thrombosis.

In **high-risk patients** with the G20210A prothrombin gene mutation or a deficiency of AT-III, protein S, or protein C, long-term anticoagulation with warfarin is recommended. Some caution must be taken in initiating warfarin therapy, especially in protein C– and protein S–deficient patients. These patients should receive full heparin anticoagulation prior to initiating the warfarin therapy, thereby preventing **coumarin-induced skin necrosis**. This condition is a rare complication that is related to an increased tendency to thrombosis of skin vessels within the first few days after beginning therapy. It may relate to the rapid reduction of the protein C (and perhaps protein S) level by the drug. In patients with **AT-III deficiency,** heparin therapy may be unpredictable. This situation reflects the lower than normal AT-III levels, or rarely, a defective AT-III protein. If full heparin anticoagulation is required, it may be necessary to provide the patient with exogenous AT-III by administration of purified AT-III (Thrombate III) or transfusion of fresh frozen plasma. Prophylactic AT-III therapy can decrease the risk of thrombosis in deficient patients undergoing surgery or childbirth.

Antiphospholipid Antibodies

Patients with antiphospholipid antibodies (lupus anticoagulant) and thromboembolic disease can represent a major therapeutic challenge. In women who experience recurrent abortions secondary to a lupus anticoagulant, aspirin therapy has been used to prevent thrombosis of the placenta and loss of the fetus. Its usefulness, however, is controversial. When the antibody is a complication of active lupus erythematosus, aggressive treatment of the primary disease can reduce the antiphospholipid titer and perhaps reduce the likelihood of thromboembolic complications. The patient with arterial thrombosis without other manifestations of autoimmune disease should receive long-term warfarin therapy with or without mini-dose aspirin. The response to this treatment is variable. Some patients seem to do very well, whereas others continue to demonstrate a thrombotic tendency. In part, this may be owing to problems monitoring the patient's level of anticoagulation. Lupus anticoagulants can interfere with the PT measurement to give inappropriately high INRs for the level of anticoagulation. Thus, many patients may be subtherapeutic. Dosing to an INR level greater than 3 to 4 may improve the clinical response but at the risk of more bleeding complications.

Arterial Thrombotic Disease

Platelet inhibitors are of proven value in the prevention of coronary artery and cerebrovascular thrombosis. Aspirin has been shown to decrease the incidence of myocardial infarction in patients with coronary artery disease. Ticlopidine has a slight advantage over aspirin in the treatment of cerebrovascular ischemia. It is suggested that a daily dietary supplement of folic acid (1 mg) and vitamin B_6 (pyridoxine 50 mg/day) may also be protective by reducing the plasma homocysteine level. However, the effectiveness of folic acid, vitamin B_{12}, or vitamin B_6 in reducing the incidence of cardiovascular disease still requires testing in randomized clinical trials. Anticoagulation with aspirin, coumadin, or both is strongly recommended in patients with atrial fibrillation to prevent arterial embolization, unless there is a major contraindication. Aspirin alone will reduce the relative risk of stroke by 22%, while adjusted-dose warfarin reduces the stroke risk by 62%. Increasing age, valvular heart disease, and congestive heart failure increase the risk of embolic disease. Younger patients with idiopathic atrial fibrillation may be managed with aspirin alone to avoid the risk of warfarin-induced hemorrhage.

In the treatment of acute arterial thrombosis, immediate thrombolysis, whether administered peripherally (rt-PA) or by catheter (urokinase), is the key to successful recanalization and prevention of end organ damage. As demonstrated in angioplasty patients, newer agents such as the GPIIb/IIIa inhibitors may be more effective than aspirin or heparin alone in the prevention of rethrombosis following thrombolysis.

Antithrombotic Therapy During Percutaneous Coronary Artery Interventions

Successful revascularization of the patient undergoing angioplasty depends on effective anticoagulation to prevent rethrombosis. Heparin and antiplatelet agents (aspirin, clopidogrel, and the GPIIb/IIIa antagonists) are the mainstays of therapy during the procedure. All patients should be preloaded with aspirin (325 mg) and clopidogrel (75 mg/day for 3 days or, for urgent cases, a single dose of 300 mg). In the case of heparin, optimal dosing during angioplasty should increase the activated clotting time (ACT) to 300–350 seconds when used alone, or 200–250 seconds when used together with a GPIIb/IIIa antagonist. Once the procedure is over, the heparin can be discontinued and the sheath removed when the ACT falls below 170 seconds. Stent patients should then be maintained on both aspirin (325 mg/day) and clopidogrel (75 mg/day) for several weeks after the procedure to prevent subacute rethrombosis.

The prominent role of platelets in the pathogenesis of rethrombosis following angioplasty, especially when a stent is placed to maintain vessel patency, has led to multiple trials looking at the added effectiveness of a GPIIb/IIIa antagonist in combination with heparin during the procedure. Three agents have been tried: abciximab (ReoPro), eptifibatide, and tirofiban. Each has shown a decrease in rethrombosis, recurrent myocardial infarction, and mortality at 3 months. The impact on mortality long-term is less clear. ReoPro has the longest duration of action and may have a greater protective effect.

BIBLIOGRAPHY

Diagnosis of Thromboembolic Disease

Birdwell BG et al: The clinical validity of normal compression ultrasonography in outpatients suspected of having deep venous thrombosis. Ann Intern Med 1998;128:1.

Buller HR et al: Deep vein thrombosis: New non-invasive diagnostic tests. Thromb Haemost 1991;66:133.

Devor M et al: Estrogen replacement therapy and the risk of venous thrombosis. Am J Med 1992;92:275.

Eikelboom JW et al: Homocyst(e)ine and cardiovascular disease: A critical review of the epidemiological evidence. Ann Intern Med 1999;131:363.

Ginsberg JS et al: Sensitivity and specificity of a rapid whole-blood assay for D-dimer in the diagnosis of pulmonary embolism. Ann Intern Med 1998;129:1006.

Ginsberg JS et al: The use of D-dimer testing and impedance plethysmographic examination in patients with clinical indications of deep vein thrombosis. Arch Intern Med 1997; 157:1077.

Goldhaber SZ: Pulmonary embolism. N Engl J Med 1998;339:93.

Heijboer H et al: A comparison of real-time compression ultrasonography with impedance plethysmography for the diagnosis of deep-vein thrombosis in symptomatic outpatients. N Engl J Med 1993;329:1365.

Hull RD et al: Diagnostic efficacy of impedance plethysmography for clinically suspected deep-vein thrombosis. Ann Intern Med 1985;102:21.

Stroke Prevention in Atrial Fibrillation Investigators: Predictors of thromboembolism in atrial fibrillation: I. Clinical features of patients at risk. Ann Intern Med 1992;116:1.

Stroke Prevention in Atrial Fibrillation Investigators: Predictors of thromboembolism in atrial fibrillation: II. Echocardiographic features of patients at risk. Ann Intern Med 1992;116:6.

Turkstra F et al: Diagnostic utility of ultrasonography of leg veins in patients suspected of having pulmonary embolism. Ann Intern Med 1997;126:775.

Primary Hypercoagulable Disorders

Alving BM, Bar CF, Tang DB: Correlation between lupus anticoagulants and anticardiolipin antibodies in patients with prolonged activated partial thromboplastin times. Am J Med 1990;88:112.

D'Angelo A, Selhub J: Homocysteine and thrombotic disease. Blood 1997;90:1.

Demers C et al: Thrombosis in antithrombin-III-deficient persons. Ann Intern Med 1992;116:754.

den Heijer M et al: Hyperhomocysteinemia as a risk factor for deep-vein thrombosis. N Engl J Med 1996;34:759.

De Stefano V, Finazzi G, Mannucci PM: Inherited thrombophilia: Pathogenesis, clinical syndromes, and management. Blood 1996;87:3531.

De Stephano V et al: The risk of recurrent deep venous thrombosis among heterozygous carriers of both factor V Leiden and the G20210A prothrombin mutation. N Engl J Med 1999; 341:801.

Koster T et al: Venous thrombosis due to poor response to activated protein C: Leiden thrombophilia study. Lancet 1993; 342:1503.

Kyrle PA et al: High plasma levels of factor VIII and the risk of recurrent venous thromboembolism. N Engl J Med 2000; 343:457.

Lane DA, Grant PJ: Role of hemostatic gene polymorphisms in venous and arterial thrombotic disease. Blood 2000;95:1517.

Love PE, Santoro SA: Antiphospholipid antibodies: Anticardiolipin and the lupus anticoagulant in systemic lupus erythematosus (SLE) and in non-SLE disorders. Ann Intern Med 1990; 112:682.

Mandel H et al: Coexistence of hereditary homocystinuria and factor V Leiden-effect on thrombosis. N Engl J Med 1996; 334:763.

Meijers JCM et al: High levels of factor XI as a risk factor for venous thrombosis. N Engl J Med 2000;342:696.

Nachman RL, Silverstein R: Hypercoagulable states. Ann Intern Med 1993;119:819.

Nygard O et al: Plasma homocysteine levels and mortality in patients with coronary artery disease. N Engl J Med 1997; 337:230.

Ridker PM: Fibrinolytic and inflammatory markers for arterial occlusion: The evolving epidemiology of thrombosis and hemostasis. Thromb Haemost 1997;78:1.

Ridker PM et al: Interrelation of hyperhomocyst(e)inemia, factor V Leiden, and risk of future venous thromboembolism. Circulation 1997;95:1777.

Ridker PM et al: Mutation in the gene coding for coagulation factor V and the risk of myocardial infarction, stroke, and venous thrombosis in apparently healthy men. N Engl J Med 1995;332:912.

Simmonds RE et al: Clarification of the risk for venous thrombosis associated with hereditary protein S deficiency by investigation of a large kindred with a characterized gene defect. Ann Intern Med 1998;128:8.

Svensson PJ, Dahlback B: Resistance to activated protein C as a basis for venous thrombosis. N Engl J Med 1994;330:517.

Thomas DP, Roberts HR: Hypercoagulability in venous and arterial thrombosis. Ann Intern Med 1997;126:638.

van Hylckama Vlieg A et al: High levels of factor IX increase the risk of venous thrombosis. Blood 2000;95:3678.

van Tilburg NH, Rosendaal FR, Bertina RM: Thrombin activatable fibrinolysis inhibitor and the risk for deep vein thrombosis. Blood 95:2855, 2000.

Management

Bauer KA: Management of patients with hereditary defects predisposing to thrombosis including pregnant women. Thromb Haemost 1995;74:94.

Hart RG et al: Antithrombotic therapy to prevent stroke in patients with atrial fibrillation: A meta-analysis. Ann Intern Med 1999;131:492.

Kearon C et al: A comparison of three months of anticoagulation with extended anticoagulation for first episode of idiopathic venous thromboembolism. N Engl J Med 1999;340:901.

Konstantinides S et al: Impact of thrombolytic treatment on the prognosis of hemodynamically stable patients with major pulmonary embolism: Results of a multicenter registry. Circulation 1997;96:882.

McConnell MV et al: Regional right ventricular dysfunction detected by echocardiography in acute pulmonary embolism. Am J Cardiol 1997;78:769.

Moll S, Ortel TL: Monitoring warfarin therapy in patients with lupus anticoagulants. Ann Intern Med 1997;127:177.

Rothrock JF, Hart RG: Antithrombotic therapy in cerebrovascular disease. Ann Intern Med 1991;115:885.

Schulman S: Optimal duration of oral anticoagulant therapy in venous thromboembolism. Thromb Haemost 1997;78:175.

Schulman S et al: Continuing anticoagulants for recurrent venous thromboembolism was better than 6-month anticoagulant therapy. N Engl J Med 1997;336:393.

Streiff MB: Vena caval filters: A comprehensive review. Blood 2000;95:3669.

Vorcheimer DA, Badimon JJ, Fuster V: Platelet glycoprotein IIbI-IIa receptor antagonists in cardiovascular disease. JAMA 1999;281:1407.

Welch GN, Loscalzo J: Homocysteine and atherothrombosis. N. Engl J Med 1998;338:1042.

Anticoagulation in the Management of Thrombotic Disorders

36

Successful management of the patient with a thrombotic disorder requires evaluation of risk factors for thrombosis, a careful assessment of the site and extent of the thrombus, and a skilled application of one or more anticoagulants. Diagnostic evaluation of the thromboembolic patient is discussed in Chapter 35. Treatment of the patient with a thrombus involves both dissolution of the clot and prevention of recurrence. Specific therapy will be dictated by the type of vessel involved, whether arterial or venous, and the clinical setting (Table 36–1). As a general rule, thrombotic disorders of arterial vessels are best managed using a combination of thrombolytic agents to rapidly dissolve the obstructing clot and antiplatelet drugs to prevent recurrence. In contrast, venous thromboembolism responds best to drugs such as heparin and warfarin that inhibit the function and formation of coagulation factors.

ANTIPLATELET DRUGS

Antiplatelet drugs act by inhibiting platelet function. They are most useful in preventing recurrent arterial thrombosis in patients with advanced atherosclerosis. Aspirin, dipyridamole, ticlopidine, and sulfinpyrazone have been used most extensively. Of these drugs, aspirin is the best studied, the most popular, and the cheapest. Newer inhibitors of platelet aggregation include abciximab (ReoPro), eptifibatide, tirofiban, sabrafiban, and clopidogrel. ReoPro has been approved by the US Food and Drug Administration (FDA) for use in patients undergoing percutaneous transluminal coronary angioplasty. The other drugs are undergoing clinical trials in patients with coronary and peripheral artery disease.

Pharmacokinetics

Aspirin acetylates prostaglandin G/H synthase, causing a loss of cyclo-oxygenase activity and an inhibition of thromboxane A_2 production and platelet aggregation. The effect is irreversible, so the impact on function is permanent for the 10-day lifespan of the platelet. A single dose of as little as 40–100 mg of aspirin is sufficient to inhibit the function of most platelets in circulation. Aspirin has no effect on platelet adhesion and does not block ADP release. **Dipyridamole** (Persantine) interferes with the platelet response to agonists by inhibiting phosphodiesterase and increasing the cell content of cAMP. It is a far less effective inhibitor than aspirin. **Sulfinpyrazone** is a weak competitive inhibitor of cyclo-oxygenase and disrupts platelet adhesion and prostaglandin synthesis.

Ticlopidine interferes with platelet aggregation by inhibiting ADP-induced GPIIb/IIIa-fibrinogen binding. Like aspirin, the effect on platelet function is irreversible. **Clopidogrel** (Plavix) is a second-generation ADP receptor inhibitor similar to ticlopidine, although its exact mechanism of action is still unknown.

Abciximab (ReoPro) is the Fab fragment of the monoclonal antibody 7E3. It binds irreversibly to the GPIIb/IIIa adhesion receptor, and by blocking fibrinogen and von Willebrand factor (vWF) binding, inhibits platelet aggregation. It is far more powerful than aspirin or ticlopidine. When given in full dose, it can completely inhibit ADP-induced platelet aggregation. Moreover, the effect lasts for the lifespan of the platelet; platelet aggregation is inhibited for more than 24 hours after treatment. Other inhibitors now under study include eptifibatide and tirofiban. **Eptifibatide** (Integrilin) is a peptide antagonist of GPIIb/IIIa with a short half-life of 2 hours. **Tirofiban** is a "small molecule" tyrosine derivative (peptidomimetic) with high specificity for the GPIIb/IIIa receptor. Both drugs also have short durations of action, 2–3 hours. Newer small molecule inhibitors (**orbofiban, xemlofiban, sibrafiban**) that can be administered orally may be useful for long-term platelet inhibition.

Table 36–1. Recommended therapy of thrombotic disorders.

Condition	Therapy
Coronary artery disease	
Stable angina/infarct prevention	Aspirin by itself or nothing
Unstable angina	Aspirin alone for outpatients; aspirin plus LMWH or UFH for hospitalized patients
Acute myocardial infarction (< 6 hours old)	Thrombolysis using intravenous streptokinase or t-PA plus full-dose heparin and aspirin
Anterior transmural infarcts (risk of mural thrombosis)	Full-dose heparin followed by warfarin therapy for 2–3 months
Reinfarction prevention	Long-term aspirin alone
Bypass graft patency	Aspirin/clopidogrel
Cerebral artery disease	
Transient ischemic attacks	Aspirin or ticlopidine
Recurring TIAs/evolving thrombotic stroke	LMWH or UFH followed by warfarin or aspirin alone (treatment debatable)
Completed thrombotic stroke	Aspirin or ticlopidine
Cerebral embolism	
Without hemorrhage on CT scan	LMWH or UFH followed by long-term warfarin therapy
With hemorrhage on CT scan	Postpone anticoagulation for 2 weeks
Vascular heart disease	
Mitral valve disease (especially stenosis) with atrial fibrillation or history of embolism	Long-term warfarin therapy
Atrial fibrillation cardioversion	Warfarin therapy for 2–3 weeks prior to and 4 weeks after cardioversion
Bioprosthetic mitral valves	Long-term moderate-dose warfarin therapy (INR 2.0–2.5)
Mechanical prosthetic valves	Long-term warfarin therapy (INR 3.0–4.0) with or without dipyridamole
Venous disease	
Deep venous thrombosis with pulmonary embolism	LMWH or full-dose UFH for 7 days followed by warfarin for 6 months or longer according to risk factors
Superficial phlebitis or limited to calf vessels	Anticoagulation not indicated unless extends proximally
Subclavian/superior vena cava thrombosis secondary to an in-dwelling catheter	Thrombolysis with streptokinase or t-PA followed by heparin, short-term warfarin, and line removal
Thromboembolism prevention	
Forced bed rest/general surgery	LMWH heparin (30 mg SC bid)
Orthopedic/elective hip surgery	LMWH heparin or moderate-dose warfarin

Clinical Applications

A. ASPIRIN:

Aspirin still enjoys the widest applicability. In general, aspirin therapy appears to work best in patients with distorted arterial anatomy, especially atherosclerotic vascular disease. This is a situation where a disruption in the endothelial surface provides a strong stimulus for platelet activation, aggregation, and subsequent clot formation.

Several clinical trials have supported the use of aspirin therapy to prevent thrombosis in patients with cerebrovascular disease, coronary artery disease, and to some extent, peripheral arterial disease seen in diabetic patients. The use of aspirin in patients with coronary artery disease is clearly established. The incidence of coronary occlusion and sudden death following acute myocardial infarction and in patients with unstable angina can be reduced by 30–60%. As for primary prevention, a single aspirin (325 mg) given every other day resulted in a 44% reduction in the incidence of myocardial infarction in a 5-year study of 22,000 male physicians. Aspirin can also reduce the risk of stroke, myocardial infarction, and sudden death by 20–30% in patients with cerebrovascular disease.

B. OTHER ANTIPLATELET DRUGS:

Clopidogrel has become the alternative drug of choice for patients who are aspirin sensitive. It is also used in combination with aspirin in angioplasty patients with implanted coronary artery stents.

The other oral antiplatelet drugs have more limited

applications. **Dipyridamole** has been used in conjunction with warfarin to prevent prosthetic heart valve embolization. It has also been used together with aspirin to provide a greater inhibition of platelet function. There is no clinical evidence, however, that this is better than aspirin alone in patients with atherosclerotic disease. **Ticlopidine** has been approved for the management of patients with cerebrovascular disease, where it has a slight advantage over aspirin. Ticlopidine therapy is associated, however, with several significant side effects, including the sudden appearance of a thrombotic thrombocytopenic purpura (TTP)–like syndrome that carries a 40% mortality. The extra expense is also an issue. Clopidogrel would appear to be a natural alternative to ticlopidine, since it is also an ADP pathway inhibitor. The CAPRIE trial supports its efficacy in reducing the event rate for stroke and vascular death when compared with aspirin. Like ticlopidine, however, rare cases of TTP have been reported with clopidogrel therapy. **Sulfinpyrazone** is not considered to be equally effective and therefore is not recommended.

Abciximab has been approved for the treatment of unstable angina patients destined for angioplasty and following angioplasty to prevent immediate reocclusion of dilated arteries. Multiple trials of ReoPro (EPILOG, EPISTENT, CAPTURE) in combination with heparin in patients undergoing angioplasty have shown significant reductions in reocclusion, myocardial infarction, and death at 30 days and 3 months. ReoPro has also been studied as an adjunct to thrombolytic therapy in acute myocardial infarction patients. ReoPro used in combination with half-dose tissue-type plasminogen activator (t-PA) (TIMI-14, SPEED) appears to be more effective than t-PA alone, achieving overall patency rates of 93%.

The peptide and peptidomimetic inhibitors (**eptifibatide, tirofiban**) show great promise in patients at high risk for platelet thrombus formation. Trials of tirofiban and eptifibatide in angioplasty patients have shown improved outcomes, with decreased rates of reocclusion, myocardial infarction, and death at 30 days. When given in combination with heparin and aspirin (PRISM-PLUS, ESPRIT) to patients with unstable angina/non-ST elevation myocardial infarction, tirofiban therapy resulted in a 30–40% reduction in rates of death, myocardial infarction, and recurrent ischemia. Moreover, since these agents have the advantage of being very short acting, they can be used as first-line therapy in unstable angina patients who are destined to go to emergency angioplasty or coronary artery bypasss graft (CABG).

Therapeutic Guidelines

A. Aspirin or Ticlopidine:

A low-dose aspirin regimen of 40 mg per day or an every other day dose of 80 mg is recommended to in-

hibit platelet function without impairing endothelial cell prostacyclin production. However, for the sake of convenience, a daily or every other day 325-mg dose can be used with equal clinical effectiveness and no greater risk of abnormal bleeding. Higher doses (900 mg or more daily) provide no greater inhibition of thromboxane metabolism and are associated with an increased incidence of gastrointestinal bleeding. For transient ischemic attack patients, 250 mg of ticlopidine twice daily taken with food may be more effective. When using ticlopidine, patients need to be closely monitored with frequent blood counts during the first several months of therapy.

B. Clopidogrel:

Trials of clopidogrel have used 75 mg once a day with a significant improvement in outcome in patients with peripheral arterial disease. At this dose, the full effect is not seen for up to a week. If more immediate blockade is required, as with emergent angioplasty, a single clopidogrel dose of 300 mg should be given initially followed by 75 mg/day. Clopidogrel can be given in combination with aspirin without a change in dose.

C. Abciximab:

The recommended dose of abciximab for angioplasty patients is 0.25 mg/kg given intravenously (IV) 10–60 minutes prior to the start of the procedure, followed by a continuous infusion of 0.125 µg/kg/minute, up to a maximum dose of 10 µg/minute, for at least 12 hours. Unstable angina patients should be maintained on a 10 µg/minute infusion until angioplasty is performed. This should be accompanied by low-dose heparin (70 U/kg), adjusted to keep the activated clotting time (ACT) between 200 and 250 seconds in order to minimize bleeding complications. Special caution should be taken in patients who have received thrombolysis prior to angioplasty. If possible, abciximab treatment should be delayed for 12–18 hours until the thrombolytic effects have been largely reversed. When studied in combination with t-PA, the dose of both t-PA and heparin was reduced (t-PA—15-mg bolus followed by a 35-mg infusion over 60 minutes; heparin—60 U/kg bolus followed by a 7 U/kg constant infusion) to avoid excessive bleeding.

D. Tirofiban or Eptifibatide:

Both tirofiban and eptifibatide are administered as a bolus followed by a continuous intravenous infusion. Effectiveness depends on the level of inhibition of platelet aggregation. The ESPRIT trial, which used a double bolus of eptifibatide, two 180-µg/kg doses 10 minutes apart, together with a continuous infusion of 2 µg/kg/minute, achieved 85–95% platelet inhibition. Tirofiban is administered as a 0.4-µg/kg/minute infusion for 30 minutes, followed by a continuous infusion of 0.1 µg/kg/minute. Both agents have very short half-lives. Once the infusion is discontinued, platelet aggregation returns to normal in 2–4 hours.

E. Oral GPIIb/IIIa Inhibitors:

Trials of the "first-generation" oral GPIIb/IIIa inhibitors (orbofiban, xemilofiban, sibrafiban) have yet to show a comparable benefit when compared with aspirin or the intravenous inhibitors. This may relate to an inability to achieve a constant blood level with oral dosing. Moreover, some of these agents may actually have a procoagulant effect.

Laboratory Monitoring

No laboratory monitoring is required with aspirin, ticlopidine, or clopidogrel therapy. Low-dose aspirin therapy (less than 325 mg per day) does not significantly prolong the bleeding time measurement. Furthermore, other coagulation tests are not affected. ReoPro and the other newer platelet aggregation antagonists can theoretically be dose adjusted using platelet aggregation studies if less than maximum inhibition is desired. However, clinical trials of these drugs have not tested the effectiveness of lower-dose regimens.

Adverse Effects

Low-dose aspirin therapy is not associated with an increased incidence of abnormal bleeding and does not pose a risk for the patient who requires an operative procedure. Patients taking aspirin who undergo coronary bypass surgery do not experience an increased amount of blood loss compared with aspirin-free patients. If the surgeon considers it important to reverse the aspirin effect prior to surgery, it is best accomplished by giving the patient a single intravenous injection of 0.3 µg/kg of desmopressin (DDAVP) just prior to surgery. Platelet transfusions will not be effective if the patient is taking large doses of aspirin, since the transfused platelets will also be affected. Similarly, clopidogrel therapy is not a contraindication to surgery.

Ticlopidine therapy is associated with adverse reactions in 50% or more of patients. Diarrhea, nausea, vomiting, and rash are the most common side effects. They usually occur during the first 3 weeks of therapy and may be severe enough to require discontinuing the drug in up to 20% of patients. The most worrisome adverse effects are the development of severe neutropenia, granulocyte counts below 500/µL, aplastic anemia, and a TTP-like syndrome that carries a high mortality. These can occur suddenly anytime during the first 3 weeks to 6 months of therapy. It is essential, therefore, to monitor the complete blood count with white cell

differential every 2 weeks for at least the first 3 months and be alert to clinical signs of TTP. With the approval of clopidogrel, which does not carry the same risk of adverse reactions, there is much less need for this drug.

Abciximab therapy in patients who are also receiving full-dose heparin is associated with a significant increase in both minor and major bleeding, most often bleeding at the femoral artery access site. Intracranial hemorrhage is rare. Predictors of bleeding include heparin and abciximab dosage, small body size, larger sheath size, female sex, and age. Bleeding may be controlled by using low-dose heparin, keeping the ACT between 200 and 250 seconds, or low-molecular-weight heparin (LMWH) without an apparent loss of effectiveness. Reduction in the dose of abciximab to lessen the aggregation defect as a way to reduce the bleeding complications has not been tested. Mild to severe thrombocytopenia can complicate abciximab therapy and require platelet transfusion. Since abciximab has a very long half-life, a demonstrable aggregation defect for up to 2–3 weeks, reversal can be difficult in the bleeding patient. If major bleeding does occur, both the abciximab and heparin should be discontinued, any obvious bleeding site such as the femoral access site controlled, and the patient given a transfusion with platelets and red blood cells as needed. Major surgery should be delayed for at least 12–24 hours after discontinuing abciximab. Better yet, if the need for an emergency CABG is anticipated, the patient should be treated with tirofiban rather than abciximab to take advantage of the shorter duration of action (4–6 hours).

Immediate, severe thrombocytopenia can occur with the initial exposure to abciximab and should be watched for. It appears to be somehow related to the presence of naturally occurring IgG antibodies to platelet GPIIb/IIIa, which are reactive with abciximab-coated platelets. Caution must be exercised in interpreting automated platelet counts. Since EDTA-pseudothrombocytopenia (Chapter 30) has been reported following abciximab therapy, a blood smear should be examined to rule out platelet agglutination.

ORAL ANTICOAGULANTS (COUMARINS)

The coumarin compounds have been recognized for more than 50 years for their value in treating thromboembolic diseases. The 4-hydroxycoumarin derivative, warfarin sodium (Coumadin), is the preferred compound for clinical use.

Pharmacokinetics

Warfarin is a mixture of equal amounts of two active racemic isomers, the R and S forms. The drug is absorbed rapidly and completely, resulting in a peak plasma level in 90 minutes. It is then gradually cleared into liver cells, where it blocks vitamin K reductase enzymes, thereby depleting the cell of **vitamin KH₂.** The latter is an essential cofactor for the required gamma carboxylation of the vitamin K–dependent coagulation proteins: prothrombin; factors VII, IX, and X; protein C, and protein S (Figure 36–1). The R and S isomers are cleared by different pathways. The S isomer is oxidized and excreted in bile, whereas the R isomer is excreted in urine.

As highlighted in Figure 36–1, several factors will influence effectiveness of warfarin therapy. Fluctuations in the dietary intake and absorption of vitamin K will influence the dose response. Vitamin K is a fat-soluble vitamin and its absorption is impaired in conditions of fat malabsorption or with ingestion of drugs such as clofibrate and oral antibiotics. Liver functional status is also important; cirrhosis or passive congestion of the liver can increase sensitivity to warfarin by decreasing synthesis of the coagulation factors.

Several **drug interactions** can affect warfarin kinetics. The most important are those drugs (phenylbuta-zone, metronidazole, sulfa drugs, disulfiram, and amiodarone) that inhibit the clearance of the more active S isomer, since this significantly prolongs the prothrombin time (PT). Drugs that inhibit R isomer clearance (cimetidine and omeprazole) have a less pronounced effect on the PT. Other drugs that have been reported as potentiating the effect of warfarin include erythromycin, the anabolic steroids, phenytoin, quinidine, tamoxifen, isoniazid, ethacrynic acid, and ketoconazole. The mechanism involved is less clear.

Resistance to warfarin therapy can be caused by an inherited trait or more likely a drug interaction that reduces absorption (cholestyramine) or increases the rate of clearance of the drug (alcohol, barbiturates, rifampin, glutethimide, griseofulvin, and carbamazepine).

Clinical Applications

Oral anticoagulant therapy has been proven effective for the treatment and prevention of venous and arterial thrombosis, pulmonary thromboembolism, and systemic embolism in patients with prosthetic heart valves

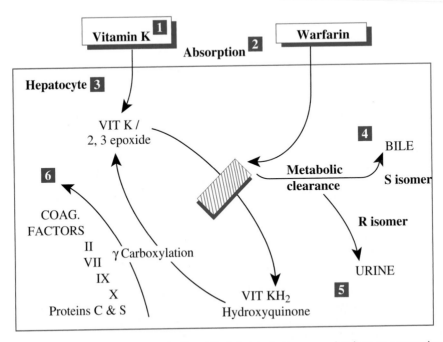

Figure 36–1. **Warfarin and vitamin K metabolism.** Warfarin blocks the normal reductase conversion of vitamin K epoxide to the hydroxyquinone (KH₂). This interferes with formation of the vitamin K–dependent factors—prothrombin; factors VII, IX, and X; and the anticoagulant proteins C and S. Therapeutic anticoagulation with oral doses of warfarin can be affected by multiple factors at several sites: (**1**) dietary content of vitamin K; (**2**) malabsorption of vitamin K; (**3**) liver function; (**4**) inhibition of S isomer clearance; (**5**) inhibition of R isomer clearance; and (**6**) coagulation-factor production (pregnancy, fever, hyperthyroidism).

or atrial fibrillation (see Table 36–1). It also has a role in the treatment of patients with acute myocardial infarction and evolving strokes. Low-dose therapy has been used to prevent venous thrombosis and pulmonary embolism after major orthopedic and gynecologic surgery, and in cancer patients with in-dwelling catheters.

Therapeutic Guidelines

Full anticoagulation with warfarin takes 3–4 days. This period reflects the relatively long half-lives of factors II (prothrombin), IX, and X in circulation once synthesis is inhibited. Therefore, a patient who requires immediate anticoagulation should be given heparin. Warfarin therapy can be started simultaneously using a dose of 5–10 mg/day for the first 2 days, then reducing the dose to 5 mg/day for maintenance. Since it is impossible to accurately predict a patient's final maintenance requirement, anywhere from 1–15 mg/day, a PT should be measured daily to make appropriate adjustments in dosage. Only after the patient's response has stabilized should the frequency of the PT measurements be reduced. For patients who are stable on chronic therapy, the PT may be measured as infrequently as once or twice a month.

In the nonurgent patient, oral anticoagulant therapy is best initiated by simply starting a daily maintenance dose of 5 mg. This dose schedule results in a smooth and balanced decline in factor levels (factors II, VII, and X and protein C), largely avoiding the risk of increased thrombotic potential for the first 48 hours because of a rapid depletion of protein C. Only patients with a congenital deficiency in protein C or S

are at significant risk of increased thrombosis, skin necrosis, or both if warfarin is initiated without heparin anticoagulation.

A. MAINTENANCE THERAPY:

Maintenance therapy requires a well-educated patient, at least monthly measurements of the PT by a reliable laboratory, and a recognized algorithm for adjusting the warfarin dose. The latter is most important if multiple members of the staff are interacting with the patient. Dose adjustments should be gradual, using modest daily changes planned over 1–2 weeks as follows:

- International normalized ratio (INR) < 2: Increase the weekly dose by 5–20%
- INR 3 to 3.5: Decrease weekly dose by 5–15%
- INR 3.6 to 4: Withhold 0–1 day's dose and decrease weekly dose by 10–15%
- INR > 4: Withhold 1 day's dose and decrease weekly dose by 10–20%

For very high INRs, one or two oral doses of vitamin K (2.5–5 mg) can be given, while continuing the warfarin therapy. This will speed the correction of the INR without reversing completely the patient's anticoagulation.

Recommended target ranges for anticoagulation are listed in Table 36–2. For most situations, an INR range of 2 to 3 is recommended. Higher-intensity anticoagulation has been reported to provide protection against recurrent myocardial infarction and stroke in patients following acute myocardial infarction. However, high-intensity regimens are associated with an increased

Table 36–2. Target ranges for warfarin therapy.

Condition	INR	Duration
Venous thrombosis		
Treatment	2.0–3.0	3–6 months
Prevention	1.5–2.5	Chronic
Atrial fibrillation		
Embolus prevention	1.5–2.5	Chronic
Myocardial infarction		
Embolus prevention postinfarction	2.0–3.0	2–3 months
Prevent reinfarction	3.0–4.5	Chronic
Mechanical heart valves		
Tissue valves	2.0–2.5	Chronic
Mechanical valves	3.0–4.0	Chronic
Arterial thrombosis		
Stroke prevention	2.0–4.0	Chronic

incidence of bleeding complications. The same is true for patients receiving chronic anticoagulation to prevent embolism from mechanical heart valves. This situation has led to recommendations for even less intense regimens, INRs of 1.5 to 2.5, and regimens that combine lower-dose warfarin with low-dose aspirin. The efficacy of these low-dose regimens appears to be comparable to that of the higher-dose approach, and bleeding complications are considerably less. Low-dose warfarin (INR of 1.5) may be as effective as low-dose heparin in preventing thromboembolism in orthopedic surgery patients. Very low-dose warfarin, 1 mg/day, can significantly reduce the incidence of catheter-related thrombosis in cancer patients.

B. MANAGEMENT OF ANTICOAGULATED PATIENTS DURING AND AFTER SURGERY:

The management of anticoagulated patients during surgery depends on the reason for the warfarin therapy and the duration of anticoagulation. Most patients who receive long-term oral anticoagulants can be managed by simply discontinuing the daily warfarin dose 4 days before surgery and then restarting it as soon as possible following the operation. Since it takes 3–4 days for the INR to fall below 1.5 and another 3 days to rise above 2.0 once the warfarin is restarted, the patient is subtherapeutic for only 3–4 days. If the INR is maintained at levels above 3, the daily warfarin dose should be stopped earlier or a small subcutaneous dose of vitamin K (1 mg) given the day before surgery.

Major surgery should be avoided for at least 1 month following a venous or arterial thromboembolism. If it is required, the patient should receive heparin perioperatively while the INR is below 2. The heparin can then be discontinued 6–8 hours prior to surgery and restarted 12–18 hours later, minimizing the period of risk. Without anticoagulation, patients run a risk of recurrent thromboembolism of 1% per day. If a patient cannot receive heparin because of the higher risk of bleeding, a vena caval filter should be considered.

After 2–3 months, preoperative full-dose heparin therapy is not recommended, since the risk of hemorrhage exceeds the risk of thromboembolism. However, these patients should receive prophylaxis with low-dose regular heparin or LMWH during the postoperative period, until their INR is greater than 2. In patients who receive anticoagulation for atrial fibrillation or a mechanical heart valve, the risk of thromboembolism with surgery is much lower. Therefore, they can be managed without perioperative heparin other than routine prophylaxis.

Laboratory Monitoring

Although several laboratory tests can be used to monitor anticoagulation, the one-stage PT is the most popular. The test is quick and quite sensitive to reductions in the levels of prothrombin and factors VII and X. The PT is not significantly prolonged by heparin given in therapeutic amounts to blood levels less than 0.5 U/mL. Therefore, it can be used to monitor therapy without interrupting a continuous heparin infusion.

The sensitivity of the PT depends, however, on the type of thromboplastin used to initiate the reaction. Different commercial thromboplastins have different sensitivities, varying over a two- to threefold range. This situation has led to the development of a system for normalizing the observed prothrombin time ratio (patient PT/control PT) to obtain a ratio that makes different thromboplastins comparable (Figure 36–2). By knowing the relative sensitivity of a commercial thromboplastin, the **International Sensitivity Index** (**ISI**), the nomogram can be used to convert a patient's prothrombin ratio to a normalized ratio (INR).

Traditionally, the PT has been measured on a venous blood sample by a local reference laboratory. However, instruments designed to do a PT on capillary whole blood, collected by finger stick, are now available for office use and patient self-testing. The CoaguChek, ProTime Monitor, and Avocet instruments have all been approved for home use. Care needs to be taken to standardize the instrument's results to those of the local laboratory to guarantee appropriate dosing. Success keeping any patient within a therapeutic range will also reflect the frequency of PT testing and the attention given to following up the patient. Many medical centers now offer an anticoagulation management service dedicated to tracking patients who receive warfarin or heparin. Studies suggest that these services do much better maintaining patients within an appropriate therapeutic range, with a significantly lower incidence of bleeding.

Adverse Events

A. ABNORMAL BLEEDING:

Abnormal bleeding is the principal adverse effect of oral anticoagulation. Risk factors that increase the likelihood of a bleed include advanced age, a pre-existing medical condition, or bleeding diathesis, concomitant use of heparin or aspirin, and the intensity of the regimen. Generally, an INR below 3 should not by itself result in an abnormal bleed, while higher INRs are associated with a significant bleeding incidence of 20–40% per year. The relative risk of bleeding can be in part predicted using the Blythe model of factoring in risk factors (age, recent stroke, cardiovascular disease, renal failure, diabetes mellitus) to derive a bleeding risk index. If a bleed occurs, the patient should be carefully worked up for an underlying medical condition. In the case of gastrointestinal bleeding, a full evaluation for

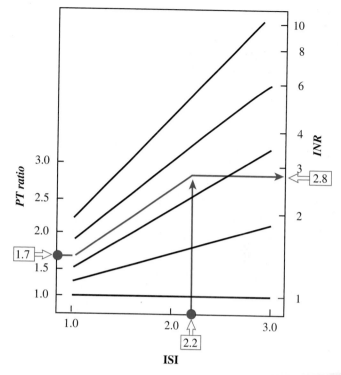

Figure 36–2. Nomogram for determining the INR. The prothrombin time (PT) needs to be corrected for the sensitivity of the thromboplastin in use in the laboratory. By knowing the published sensitivity of the commercial thromboplastin (ISI), the nomogram is used to convert the measured PT ratio (patient's PT/control PT) to an INR. The figure shows the example of converting a PT ratio of 1.7 for a thromboplastin with an ISI of 2.2.

ulcer disease or an occult neoplasm in the large bowel is required.

B. Contraindication of Warfarin During Pregnancy:

Warfarin is contraindicated during pregnancy, especially during the first trimester. The drug freely crosses the placenta and can cause skin, bone, and central nervous system abnormalities in the fetus. Risk estimates for first trimester exposure are as high as 30%. Warfarin therapy at term will effectively anticoagulate the fetus with the risk of a significant fetal hemorrhage at delivery. If anticoagulation is required during pregnancy, heparin must be used.

C. Reversal of Warfarin Anticoagulation:

Warfarin anticoagulation can be reversed with vitamin K or the administration of fresh frozen plasma (FFP) to directly replace vitamin K–dependent coagulation factors. The latter should be reserved for emergency situations, as for example an anticoagulated patient who must undergo immediate surgery. To reverse an INR of 3 or greater in preparation for emergency surgery, the patient should receive 10–20 mL/kg of FFP (at least 1000 mL) to increase levels of factors II, VII, IX, and X to at least 30% of normal. Vitamin K should also be

given to correct factor production; otherwise, the PT will again rise as the infused factors, especially factor VII, which has a half-life of only 3–4 hours, are cleared.

When there is less urgency, vitamin K given orally or by injection will effectively reverse the warfarin effect within a matter of hours. An INR greater than 5 can be brought into the therapeutic range within 24–48 hours by withholding the warfarin for 2 days and orally administering a single vitamin K dose of 2.5 mg. Several days of vitamin K therapy plus withdrawal of warfarin are required to completely reverse anticoagulation. Patients who have liver disease or have taken an overdose of warfarin can be resistant to therapy.

Vitamin K_1 (phytonadione) is the recommended preparation. It is available as 5-mg tablets, a liquid formulation containing 5–10 mg/mL for oral use, and a viscous liquid for injection (AquaMEPHYTON). A dose of 2.5–5 mg of vitamin K_1 given orally, subcutaneously (SC), or IV, is usually sufficient to reverse therapeutic levels of warfarin anticoagulation. With marked overdose or ingestion of rat poisons containing coumarin derivatives with extremely long half-lives, much larger and repeated doses of vitamin K will be required together with plasma infusions. Patients who have ingested rodenticides can require daily doses of 50–200 mg of vitamin K for months to counteract the coumarin effect.

UNFRACTIONATED HEPARIN

Unfractionated heparin is a heavily sulfated, complex polysaccharide that is naturally found in mast cell secretory granules. **The commercial drug heparin** is a mixture of glycosaminoglycan chain fragments of varying sizes (3000–30,000 daltons) extracted from bovine lung or porcine intestine. It is a highly effective anticoagulant for several clinical purposes.

Pharmacokinetics

Heparin acts by binding to and potentiating antithrombin III 1000-fold to inactivate thrombin and activated factor X (Xa) (Figure 36–3). Only the larger heparin molecules, those with at least 18 saccharide residues, are capable of inhibiting thrombin. Smaller heparin fragments have little effect on thrombin but do inhibit factor Xa. This difference in activity has been applied in development of LMWH preparations.

Heparin can only be administered by intravenous or subcutaneous injection. Given IV, its anticoagulant effect is immediate and easily monitored with clotting tests such as the thrombin time and partial thromboplastin time (PTT). The dose response is not directly proportional to the dose administered. The clearance is biphasic, reflecting a rapid but saturable binding/uptake by plasma proteins, endothelial cells, macrophages, and hepatocytes, followed by a slower renal clearance phase. With increasing doses, the half-life of the drug in circulation lengthens significantly from one to several hours. Final degradation and elimination of heparin appears to involve endothelial cell and monocyte removal, hepatic metabolism, and renal clearance. Unlike the oral anticoagulants, the response to heparin is less affected by liver disease.

Heparin binding to plasma proteins can reduce its anticoagulant activity, whereas binding to platelets, vWF, and endothelial cells can lead to microvascular bleeding. Since some of the plasma proteins responsible

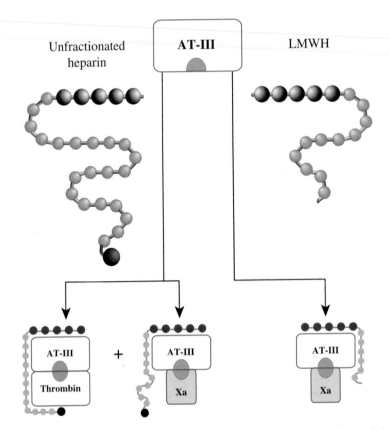

Figure 36–3. **Thrombin and factor Xa binding by unfractionated and low-molecular-weight heparin.** Both heparins are capable of binding to antithrombin III to catalyze the inactivation of factor Xa. Unfractionated heparin, because of its longer chain size, can also inactivate thrombin.

for heparin binding are acute phase reactants, ill patients can demonstrate heparin resistance. This is often seen in patients with pulmonary embolism or a large volume of thrombus. A significant decrease in antithrombin III levels secondary to liver or renal disease, or an inherited deficiency, will also interfere with the heparin response, since antithrombin III is required for its action.

Clinical Applications

Heparin is the drug of choice whenever a patient requires immediate anticoagulation, and it is a mainstay in the treatment and prevention of venous and arterial thromboembolic disease (Table 36–3). It is also widely applied in the treatment of patients with unstable angina or acute myocardial infarction, and as adjunctive therapy following thrombolysis to prevent rethrombosis. Heparin is the recommended agent for anticoagulation during pregnancy, since it does not cross the placenta and pose a risk to the fetus.

Heparin is routinely used to prevent thrombosis when patients undergo bypass surgery or hemodialysis. Low-dose heparin therapy can be used to prevent venous thrombosis and embolism following orthopedic surgery and in patients who are required to be at complete bed rest. Finally, heparin is a ubiquitous additive to intravenous fluids in order to prevent line clotting.

Therapeutic Guidelines

Heparin may be administered by continuous intravenous infusion or intermittent intravenous or subcutaneous injection. The intravenous route is preferred when immediate anticoagulation is desired, since the subcutaneous route is less dependable in time of onset

and dose response. Intravenous heparinization should begin with a loading dose of 5000 U (75 U/kg body weight) followed by a continuous infusion of 1000–1500 U per hour (28,000–40,000 U over the first 24 hours). An alternative approach is to use one of the published weight-based nomograms where 80 U/kg is given as a loading dose, followed by a continuous infusion of 18 U/kg/hour. Although overweight patients are more likely to achieve a therapeutic PTT within the first 24 hours by this approach, the PTT still needs to be closely monitored and the dose adjusted accordingly.

A. DOSE ADJUSTMENT:

For the first 48 hours, a PTT should be measured at 6- to 12-hour intervals and the rate of infusion adjusted to achieve a prolongation of between 1.5 and 2.5 times normal. Table 36–4 lists guidelines for dose adjustment according to the PTT measurement. The most common failure is achieving a therapeutic range within the first 12–24 hours. Therefore, close attention should be paid to the first few PTT measurements and the infusion rate adjusted appropriately. Regardless of the method used to dose adjust, weight-based nomogram or non–weight-based PTT-guided adjustment, only 50% of patients will reach the target range for the PTT by 24 hours. The rest will fall below or above the 1.5 to 2.5 times normal therapeutic range.

Dosing is more difficult when the drug is given IV or SC on an intermittent schedule every 4, 6, 8, or 12 hours. This situation results in very high heparin blood levels immediately after injection, followed by a return of the PTT to near normal just prior to the next injection. To monitor therapy, the PTT should be obtained the hour prior to the next scheduled injection and the heparin dosage adjusted to keep it at levels greater than 1.5 times normal. When a 12-hour schedule is used,

Table 36–3. Target ranges for heparin therapy.

Recommended Dosage	PTT (times normal control[a])
Venous thrombosis/pulmonary embolism	
Treatment: 5000-U bolus, 1000–1500 U/h continuous infusion (28,000–40,000 U/24 h)	2.0–2.5
Prevention: 5000 U SC 8–12 h	< 1.5
Acute myocardial infarction	
With thrombolytic therapy: 5000-U bolus, 1000 U/h (to prevent rethrombosis): infusion (24,000/U/24 h)	1.5–2.5
Mural thrombus 8000 U SC every 8 hours for prevention and to initiate warfarin	1.5–2.0
Unstable angina	
Treatment: 5000-U bolus, 1000 U/h continuous infusion (24,000 U/24 h)	1.5–2.5

[a] Assumes PTT has been standardized against by heparin titration so that therapeutic range (1.5–2.5 times control) is equivalent to a heparin blood level of 0.2–0.4 U/mL.

Table 36–4. Heparin dose adjustment.

PTT(s) (normal 27–35 s)	Start: 5000-U bolus; 1300 U/h continuous infusion
< 50	Rebolus 5000 U; increase infusion rate by 100 U/h
50–60	Increase infusion rate by 100 U/h
60–85	No change
85–100	Decrease infusion rate 100 U/h
100–120	Stop infusion for 30 min, decrease rate 100 U/h
> 120	Stop infusion for 60 min, decrease rate 200 U/h

there is a definite risk that the PTT will return to normal for some hours prior to the next treatment, thereby breaking the continuity of anticoagulation.

In general, patients receiving intermittent intravenous injections will require more heparin per 24 hours than those receiving continuous infusion (36,000 U versus 30,000 U per 24 hours on the average). Subcutaneous injection patients will also require higher 24-hour dosages of heparin. Moreover, they run the risk of erratic absorption from injection sites, which can lead to a loss of control, either too little or too great a PTT response.

B. Low-Dose Heparin and Other Therapies:

Low-dose heparin, 5000 U every 8 or 12 hours administered SC, will reduce the risk of venous thrombosis and pulmonary embolism in medical and surgical patients. The PTT is not prolonged and the risk of major bleeding is not increased, even when patients undergo major orthopedic surgical procedures. However, for the latter purpose, LMWH or low-dose warfarin therapy may be more effective. Full-dose heparin therapy can be safely given to cardiac patients as part of their treatment for an acute myocardial infarction and as an adjunct to thrombolytic therapy. Combination therapy with aspirin, 300 mg or less per day, is also safe and may be more effective in preventing coronary rethrombosis.

C. Addition of Warfarin for Chronic Anticoagulation:

When chronic anticoagulation is indicated, warfarin therapy should be initiated at the same time the patient receives heparin. This approach should permit discontinuation of the heparin by the fourth to sixth day, once full anticoagulation with warfarin is achieved. Delays in starting warfarin increase the risk of complica-

tions from heparin anticoagulation, whether abnormal bleeding or the development of heparin-induced thrombocytopenia (HIT)/thrombosis.

D. Treatment of Thromboembolic Disease During Pregnancy:

An obvious exception to this rule is the treatment of thromboembolic disease during pregnancy. For prophylaxis, low-dose heparin 5000 U SC twice a day escalating to 10,000 U SC twice a day during the third trimester or an equivalent dose of LMWH is recommended, followed by 4–6 weeks of warfarin anticoagulation postpartum. Full-dose unfractionated heparin or LMWH can be used safely in women with symptomatic thromboembolic disease. Long-term heparin therapy is associated with a 5–7% loss in bone mass. Women with a history of an antiphospholipid antibody complicated by a thromboembolic event or previous miscarriage should be treated with aspirin plus low-dose heparin or LMWH for the first 34 weeks of gestation. This therapy is well tolerated and significantly increases the chance for a live birth.

Laboratory Monitoring

The **activated PTT** is the preferred laboratory test for monitoring heparin therapy. It is readily available in most hospital laboratories and will reflect heparin blood levels with considerable precision if well standardized. The reagents used in the PTT do influence the responsiveness of the test. Therefore, each laboratory should establish the therapeutic range in seconds for its own PTT method to correspond to a plasma heparin level of 0.2–0.4 U/mL.

Measurements of the plasma heparin level, the ACT (**recalcification time**), and the thrombin time have applications in the management of patients receiving heparin for coronary bypass surgery. In this situation, the issue is one of guaranteeing full reversal of heparinization following surgery. The ACT can be performed in the operating room as a part of protamine reversal therapy. However, its sensitivity is affected by thrombocytopenia and platelet dysfunction. The thrombin time can provide a very sensitive measurement for trace amounts of residual heparin. Finally, a direct measurement of heparin levels is now becoming possible using automated equipment.

Adverse Effects

A. Sudden, Severe Bleeding:

The principal adverse effect of heparin is sudden, severe bleeding. Factors that increase risk of hemorrhage include dose and route of administration, reduced levels of key coagulation proteins, the concomitant use of other anticoagulants or drugs that inhibit platelet function, and the presence of a medical or surgical illness that increases the risk of bleeding. As regards dosing, the incidence of major bleeding is increased in patients receiving larger 24-hour doses of heparin and in those given intermittent intravenous or subcutaneous injections. When used in conjunction with thrombolytic therapy, marked hypofibrinogenemia increases the risk of bleeding spontaneously or with invasive procedures. Patients with renal failure or severe liver disease also have a greater risk of bleeding when they receive heparin.

B. Heparin-Induced Thrombocytopenia (HIT) and Platelet Thrombosis:

HIT (type II) and platelet thrombosis is the other major adverse effect. HIT would appear to be a reaction to the larger heparin fragments in the commercial preparation. When exposed to heparin for more than 5 days, patients can form IgG antibodies that are capable of binding a heparin/PF4 complex to the platelet surface, resulting in activation, aggregation, the release of thrombogenic platelet microparticles, and removal of platelets from circulation. An incidence of HIT of 10–15% has been reported in patients who receive bovine heparin, whereas the incidence with porcine heparin is 4–6%. Risk is related to the dose of heparin and the duration of therapy. Patients receiving full-dose heparin for more than 5 days are at greatest risk. Patients who are exposed to heparin on more than one occasion are also at increased risk and can develop thrombocytopenia more rapidly with reexposure.

Heparin antibody–induced platelet aggregates tend to form tightly bound white thrombi/emboli that can cause significant tissue damage and even death. The frequency of arterial or venous thrombosis in patients receiving unfractionated heparin for more than 5 days depends on the clinical situation. While it may be no more than 1% in otherwise healthy patients, it can reach incidences of 40–50% in postoperative patients with high levels of circulating thrombin. Therefore, the **platelet count** should be monitored as frequently as every or every other day when a patient is treated for longer than 5 days. Even a modest decrease in the platelet count to levels below 150,000/μL can indicate the appearance of the antibody.

If there is no other obvious explanation for the thrombocytopenia, the heparin should be discontinued and an oral agent substituted if long-term anticoagulation is required. To continue the heparinization in the face of a falling platelet count is to risk the chance of a significant thromboembolic event. In situations where full anticoagulation is required (coronary artery bypass surgery, dialysis, etc), recombinant hirudin (Lepirudin) or danaparoid (Organan), a mixture of glycosaminoglycans with predominant antifactor Xa activity, should be used. Hirudin is preferred. It is more easily monitored using the standard PTT. Danaparoid monitoring requires a more difficult factor Xa assay. Moreover, the in vitro cross-reactivity of danaparoid with heparin antibody IgG is 10–20%, although this does not appear to be clinically significant.

C. Other Side Effects:

Several less common side effects include hypersensitivity reactions, skin reactions, hypoaldosteronism with hyperkalemia, and osteoporosis. Urticaria, erythematous plaques, and even skin necrosis can occur at the site of injection. In these patients LMWH and danaparoid can be reaction-free alternatives.

D. Reversal of Heparin Anticoagulation:

Heparin anticoagulation can be reversed by the intravenous infusion of protamine sulfate, a low-molecular-weight protein derived from fish sperm. One milligram of protamine neutralizes approximately 100 units of heparin. The treatment dose must be estimated according to the status of the heparin regimen and the predicted half-life of residual heparin in the patient. The calculated dose of protamine sulfate is then infused IV at a rate no greater than 5 mg per minute. Rapid infusion can result in marked hypotension, dyspnea, bradycardia, and even anaphylaxis. In light of these side effects, it is best to allow the heparin anticoagulant effect to naturally dissipate. This should occur within a matter of hours, unless very large amounts of heparin have been administered.

LOW-MOLECULAR-WEIGHT HEPARIN (LMWH)

Heparin molecules with fewer than 18 saccharides can be prepared chemically or enzymatically from natural heparin. Because of the smaller molecular size (average 5000 daltons), LMWH is less able to bind to antithrombin III and thrombin simultaneously but does retain its ability to inhibit factor Xa (see Figure 36–3). LMWH does not inhibit platelet function or increase microvascular permeability to the same extent as heparin.

The lower molecular size also affects the pharmacokinetics. LMWH has a lower binding affinity for endothelial cells and several plasma proteins, including platelet factor 4, fibronectin, and vWF. This translates into a better dose-response relationship for therapeutically administered LMWH preparations. LMWH has a dose-independent plasma half-life that is two to four times longer than unfractionated heparin when given IV and three to six times longer when given SC at therapeutic doses, making it possible to administer LMWH on a less frequent schedule. Clinical trials of LMWH (enoxaparin) for the prevention of thrombosis during surgery have successfully used twice-a-day dosing regimens. Dalteparin, a longer-acting LMWH, can be administered once a day. The extremely reliable dose response to LMWH makes laboratory testing unnecessary except in patients who weigh more than 80 kg or have renal failure.

Clinical Applications

LMWH has now been studied in several randomized clinical trials aimed at the prevention and treatment of venous thrombosis in high-risk patients. In general, it appears with be a more effective anticoagulant when compared with unfractionated heparin, while reducing the incidence of microvascular bleeding. LMWH is the recommended prophylactic therapy for patients over age 40 who are undergoing a major surgical procedure, especially if they have a history of previous thromboembolic disease, a malignancy, a fracture, or spinal cord injury. Untreated, this group of patients has a 40–80% incidence of deep venous thrombosis (DVT) and a 4–10% risk for a pulmonary embolus (PE). LMWH prophylaxis reduces the risk of DVT by 75–80%. In patients undergoing hip or knee surgery or long bone fracture repair, LMWH reduces a 50% untreated incidence of DVT by 60–70%. It has also been shown to be more effective than warfarin in patients undergoing knee surgery.

In medical patients, LMWH is strongly recommended in ischemic stroke and multiple trauma patients to prevent DVT. Patients with complicated medical illness admitted to hospital for extended stays of 5 days or more can benefit from low-dose LMWH (40 mg enoxaparin SC once a day) without an increase in bleeding complications. LMWH is comparable to or better than unfractionated heparin in unstable angina patients but so far appears to provide no advantage over unfractionated heparin in angioplasty patients. Finally, LMWH is the preferred anticoagulant for the initial treatment of patients with DVT or PE. It is more effective in preventing a subsequent embolus, while causing fewer bleeding complications. It also has the advantages of easier administration and a more reliable dose response. This makes laboratory testing unnecessary and opens the door to earlier discharge from the hospital or even treatment from day one with home therapy.

Overall, LMWH is a safer drug. It is more effective than standard heparin, with a lower risk of significant bleeding. This reflects the reduced binding to platelets, vWF, and endothelial cells. The incidence of HIT and thrombosis is also significantly lower with LMWH. However, since there is cross-reactivity, LMWH cannot be automatically substituted for standard heparin in HIT patients. Unresolved issues include the risk of osteoporosis with long-term use and the effectiveness of protamine in reversing the LMWH anticoagulant effect. Protamine sulfate does not bind as well to low-molecular-weight fragments of heparin but will partially neutralize its effect.

Therapeutic Guidelines

In the United States, several LMWH preparations (enoxaparin, dalteparin, and ardeparin) have been approved for use in thrombosis prevention in surgery patients and in the treatment of thromboembolic disease (Table 36–5). Given in a dose of 30 mg (3000 antifactor Xa IU) SC twice a day (40 mg once a day for general medical and surgical patients), enoxaparin is more effective than standard heparin and has a lower inci-

Table 36–5. LMWH dose recommendations.

Indication	Recommended Dose and Schedule
Prophylaxis	
General surgery	
Low risk	Enoxaparin 4000 U before and then daily or dalteparin 2000–3000 U SC just before and then daily after surgery
High risk	Enoxaparin 3000 U SC before and then bid or dalteparin 5000 U SC before and then daily
Orthopedic surgery	Enoxaparin 3000 U SC before and then bid or dalteparin 5000 U SC before and then daily
Trauma/spinal injury	Enoxaparin 3000 U SC bid
Immobility (bed rest secondary to medical illness: stroke, CHF, etc)	Enoxaparin 4000 U SC or dalteparin 2000–3000 U SC daily
Treatment	
DVT or PE	Enoxaparin or dalteparin 100 U/kg SC bid
Unstable angina	Enoxaparin or dalteparin 100 U/kg SC bid

dence of bleeding complications. The longer-acting preparation, dalteparin (Fragmin), can be given once a day in doses of 2500 or 5000 U, depending on the severity of the surgery. Orthopedic surgery patients who receive LMWH prophylaxis for 4–10 days while in the hospital can be discharged off anticoagulants with little risk of subsequent symptomatic DVT or pulmonary embolism. Patients with an inherited thrombophilia or history of recurrent thrombotic disease may be maintained on an oral anticoagulant for up to 1 month following discharge to minimize the risk of late-occurring thromboembolism.

Full-dose LMWH, 1 mg/kg (100 U/kg) of enoxaparin given SC twice a day, is the preferred therapy in the treatment of DVT or PE. To guarantee effectiveness, dalteparin should also be given in a dose of 100 U/kg twice a day. LMWH can be used safely in patients with CT scan–proven ischemic stroke to prevent paralysis/bed rest–induced phlebothrombosis. It can also be used in full dose for unstable angina with comparable efficacy to unfractionated heparin. LMWH can be used in the treatment of angioplasty patients to prevent restenosis but holds no particular advantage over unfractionated heparin.

New formulations of LMWH, as well as unfractionated heparin, which facilitate at least limited absorption by the gastrointestinal system, have recently been introduced. These compounds use synthetic amino acids to promote absorption, sufficient to prolong the PTT. Studies of heparin prophylaxis in hip and knee surgery patients are under way.

Cost-effectiveness

LMWH is currently 10–20 times more expensive than unfractionated heparin. For this reason alone, its use cannot be justified when unfractionated heparin is equally efficacious, as with low-dose prophylaxis in routine medical and surgical patients. However, a case can be made for LMWH as the more effective agent in orthopedic surgery patients and in the treatment of patients with venous thrombosis/thromboembolism. With orthopedic surgery, the lower incidence of post-operative thromboembolic disease provides a significant cost saving by preventing prolonged hospital stays for a complicating DVT or PE. In the treatment of the medical patient with venous thrombosis/thromboembolism or unstable angina, the elimination of the need for the heparin-infusion pump and laboratory testing (PTTs two to four times per day) makes the cost of unfractionated heparin and LMWH equivalent. An earlier discharge from the hospital, or even total treatment as an outpatient, makes LMWH an even more cost-effective treatment strategy.

Adverse Effects

Just as with unfractionated heparin, the principal adverse effect of LMWH is bleeding. Although the risk at recommended dosages is somewhat less with LMWH, there is a dose relationship. Patients given more than 1 mg/kg twice a day have a higher incidence of bleeding. Renal failure patients are at special risk, since LMWH is primarily cleared through the kidney. In this situation, laboratory monitoring of antifactor Xa activity is needed to adjust the LMWH dose. There have also been reports of spinal cord bleeds in patients receiving LMWH who have had epidural catheters placed.

DANAPAROID

Danaparoid (Orgaran) is a mixture of glycosaminoglycans (heparan, dermatan, and chondroitin sulfates) that has selective antifactor Xa activity and low affinity for AT-III. Given in a dose of 750 U SC two or three times a day, danaparoid is as effective as either unfractionated heparin or LMWH in DVT prophylaxis in orthopedic surgery. In the treatment of venous thromboembolic disease, a danaparoid dose of 1250 U SC twice a day is equivalent to full-dose heparin in preventing recurrence, whereas 2000 U twice a day appears to be even more effective than heparin. Danaparoid can also be administered by infusion in patients undergoing hemodialysis or bypass surgery or by bolus intravenous injection for cardiac catheterization and angioplasty. Like LMWH, danaparoid is primarily cleared by the kidney. Therefore, renal failure patients need to be monitored by antifactor Xa assay to adjust the dose.

The principal indication for danaparoid is in patients with known or suspected HIT. Because it has only a 10–20% cross-reactivity with heparin-induced IgG antibodies, danaparoid is a reasonable drug for the treatment of HIT patients. When danaparoid treatment is initiated during an episode of HIT, the platelet count recovers to normal levels within 5–7 days and the risk of thromboembolism is markedly reduced. The cost of danaparoid therapy is some six to seven times that of either unfractionated heparin or LMWH, making routine use of the drug prohibitive.

Complications with danaparoid therapy are similar to those seen with unfractionated heparin or LMWH. The risk of bleeding is no greater and may be somewhat less. Like LMWH, danaparoid is given as a fixed dose without monitoring. Plasma anti-Xa activity can be measured in grossly under- or overweight individuals and in renal failure patients in order to adjust the dose. Reversal of danaparoid anticoagulation is an issue; protamine, DDAVP, epsilon aminocaproic acid, and FFP or platelet transfusions are of little or no value.

RECOMBINANT HIRUDIN

Lepirudin (Refludan), a recombinant hirudin derived from yeast, is a highly specific direct inhibitor of thrombin, binding to thrombin without AT-III as a cofactor. It was initially studied in combination with t-PA in order to prevent the reocclusion of coronary arteries following successful thrombolysis. However, it did not appear to add significant value to the treatment outcome and there was a greater incidence of bleeding requiring transfusion. Lepirudin is FDA approved for the treatment of HIT. It is also as least as good as, if not better than, LMWH in the prevention of DVT in postoperative patients, when given in a dose of 15 mg SC twice a day.

Lepirudin is considered by many to be the drug of choice for the treatment of HIT. It completely avoids the issue of cross-reactivity and is easier to manage, since the PTT or, in the catheterization lab, the ACT can be used to adjust the dose. After the clinician documents a baseline PTT in the normal range, the drug is administered IV in a bolus of 0.4 mg/kg followed by continuous infusion at a rate of 0.15 mg/kg/hour. The dose should then be adjusted to keep the PTT between 1.5 to 2.5 times normal. Renal failure patients will require a dose reduction of 30–50%, since hirudin is primarily cleared through the kidney. If oral anticoagulation is initiated, the dose should be reduced to keep the PTT at 1.5 times the control. As with danaparoid, the platelet count should show a rapid recovery, indicating a reversal of the HIT process of platelet activation and consumption.

Lepirudin is generally well tolerated. The most common adverse effect is bleeding, usually minor bleeding from puncture sites. However, blood loss sufficient to require transfusion is seen in up to 15% of patients. The formation of antihirudin antibodies has been observed in some 40% of treated patients. This can increase the anticoagulant effect, probably by slowing renal clearance.

Bivalirudin is a semi-synthetic analogue of hirudin that produces a much more transient inhibition of thrombin. This enhances its safety when used in situations like angioplasty, where hirudin use has been associated with a greater incidence of bleeding complications.

ARGATROBAN

Argatroban (Novastan), a substituted derivative of arginine, is a reversible inhibitor of both soluble and fibrin-bound thrombin. It can be used clinically in any situation where heparinization is indicated. Like heparin, it is best administered as a continuous intravenous infusion (2.0 μg/kg/minute), titrated to achieve an acti-

vated PTT of 1.5 to 3 times baseline. Advantages of this new agent include its rapid reversibility, a half-life of 30 minutes, and its lack of cross-reactivity with heparin-induced antibodies. It may, however, be associated with a high incidence of major bleeding, especially in patients with heparin-induced thrombosis.

A new orally absorbed drug—**H376/95,** which is rapidly metabolized to the thrombin inhibitor melagratan, is now being tested for its efficacy in the treatment and prevention of venous thromboembolism.

NEW ANTICOAGULANTS

Several new anticoagulants are currently being developed and are undergoing clinical trials as alternatives to warfarin and heparin. They include inhibitors of factors IXa, Xa, and VIIa/tissue factor (recombinant tissue factor pathway inhibitor and recombinant nematode anticoagulant peptide), as well as anticoagulant enhancers—recombinant protein C and activated protein C concentrates, soluble thrombomodulin, thrombin variants that promote protein C activation, and allosteric modulators of thrombin.

THROMBOLYTIC DRUGS

Intravascular thrombi can be dissolved by thrombolytic drugs, such as streptokinase, urokinase, and t-PA. These agents are of greatest use in the treatment of patients with arterial thrombosis, including coronary artery thrombosis.

Pharmacokinetics

Streptokinase binds to and activates plasminogen to form free plasmin. When given in doses of 250,000–1.5 million units IV, the active streptokinase-plasminogen complex is not inhibited by α_2-antiplasmin, and both fibrin and fibrinogen destruction occur. This situation continues as long as the drug is infused or for about 80 minutes after a single bolus dose. **Urokinase** is a serine protease that also lacks fibrin specificity. It is most often used as a continuous infusion by catheter to the site of a peripheral arterial thrombosis.

t-PA is also a serine protease. However, it is selective for plasminogen bound to fibrin clot, making it more clot specific. t-PA is naturally produced by endothelial cells to inhibit clot propagation. As a part of this natural cycle, only small amounts are released and this is inactivated rapidly by plasminogen activator inhibitor I so as to prevent any effect on circulating plasminogen and fibrinogen. When **recombinant t-PA** (rt-PA) is administered to patients with coronary thrombosis, a loading dose is given, followed by a continuous infusion over 3–4 hours to a total of 100–150 mg of rt-PA. This situation results in plasma concentrations of t-PA that are several thousand times greater than physiologic levels. It is common, therefore, to see partial breakdown of circulating fibrinogen as well as clot lysis.

Clinical Applications

The principal application of the thrombolytic agents is to dissolve arterial thrombi to prevent irreversible organ damage. In the case of a thrombus or embolus in large arterial vessels, direct infusion of a lytic agent by catheter can result in effective clot lysis with little systemic fibrinogen destruction. With thrombosis of smaller arterial vessels, especially acute coronary artery occlusion, intravenous administration of either streptokinase or rt-PA can result in dissolution of the offending thrombus and return of blood flow. However, new clot formation may occur shortly after thrombolysis unless effective anticoagulation is maintained with heparin and aspirin.

Most patients with iliofemoral DVT will develop post-phlebitic syndrome with objective signs and symptoms of venous insufficiency, including skin thickening (nonpitting edema) and discoloration and, in some, unhealing leg ulcers and venous claudication. Thrombolytic therapy for iliofemoral venous thrombosis has had variable success in decreasing the severity of post-phlebitic venous insufficiency. However, if and when clot lysis is complete, morbidity is reduced. Both catheter-directed urokinase therapy and venous t-PA have been used effectively. Thrombolytic drugs are also used to clear thrombosed intravenous catheters and in treatment of life-threatening PE.

Adverse Effects

Thrombolytic agents not only dissolve intravascular clots but also will interfere with the normal coagulation sequence required for wound healing. Therefore, contraindications to thrombolytic therapy include recent surgery or an invasive procedure involving arterial puncture, a history of a previous cerebrovascular accident, significant hypertension, recent gastrointestinal bleeding, or a history of a hemorrhagic diathesis. The incidence of complicating hemorrhage following intravenous streptokinase or rt-PA is directly related to the drug dosage, the concurrent use of heparin, and an undetected contraindication to therapy.

Protocols used by cardiologists in the treatment of coronary artery thrombosis usually involve the administration of a fixed dose of streptokinase or rt-PA without regard for body size. It is not surprising, therefore, that women of lower body weight show a higher incidence of fibrinogen destruction and complicating hem-

orrhage. When thrombolytic agents are infused over many hours, as has been used for peripheral arterial or venous disease, fibrinogen destruction to levels less than 100 mg/dL with accompanying hemorrhage is much more common. Severe bleeding immediately following fibrinolytic therapy should be managed by discontinuing the heparin and administering fibrinogen (cryoprecipitate or FFP) if the measured fibrinogen level is less than 100 mg/dL. Finally, late-onset bleeding occurring hours or days after thrombolysis is invariably the result of concurrent heparin therapy, not the lytic agent.

Patients who have previously received streptokinase or have antistreptokinase antibodies resulting from a prior streptococcal infection are at risk of an adverse reaction to the drug. This includes an IgE-mediated acute allergic reaction and on occasion severe anaphylaxis. This is not true for rt-PA, which is a recombinant human protein. At the same time, the cost of rt-PA is far greater than that of streptokinase.

BIBLIOGRAPHY

Principles of Management

Goad KE, Gralnick HR: Coagulation disorders in cancer. Hematol Oncol Clin North Am 1996;10:457.

Kearon C, Hirsh J: Current concepts: Management of anticoagulation before and after elective surgery. N Engl J Med 1997;336:1506.

Vongpatanasin W, Hillis LD, Lange RA: Prosthetic heart valves. N Engl J Med 1996;335:407.

Antiplatelet Drugs

Berkowitz SD et al: Acute profound thrombocytopenia after c7E3 Fab (abciximab) therapy. Circulation 1997;95:809.

Creager MA: Results of the CAPRIE trial: Efficacy and safety of clopidogrel. Vasc Med 1998;3:257.

Epilog Investigators: Platelet glycoprotein IIb/IIIa receptor blockade and low-dose heparin during percutaneous coronary revascularization. N Engl J Med 1997;336:1689.

Hass WK et al: A randomized trial comparing ticlopidine hydrochloride with aspirin for the prevention of stroke in high-risk patients. N Engl J Med 1989;321:501.

Madan M, Berkowitz SD, Tcheng JE: Glycoprotein Iib/IIIa integrin blockade. Circulation 1998;23:2629.

O'Neill WW et al: Long-term treatment with a platelet glycoprotein-receptor antagonist after percutaneous coronary revascularization. N Engl J Med 2000;342:1316.

Patrono C: Aspirin as an antiplatelet drug. Ann Intern Med 1994;330:1287.

PRISM PLUS Study Investigators: Inhibition of the platelet glycoprotein IIb/IIIa receptor with tirofiban in unstable angina and non-Q-wave myocardial infarction. N Engl J Med 1998;338:1488.

PURSUIT Trial Investigators: Inhibition of platelet glycoprotein IIb/IIIa with eptifibatide in patients with acute coronary syndromes. N Engl J Med 1998;339:436.

Sharis PJ, Cannon CP, Loscalzo J: The antiplatelet effects of ticlopidine and clopidogrel. N Engl J Med 1998;129:394.

Topol EJ, Byzova TV, Plow EF: Platelet GPIIb-IIIa inhibitors. Lancet 1999;353:227.

Topol EJ et al: Outcomes at 1 year and economic implications of platelet glycoprotein Iib/IIIa blockade in patients with coronary stenting: Results from a multicentre randomized trial. Lancet 1999;354:2019.

Oral Anticoagulants

Blythe BJ, Quinn L, Landefeld C: Prospective evaluation of an index for predicting the risk of major bleeding in outpatients treated with warfarin. Am J Med 1999;195:91.

Chiquette E, Amato MG, Bussey HI: Comparison of an anticoagulation clinic and usual medical care: Anticoagulation control, patient outcomes, and health care costs. Arch Intern Med 1998;158:1641.

Clagett GP et al: Prevention of venous thromboembolism: Fourth ACCP consensus conference on antithrombotic therapy. Chest 1995;180(4):312S.

Gosselin R et al: A comparison of point-of-care instruments designed for monitoring oral anticoagulation with standard laboratory methods. Thromb Haemost 2000;83:698.

Harrison L et al: Comparison of 5-mg and 10-mg loading doses in the initiation of warfarin therapy. Ann Intern Med 1997;126:133.

Hirsh J: Oral anticoagulant drugs. N Engl J Med 1991;324:1865.

Pritchett ELC: Management of atrial fibrillation. N Engl J Med 1992;326:1264.

Weibert RT et al: Correction of excessive anticoagulation with low-dose oral vitamin K_1. Ann Intern Med 1997;126:959.

Wells PS et al: Interactions of warfarin with drugs and food. Ann Intern Med 1994;121:676.

Heparin/LMWH

Becker RC et al: A randomized, multicenter trial of weight-adjusted intravenous heparin dose titration and point-of-care coagulation monitoring in hospitalized patients with active thromboembolic disease. Am Heart J 1999;137:59.

The Columbus Investigators: Low-molecular-weight heparin in the treatment of patients with venous thromboembolism. N Engl J Med l997;337:657.

Greinacher A et al: Heparin-induced thrombocytopenia with thromboembolic complications: Meta-analysis of 2 prospective trials to assess the value of parenteral treatment with lepirudin and its therapeutic aPTT range. Blood 2000;96:846.

Heit JA et al: Ardeparin sodium for extended out-of-hospital prophylaxis against venous thromboembolism after total hip or knee replacement. Ann Intern Med 2000;132:853.

Hirsh J: Heparin: Mechanism of action, pharmacokinetics, dosing considerations, monitoring, efficacy, and safety: Fourth ACCP consensus conference on antithrombotic therapy. Chest 1995;108(4):258S.

Hirsh J, Levine MN: Low molecular weight heparin. Blood 1992;79:1.

Hommes DW et al: Subcutaneous heparin compared with continuous intravenous heparin administration in the initial treatment of deep vein thrombosis. Ann Intern Med 1992;116:279.

Hull RD et al: A comparison of subcutaneous low-molecular-weight heparin with warfarin sodium for prophylaxis against deep-vein thrombosis after hip or knee implantation. N Engl J Med 1993;329:1370.

Hull RD et al: Subcutaneous low-molecular-weight heparin compared with continuous intravenous heparin in the treatment of proximal-vein thrombosis. N Engl J Med 1992;326:975.

Januzzi JL, Jang I: Heparin induced thrombocytopenia: Diagnosis and contemporary antithrombin management. J Thrombosis Thrombolysis 1999;7:259.

Levine M et al: A comparison of low-molecular-weight heparin administered primarily at home with unfractionated heparin administered in the hospital for proximal deep-vein thrombosis. N Engl J Med 1996;334:677.

Levine MN et al: Prevention of deep vein thrombosis after elective hip surgery: A randomized trial comparing low molecular weight heparin with standard unfractionated heparin. Ann Intern Med 1991;114:545.

Raschke RA et al: The weight-based heparin dosing nomogram compared with a "standard care" nomogram. Ann Intern Med 1993;119:874.

Samama MM et al: A comparison of enoxaparin with placebo for the prevention of venous thromboembolism in acutely ill medical patients. N Engl J Med 1999;341:793.

Simonneau G et al: A comparison of low-molecular-weight heparin with unfractionated heparin for acute pulmonary embolism. N Engl J Med 1997;337:663.

Spiro TE et al: Efficacy and safety of enoxaparin to prevent venous thrombosis after hip replacement surgery. Ann Intern Med 1994;121:81.

Warkentin TE et al: Heparin-induced thrombocytopenia in patients treated with low-molecular-weight heparin or unfractionated heparin. N Engl J Med 1995;332:1330.

Weitz JI: Low-molecular-weight heparin. N Engl J Med 1997;337:688.

Other Thrombin Inhibitors

Eriksson BI et al: A comparison of recombinant hirudin with low-molecular-weight heparin to prevent thromboembolic complications after total hip replacement. N Engl J Med 1997;337:1329.

Fareed J: Antithrombin agents as anticoagulants and antithrombotics: Implications in drug development. Clin Appl Thromb Hemost 1998;4:227.

Matsuo T, Koide M, Kario K: Development of argatroban, a direct thrombin inhibitor, and its clinical application. Semin Thromb Hemost 1997;23:517.

Schiele F et al: Subcutaneous recombinant hirudin (HBW 023) versus intravenous sodium heparin in treatment of established deep venous thrombosis of the legs: A multicentre prospective dose-ranging randomized trial. Thromb Haemost 1997;77:834.

Thrombolytic Drugs

Collen D, Lijnen HR: Basic and clinical aspects of fibrinolysis and thrombolysis. Blood 1991;78:3114.

Hyers TM et al: Antithrombotic therapy for venous thromboembolic disease. Chest 1998;114:561.

Popma JJ, Topol EJ: Adjuncts to thrombolysis for myocardial reperfusion. Ann Intern Med 1991;115:35.

PART IV
Transfusion Medicine

Blood Component Therapy 37

Blood transfusion became practical early in the twentieth century with the discovery of blood group antigens and methods for typing and matching donor to recipient. Subsequently, with development of fortified anticoagulants to improve red blood cell preservation, the biocompatible plastic bag system that allows blood fractionation, and expanded testing to prevent disease transmission, modern concepts of blood component therapy gradually evolved. Transfusion practice is now a complex therapeutic discipline, requiring all the skills of a trained clinician. The transfusion of a blood component can never be taken lightly; it should only be given for a good reason after careful evaluation of the clinical situation.

Transfusions should always be targeted to the clinical problem, whether blood loss, anemia, or both; thrombocytopenia; or a coagulopathy. Only the most appropriate blood component(s) should be ordered and transfused (Table 37–1). It is also essential to take into account any special needs of the patient, for example, as in the immunosuppressed patient who should receive only irradiated products to avoid graft-versus-host disease (GVHD). Great care must be taken to prevent mistakes in matching donor product to recipient, and also in recognizing and treating transfusion reactions. All these items are the responsibility of the physicians and nurses involved in the patient's care.

WHOLE BLOOD

The practice of whole blood transfusion has largely been replaced by component therapy. However, some blood centers do offer "modified" whole blood (whole blood minus the platelet component) for the treatment of large-volume blood loss. Its use can save time, cost less, and expose the recipient to fewer donors. In the patient with massive blood loss, modified whole blood will sustain the levels of coagulation factors in plasma, with the exception of platelets, which will need to be replaced separately.

RED BLOOD CELLS

Packed red blood cells are used to treat most anemias, regardless of cause, to improve oxygen delivery to tissues. A unit of "packed cells" contains all of the red blood cells from a 450-mL unit of whole blood (~200 mL of red blood cells) suspended in 130 mL of plasma/acid citrate dextrose (ACD) solution to give a hematocrit of about 60%. A red blood cell unit also contains sufficient white blood cells and platelets to induce alloimmunization to HLA antigens, and with storage, to increase levels of cytokines capable of producing a febrile transfusion reaction. Blood banks offer several other red blood cell products for specific purposes:

- **Leukodepleted red blood cells:** These cells are similar to packed red blood cells but are passed through a microfiber filter to remove most white blood cells (99.9% of leukocytes with a loss of 15–20% of the red blood cells). This step reduces the risk of HLA alloimmunization, cytomegalovirus (CMV) transmission, and if the cells are filtered prior to storage, cytokine-induced febrile reactions. This product should always be used in a patient with a history of febrile reactions.
- **Washed red blood cells:** These are red blood cells suspended in saline, following repeated saline washes. This procedure removes 85% of the leukocytes and 99% of the original plasma. Washed red blood cells are indicated for patients with paroxysmal nocturnal hemoglobinuria and

Table 37–1. Blood components for transfusion.

Red blood cells
"Packed" red blood cells
Leukodepleted red cells
Washed red cells
Irradiated red cells
Frozen (deglycerolized) red cells
CMV-negative red cells
Platelets
Pooled random donor platelets
Single donor pheresis platelets
HLA-matched single donor platelets
Coagulation factors
Fresh frozen plasma
Cryoprecipitate, factor VIII, and fibrinogen

cold agglutinin disease (IgM cold antibody hemolytic anemia), where transfused complement could exacerbate the disease process. They are also used to transfuse IgA deficient patients who because of the formation of anti-IgA antibodies are at risk for an anaphylactic reaction when receiving a transfusion of normal plasma.

- **Frozen (deglycerolized) red blood cells:** Like washed cells, cryopreserved red blood cells, once deglycerolized, are suspended in saline for transfusion. Therefore, they can be used for the same indications as washed cells. The principal use of frozen red blood cells, however, is the treatment of patients with rare blood types who are difficult to crossmatch.
- **Irradiated red blood cells:** Red blood cells are exposed to a minimum dose of 2500 rads prior to transfusion. This product is indicated when, because of marked immunosuppression, the recipient could accept a transplant of donor lymphocytes and develop GVHD.
- **CMV-negative red blood cells:** This is a preferred product for CMV-negative recipients, especially those who are undergoing bone marrow transplantation.

Red Blood Cell Transfusion Therapy

A transfusion of red blood cells is not without risk and, therefore, should only be performed when clearly indicated. Hospitals have strict transfusion guidelines that spell out when red blood cell transfusions are indicated—whether for blood loss related to a procedure, significant anemia (hemoglobin level less than 7–8 grams per deciliter unless age, illness, or cardiopulmonary disease mandates a higher hemoglobin level), or ongoing hemorrhage. Red blood cells are used to im-

prove oxygen delivery to tissues, not to treat hypovolemia (Chapter 10). Although red blood cells do provide some volume expansion, actively bleeding patients will require further volume support with electrolyte, colloid, or plasma transfusions. Each unit of packed red blood cells given to an average-sized adult will increase the hemoglobin level by 1 gram per deciliter (~3% hematocrit rise).

Patients can only receive transfusions with red blood cells of the same or a compatible ABO and Rh blood type. Furthermore, plasma antibodies to any one of several minor blood group antigens can make matching difficult or even render the patient untransfusable. It is important, therefore, to have a basic understanding of the blood group antigen system.

A. Blood Group Antigens:

Blood group antigens are inherited amino acid and carbohydrate moieties on the surface of the red blood cell that define the immune potential of the cell. When a person lacking an antigen receives antigen-positive blood, alloantibodies may form, resulting in a transfusion reaction with destruction of the transfused cells. Over 250 antigens, assigned to 23 blood groups, have been identified. However, only the ABO and Rh systems and a handful of so-called minor blood group antigens (Kell, Duffy, Kidd, and the MNSs systems) are of primary importance in transfusion practice. More extensive genotyping of minor blood group antigens is of value in tissue typing, paternity testing, and the genetic localization of diseases whose genes are close to a blood group antigen locus.

1. ABO system—Historically, the naturally occurring isoagglutinins, anti-A and anti-B, were used to define the major blood types: A, B, AB, and O. The frequency of each blood type in Caucasian populations is listed in Table 37–2. Genetic analysis has since revealed many subgroups in the ABO system (A_2, A_8, *cis* AB, B_m, etc), which has helped explain the variable expression of the A and B antigens.

Table 37–2. ABO and Rh phenotype frequencies (Caucasians).

Phenotype	Frequency (%)
O	43
A	44
B	9
AB	4
Rh (D)⁺	85

To avoid a major adverse reaction, transfused blood must be type specific. Type O patients have both anti-A and anti-B in their serum and, therefore, must receive type O blood. Type B patients carry anti-A, and type A patients carry anti-B. Only type AB patients can accept red blood cells of any type without risk. Type O red blood cells, because they are antigenically silent, can be given to A and B patients in an emergency. Life-threatening hemolytic transfusion reactions are generally associated with transfusions of type A blood to type O recipients, especially those who carry a high-titer hemolytic anti-A alloantibody.

2. Rh system—The Rh blood group system includes five important antigens—D, C, c, E, and e, coded by two highly homologous genes on chromosome 1. The prevalence of Rh-negative (D-negative) people varies by race, from as high as 15% in Caucasians to less than 1% in Asians. D-negativity is most often due to a deletion of the entire RHD gene, setting the stage for a strong immune response upon exposure to D antigen with transfusion or pregnancy. Still, formation of anti-D is not a certainty; naive Rh-negative women come to term without sensitization by a D-positive fetus more often than not. Moreover, the risk of Rh immunization can be reduced to near zero by the administration of hyperimmune anti-D serum (Rh immune globulin) postpartum or following a mismatched transfusion. Much less commonly, hemolytic disease of the newborn can result from antibody formation to C, c, E, and e or a minor blood group antigen.

3. Kell system—The Kell antigens are coded by a gene on chromosome 7. Antibodies to the Kell blood group system (**anti-K**) have been associated with rapid destruction of Kell-positive red blood cells following transfusion and an anemia of the newborn secondary to marrow suppression, not hemolysis.

4. Duffy system—The Duffy system consists of two polymorphic antigens—Fy^a and Fy^b, reflecting a single amino acid difference. Most African Americans (and 100% of West Africans) are $Fy^{(a-b-)}$, perhaps through natural selection inasmuch as the Duffy antigen is an obligate receptor for *Plasmodium vivax* and *Plasmodium knowlesi*. Patients with this phenotype may form anti-Fy^a after transfusion but not anti-Fy^b because the $Fy^{(a-b-)}$ recessive gene still encodes normal amounts of Fy^b protein in nonhematopoietic tissues.

5. Other minor blood group antigens—Other minor blood group antigens of importance include the following:

- **The Kidd gene,** located on chromosome 18, codes for two antithetical antigens—Jk^a and Jk^b—as well as Jk3. Anti-Jk^a and jk^b are potent antibodies capable of delayed hemolysis after transfusion.

- **The Diego antigens,** Di^a and Di^b, have also been implicated as a cause of hemolytic disease of the newborn. Deficiency in band 3, which carries both the Diego and Wright antigens, has been associated with hereditary spherocytosis.
- **The MNSs system** is expressed on the red blood cell surface as two homologous proteins, glycophorin A (M and N antigens) and glycophorin B (S and s antigens). S and s antibodies have been associated with hemolysis, while M and N antibodies have not.
- **Lewis antigens** (Le^a and Le^b), P antigen, and the Ii antigen system are targets for IgM cold-reacting antibodies seen with cold agglutinin disease, Epstein-Barr virus and mycoplasma infections, and lymphomas. The rare P- or I-negative patient can form strong alloantibodies with transfusion.

B. TYPING AND CROSSMATCH:

Each unit of donated blood is routinely typed prior to storage for both ABO and Rh (D) antigens. In addition, the plasma from the unit is tested for the presence of anti-A and anti-B and for other minor blood group antibodies using the **indirect antiglobulin test** (Chapter 11). For the purpose of screening, the test uses a standard set of red blood cells, which express a full range of blood group antigens, to detect plasma IgG antibodies against minor blood group antigens. Approximately 0.5% of donated units will test positive. Even when present, these antibodies pose little risk to the recipient, since the amount of donor plasma transfused with a unit of red blood cells is only ~20 mL. They do need to be recognized, however, when it comes to the preparation of platelets and fresh frozen plasma (FFP), where the amount of donor plasma transfused is considerably greater.

Donor blood is also tested for several transmissible diseases (Table 37–3), and all components are quarantined until the test results are available. This approach together with prescreening of all donors prior to phlebotomy has made the US blood supply extremely safe. For example, since the hepatitis C (HCV) enzyme immunoassay for viral antibody was introduced in 1990, the risk of HCV transmission has decreased from 1 in 500 to 1 in 100,000 units transfused. Blood centers also routinely offer an **autologous blood service,** where patients can store their own blood in preparation for surgery. This further reduces, but certainly does not eliminate, the risk of disease transmission and transfusion reactions. Errors can still occur because of mishandling of the blood at the time of transfusion.

Red blood cells can be stored for up to 42 days at 4°C. Washed cells have to be used within 24 hours of preparation to guarantee sterility. Prior to transfusion, the donor and the recipient must be matched for

Table 37–3. Transmissible disease tests.

Agent	Test
T pallidum (syphilis)	Antibody
Hepatitis B (HBV)	HBsAg
Hepatitis C (HCV)	Viral protein antibody, nucleic acid testing
CMV	Viral antibody
HIV-1 and -2	Viral antibodies, nucleic acid testing
HTLV-1	Viral antibody

compatibility. This process includes selecting ABO and Rh type-specific blood, screening the recipient for serum antibodies, and performing a "major" crossmatch (testing donor cells against patient serum for ABO compatibility). This process is made much more difficult if the patient has a positive indirect antiglobulin test for minor blood group antibodies. In this situation, the antigen specificity of the antibodies must be identified to permit selection of donor units that lack the target antigen.

Compatibility testing can be both costly and time consuming. This is especially true for the large amount of blood that must be selected and put aside each day in support of surgical procedures that may or may not require transfusion. There is also the issue of the time required for crossmatch when blood is needed urgently. These factors have led to a standard approach to ordering that addresses these logistical problems:

- **Fully crossmatched red blood cells:** Patients requiring an elective transfusion of red blood cells should receive fully crossmatched blood. This includes typing, screening for antibodies, and performing a major crossmatch of each unit. Depending on the workload in the blood bank, several hours may be required before blood will be available for transfusion.
- **Type and screen:** For surgical procedures where blood is only occasionally needed, it is common practice to determine the patient's ABO and Rh type and test the serum for red blood cell antibodies. If none are detected, type-specific blood is set aside but the major crossmatch is not performed. Then, if the patient requires transfusion, crossmatched red blood cells can be made available within 15 minutes, or if it is an emergency, the type-specific blood can be transfused and the crossmatch performed post facto to detect any mismatch.

- **Emergency crossmatch:** When blood is needed urgently, the blood bank can type and crossmatch red blood cells in 15–30 minutes, once a sample of the patient's blood is available. For patients who have already received transfusions, the blood bank usually has a sample on hand. If not, an extra delay can result. Antibody screening results will generally not be available prior to transfusion, but this poses almost no risk to the patient.
- **Uncrossmatched/type-specific red blood cells:** If a patient cannot wait the 15–30 minutes required to obtain crossmatched blood, ABO type-specific or, in a situation where the patient's blood type is unknown, type O-(Rh)negative red blood cells can be transfused. When the supply of O-negative cells is exhausted, O-positive red blood cells can be substituted with little risk to the recipient. The chance of a reaction to Rh-positive cells is very small; less than 0.5% of patients will both be Rh negative and have an anti-D antibody. Moreover, the risk of inducing an antibody is only of importance in young women with childbearing potential. A tube of the patient's blood should always be drawn prior to transfusion to avoid confusion and allow the blood bank to start crossmatching additional units. Since the supply of O-negative red blood cells is always limited, conversion of the patient to type-specific, crossmatched blood should occur as soon as possible.

C. ADMINISTRATION:

Red blood cells should never be administered without the informed consent of the patient. The risks involved and the alternatives to transfusion need to be explained, and the patient's consent needs to be documented. It is essential that any transfusion be taken very seriously. It is estimated that 1 in every 10,000–40,000 red blood cell transfusions given in the United States is ABO incompatible, not because of an error in crossmatching, but because of a clerical/management error. The most common are mislabeling of the patient's blood sample for typing and crossmatch and failure to match the unit to be transfused with the right patient at the time of transfusion. Hospitals have written procedures for both sample collection and blood administration. If followed meticulously, they can go a long way toward eliminating transfusion errors.

Red blood cells are administered intravenously using one of several types of **filter sets.** The traditional filter set traps clots and any large particulate debris. Microaggregate filters have been used to exclude platelet, leukocyte, and fibrin microemboli, which may play a role in acute respiratory distress syndrome and complications of cardiovascular surgery. However, microfiber leukodepletion filters have largely replaced the use of microaggregate filters. They have the added benefit of reducing the incidence of febrile reactions to leukocyte products and preventing CMV transmission.

The **rate of administration** will vary with the clinical situation. When red blood cells are given electively to treat a chronic anemia, the first 25–50 mL of each unit should be administered slowly over 10–15 minutes, while closely monitoring the patient. If no immediate adverse reaction is observed, the rate can then be increased. The overall rate will vary depending on the patient's cardiovascular status, the number of units to be transfused, and the patient's tolerance. Signs of volume overload or the appearance of a delayed transfusion reaction, such as fever and chills, will necessarily cut short the transfusion event.

Red blood cells should never be diluted to decrease viscosity and improve the rate of infusion. The use of fortified anticoagulant solutions (Adsol, etc) for storage maintains the unit's hematocrit at about 60%, so infusion flow rates should not be a problem. If red blood cells are piggybacked to an existing in-dwelling catheter, only isotonic saline solution should be used in the main line. Exposure to even small amounts of dextrose in water or hypotonic saline can result in clumping and hemolysis; lactated Ringer's solutions can cause clot formation. When a higher rate of infusion is required, as with massive blood loss, a pressure bag or cuff can be used to speed delivery. However, flow will not significantly increase unless a large-bore catheter or needle (18 gauge or higher) is in place.

Warming is rarely necessary when red blood cells are given slowly. It is recommended when multiple units are given at rates exceeding 50 mL per minute, the patient has a high-titer cold agglutinin, or a newborn receives an exchange transfusion. Warming should always be done using an approved device designed specifically for blood warming. Never use a microwave to warm blood! Hypocalcemia secondary to citrate toxicity is rarely seen with red blood cell transfusions, even when multiple units are given in cases of massive blood loss. It is seen in adults undergoing pheresis procedures and newborns needing exchange transfusion.

Transfusion Complications and Adverse Reactions

Several adverse reactions can complicate a red blood cell transfusion (Table 37–4). Some are relatively frequent, such as febrile (cytokine-induced) reactions, alloimmunization to HLA antigens, IgE-histamine–driven allergic reactions, and induction of minor blood group antibodies. Others are rare, but can be devastating. The most dreaded is an ABO-incompatible hemolytic transfusion reaction. The severity of reaction to

Table 37–4. Adverse effects of blood transfusion.

Hemolytic reactions
  ABO-incompatible, intravascular hemolysis
  Delayed, extravascular hemolysis
Febrile reactions
  Cytokine-induced fever
  HLA alloimmunization reactions
Allergic reactions
  Alloimmunization, decreased platelet survival
  IgE-related histamine reactions
  IgA-deficient anaphylaxis
  Acute lung injury—leukocyte antibodies
Immune compromise
  Transfusion-associated GVHD
  Post-transfusion immunomodulation
Infectious agent transmission
  Bacterial contamination
  Cytomegalovirus
  EBV seroconversion
  Viral hepatitis (B, C, other)
  HIV and HTLV-1
Other adverse effects
  Circulatory overload
  Iron overload

an ABO-mismatched unit of red blood cells varies depending on the type of mismatch, with type A red blood cells administered to a type O patient expressing a high-titer anti-A antibody being the worst. The most severe involve sudden intravascular hemolysis, which may go unrecognized until a large volume of cells has been infused. This reaction can result in acute renal failure or, when severe, even cardiovascular collapse and death.

The key to preventing a life-threatening reaction to transfusion is to closely monitor the patient during the act of transfusion. The **most frequent signs and symptoms** that accompany a hemolytic reaction include fever, chills, chest and low back pain, hypotension, and often a feeling of impending doom. The transfusion must be discontinued immediately and a venous blood sample drawn to look for intravascular hemolysis and to repeat the crossmatch. The further workup and management of the patient with intravascular hemolysis is discussed in Chapter 11.

A. TYPES OF REACTIONS:

Delayed hemolytic transfusion reactions are seen in patients who develop antibodies to one of the minor blood group antigens, most often to the Rh system (E or c), Kell, Fy^a, or Jk^a. Generally, this occurs in a patient who has already been immunized from a past pregnancy or transfusion but is not detected by the routine serum antibody screen. The extravascular red blood cell hemolysis that results is usually clinically silent, other than a surprising fall in the hematocrit within a few days or a week or two. If this happens, a repeat of the serum antibody screen will usually detect the antibody.

Patients who have had multiple transfusions and **patients receiving red blood cells that have been stored for long periods without leukodepletion** often experience fever and chills or fever alone, beginning during or several hours after the transfusion. This effect is not a hemolytic reaction. It is caused by cytokines released by contaminating leukocytes or alloantibodies to leukocyte and platelet HLA antigens. Transfusion with leukodepleted red blood cells, together with premedicating the patient with hydrocortisone and acetaminophen (Tylenol), can greatly ameliorate this reaction. Patients who have had several febrile reactions to blood should receive only leukodepleted red blood cells, preferably cells leukodepleted at the time of donation.

Simple **allergic reactions** are common with transfusion. The incidence of hives and mild bronchospasm, perhaps related to IgE-related histamine response to infused plasma proteins, cytokines, or both, has been estimated to occur in 2–10% of transfusions. **Atopic individuals** may be at greater risk. Treatment of affected patients with diphenhydramine HCl (Benadryl) 25–50 mg orally or intravenously will usually ameliorate this reaction, so that transfusion can be completed.

IgA-deficient patients are at considerable risk for a severe anaphylactic reaction, if they have formed anti-A antibodies. Once identified, they should only receive a transfusion of washed or deglycerolized red blood cells. Any plasma component transfusion should be with product from an IgA-deficient donor. **Transfusion-related acute lung injury,** a severe, sometimes fatal pulmonary reaction characterized by noncardiogenic pulmonary edema and hypotension, has been described in association with leukocyte or HLA-specific complement-activating antibodies in transfused plasma. The passive transfer of these antibodies to the donor's leukocytes results in aggregation, activation, and microvascular pulmonary damage.

Red blood cell transfusions carry a special risk for the severely **immunocompromised patient.** Only irradiated red blood cells and, if the patient is CMV negative, CMV-negative units should be used. Unirradiated red blood cells contain enough viable lymphocytes to cause GVHD. Red blood cell transfusions are also believed to modulate the immune system. They have been used to induce tolerance in patients receiving renal transplants and may be associated with a higher incidence of postoperative infection and second cancers. Finally, although the risk of disease transmission is very small, **bacterial and viral infections secondary to transfusion** still do occur. The risk of infection for hepatitis B, HCV, and HIV from well-screened, fully tested blood is approximately 1 in 50,000 to 1.5 million units/components transfused.

Red Blood Cell Transfusion Alternatives

Many of the risks of transfusion can be reduced, but certainly not eliminated, by the use of **autologous blood.** The opportunity for a clerical error or a mistake in patient-unit identification is still there. Bacterial contamination can still occur. There is also a limited set of circumstances when autologous blood storage makes sense, such as in an elective surgery procedure where transfusion of 2–4 units of red blood cells is predictable and sufficient. Orthopedic procedures such as total hip and major knee operations are another example. Autologous blood storage is unnecessary in elective surgeries where blood loss is usually minimal (less than 1–2 units) or major procedures requiring more than 4 units. Red blood cell savers have also been used in major surgical procedures to reduce the need for transfusion.

Perioperative erythropoietin therapy, while expensive, can reduce the need for transfusion. It has been used to increase the amount of autologous blood donated and stored. It has also been shown to increase in vivo erythropoiesis pre- and postoperatively. When erythropoietin is given a week or more before and continuing for up to 10 days after major elective surgery, the immediate postoperative anemia is less and a 5–6% rise in the hematocrit level can be seen by the tenth postoperative day (Chapter 10). The number of units of red blood cells transfused is also less. Success, however, is very much dependent on the level of iron supply during treatment, so aggressive iron supplementation is essential.

Red blood cell substitutes have been a dream for a long time. Perfluorocarbon emulsions have been studied for the past 50 years with little success. Second-generation compounds carry more oxygen and have fewer side effects but are still in the testing stage of development. Polymerized hemoglobin solutions are also under investigation.

PLATELETS

Platelet concentrates can be prepared from individual units of donated blood (**random donor platelets**) or harvested from a single donor by cytapheresis (**pheresis platelets**). In the United States, where blood is routinely collected using a multibag system (Figure 37–1), platelet rich plasma (PRP) is separated from red blood cells by centrifugation at a low G force. The PRP is then transferred to a smaller connected bag, where following a second spin at a higher G force to further concentrate the platelets, excess supernatant plasma is

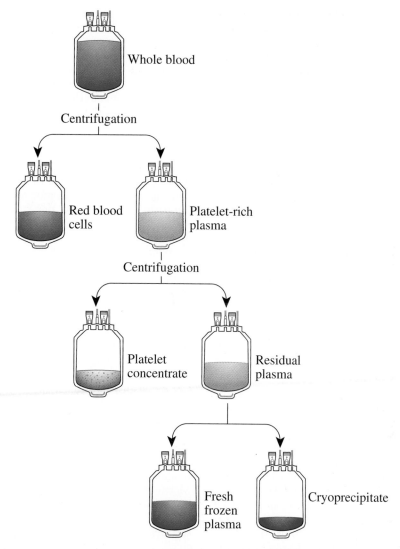

Figure 37–1. **Blood component preparation.** Diagram of the separation of whole blood into "packed" red blood cells, platelet concentrate, and FFP or cryoprecipitate, using the multibag system.

transferred to a third bag. About 50 mL of plasma/ACD solution is left behind. This method recovers about 60–70% of the platelets from the original unit of blood, together with a portion of the leukocytes and a few red blood cells. Most platelet concentrates contain 10^8 or more leukocytes, which is enough to induce alloimmunization and cause febrile transfusion reactions and traces of red blood cells (< 0.3 mL).

Random donor platelet concentrates can be stored for up to 5 days at 20–24°C, though with a progressive decrease in viability. The normal survival of platelets is 10 days, so by the fifth day of storage, recovery after transfusion is predictably reduced by 25% or more. At the time of transfusion, 4–8 units of random donor platelets are pooled. When transfused into an average-sized adult, 6 units (a "six-pack") of random donor pooled platelets will increase the platelet count by ~50,000/μL, usually enough to control any bleeding tendency. If the final total volume of plasma is too large, the pooled unit can be centrifuged and excess plasma removed. However, this can result in a further loss of 15–50% of the platelet component.

Platelets in amounts equivalent to 6–10 pooled random donor units can be harvested from a single donor by cytapheresis. Each plateletpheresis unit has a volume of 200–500 mL and contains ~3 × 10^{11} platelets. Like random donor units, apheresis platelets can be stored for up to 5 days at 20–24°C. Single donor apheresis platelet units are processed like a unit of whole blood. They are ABO and Rh typed and tested for transmissible disease and, therefore, are only available for transfusion once testing results are known, usually 24 hours. Most blood centers also provide single-donor apheresis platelets drawn from a registry of HLA-typed donors, as a strategy to improve platelet recoveries and survivals in the patient who has become alloimmunized.

Platelet Transfusion Therapy

The routine availability of platelet concentrates for transfusion has revolutionized the management of thrombocytopenia. Myeloablative chemotherapy for hematologic malignancies and bone marrow transplantation are two situations where platelet transfusions are an absolutely essential part of the therapeutic regimen. Platelet therapy is used both to prevent bleeding and to treat the actively bleeding patient with thrombocytopenia. Guidelines for platelet transfusions in various platelet disorders are discussed in Chapter 30.

A. TYPING AND CROSSMATCH:

As with red blood cell transfusions, platelets should be ABO type-specific if possible. A-antigen is present on the surface of platelets of type A patients, so a transfusion of incompatible platelets may result in a somewhat shortened survival. However, since this is a relatively minor issue, ABO-incompatible platelets can be given when the supply of type-specific platelets runs short, without risk to the patient. If large volumes of type-O donor plasma (> 500 mL), containing anti-A and anti-B, are transfused to a type A, B, or AB patient, the direct antiglobulin test may turn positive and both transfused platelet and patient red blood cell survivals may be reduced. Rh antigens are not present on the platelet surface, so the Rh type need not be considered. However, the small number of red blood cells present in the platelet preparation can induce anti-D antibody in the Rh-negative patient given platelets from Rh-positive donors. This effect will not affect platelet survival and is of no other consequence unless the patient is of childbearing age.

Patients receiving transfusions of multiple units of platelets are likely to become "**refractory**," defined as a failure to get a respectable platelet count increment immediately following transfusion or little or no improvement in the platelet count at 24 hours, or both. Depending on the clinical illness, the cause may be multifactorial. Antiplatelet antibodies in the patient with idiopathic thrombocytopenic purpura or nonimmune factors such as sepsis, disseminated intravascular coagulation, and hypersplenism can all be responsible. However, alloimmunization to platelet and leukocyte HLA antigens must also be considered, especially for the aplastic anemia patient who receives transfusions over a long period. Patients markedly immunosuppressed by high-dose chemotherapy are much less likely to become alloimmunized. In addition, patients receiving transfusions primarily with single-donor apheresis platelets may be at lower risk, perhaps because the exposure to multiple donors is less.

To rule in alloimmunization, patients should receive transfusions with 24-hour-old ABO identical, HLA-matched platelets, drawn from a matched sibling or an HLA-matched unrelated community donor(s). If this approach gives improved post-transfusion recoveries and survivals, a significant component of alloimmunization can be assumed. Platelet crossmatching using a solid-phase red blood cell adherence assay has also been used to identify compatible donors and may be superior to HLA matching. When crossmatched or HLA-matched platelets fail, continued transfusion of random donor platelets may be of clinical benefit even though there is no apparent improvement in the platelet count.

B. PLATELET ADMINISTRATION:

Like red blood cells, platelets should be transfused using a standard filter set to exclude fibrin clots and debris. Microfiber filters are available to leukodeplete the platelet unit at the time of transfusion at the cost, however, of a 20–25% loss of platelets. Leukodepletion also helps prevent CMV transmission and alloimmunization, whether random or apheresis platelets are used. Sensitized patients should always receive leukodepleted products to reduce the severity of the fever and chills. Moreover, these patients should be premedicated and infused at a slower rate. Even in the face of severe fever and chills, platelet recoveries and survivals may be respectable. Severely immunocompromised patients should receive irradiated platelets.

The effectiveness of a platelet transfusion can only be determined by its impact on the patient's platelet count and the control of ongoing hemorrhage (Chapter 30). Measurement of the patient's platelet count at 1, 4, and 24 hours following transfusion can be used to assess **immediate recovery** (the incremental rise in the platelet count at 1 hour), and **survival** (the fall in the platelet count at 4 and 24 hours). This information is essential for planning subsequent platelet transfusions. The pattern of the response may also help identify the cause of apparent refractoriness (see discussion in Chapter 30).

C. COMPLICATIONS:

Because platelets are stored at room temperature, the risk of bacterial contamination is significantly increased. The rate of contamination of platelets is estimated to be as high as 0.1% of units transfused, although apheresis platelets generally pose a lower risk. Sepsis or persistent fever following transfusion should be reason to draw blood cultures and, if available, culture the remnant of the transfused unit.

COAGULATION FACTOR COMPONENTS

As an integral part of blood component therapy, blood centers prepare FFP and cryoprecipitate as a source of both factor VIII and fibrinogen. These components are used in the patient with massive blood loss, where factor depletion can result from inadequate replacement of plasma coagulation components, and in individual factor deficiencies secondary to an inherited coagulopathy (hemophilia, von Willebrand disease, etc) or a consumptive coagulopathy.

Fresh Frozen Plasma (FFP)

FFP can be harvested from donated whole blood as part of the preparation of platelet concentrates. Using a three-bag system, the excess plasma/ACD solution left after the platelet concentrate centrifugation step (~250 mL) is transferred to the third bag, separated, and frozen within 8 hours of collection. FFP can then be stored for up to 1 year at −20°C. At the time of transfusion, it is thawed at 37°C, a process that takes 30–60 minutes. Once thawed, FFP should be transfused within 12 hours to guarantee adequate coagulation factor levels and sterility. FFP should be ABO compatible with the patient's red blood cells.

FFP is used in several clinical situations (Table 37–5). The dose will depend on the type and severity of the coagulation abnormality. To sustain factor levels in a patient with massive blood loss, the number of

Table 37–5. Indications for coagulation factor replacement.

Fresh frozen plasma
Massive blood loss/transfusion
Emergency reversal of warfarin therapy
Factor replacement in DIC
Treatment of hereditary coagulopathies
Liver disease
Cryoprecipitate
Treatment of von Willebrand disease
Fibrinogen replacement
Factor VIII replacement–hemophilia
Purified and recombinant factor preparations
Inherited factor deficiencies

FFP units transfused will be determined by the clinical setting, the type of red blood cells used to resuscitate the patient (whether whole blood, packed cells, washed cells, or cell saver blood), and the results of coagulation tests [platelet count, prothrombin time (PT), partial thromboplastin time (PTT), and fibrinogen levels]. Microvascular bleeding is most often related to thrombocytopenia or platelet dysfunction and should be treated with platelet transfusions. As a general rule, a six-pack of platelets should be transfused for every 6–10 units of red blood cells transfused, with additional platelets given according to the clinical situation (Chapter 30).

When FFP is used to treat a PT or PTT greater than 1.5 times control (factor levels below 15% of normal), at least 6 units must be given to achieve factor levels of greater than 30%. Each FFP unit will increase coagulation factor levels by only 2–3%. This involves the transfusion of close to 1500 mL of plasma/ACD solution, and unless the patient is actively bleeding, can result in volume overload and congestive failure. Certainly, any additional FFP infusions will be limited by the large volumes required for an appreciable impact on factor levels. In addition, any sustained benefit from FFP therapy requires a normal level of coagulation factor production by the liver. Patients with severe liver disease will benefit only briefly, no more than a day, before the transfused coagulation factors, especially factor VII, decline and the PT rises once again.

Allergic reactions to FFP are similar to but frequently more intense than those seen with red blood cells and platelets. Urticaria, bronchospasm, and laryngeal spasm are common. An immediate and impressive leakage of oncotic protein out of the intravascular space can result in a fall in blood pressure and a rise in hematocrit level. This effect can add considerable confusion to the management of a surgery patient or a patient experiencing a major blood loss. Infusions of FFP have also been associated with sudden marked symptomatic thrombocytopenia, so-called post-transfusion purpura (see Chapter 30). Febrile reactions are uncommon, since FFP is free of leukocytes, platelets, and cytokines.

Cryoprecipitate

Cryoprecipitate is prepared by flash freezing fresh plasma and then thawing it at 4°C. This process leaves a residual precipitate, once the plasma/ACD supernatant is removed, of cryoproteins, including fibrinogen, von Willebrand factor (vWF), and factor VIII. The procedure recovers 150–200 mg of fibrinogen and 80–100 units of factor VIII/vWF in 15 mL of residual plasma, a 10-fold concentration over FFP. Cryoprecipitate units can then be stored for up to 1 year at −20°C. In treating a patient, several units are thawed, pooled, and transfused within 4 hours. Indications for cryoprecipitate therapy are listed in Table 37–5.

Each unit of cryoprecipitate will raise a patient's fibrinogen level by only 5–7 mg/dL. Thus, when it is used to treat hypofibrinogenemia (fibrinogen levels < 100 mg/dL), 10–20 units need to be pooled, sufficient to increase the circulating fibrinogen level in an average-sized adult by at least 100 mg/dL. Following transfusion, the fibrinogen level should be monitored and repeated infusions given to maintain levels above 100 mg/dL. The amount required will vary with the rate of fibrinogen consumption.

The treatment of von Willebrand disease is very empirical and depends on the disease subtype. Doses can range from 20 to 30 pooled units/day in an adult with severe type 1 or 3 disease to less than 10 units/day with mild disease (Chapter 31). With the development of highly purified factor VIII and recombinant VIII products, cryoprecipitate is no longer the product of choice in the treatment of hemophilia A. Cryoprecipitate is used for the preparation of fibrin glue for topical surgical hemostasis.

Like FFP, cryoprecipitate infusions can cause an immediate IgE-histamine-driven allergic reaction. In the past, hemophiliac children who received large volumes of cryoprecipitate were frequently exposed to HCV.

Human parvovirus B19 also can be transmitted by cryoprecipitate. Although parvovirus infection is characterized by little more than transient polyarthritis and an exanthema in children and young adults, pregnant women and patients with hemolytic anemias are at special risk, such as for the development of severe red blood cell aplasia. Testing for the presence of HPV-B19 viremia in the donor is not yet possible.

Purified & Recombinant Factor Preparations

The treatment of the inherited coagulopathies has changed dramatically first with the purification of individual factors from pooled plasma and now with the synthesis of recombinant factors and growth factors, especially thrombopoietin. Recombinant technology has opened the door to a highly sophisticated approach to the management of both bleeding disorders and some thrombopathies. See Chapters 30, 32, 33, and 35 for a full discussion.

BIBLIOGRAPHY

McCullough J: *Transfusion Medicine.* McGraw-Hill, 1998.

Speiss BD, Counts RB, Gould SA: *Perioperative Transfusion Medicine.* Williams & Wilkins, 1997.

Index